The Concordant Clinical Homeopathic Repertory

Robert Medhurst BNat DHom

ISBN 978-0-9580798-2-2

Printed and bound by Lightning Source

For correspondence and the purchase of copies of this book, please contact the author:

Robert Medhurst
Address
P.O. Box 485
Hahndorf
South Australia
Australia, 5245
Phone
(Australia) 0435 487 400
Email
medhurstr@yahoo.com

Index

Introduction

The practice of homeopathy is based on Samuel Hahnemann's primary guiding principle, Similia Similibus Curantur. This is a perfectly reasonable, feasible and effective proposition.

Inherent in this proposition is the notion that every living entity, when in a state of dis-ease, expresses the signs and symptoms of this state in its own idiosyncratic way. That is to say that no two individuals suffering from the same clinical condition will express this condition in the same way. For example, no two sufferers of the common cold will have the same level of thirst, fever or appetite, their speed of symptom development will differ, their aggravating and ameliorating factors will differ, and so on. Once again, this is perfectly reasonable.

The job of the homeopath, in accordance with the principle stated above, is to define the patient's individual symptoms, match these against the proving symptoms of the full range of homeopathic remedies available and arrive at the correct remedy for that patient at that time, otherwise known as the similimum. Again, a perfectly reasonable proposition, but it's at this point that problems start to arise, the biggest of which relates to provings and the information derived from them.

Provings and the information derived from them form the primary tools of homeopathic practice. Unfortunately, the methodology used to carry out provings, particularly many of the older ones, leaves a lot to be desired. For example, toxicology trials on Secale performed by Strahler, as reported in Hughes and Dakes' *Cyclopedia of Drug Pathogenesy* (Jain, New Delhi, 2000, 76 et seq) were done on dogs using powders or infusions of Secale. The same text carries reports from Wernich performing toxicology trials on frogs. Page 52 of the text reports the results of human provings by Dr Hooker using oil of ergot (Secale), obtained by macerating powder in sulphuric ether. Other provers swallowed infusions, some swallowed powders and some had Secale spread on bread. This is far from being an isolated case and all of the results from these studies have gone into the materia medicas and repertories, unqualified, for Secale, despite the different dose forms used and the substances that they were potentially contaminated with, and despite the different dose volumes used, different levels of supervision, different proving durations used and the different life forms with their varying physiologies that were given the drug. This is but one of many examples that could be used to illustrate the point that much of the data that's gone into proving reports and subsequently into material medicas and repertories is questionable and may have a considerable influence on the accuracy of individualised homeopathic prescribing. This may be one of the reasons why even the best prescribers rarely manage to pick the similimum, particularly at the first consultation. For example, in a discussion with US homeopathic educator Dana Ullman and noted US homeopath Edward Whitmont, reported by Dana on an internet discussion list in 2005 (Lyghtforce, 28 October 2005), Whitmont stated that, using a standard repertory and materia medica, he only managed to find the similimum, at least initially, around 30% of the time.

Sadly, even if all of the homeopathic provings that had ever been recorded were completely reliable, few prescribers of homeopathy use these as their primary data sources when selecting the similimum. In most cases, the first text selected is the standard repertory. Most repertories contain information gleaned from sometimes hundreds of different authors; some of this information is derived from provings, some from toxicology studies and some from clinical experience. A large repertory can contain hundreds of thousands of pieces of information, all of which are placed there by the well-intentioned author in an effort to guide the prescriber to the similimum. Most repertories are based on the homeopathic repertory written by James Tyler Kent and published in 1897, and use his remedy listings as the basis for their repertory data. The first edition of this repertory was found to contain a substantial number of errors and while subsequent editions attempted to correct these, the final version may still be far from perfect and therefore may, in the case of entries derived from provings, be slightly less reliable than the provings themselves, many of which, again, are questionable. Most homeopaths, after being guided in the direction of a handful of possible remedies by the repertory, will then do further research on these with the help of a materia medica, which again may contain a mixture of proving, toxicological and clinical information, and again may be inaccurate and contain entries of questionable provenance.

I've struggled with this problem for decades and after many successes and failures in my homeopathic practice came to rely far more on the remedies that had clinical confirmation for the rubric in question than on the guidance provided by the traditional reportorial or material medica texts. This is not to say that one should completely abandon the use of these latter materials, simply that while the remedies they indicate should be studied with all diligence, there's also a case to be made for the consideration of remedies that have shown consistent results for specific clinical conditions, and an even greater case to be made for a text that operates in the same way as any other repertory, but is arranged on the basis of clinical conditions, using remedies that have been clinically confirmed for that condition.

My aim with this book has been to address this problem by constructing a text that will provide competent guidance towards the remedies that have had consistent and reliable clinical confirmation for specific clinical conditions. The issue of whether or not this approach is consistent with Hahnemann's guiding principle of individualized prescribing will be discussed later, but it should be clearly understood that this is a repertory, not a collection of homeopathic specifics for defined clinical conditions.

About this book

This being a concordant clinical repertory, it's important to briefly discuss the issue of concordance. Some authors, recounting their clinical experiences in homeopathy, recommend one or two remedies for a clinical condition, yet others do not support the same recommendations. Some authors recommend dozens of remedies for a specific clinical condition and others only one. Some authors vigorously recommend one remedy and give a passing nod to another twenty.

It's for this reason that this text uses a system of tables detailing suggested remedies assembled using concordance or agreement among authors on what, in their clinical experience, constitutes a reliable homeopathic recommendation for the condition. The extent of concordance can be seen in the position that the various remedies take in the tables; with those most commonly recommended on the left of the table and those least so on the right. Where there is an equal level of concordance for more than one remedy, these are arranged alphabetically from left to right. Where an author graded the strength of the recommendation, the extent of this grading is reflected in the remedy grading within the table and this affects the positioning of the remedy in the table. Remedy grading is discussed in more detail below.

In regard to the entries in the tables, the recommended remedies appear along the top row and the author making the recommendation is referred to by the author's number in the far left column, with their remedy recommendations appearing in their corresponding row and entered by the use of an X where the remedy column and the author row intersect. In the body of the table, "X" denotes a standard entry with a mathematical value in the table of 1. "**X**" in bold type denotes a remedy that has a moderately strong grading or recommendation from that author and is given a mathematical value in the table of 1.5. "**<u>X</u>**" in bold and underlined type denotes a remedy that has a very strong recommendation from that author and is given a mathematical value in the table of 2. "***<u>X</u>***" in bold, underlined and italicized type denotes a remedy that has the highest recommendation from that author and is given a mathematical value in the table of 2.5. The reader may note that many of the tables in the text contain columns that are empty of remedy suggestions. This has occurred because for many clinical rubrics there were more remedies recommended than there was space available for. For example, a clinical entity may have 60 remedy recommendations; 5 of these recommended were made by 10 authors, 3 by 9 authors, 15 by 5 authors and another 20 by 4 authors and 17 by 1 author. In this case, because there is insufficient space to carry the remedies with 4 or less recommendations, the columns will be empty after the 15 remedies recommended by 5 authors.

Clinical trials that have involved the use of homeopathy for specific clinical conditions have also been included in the tables and unless a remedy was found to be particularly efficacious in alleviating the condition, in which case the remedy is given a numerical value of 1.5, all remedies that were successful in the trial are given a numerical value in the table of 1.

It should be noted that the books used as data sources have been used in their entirety. That is, the remedy recommendation may be taken from anywhere in that book, not just in the author's formal remedy listing for the specified clinical condition. One of several issues that had to be dealt with in constructing this text was what to do with the clinical conditions where there was no agreement among authors. Given that this work attempts to focus on concordance, where there was none, i.e. there was only one author recommending remedies for the disease, there was a case for omitting mention of the disease. However, for the sake of completeness and for the purpose of allowing those with a favourite author to see what that author's advice may have been, it was decided to retain these entries, but in most cases only where some form of grading had been applied by that author. The reader is advised to be cautious about remedy recommendations that rely on the advice of too few authors. For those clinical rubrics where a large number of remedies were recommended, such as fever, diarrhoea or constipation, obviously not all of the remedies recommended could be used and the number is limited by the size of the table and the concordance thresholds for the remedies recommended.

It's also important to be aware that many of the texts used in the construction of this repertory use medical terms that have fallen from common use. Where the preponderance of data makes reference to a particular term to describe a clinical condition, this is the term that is used. For example, when dealing with urinary tract infections, the reader will find that the predominance of remedy recommendations appear under the clinical rubric, nephritis. Where there is general disagreement, the most contemporary term is used. For example, it was decided that terms such as Bronze John, Bone Shave and Bloody Flux may create some difficulties, and so the more contemporary names of yellow fever, sciatica and dysentery, respectively, have been used. The reader may note that, with a few exceptions, most of the subjective symptoms found in repertories have been ignored and the reader is encouraged to use the standard repertory for the purpose of cross-referencing these against the entries herein.

At this point it should be stressed that a particular position on the table does not necessarily imply that one remedy is better than another for a defined clinical condition, but simply that this is where it appeared in the concordance ranking. Given the individual nature of disease, while it may be tempting to do so, the reader is strongly advised to consider all of the remedies in the table and to do this without reference to the position of the remedy in the table. For example, it may be seen that under the clinical rubric, oedema, Digitalis ranks quite highly and from this one may assume that it's useful in most cases of oedema. This assumption would be misplaced because Digitalis is predominantly a cardiac remedy and as such is of most use in oedema of cardiac origin. Similarly, it's important to understand that while, for example, Aconite might be very useful for shock, Aconite will only be useful for those in whom the totality of the symptoms they express, and the causative agent or agents of the shock, are consistent with the proving picture for Aconite. In effect, Aconite, used for shock, will generally be of most use only in an Aconite shock, i.e. where the symptoms are consistent with the proving symptoms for Aconite. Arnica is commonly used for stroke, but normally only stroke that's occurred in response to injury; Nux vomica is very useful for atrophy of the optic nerve, but usually only when that atrophy is secondary to the effects of alcohol abuse. While Cina appears in many of the clinical rubrics herein, it's primarily a worm remedy and so should generally only be considered for use where the clinical rubric has an association with worm infestation. Therefore, each remedy needs to be carefully researched in reference to the totality of the sufferer's symptoms before being used.

The reader is also advised not to look at one disease state in isolation. For example, when considering remedies for constipation, as well as examining this rubric it's useful to venture into associated areas such as Digestion, Slow; Paralysis, Intestines; Mucous Membranes, Dryness Of, and so on. This text should be used in the same way as any other homeopathic repertory in that while one may see a list a remedies noted for use in cystitis, the reader should also look at the remedies listed under fever, dysuria, lower back pain, etc and any concomitant symptoms associated with the disruption of the sufferer's vital force, to derive the full value from this work.

Data Sources

The aim of this work has been to identify and record areas of concordance and highlight those remedies about which most of the notable authorities on homoeopathy agree. It should be mentioned here that while there now exist "medical repertories", the relative lack of provenance for the recommendations made by these texts makes the value of that advice questionable, and as such these medical repertories have not been used as sources of information for this text.

As to the data sources that have been used, the clinical texts that are currently accessible through computer programs such as MACREP and RADAR, with a few exceptions, have been avoided because this information is already available via these programs, and while the data produced by these programs is not as refined as that provided by this text, there's little point in duplicating this information. In addition, many of my most useful data sources are somewhat less than mainstream. It should also be noted that some of the data sources used here employ relatively few remedies. This is particularly the case with authors such as Joseph Laurie, who, because of the age in which he practiced, was limited to a materia medica of 68 remedies. So while his suggestions certainly have merit, he may well have chosen something more specific had a wider choice of remedies been available to him.

As mentioned previously, the numbers down the far left column in each table indicate author whose remedy recommendations are recorded along that row and an X is marked under that remedy recommended by that author where the remedy column and the author row intersect. Details on these authors follow. Row 29 in the tables is reserved for clinical trial entries.

1. Rai Bahadur Bishambur **Das**- *Select Your Remedy.* 1992, 14th Edition, B Jain, New Delhi, India. Das was a prominent New Delhi homeopath of 35 years experience and for many years operated a free clinic in this area. It is possible that some of his suggestions, not attributed to other authors, are actually borrowed from other authors, in particular, WA Dewey, although these borrowed remedies appear to have had Das's clinical confirmation.

2. John Henry **Clarke**- *A Clinical Repertory to the Dictionary of the Materia Medica.* 1979, Health Sciences Press, England, ISBN 0 85032 061 5. This book was originally published in 1904. One of most important of the English homeopaths and author of the *Dictionary of Materia Medica*, Clarke was also Honorary President of the International Homeopathic Congress. Note that remedies shown in bold are the remedies that also appear in Clarke's "Prescriber", and are assumed to be his preferred remedies for the conditions listed. Where Clarke lists two separate rubrics for what appears to be the same clinical condition (for example, Throat, Sore and Sore Throat) these rubrics have been combined. Where a large number of remedies are listed (e.g. diarrhoea) only Clarke's italicised remedies were used. Note also that only the remedies from the clinical repertory section of this book were used.

3. JN **Shinghal**- *Quick Bedside Prescriber*. 1991, 6th Edition, B Jain, New Delhi, India. Shinghal was an Indian medical homeopath with over 50 years' clinical experience. On occasions Shinghal quotes other authors whose remedy suggestions appear in his text. Where this occurs, the remedy has not been used. It is possible that some of his suggestions, not attributed to other authors, are actually borrowed from other authors, in particular, Das and Clarke, although these appear to have had Shinghal's clinical confirmation.

4. Willis Alonzo **Dewey**- *Practical Homoeopathic Therapeutics.*1991, 2nd Edition, B Jain, New Delhi, India. This book was first published in the early 20th century. Dewey was Professor of Materia Medica and Therapeutics and Clinical Professor of Nervous Diseases at the Homeopathic Medical Department of the University of Michigan during the early 1900's. He was a graduate of the New York Homeopathic Medical College in 1880, and taught at the Hahnemann Medical College in San Francisco.

5. Michael **Bouko Levy**- *Homeopathic and Drainage Repertory.* 1992, Editions Similia, France, ISBN-2-904928-70-7. Bouko Levy is a medically qualified homeopath and has been practicing homeopathy since 1977, is the founder of the Israeli Institute of Homeopathy, founder and chairman of the Institute of Homoeopathy of Provence. He taught homoeopathy at the Medical Faculty of Marseille and at many other places around the world.

6. Charles Godlove **Raue**- *Special Pathology and Diagnostics with Therapeutic Hints*, 1981, 4th Edition, B Jain, New Delhi, India. First published in 1896. Born in Nieder-Kunnersdorf, Saxony, in 1820, Raue graduated from the Philadelphia Medical College in 1850. From 1864 till 1871 he was the Professor of Pathology and Practice at the Homoeopathic College of Pennsylvania, and at Hahnemann Medical College in Philadelphia. Raue was a student of Constantine Hering, and in this work he draws from his own clinical experience as well as that of Virchow, Rokitansky, Vogel, Griesinger, Hasse, Wintrich, Bamberger, Simon, Neimeyer, Bock, Bednar, Hubner, Kuttner, Wagner, Skoda, Hebra, Wilson, DaCosta, Hughes, Barclay, Bryan, Hammond, Hahnemann, Hering, Boenninghausen, Ruckert, Oehma, Hartmann, Jahr, Grauvogl, Muller, Meyer, Baehr, Kafka, Ludlam, Hale, Wells, Dunham, Lilienthal and others, albeit with his own clinical confirmation.

7. Kalvin B **Knerr**- *Repertory of Hering's Guiding Symptoms of our Materia Medica.* 1997, B Jain, New Delhi, India. This book was first published in 1896. Knerr was Constantine Hering's pupil, son-in-law, and one of the people responsible for the conclusion of Hering's *Guiding Symptoms,* completed after the latter's death. This work has been used because of the value of the clinically confirmed symptoms in Hering's *Guiding Symptoms.* Only those remedies with Knerr's one and two bar grading have been used, with the two bar remedies given bold status in this text. In addition, only the remedies listed in undifferentiated disease/symptom rubrics and those remedies that appear more than once in the sub rubrics have been used.

8. Samuel **Lilienthal**- *Homoeopathic Therapeutics.* 2001, 4th Edition, Indian Books and Periodicals Syndicate, New Delhi, India. First published in 1915. Lilienthal taught at the New York Homeopathic College and then Hahnemann Medical College of the Pacific in San Francisco. He was editor of the North American Journal of Homoeopathy and held professorships at the New York Homeopathic Medical College and the New York College Hospital for Women. It's thought that Lilienthal's remedy selection may have been influenced by Jahr and while this does appear to be the case, it's assumed that Lilienthal listed these remedies because of his own clinical confirmation of them.

9. Anton **Jayasuriya**- *A Compete Course on Clinical Homoeopathy.* 1991, 3rd Edition, B Jain, New Delhi, India. Book Code B-2300. Jayasuriya is an acupuncturist, homoeopath, senior consultant rheumatologist to the Sri Lankan Ministry of Health and the author of 19 books on acupuncture, homoeopathy, oriental philosophy and neurophysiology. At the time of writing this book it's claimed that Jayasuriya had treated over 1 million people at the free clinic in the Colombo South General Hospital over a period of 32 years.

10. TS **Iyer**- *Beginners Guide to Homoeopathy.* 1952, 2nd Edition, B Jain, New Delhi, India. Iyer was not originally qualified in medicine or homoeopathy, but was a mathematician and economist who made a study of homoeopathy. He spent 40 years studying and practicing homoeopathy throughout Southern India, and became widely renowned as a master homoeopath. The remedies noted are apparently his own suggestions, with possible influences by Raue, Dewey, and others.

11. Kamal **Kansal**- *Practice of Medicine, with Homoeopathic Therapeutics.* 1999, 1st Edition, B Jain, New Delhi, India. Kansal was a well known Indian homeopath, being a former examiner, Board of Homoeopathic System of Medicine, Delhi, the former editor of Homoeopathic Up-date, and Directorate of Health Services, Govt of NCT, Delhi.

12. E Harris **Ruddock**- *The Homoeopathic Vade Mecum.* 1914, The Homoeopathic Publishing Company, London. The author of a number of important texts on homeopathy, Ruddock was a member of the Royal College of Physicians, Royal College of Surgeons, a licensed Midwife and consulting physician to the Reading and Berkshire Homeopathic Dispensary.

13. Constantine **Lippe**- *Repertory to the More Characteristic Symptoms of the Materia Medica.* 2001, B Jain, New Delhi, India. This was originally published in 1880 and draws on the clinical experiences of Lippe and the works of Hering, Jahr, Guernsey, Bell and Boenninghausen, conceivably with Lippe's clinical confirmation. Entries are taken from undifferentiated rubrics, or where they are differentiated, only those remedies that are shown in italics are used.

14. RK **Tandon** and VR **Bajaj**- *Homoeopathic Guide to Family Health.* 1994, Rajendra Publishing House, 205, Neelam, Worli Seaface Rd, Bombay, India, ISBN 81-900085-0-1. VR Baja holds a doctorate in medicine from Punjab University, Chandrigarh, and was formerly the chief physician in the Dept of Skin and Sexually Transmitted Diseases at Medical College Amristar. RK Tandon has a 10 year history of study in homeopathy.

15. Joseph **Laurie**- *An Epitome of the Homoeopathic Domestic Medicine*. 1976, B Jain, New Delhi, India. Laurie wrote this book in the early 19th century. He was a member of the Royal College of Surgeons, Edinburgh, a graduate of the Homeopathic Medical College of Pennsylvania, as well as being the Physician to the Westminster and Lambeth Medical Institution and Dispensary.

16. Frederick L **Compton**- *Homoeopathic Preventive Medicine*. 1993, B Jain, New Delhi, India. First written in 1981. A prominent American homeopath, in this text Compton's inspirations were predominantly the works of Boericke, Shephard, Grimmer and Royal whose recommendations it can be assumed he confirmed in his own practice. In the areas where he mentions remedies used by Clarke and Dewey and other texts already used in this book, these suggestions have been ignored.

17. Prakash **Vakil** - *A Textbook of Homoeopathic Therapeutics for Students and Practitioners*. 1999, 3 Volumes, Indian Books and Periodicals Publishers, New Delhi, India. First published 1977, this 3 volume set covers diseases of the central nervous system, cardiovascular diseases and diseases of the ears, nose and throat. Prakash Vakil is listed as an LCEH (Bom), Honorary Physician and Professor, Govt Homoeopathic Hospital, Bombay, Examiner for LCEH, DHMS and BHMS, Court of Examiners, Maharashtra, Gujurat, Delhi. Ex-Convener, Research Standing Committee of Homoeopathic Medical Association of India.

18. Jacques **Jouanny**, Jean-Bernard **Crapanne**, Henry **Dancer**, Jean Louis **Masson**- *Homeopathic Therapeutics- Possibilities in Acute Pathology, Possibilities in Chronic Pathology*, (2 Volumes). 1996, Editions Boiron, France. Jouanny is one of France's most prominent teachers of homeopathy and his co-authors are specialists in this field.

19. Roger **Morrison**- *Desktop Companion to Physical Pathology*.1998, Hahnemann Clinic Publishing, California USA. ISBN 0-9635368-2-6. Morrison is one of America's most prominent medical homeopaths, is a graduate of George Vithoulkas' Athenian Centre for Homeopathic Medicine, and the author of countless articles and many excellent books on homeopathy.

20. Stephen **Cummings** and Dana **Ullman**, *Everybody's Guide to Homeopathic Medicines.* 1984, Tarcher, USA. ISBN 0-87477-337-7. Dana Ullman is widely recognized as the foremost spokesperson for homeopathic medicine in the U.S. To date he has authored nine books, published many more and authored countless articles on homeopathy. He has taught homeopathy and integrative health care, served as an instructor in homeopathy at the University of California at San Francisco, and as member of the Advisory Council of the Alternative Medicine Center at Columbia University's College of Physicians and Surgeons. In previous years he has been the chairperson for the National Center for Homeopathy's Annual Conference, and has been consulted by Harvard Medical School's Center to Assess Alternative Therapy for Chronic Illness. Stephen Cummings is a psychiatrist and began practicing homeopathy during the 1970s and previously co-edited the Journal of Homeopathic Practice. He is currently Medical Director of Psychiatry at San Mateo Medical Center, a public hospital serving people with limited resources in San Mateo County, California. He is also the attending psychiatrist at the San Mateo County AIDS Program, a centre for HIV AIDS -related clinical care and research.

21. Andrew **Lockie**- *The Family Guide to Homeopathy.* 1989, Guild Publishing, UK. ISBN: 0241135729. Andrew Lockie was a medically qualified homeopathic physician, a member of the Royal College of General Practitioners and the Faculty of Homeopathy. He practiced as a homeopathic physician for several decades and was a founding member of and teacher at the Homeopathic Physicians Teaching Group in Oxford, where homeopathy is taught to doctors and other healthcare practitioners.

22. Maesimund B. **Panos** and Jane **Heimlich**, *Homeopathic Medicine at Home*. 1980, JP Yarcher, Los Angeles, USA. ISBN 0-87477-119-6. Panos was a prominent US medical homeopath who trained with Julia Green and brought George Vithoulkas out to the US in 1974.

23. Alexander L **Blackwood**- *A Manual of Materia Medica Therapeutics and Pharmacology.* 2002, B Jain, New Delhi, India. ISBN 81-7021-733-4. This book was first published in 1906. Blackwood was Professor of Clinical Medicine and Therapeutics at the Hahnemann Medical College, Chicago, Attending Physician to the South Chicago Hospital, and Fellow of the American College of Physicians.

24. Surinder R **Verma**- *Practical Handbook of Surgery with Homoeopathic Therapeutics.* 1983, B Jain, New Delhi, India. Verma is a prominent Indian homeopath and is listed as Assistant Director (Homoeopathy), Directorate of ISM & Homoeopathy, Govt. of NCT of Delhi.

25. Trevor **Smith**- *Homeopathic Medicine, A Doctor's Guide to Remedies for Common Ailments.* 1989, Healing Arts Press, Vermont USA, ISBN 0-89281-293-1. Trevor Smith is a renowned medical practitioner specialising in homeopathy and psychiatry. He's written widely on this subject in several books and numerous articles.

26. George Heinrich Gottleib **Jahr**, Translated by Charles J Hempel- *Therapeutic Guide; The Most Important Results of more than Forty Years Practice.* 1999, B Jain, New Delhi, India. ISBN 81-7021-005-4. Originally written in 1869. Jahr worked as an assistant to Hahnemann before completing his medical degree, later going to Paris with Hahnemann to work as his colleague. He taught and wrote widely on homeopathy and was a pivotal figure in its development in Europe. Note that some of the remedy suggestions here are from Hempel alone, not Jahr.

27. Steve **Smith**- *Medical Homoeopathy.* 2007, Winter Press, UK. ISBN (13)9781874581901. Smith is a renowned UK homeopathic practitioner, psychologist, lecturer in homeopathy and clinic supervisor at the South Downs College of Homeopathy in the UK.

28. Robert **Medhurst**- The recommendations here are taken from cured cases from the authors' case files, compiled from several decades of practice. The author is a naturopath specialising in homeopathy, was formerly the inaugural Expert Advisor on Homeopathy to the Australian Federal Government's Dept of Health and Ageing, Tutor in Homoeopathy at the National Institute of Health Sciences in Canberra, and course reviewer for the course, Homeopathy For Community Pharmacy, conducted by the Pharmacy Guild of Australia. He's also acted as an advisor on homoeopathy to the South Australian Crown Solicitors Office, was a member of the Homeopathy Reference Group, Australian Complementary Healthcare Council, was formerly the Head of Department of Homeopathy for the Australian Traditional Medicine Society, Australia's largest association of complementary healthcare providers, has been a member of several doctoral thesis advisory committees on homeopathy, has taught homeopathy across Australia and in the US since 1995 and has written countless articles on this subject. Prior to this Medhurst was involved in private pathology practice, and teaching as well as research within the Medical Faculty at the University of Sydney.

On Specifics in Homeopathy

The notion that there are specific homeopathic medicines for specific diseases has been derided as being both inconsistent with Hahnemann's guiding principle and, if widely promoted, capable of damaging the capacity of homeopathy to persist in its original form. The use of specifics is certainly inconsistent with Hahnemann's guiding principle of individualised prescribing and while it can be argued that the widespread use of specifics, in the hands of non-homeopaths could be detrimental to the long-term health of homeopathy, there is certainly a case to be made for their consideration within a group of possible homeopathic similimums. The fact is that in the majority of cases, people use homeopathic medicines and consult prescribers of homeopathic medicines because they're seeking relief from hay fever, headaches, eczema or some other defined clinical condition. The condition has been defined as such because its combined signs and symptoms are consistent with the accepted constellation of signs and symptoms described for that clinical condition. The proper homeopathic repertorisation of those undifferentiated signs and symptoms will result in the discovery of a number of remedies, any of which may be capable of relieving the sufferer of their symptoms.

The problem is that the disease-specific remedy is just that; specific to the disease, not to the person suffering from it and it's the person who's treated in homeopathy, not the disease. This is because no one person experiences the same disease in exactly the same way as the next person and it's this idiosyncratic symptom expression that should lead the prescriber to the similimum. So while there may be disease specifics, they're not necessarily specific to the person suffering from that disease and if used without any reference to Hahnemann's original principles, may fall well short of relieving the sufferer of the susceptibility to the disease and the disruption of the vital force that caused it. It's for this reason that so-called specifics in homeopathy should only be used within the paradigm of orthodox homeopathy. When used in this context, these remedies form extremely valuable additions to the remedies found by the traditional method of repertorisation.

While the concept of specifics has been pilloried by the majority of those responsible for the foundation and development of homeopathy, the extent to which they were recommended by those same people is interesting. For example, in the Materia Medica Pura, Hahnemann himself promoted the use of specifics such as Belladonna for scarlet fever, Spongia for goitre, Hepar sulph and Spongia in croup and Drosera in whooping cough. Boenninghausen's article, *My Treatment of Membranous Croup*, in his *Lesser Writings*, makes mention of his "croup powders", composed of 3 homeopathic remedies in sequence: Aconite, Hepar Sulph, and Spongia. James Tyler Kent, to use another example, has been quoted as recommending the use of Hepar sulph 9X three times daily for nasal abscesses. Steve Smith (the 27th reference mentioned above) on page 124 of his book, quotes famed Greek homeopath George Vithoulkas as saying for sinusitis, "use kali bic unless another remedy is better indicated." GHG Jahr, reference 26 above, mentions on page 228 of his book for the treatment of Lumbago, "The specific remedy for this disease…is Rhus t".

The salient point here is that while these read like mechanical prescriptions, they're far from it. They were prescriptions that were made with the full understanding of the remedy and the implications of its use in this way, and while they were recommendations, they were not always rigidly adhered to. For example, Arnica is often thought of as a specific remedy for injury, but the experienced prescriber will know that while a great many injury cases will respond well to Arnica, many will not, and a complete cure from the effects of the injury will only occur if the signs and symptoms generated by the injured person are synonymous with those exhibited in a properly conducted proving of that remedy.

My hope is that while this book contains a vast number of recommendations, that they're taken exactly as that- recommendations to be considered with all other remedies that are arrived at by properly reasoned repertorisation, and used according to traditional homeopathic principles.

Robert Medhurst 2013

Abdomen, Diseases Of

	CHINA	ANT C	ARS	ASAF	CALC	CAPS	COCCUL	HEP	LACH	LYC	NAT M	NUX V	PHOS	PULS	SULPH
7				X				X	X						
8	X	X			X	X	X			X	X	X	X	X	X
9	X		X												

Abortion/Miscarriage, Threatened

	SABIN	SEC	ARN	CAULO	VIB OP	ACON	CHAM	IPEC	PULS	SEP	CIMICI	BELL	CHINA	CINNAM	CROC	CALC	ALET	APIS	SIL	HELL	KREO	NUX V	OP	PHOS	PLAT	TRILL P	VIB P	FERR
1	X	X	X			X		X	X	X					X	X	X				X				X		X	X
2	**X**	X	**X**	X	X	**X**	**X**								X	**X**			**X**								X	
3	X	X	X	X	X	X	X	X	X	X	**X**			X		X			X	X	X		X	X			X	
4	**X**	**X**		X	**X**	X	X		X	X	**X**	X		X						X								
6	X			X													X											
7	X	X	X	X	X		X	X	**X**	X		X	X	X		X		X	X	X		X	X			X		X
8	X	X	X	X	X	X	X	X	X	X	X	X	X	X	X	X	X	X	X	X	X	X	X	X	X	X	X	X
9	X	X	X	X	X	X	X		X	X	X	X	X	X		X		X						X				
10	**X**	X	X				X	X		X		X	X	X	X	X						X			X			
13	X	**X**	X	X	X	X	X	**X**	X	**X**		X	X		**X**	**X**	X	X	**X**		X	X	X	X	X			**X**
14	X		X	X	X										X		X									X		
15		X	X				X	X					X															
16	X	X	X	X	X	X	X	X		X	X	X	X	X	X	X		X			X	X	X		X	X		
19	**X**	X			X	X		X	X			X	X	X	X		X							X				
21	X	X	X			X		X	X	X		X																
22	X																											
23	X			X							X									X						X	X	
25	X	X	X		X				X				X	X				X										
27	X			X																								
28	X	X				X																						
29*				X																								

29* Day C. Control of Stillbirths in Pigs Using Homeopathy. Veterinary Record, 114, March 3, 1984: 216 reprinted in American Institute of Homeopathy, 779, December 1986, 146-147.

Abortion/Miscarriage, Threatened, 1st Month

	CROC	SEC	VIB OP
16	X		X
25		X	

Abortion/Miscarriage, Threatened, 2nd Month

	KALI CAR	APIS	SABIN	VIB OP	CIMICI	CROC	IPEC	THUJA	TRILL P
1			X						
4				X					
7	**X**	X					X		
8	X		X		X	X		X	X
16	X	X		X					

Abortion/Miscarriage, Threatened, 3rd Month

	SABIN	SEC	APIS	KALI CAR	CROC	VIB OP	KREO	NUX V	THUJA	MERC	TRILL P
1	X										
3		X					X				
4	**X**	X				**X**					
6	X										
7	X	X	X	**X**	X			X		X	
8	X	X	X	X	X				X		X
9	X	X	X								
14	X										
16	X	X	X	X	X	X	X	X	X		
21	X										
25	X	X	X								

Abortion/Miscarriage, Threatened, 4th Month

	APIS
7	**X**

Abortion/Miscarriage, Threatened- From the 5TH Month

	SEP	APIS	RUTA	SEC	VIB P
1	X	X			X
4				**X**	
7	X		X		
8	X	X			
16	X		X		

Abrasions

	CALEND	HYPER	ARN	HEP	PETR
3				X	X
14	E				
16	E	E			
22	X				
25		B	X		

E- External B- Both Internal and External use

Abscesses

	SIL	HEP	MERC	BELL	LACH	ARN	SULPH	ARS	CALC	APIS	CALC SUL	PYROG	RHUS T	ANTHRAC	PHOS	TAR C	CALEND	ASAF	CARB V	ACON	CHINA	BRY	CHAM	KALI IOD	LYC	NIT AC	PULS	ECHIN
1											X		X			X												
2	**X**	**X**	**X**	**X**		**X**		**X**		**X**	X	X					**X**				**X**							
3	X	X	X	X	X	X	X	X		X	X	X	X	X										X				
4	**X**	**X**	X	**X**	**X**	**X**	**X**	X	X		X	**X**	**X**				X	X	X				X	X	X			**X**
5	X	**X**		X	X		X			X		X		X														X
6	X																											
7	**X**	**X**	**X**	X	X	X	X			X			X	X	X			X	X			X	X			X	X	
8	**X**	**X**	**X**	X	X	**X**	X	X	X	X			X		X	X	X	X	X			X	X		X		X	
9	X	X	X	X																								
10	X	X	X	**X**	X	X	X		X						X					**X**								
12	X	X	X	X			X	X	X								E			X	X							
13	**X**	X	X		X		X		X									X								X	X	
14	**X**	**X**	X			X			X							X												
15	X	X	X	X	X	X														X								
16			X																									
18		X	X	X	X			X		X		X		X		X												
19	**X**	**X**	X	X	X	X	**X**	X	X		**X**	X		X	X	X								X		X		
20	X		X	**X**	X			X																				
21	X	X	X	X																								
23		X									X																	
24	X		X	X	X	X															X							
26	**X**	X	X	X	X		X		X						X				X			X			X			
28	X																											

E- External

Abscess, Ankle Joint

	ANGUST
6	X
8	X

Abscess, Anus

	CALC SUL	SIL	BAR M	CALC	HEP	MERC	PAEONIA
1	X						
2			X				
3	X						
7	X	X		X	X	X	X
11	X						
21	X	X					

Abscess, Arm

	ANANTH	BUFO
7	X	
19		X

Abscess, Axilla

	HEP	RHUS T	SIL	TAR C	NIT AC	IRID	JUG R	MERC	PHOS	SULPH	THUJA
1				**X**							
2	X					X					
4		X			**X**						
7	X	X	X								
8	X										
19	X		X				X	X	X	X	X

Abscess, Back

	SIL	SULPH	KALI IOD	STAPHYS
13	**X**	X		X
19	X	X	X	

Abscess, Bones

	SIL	AUR	ASAF	CALC FL	CALC PH	MANG	PHOS	PULS
1	X							X
4		X	X	X	X	X	X	
12	X							

Abscess, Brain

	ARN	BELL	CROT H	CUPR	HEP	IOD	LACH	MYRIST	OP	VIP
7				X						
14	X	X	X		X			X		
17	X	X	X			X	X		X	X

Abscess, Breast

	HEP	PHYTO	SIL	BELL	BRY	PHOS	MERC	ACON	CALC	CAMPH	CON	GRAPH	HYDRAST	LACH	MERC SU	SABAL
1		X	X		X									X		
2						X										
3	X	X		X			X				X		X			X
5									X							
7	X	**X**	**X**			X	X			X						
8	X		X						X							
9	X	X		B	X		X	X							X	
14		X			X											
13	**X**		X													
19			X	X		X	X					X				
21				X	X											
25	X	X		B	X			X								
26			X			X										

B- Both External and Internal use

Abscess, Buttocks

	SULPH	GRAPH	THUJA
19	**X**	X	X

Abscess, Cornea

	HEP	CALC M	CALC SUL	KALI SUL	SIL
1	X	X			X
3		X			
4	**X**		X	X	
8	X				

Abscess, Dental

	SIL	MERC	HEP	BELL	AMM C	CALC	CALC FL	CAUST	GUNPOW	HECLA	MYRIST	PHOS	PYROG	SULPH	ZINC
1	X														
3	X														
4	**X**	**X**	X	**X**											
5			X								X				
8	X														
9	X														
10		X													
14	X	X													
18		X													
19	X	X	X		X	X	X	X		X		X		X	X
21	X	X		**X**					X						
25	X														
28			X										X		

Abscess, Ear

	BAR M	CALC	CAUST	HEP	MERC	PIC AC
1				X		
7	X	X			X	
19			X			X

Abscess, Eye (Includes Abscess, Eye, Inner Angle)

	RHUS T	APIS	BELL	HEP	PULS	SIL
4	X					
6	X	X	X	X	X	
14						X

Abscess, Eyelid

	PHOS	PULS	SIL
19	X		X
27		X	

Abscess, Face

	BELL	HEP	KALI IOD	SIL	MERC
7	X	X	X	X	**X**
19	X	X	X	X	

Abscess, Glands

	MERC	RHUS T	CALC	ARS	BELL	CALC IOD	HEP	MERC I F	PHOS
1								X	
4	X	X	X			X			
7		X							
8		X			X				
19	X		X	X			X		X
24	X								

Abscess, Groin

	NIT AC	HEP	MERC	SIL	SULPH	THUJA
3				X		
4	**X**					
19		X	X		X	X

Abscess, Gums

	SIL	CAUST	HECLA	HEP	MERC	NUX V	BAR C	BELL	CALC	LYC	NAT M	PETR	STAPHYS
1	X		X	X									
7	X			X		X	X						
8	X	X							X	X	X	X	X
14			X		X								
26		X			X	X		X					

Abscess, Hand

	ANANTH	BUFO
7	X	
19		X

Abscess, Jaw, Lower

	HECLA	SULPH
7	X	X
19	X	

Abscess, Kidney

	HEP	ARS	MERC	SIL	ARN	BELL	BERB V	CROT H	LYC
7	X	X	X	X					
10	X	X	X	X				X	
15	X				X	X			
24							X		X

Abscess, Knee

	SIL	HEP	TAXUS	BELL	BRY	CALC HP	LACH	MERC	SULPH
2			X						
3			X			X			
7	**X**	X		X					X
26	X	X			X		X	X	

Abscess, Labia

	GOSSYP	HEP	SIL
2	X		
14		X	X

Abscess, Leg

	ANANTH	BELL	GRAPH	HEP	SIL
7	X				
19		X	X	X	X

Abscess, Liver

	SIL	HEP	LACH	MERC	BELL	KALI C	ARS	BRY	THERID	CHINA	MEDO	NUX V	RAPH	RHUS T	VIP	CHIN ARS	LYC	PHOS	PULS	RUTA	SEP
1			X						X												
2									X		X		X	X							
3		X																			
6	X		X			X															
7	X	X	X	X	X	X			X		X	X					X				
8	X	X	X	X	X	X		X		X		X							X	X	X
11	**X**	**X**	X	**X**	X		X	X					X	X	X	X		X			
13	X		X																		
14	X	X																			
15	X	X			X		X														
17				X		X															
24	X	X	X	X	X	X	X	X		X					X						

Abscess, Lung (Note that only main remedies are used from 17)

	HEP	SIL	PHOS	ARS IOD	CALC	KALI C	MANG	MERC	ACON	BELL	CHINA	CROT H	HIPPOZ	LACH	LED	LYC	PLUM	PSOR	PULS	STAPHYS	SULPH	TUB
3	X																					
7	**X**	X					X															
11	X	X	X		X																	
12			X																			
13						X																
14				X																		
17	X	X	X	X	X	X	X	X			X	X	X	X	X	X	X	X	X	X	X	X
21	X								X	X												
24	X	X						X														

Abscess, Lymphatics

	SIL	PHOS
8		X
19	**X**	

Abscess, Mastoid

	CAPS	AUR	NIT AC	SIL
3	X	X	X	
6	X			
8	**X**	X	X	X

Abscess, Nose

	HEP	SIL	AUR	CAD S	CAUST	MERC	PIC AC
1				X			
3	X		X				
7	X	X			X	X	
19		X					X

Abscess, Ovaries (Includes Ovaries, Suppuration)

	LACH	MERC	ARS	HEP	PYROG	SIL
2					X	
7	**X**	X	**X**	X		X
8	X	X				

Abscess, Peritonsillar- See Quinsy

Abscess, Psoas

	PH AC	SIL	ARS	ASAF	AUR	BELL	CALC	CUPR	HEP	IOD	LAPIS	LYC	MEZ	STAPHYS	SULPH	SYMPH	SYPH
2	X	X												X		X	X
7	X	X						X									
8	X	X	X	X	X	X	X		X	X	X	X	X		X		

Abscess, Retropharyngeal

	HEP	SIL	APIS	ARN	ASAF	AUR	BELL	BRY	CALC	LACH	LYC	MERC	MEZ	NIT AC	PHOS	PULS	RHUS T	SULPH
4	X																	
6	**X**	**X**	X	X	X	X	X	X	X	X	X	X	X	X	X	X	X	X

Abscess, Scrotum

	HEP	MERC	SIL	STILLING	STRYCHN
2					X
27	X	X	X	X	

Abscess, Slow to Heal

	SIL	GRAPH	MERC	THYROID
2				X
7			X	
12	X			
19		X		
20	X			

Abscess, Tonsil- See also Quinsy

	HEP	LACH	MERC	SIL	BAR C	CALC SU	ANAC	APIS	BELL	GUIAIA	KALI BIC	LAC C	LYC	MERC I F	PLUM	SABAD
4	X	X		X												
7	X	X	X	X	X	X	X	X	X		X	X	X	X		X
9	X															
10			X	X												
13															X	
14		X														
18			X													
19					X											
21	X					X										
24		X								X						
25	X															

Abscess, Tongue

	CALC	MERC
1	X	
7		X

Acetoneaemia

	CARB AC	LYC
2	X	
18		X

Achalasia

	CIMICI	ALUM	PHOS
21	X	X	X

Achalasia Cardia (AKA Cardiospasm)

	ABIES N	BAPT	BELL	CARB V	IGN	NAJA	VER V
11		X	X		X	X	X
14	X			X			

Achlorhydria- See Hypochlorhydria

Achromatopsia

	CARB S
1	X
2	X

Acne

	SULPH	HEP	KALI BR	PULS	SIL	ANT C	THUJA	GRAPH	NAT M	PSOR	SEP	CALC SUL	ARS	CARB V	SUL IOD	ARS BR	BELL	EUGEN	NUX V	PH AC	MERC	NIT AC	RHUS T	SANG
1	X	X	X	X			X																	
2	X		X	X	X			X		X				X	X	X	X	X		X				
3	X	X	X	X		X	X		X					X	X		X					X		X
4	**X**		**X**						X			X	X			X								**X**
5			X		X	X	X	X	X		X				X	X		X		X			X	
6	X	X																						
7	X	X		X	X	X		X	X		X										X	X	X	
8	X	X					X	X	X				X			X								
9	X	X	X	X	X	X				X		X	X											
10	X													X					X	X				X
11		X	X		X	X	X			X	X	X		X					X					
12	X	X				X											X			X				
13	X	X		**X**	X	X	X	X	X		X		X	X			X		X	B	X	**X**	**X**	
14	X	X			X			X																
15	X	X									X										X		X	
16			X																					
18	X	X	X	X	X	X	X		**X**		X				X			X	X					
19	**X**	**X**	**X**	X	**X**		**X**	X		X	X	**X**	X				X	X	X		**X**			
20	X	X																						
21	X	X	X	X	X	X						X			X									
22	X	X	X																					
23	X	X	X				X			X					X	X		X						
24				X																				
25	X		X	X		X				X		X	X											
26																						X		
27	X									X				X										
28	X	X			X			X																

B- Both External and Internal

Acne, Back

	KALI BR	GRAPH	IOD	KALI IOD	LACH	NIT AC	THUJA
5		X		X	X	X	X
9	X						
12			X				
18	X						
19	X	X					
25	X						

Acne, Chin

	SEP	HYDRAST	VIOL T
5	X	X	X
19	**X**		

Acne, Facial

	KALI BR	SULPH	HEP	PH AC	LED	CALC	NAT M	NUX V	ANT C	AST R	BELL	CARB V	NIT AC	ARS	ARS IOD	EUGEN	PULS	SEP	SULPH IO	AMBRA	ARS BR	CLEM	SIL	THUJA
1		X								**X**					X		X		X					X
2					**X**															**X**		**X**		
3	**X**									**X**					X				X			X		
4									**X**															**X**
6		X	X			X								X			X							
7	X	X	**X**	X	X	X	X	X	X		X	X	X	X		X					X		**X**	
8	X	**X**	**X**	X	X	X	X	**X**			**X**	**X**	X	X	X	X	X		X		**X**			
9	X																							
10		X		X	X	X		X			X	X						X						
12									X															
13				X			X						**X**			X		X		X				
15				X																				
18	X						X																	
19																		X					X	
25	X																							

Acne, Forehead

	CAUST	HEP	KALI BR	ARS	NAT M	PSOR	SULPH	THUJA
5	X	X		X	X			
7	X						X	
19	X	X	**X**			X		X

Acne, Legs

	MERC
6	X
24	X

Acne, Nose

	CAUST	CAPS	LACH	AMM C	CALC PH	CLEM	EUPHR	KALI C	OL AN	OX AC	PALL	PETR	PLUM	PSOR	SIL	SULPH
2	X															
5	X	X		X												
13	X	X	X		X	X	X	X	X	X	X	X	X	X	X	
17			X													
19	**X**															X

Acne Rosacea

	RHUS T	ARS	CARB A	LACH	NUX V	CAUST	SEP	CARB V	RUTA	SULPH	CALC	EUGEN	KREO	LED	AGAR M	AUR MUR	MEZ	PETR	SULPH AC	CIC	SANG	VER A	HYDR AC	VIOL T
2	**X**	X	X		**X**	X						X			**X**				**X**					
3																X								
5				X	X									X					X		X			
6	X	X	X	X	X	X	X	X	X	X	X			X			X	X						
7	**X**	X	X	**X**		X	X	X	X	X	X	**X**	X			X	X	X		X		X	X	X
8	**X**	**X**	**X**	X		X	X	**X**	**X**	X	**X**		**X**	X		**X**	**X**	**X**	X	X		X	**X**	**X**
5															X									
12	X				X			X							X									
13	X	X	X	X		X	X		X				X	X										
14			X																					
18				X			X	X		X		X									X			
19					X	X	X			**X**		X												
21	X	X		X	X																X			
26	X	X	X						X		X		X							X		X		

Acrocyanosis

	CARB V	PULS	AGAR M	ARS	HAM	SEC	ARN	CACT	CUPR AR	FERR PH	LACH	NAT M	NIT AC	PHOS	TUB	VER A
5		X	X		X	X			X		X					
14	X			X									X			X
18	X	X	X		X		X					X		X	X	
21	X	X		X		X		X		X						

Acromegaly

	THYROID	CHRYS A	PITUIT	SPONG
2	X			
8				X
9	X			
11	X	X	X	

Actinomycosis

	NIT AC	HECLA	KALI IOD	HIPPOZ
2	**X**		X	
9	X	X		
24	X	X	X	X

Addison's Disease (AKA Morbus Addisonii)

	NAT M	PHOS	ARS	ARG N	CALC	IOD	BELL	NIT AC	SIL	ADRENAL	SPIG	ANT C	ARS I	CARB V	CHINA	FERR	FERR IOD	KALI CAR	KREO	OL JEC A	SEC	SULPH	TUB	BACILLIN
2	**X**			**X**						X										X				**X**
4	X	X	**X**	X	X	X	X	X			X	X	X								X		X	
6	X	X	X	X		X	X						X	X	X	X			X	X				
7	**X**	**X**	X		**X**	**X**	X	X	X		X					X	X	X				X		
8	X	X	X	X	X	X	X	X	X		X	X		X	X		X	X			X	X		
9		X	X		X																			
11	X	X			X	X		X		X									X				X	
14		X	X																					
17	X	X	X	X			X		X	X														
21	X			X					X															

Adenitis (Includes Lymphadenitis)

	SIL	BELL	PHYTO	HEP	RHUS T	CARB A	CIST C	DULC	CALC	CAMPH	GRAPH	HIPPOZ	IOD	PULS	KALI C	MERC	PHOS	SULPH
1	X				X							X		X				
2					X			X				X						
4		X																
5	X		X				X	X			X							
7	X	X	X	X		X	X		X	X								
8	X	X	**X**	X		X		X			X		X					
9	X	X		X									X					
13	X	**X**	X	X	**X**	X			X	X				X	**X**	**X**	**X**	**X**
17							X											

Adenoids, Diseases Of

	CALC	CALC PH	BAR C	SULPH	AGRAPH	BACILL	HYDRAST	BAR IOD	BROM	CINA	CIST	COR R	KALI BIC	LEM MIN	LYC	MERC I F	MEZ	NAT M	PHOS	PSOR	SAMB	SIL	STICTA	SULPH IO	TEUCR	THUJA	TUB
3	X	X		X	X	X									X	X						X					
5	X	X	X		X		X		X	X		X	X	X			X				X		X	X	X	X	
12	X		X	X														X	X	X							
14				X																							
16	X	X	X			X	X				X																X
18	X	X																									
24		X	X					X																			

Adenoids, Vegetations

	HYDRAST	CALC PH	CIST C	BAR C	KALI BIC
4	X	X	X	X	X

Adenoma, Breast- See also Tumor, Breast; Cancer, Breast

	SCROPH
4	X
11	X
24	X

Adhesions

	THIO	CALC FL	GRAPH	KALI BIC	PULS
1	X				
2	X				
5		X			
9			X	X	X
19	X				
27	X				
28	X				

Adhesions, Pleuritic

	RAN B	CARB A	HEP	SULPH
1	X			
2	X			
7	X			
13	X			
17		X	X	X

Aerophagia

	ASAF	ARG N	IGN	KALI C
5	X	X		
18			X	X

Agalactia- See also Lactation, Deficient

	AGNUS	**URT U**	**CHAM**	**ASAF**	**LAC D**	**PULS**	**ACON**	**CALC**	**CAUST**	**IGN**	**RICIN**	**DULC**	**ZINC**	**BRY**	**COFF**	**FORMICA**	**MILL**	**BELL**	**CALC PH**	**CHEL**	**CHINA**	**NAT M**	**SABAL**	**SEC**	**FRAG**			
2	X	X							X				X			X	X											
3																	X											
4	X	X	X			**X**			X		**X**																	
5					X																							
7		**X**	**X**	X	X			X	X	X		X	**X**	X	X	X	X	X		X	X							
8	X	**X**	X	X	**X**	X	X	X	X		**X**		X	X	X	X		X		X	X			X	**X**			
9	X	X	X	X	X		X	X											X			X	X	X				
14	X			X							X																	
21	**X**		X			X	X			X		**X**			X													
22										X									X									
24		X				X																						
25	X		X	X			X															X	X					
26				X		X	X	X		X		X		X														
28		X			X																							

Ageing

See Arteriosclerosis, Senile; Asthma, Senile; Atrophy, Brain, Senile; Catarrh, Senile; Constipation/ Diarrhoea Alternating, Senile; Constipation, Senile; Cough, Senile; Deafness, Senile; Dementia, Senile; Diarrhoea, Senile; Dyspepsia, Senile; Emaciation, Senile; Erysipelas, Senile; Heart, Diseases of, Senile; Impotence, Senile; Incontinence, Urinary, Senile; Indigestion, Senile; Insomnia, Senile ; Memory, Deficient, Ageing Related, Senile; Ophthalmia Senilis; Paralysis, Senile; Pleuritis, Senile; Prostate, Benign Hypertrophy, Senile; Pruritis, Senile; Senility; Tremor, Senile; Vertigo, Senile; Weakness, Digestion, Senile; Weakness, Mind, Senile; Weakness, Senile.

Ageing, Premature/Effects Of

	BAR C	**AMRA**	**CON**	**OP**	**FL AC**	**AMM C**	**ARG N**	**AUR**	**BAR M**	**CAUST**	**KALI C**	**LYC**	**NAT M**	**SEC**	**AGNUS**	**ANAC**	**CALC PH**	**CARB V**	**COCA**	**CRAT**	**IOD**	**PHOS**	**SIL**	**TEUCR**				
1	X	X																										
3	X	X													X													
4			X										X				X											
5	X	X		X	X			X		X	X	X		X														
6		X	X			X	X							X				X										
7	**X**	X	X	**X**				X					X		X	X			X		X			**X**				
8	X	X	X																X									
9	X	X	X	X	X		X	X				X						X					X					
10	X	X	X	X	X	X	X		X	X	X	X	X				X			X	X	X	X					
11						X																						
12				X																								
13		X	X	X	X					X	X			X								X						
14																X												
16	X								X											X								
17	X		X		X				X																			
24	X																											

Ageing, Premature Effects Of, Skin

	PHOS	ARG N	SEC
3			X
5	**X**		
9		X	

Ageusia

	NAT M	PULS	SIL	PHOS	MAG M	ANAC	BELL	VER A	ANT C	ARS	HEP	HYOSC	NAT CAR	STRAM	AMM M	AUR	BRY	CALC	CANTH	KALI SUL	LYC	MAG C	MERC	RHOD	SANG	SEC	SEP	SULPH
1		X						X						X		X												
2	**X**	X																										
3	X				X				X													X						
4	X	X			X																							
6	X	X	X			X				X			X															
7	**X**	X	X	**X**		X			X	X	X	X	X	X		X	X		X				X		X		X	
8	**X**	X	**X**	X	X	X	X	X			X	X			X			X			X			X		X	X	X
10	X	X																										
11	X	X			X				X		X	X																
13	**X**	X	**X**	X	X	**X**	**X**	**X**		X				X	X		X	X	X		X	X	X	X		X		X
14	X	X																										
15		X																										
17	X	X		X			X													X					X			
18		X																		X								
20	X																											
21	X																											
22	X																											
24	X	X	X										X															
25		X																										

Agoraphobia

	ARG N	ACON	ARS	SULPH	ARN	BAR C	CON	GELS	HEP	KALI PH	LYC	NAT M	STRAM
2										X			
8	X	X					X						
19	X	X	X			X			X		X		X
21		X	X	**X**	X								
25	**X**							X				X	
28	X												

Ague- See also Fever

	CEDRON	CHINA	EUP PER	MALAR	NAT M	PLANTAG	SULPH	TARAX	VERBEN
2			X	X		X	X	X	X
4	X								
9		X			X				

AIDS

	CALC	PHOS	PULS	SULPH	DNA	LACH	LYC	NAT M	NUX V	PLAT	RNA	STAPHYL
11	X	X	X	X	X	X		X		X		
28											X	
29[1]												X
29[2]	X	X	X	X			X		X			

29[1] Danninger T, et al. Immunological Changes in Healthy Probands and HIV Infected Patients after Oral Administration of Staphylococcus aureus 12C: A Pilot Study. Brit Hom J, 2000, 89, 106-115.
29[2] Rastogi DP, et al. Homeopathy in HIV infection. Brit Hom J, 1999, 88, 49-57.

Ailments From- Apart from the below also see entries for the specific allergen related to the disorder and allergies to the same.

Ailments from Abortion

	AUR	BELL	CAULO	CHAM	COFF	CROC	ERIG	IPEC	KALI C	NIT AC	PLAT	PLUM	PULS	RHUS T	SABIN	SEC	TRILL P
1	X																
3					X				X				X			X	
6		X	X	X		X	X	X		X	X	X		X	X		X

Ailments from Acids

	ANT C	ARS	HEP	NUX V	SULPH	ACON	BELL	CARB V	LACH	PH AC	SEP	CAUST	FERR	IPEC	NAT M	PHOS	STAPHYS
1	X																
7	X	X			X		X				X						
8	X	X	X	X	X	X		X	X	X		X	X		X	X	
13	X	X	X	X	X	X	X		X	X	X		X	X	X	X	X
15		X	X	X				X		X							
19	X																
21	X																
24														X			
26	X	X	X	X	X	X	X	X	X		X	X					X

Ailments from Alcohol- See also Alcoholism (Includes Whiskey, Brandy, Spirits etc)

	NUX V	ARS	OP	CARB V	SULPH	CHINA	LACH	LYC	RAN B	IGN	AGAR M	BELL	CALC	COCCUL	COFF	SEL	VER A	ZINC	ANT C	LED	NAT M	PULS	RHUS T	STRAM	SULPH AC	NAT CAR		
1	X																											
2													X															
3											X																	
4	X																											
5	X										X														X			
6	X	X	X	X	X		X	X				X			X		X					X						
7	**X**	**X**	**X**	X	X	**X**	**X**	**X**	**X**	X	X	X	X	X	**X**	**X**	X	X	X	X	X	X	X	**X**	X	**X**		
8	X	X	X	X	X	X	X	X	X	X		X	X	X	X	X	X		X	X	X	X	X	X		X		
9	X				X													X	X									
10	X		X									X																
11	X	X																								X		
12	X																											
13	**X**	**X**	**X**	X	X	X	X	X	X	X	X	X	X	X	**X**	**X**	X	X	X	X	X	X	X	**X**				
14	X	X								X	X																	
15	X	X	X			X				X				X														
16	X																											
17	X	X	X	X	X	X	X	X	X							X	X	X		X	X		X		X			
18	X			X			X											X							X			
19	**X**								X					X														
20	X																											
21	X																											
22										X																		
24								X																				
26	X	X		X	X	X							X															
28	X																											
29*	X																											

29* Sukul, S. Reduction of Alcohol induced Sleep time in Albino Mice by Potentised Nux Vomica prepared with 90% Ethanol. Brit Hom J, 1999, 88, 58-61.

Ailments from Altitude, High

	ARS	COCA																										
1		X																										
3	X																											
14	X																											
17	X																											
28		X																										

Ailments from Anaesthetics- See also Ailments from Narcotics/Opiates

	PHOS	ACET AC	IPEC	NUX V	OP
2		X			
5	X				X
19	X				
21	X				
22	X				
24	X		X	X	

Ailments from Antibiotics

	NIT AC	ALOE	CAND A	CROT T	SULPH
3	**X**				X
5		X	X		
18				X	

Ailments from Arsenic (Includes Ailments from Arsenic Vapours)

	ARS	IPEC	MERC	CAMPH	SAMB	VER A	CHINA	CUPR	FERR	GRAPH	HEP	IOD	KALI BIC	NUX V
11		X												
13		**X**	**X**	X	X	**X**	X		X	X		X		X
17		X	X	X	X			X			X		X	
29[1]	X													
29[2]	X													
29[3]	X													
29[4]	X													
29[5]	X													
29[6]	X													
29[7]	X													
29[8]	X													
29[9]	X													
29[10]	X													
29[11]	X													

29[1] Belon P, et al. Can administration of a homeopathic remedy, Arsenicum album, alter antinuclear antibody (ANA) titre in people living in high-risk arsenic contaminated areas? A correlation with certain haematological parameters. Evid Based Complement Alternat Med, 2006, Mar, 3, 1, 99-107.
29[2] Datta S, et al. Efficacy of a potentized homoeopathic drug (Arsenicum Album-30) in reducing genotoxic effects produced by arsenic trioxide in mice: II. Comparative efficacy of an antibiotic, actinomycin D alone and in combination with either of two microdoses. Complement Ther Med. 1999 Sep;7(3):156-63.
29[3] Datta S et al. Efficacy of a Potentised Homoeopathic Drug (Arsenicum album -30) in reducing Genotoxic Effects Produced by Arsenic Trioxide in Mice. Complement Ther Med, 1999, Jun, 7, 2, 62-75.
29[4] Kundu SN, et al. Efficacy of a Potentised Homoeopathic Drug (Arsenicum album 30C) in Reducing Cytotoxic Effects produced by Arsenic trioxide in Mice III Enzymatic Changes and Recovery of Tissue Damage Complement Ther Med, 2000, Jun, 8, (2), 76-81.
29[5] Mitra K, et al. Efficacy of a Potentised Homoeopathic Drug (Arsenicum album -30) in reducing Genotoxic Effects Produced by Arsenic Trioxide in Mice. Complement Ther Med, 1999, Jun, 7, 2, 24-34.
29[6] Kundu SN, et al. Efficacy of a Potentised Homoeopathic Drug (Arsenicum album 30C) in Reducing Cytotoxic Effects produced by Arsenic trioxide in Mice IV.- pathological changes, protein profiles, and content of DNA and RNA. Complement Ther Med, 2000, Sep, 8, (3), 157-65.
29[7] Wiegant FAC, et al. Mild Step-Down Arsenite Treatment causes Increased Levels of Heat-Shock Proteins and Enhances Development of Tolerance. Brit Hom J,1994, 83, 84-100.
29[8] Fontes, OL, et al. A Study on the Comparative Effects of different doses of Arsenicum album 6C on the intoxication of Rats with Arsenic. Int J High Dil Res, 2006, 5, 17, 6-8.
29[9] Banerjee P, et al. A potentized homeopathic drug, Arsenicum Album 200, can ameliorate genotoxicity induced by repeated injections of arsenic trioxide in mice. J Vet Med A Physiol Pathol Clin Med. 2007 Sep;54(7):370-6.
29[10] Banerjee P, et al. Comparative efficacy of two microdoses of a potentized homeopathic drug, arsenicum album, to ameliorate toxicity induced by repeated sublethal injections of arsenic trioxide in mice. Pathobiology. 2008;75(3):156-70.
29[11] Khuda-Bukhsh AR, et al. Can Homeopathic Arsenic Remedy Combat Arsenic Poisoning in Humans Exposed to Groundwater Arsenic Contamination?: A Preliminary Report on First Human Trial. Evid Based Complement Alternat Med. 2005 Dec;2(4):537-48.

Ailments from Beer

	KALI BIC	NUX V	CHINA	SULPH	FERR	PULS	RHUS T	ARS	COLOC	LYC	MEZ	VER A	ANT C	ASAF	BAPT	BELL	CON	CYCL	EUPHR	GAMBOG	IGN	KALI CHL	MUR AC	SEP	STANN	TEUCR	THUJA	
5																		X										
7		**X**	X	X	X	X			X	X	X	X																
8	X		X	X																X			X					
9		X					X																					
11	X														X													
12	X																											
13	X	X	X	X	X	X	X	X	X	X	X	X		X		X	X		X			X		X	X	X	X	
15	X	X				X															X							
16		X																										
18	X																											
19			X	X																								
21	X																											
24			X																									
26		X	X		X		X	X					X															

Ailments from Blood, Loss Of

	CHINA	CALC	CARB V	CINA	COCCUL	FERR	HELON	HYDRAST	NAT M	NUX V	PH AC	SIL	STAPHYS	SULPH	TRILL P													
5	X				X	X			X			X			X													
8	X	X	X	X			X	X		X	X		X	X														

Ailments from Bread- See also Ailments from Farinaceous Foods

	CHINA	BRY	PULS	PH AC	RHUS T	SEP	SULPH	CAUST	HYDRAST	MERC	NAT M	NIT AC	NUX V	PHOS	SARS	STAPHYS	ZINC	ANT C	BAR C	CINA	COFF	CYCL	KALI C	LYC	RAN S	VER A		
5	X								X													X						
8	X	X	X	X	X	X	X	X	X	X	X	X	X	X	X	X	X		X	X	X			X		X		
13	X	X	**X**	X	X	X	X	X		X	X	X	X	X	X	X	X						X		X			
15	X	X	X	X																								
19																		X										
26	X	X			X	X	X																					

Ailments from Buckwheat

	PULS	IPEC	PHOS	SEP																								
7	**X**																											
8	X	X	X	X																								

Ailments from Butter

	CARB V	PULS	CHINA	ARS	CYCL	IPEC	NAT ARS	SEP	TARAX
1	X						X		
7	X	**X**		X	X			X	X
9	X								
13						X			
14	X	X							
15	X	X	X						
17	X								
19			X						

Ailments from Cabbage

	BRY	PETR	MAG CAR	LYC	CHINA	PULS
1		X				
5			X			
7	**X**	**X**	X	**X**	X	X
18	X					
19	X					
26	X					

Ailments from Cadmium (Includes Cadmium, Ailments from, Prophylaxis)

	CAD	CAD S
29[1]	X	
29[2]	X	
29[3]	X	
29[4]	X	
29[5]		X

29[1] Delbancut A, et al. New in-vivo tools to study protective effect of very low cadmium concentrations against cytotoxic cadmium doses. Brit Hom J, 1995, 84, July, 176.
29[2] Delbancut A, et al. Mechanistic Approach to the Effect of High Dilutions of Cadmium to Protect from Cytotoxic Cadmium doses in Renal Tubular Cell Cultures. Brit Hom J, April, 1994, 83, 84-100.
29[3] Herkovits J, at al. Potentised Microdoses of Cadmium Reduce the Lethal Effect of this Heavy Metal in Amphibian Embryos. Berlin J on Res In Hom, 1, 2, March 1991, 93-97.
29[4] Herkovits J, et al. Could Potentised Microdoses of Cadmium change the Toxicological Effect of this Heavy Metal? Berlin J on Res in Hom, 1, 3, 1991, 171, Congress Report Poster.
29[5] Datta S, et al. Comparative efficacy of two microdoses of a potentized homoeopathic drug, Cadmium Sulphoricum, in reducing genotoxic effects produced by cadmium chloride in mice: a time course study. BMC Complement Altern Med. 2001;1:9.

Ailments from Carbon Monoxide

	ARN	ARS	BAPT	NAT M	PYROG
3				X	
17	X	X	X		X

Ailments from Chemotherapy

	SEP	CAD S	PROTEUS
19	<u>X</u>		
27		X	X

Ailments from Chlorine

	OCIMUM
29*	X

29* Chirila M, et al. Effect of Ocimum basilicum 5X in Workers exposed to Chlorine. Brit Hom J, April, 1994, 83, 84-100.

Ailments from Chocolate

	LITH C	PULS	BOR	BRY	CAUST	LYC
1	X	X				
7	X	X	X			
8		X		X	X	X
13	X		X			

Ailments from Coffee

	NUX V	IGN	CHAM	COCCUL	CARB V	CANTH	BELL	COFF	MERC	PULS	SULPH	CAUST	RHUS T	ARS	CAMPH	CHINA	CIST	CYCL	HEP	IPEC	GUARAN	PHOS						
1	X	X		X	X																X							
2			X																									
4	X																											
5	X							X										X										
6	X	X	X	X	X		X		X	X	X		X															
7						X	X					X																
8	X	X	X	X	X	X	X		X	X	X	X	X		X	X	X	X	X	X	X	X						
9	X																											
10	X		X																									
12	X																											
13	**X**	**X**	X	X		**X**			X	X	X	**X**	X	X	X		X		X									
14		X			X																							
15	X	X	X	X						X						X				X								
17	X							X																				
18	X																											
19	X		X																									
20	X																											
21	X		X					X																				
22		X			X																							
24		X				X																						
25	X							X																				
26	X	X	X	X			X		X		X			X								X						

Ailments from Cold Air/Cold Weather

	HEP	ACON	DULC	ARS	CAUST	RHUS T	NUX V	SIL	PHOS	BELL	CALC	CARB V	CHAM	MERC	BRY	KALI CAR	PULS	RUMEX	AGAR M	BAR C	CAMPH	COLCH	CON	LYC	SEP	SPIG	CIST	MOSCH
1	X			X	X			X				X				X					X		X		X		X	
5						X	X	X	X		X						X						X	X	X			
6	X	X	X	X	X	X	X	X	X	X	X	X	X	X	X		X	X				X						
7	**X**		**X**	**X**	**X**	X	**X**	**X**	X	X	X	X		X	X	**X**		**X**	X	X	**X**	X	X	X	X		**X**	**X**
8	X	X	X	X	X	X	X	X	X	X	X	X	X	X	X	X	X			X	X	X	X	X	X	X		X
9	X	X		X	X	X						X							X	X								X
10	X	X	X	X	X	X	X	X	X	X	X		X	X	X		X		X			X			X			
11		X	X					X																		X		
12	X	X	X	X					X	X			X	X	X		X	X								X		
13	**X**	X	X	**X**	**X**	**X**	**X**	X	**X**	X	X	X	X	X	X	**X**	X	X	X	X	**X**	X	X	X	X		X	
14	X	X	X	X	X	X	X	X		X								X	X								X	
15	X	X	X	X			X			X			X	X	X		X									X		
16					X																							
17	X	X	X				X												X					X		X		X
18		X	X		X																		X					
19	X	X	X	X	X	X	X	X	X		X		X	X		X											X	
20	X	X	X	X	X	X	X	X	X							X		X						X		X		
21	X	X	X	X	X	X				X	X	X	X		X						X							X
22	X	X	X	X			X											X		X								
24	X	X				X											X											
25	X	X				X						X								X								
26	X		X	X	X	X	X		X			X	X	X								X						
27					X	X										X												

Ailments from Cold Drinks

	ARS	NUX V	BRY	HEP	LYC	PULS	SIL	NAT M	BELL	CARB V	MERC	ACON	CANTH	CHAM	DULC	NUX M	RHUS T	SPIG	STAPHYS	SULPH
7	**X**	**X**			**X**		X	X	X		X		**X**			X	**X**	X		X
8	X	X	X	X	X	X	X	X			X	X		X		X			X	X
9				X																
10	X		X	X											X					
12			X			X			X		X	X		X	X				X	
13	X	X	X	X	X	X	X	**X**	X	X			**X**		X	X	**X**	X	X	X
14	X		X				X					X								
15	X	X				X				X	X			X				X		
17				X			X	X		X										
18	X																			
19				X																
20	X																			
21					X	X														
22	X				X															
24	X																			
26	X	**X**	X						X	X										

Ailments from Cold Food

	ARS	LYC	PULS	NUX V	RHUS T	BRY	CHAM	SULPH	ARG N	CARB V	GRAPH	HEP	MERC	NUX M	RHOD	SPIG	STAPHYS	VER A	ACON	BELL	CALC	CALC PH	CON	GLON	KALI IO	KREO	MANG	
7	**X**	**X**		**X**	**X**			X			X			X	X	X		X					X			X	X	
8	X		X	X	X	X	X	X	X								X				X							
9			X																									
10	X					X						X																
12			X				X						X				X		X	X				X				
13	X	X	X	X	X			X		X	X			X	X	X		X										
14	X					X			X																			
15	X						X			X			X															
18	X																											
19		X										X										X						
20	**X**																											
21		X																							X			
24	X																											

Ailments from Cold Water or Cold Wind

	ACON	RHUS T	ANT C	BELL	CAUST	HEP	NUX V	ARS	BRY	DULC	PULS	CALC	MERC	NAT SUL	NIT AC	NUX M	STAPHYS	SULPH										
5			X																									
6	X	X		X	X	X	X	X	X		X	X	X	X		X	X	X										
8		**X**	X	X	X			X		X	X	X	X		X	X		X										
10	X						X			X																		
12								X									X											
13		X	X	X											X													
14	X		X	X		X																						
15							X		X																			
17	X	X					X		X																			
18					X					X																		
19	X	X	X		X	X																						
20	X																											
24														X														
25	X	X				X					X																	

Ailments from Eggs

	COLCH	FERR	CARB V	CHINA	CHIN ARS
1			X		
5		X			
7	X	X		X	
13	X				
16					X
17			X		
18	X				
19		X			
26	X	X			

Ailments from Exertion, Mental

	NUX V	CALC	PHOS	NAT C	SIL	BELL	NAT M	ANAC	PULS	ARN	COFF	GELS	IGN	KALI PH	LACH	PIC AC	SEP	SULPH	AUR	SABAD	ARG N	CHINA	COLC	LYC	PH AC	PARIS
6	X	X	X		X	X	X		X	X					X	X	X	X								
7	**X**							X																		
8	X	X	X	X	X	X	X	X	X	X	X		X		X	X	X	X	X	X	X	X	X	X	X	
9	X			X				X			X	X		X		X				X	X			X		
10	X	X		X		X					X	X		X								X				
11	X	X																			X					
12	X										X															
13	**X**	**X**	X	**X**	**X**		X	**X**	**X**	X			X		X		X	X	**X**	**X**		X	X	X	X	**X**
14	X	X	X	X																						
15	X					X																				
17		X	X	X			X																			
18														X												
19	**X**	X	X				X					X	X												X	X
20	X				X																					
21	X																									
22	X		X									X														
24	X		X																							
25	X																									
26	**X**	X	X	X	X	X			X	X			X		X		X	X	X				X			
27													X			X										

Ailments from Exertion, Physical- See also Ailments from Labour; Ailments from Over-Lifting

	RHUS T	ARN	CALC	ARS	NAT M	NUX V	PHOS	BRY	CHINA	GELS	PH AC	ARG N	CAUST	COCCUL	PULS	RUTA	SIL	ACON	LYC	SPIG	SULPH	VER A	AMM C	CACT	DIG	DULC	IOD	
5	X	X												X		X												
6	X	X	X					X	X			X		X		X								X				
7	X	X	**X**	X	X		X		X		X	X	X	X			X		X		X							
8	X	X	X		X	X		X	X			X	X	X		X	X	X	X		X	X	X				X	
9	X					X				X	X	X								X				X	X		X	
10	X	X	X	X		X		X	X	X										X								
11										X													X			X	X	
12		X	X							X																		
13	**X**	**X**	X	**X**	**X**	**X**	X	**X**	X		X		X	**X**	X	X	X	**X**	**X**	**X**	**X**	**X**	X		X	X		
14	X	X	X	X	X		X								X							X						
15	X		X				X				X							X										
17	X	X	X	X		X	X	X	X	X												X		X	X	X	X	
18	X																											
19	X	X	**X**	X	X	X				X		X	X		X	X	X			X			X	X				
20	X														X													
21	X		X		X																				X	X		
22		X					X																					
24	X						X																					
25											X																	
26	X	X	X	X	X	X		X							X		X	X	X		X							
27	X	X									X																	

Ailments from Farinaceous Foods- See also Ailments from Pastry

	NAT SUL	PULS	NAT M	NUX V	SULPH	CAUST	CHINA	LYC	NAT CAR	BRY	NIT AC	PH AC	RAN S	KALI BIC	RHUS T	SARS	SEP	VER A	ZINC									
5	X		X	X		X			X																			
6				X		X																						
7	X	**X**	**X**	X	X		X	X		**X**	**X**	**X**	**X**		X	X	X	X	X									
8	X		X		X		X	X	X					X														
9		X																										
13	X				X																							
25		X																										

Ailments from Fatty/Oily/Rich Foods

	PULS	CARB V	SEP	ANT C	ARS	COLCH	FERR	IPEC	NAT M	NIT AC	SULPH	CYCL	BRY	CHINA	DROS	HELL	MAG M	TARAX	ASAF	SPONG	THUJA
1	X	X																			
5	X	X	X			X	X	X													
6	X							X													
7	X		X		X	X	X		X	X	X	X			X	X	X	X	X	X	
8	X	X	X	X	X	X	X		X	X	X	X	X	X	X	X	X	X			X
9	X	X																			
10	X																				
12	X																				
13	**X**	**X**	X	X	X	X	X		X	X	X	**X**			X	X	X		X	X	X
14	X	X		X				X													
15	X	X	X											X							
17		X																			
18	X									X											
19	X													X							
20	X																				
21	X												X								
22	X												X								
25	X																				
26	X	X	X	X	X			X	X		X							X			

Ailments from Fish- See also Ailments from Seafood

	CARB V	ARS	CARB A	CHINA	COLCH	KALI BIC	KALI C	PLUM	PULS	RHUS T
1		X								
13			X				X	X		
15	X					X				
17	X									
18					X					
26	X			X					X	X

Ailments from Fish, Spoiled

	CARB V	PULS	CHINA	RHUS T	ALL C	KREO
8	X	X		X	X	
13	X	X				
15	X		X			X
17	X					
26	X	X	X	X		

Ailments from Fluid, Loss Of

	CHINA	PH AC	CARB V	PHOS	CALC	ARS	NAT M	NUX V	PULS	SEP	CALAD	CARB A	FERR	SEL	SULPH	VER A	STAPHYS
5	X	X											X				
7	X	X	X	X	X						X	X					
9	X							X									
10	X		X														
12	X	X		X													
13	**X**	X	X	X	**X**	X	X		**X**	**X**	X			X	X		**X**
14	X	X	X				X										
15	X																
17	X	X		X								X		X			
18	X					X	X	X					X			X	
19	X																
21	X																
22	X																
24	X			X													
25	X																
26	**X**	X	X		X	X		X	X	X					X	X	

Ailments from Fruit

	CHINA	PULS	ARS	BRY	VER A	SEL	NAT CAR	BOR	IPEC	MAG M	SEP	CARB V	CROT T	LACH	LYC	MAG CAR	MERC	RHOD
1	X	X	X			X												
5	X		X						X									
6	X														X			
7	**X**	**X**	**X**	X	**X**	X	X	X	X	X	X	X			X			
8	X	X	X	X	X	X	X	X	X	X	X		X	X		X	X	X
9		X																
10	X	X											X					
11	X																	
13	**X**	**X**	**X**	**X**	X	X	**X**	X		X	X	X		X			X	X
14		X																
15	X	X	X	X														
19	X																	
22			X															
24	X	X			X											X		
26		X	X	X	X													

Ailments from Fruit, Over-ripe

	ARS
1	X
21	X

Ailments from Fruit, Unripe

	RHEUM	CHINA	COLOC	IPEC	ARS	BRY	SULPH AC
1	X		X				
6	X			X			
7	X						X
9		X					
10					X		
12			X				
18	X						
21						X	
24				X			
25		X					

Ailments from Hair, Cutting Of

	BELL	BRY
6	X	X
21	X	
24	X	

Ailments from Hair, Washing Of

	BELL
21	X
22	X

Ailments from Heat (Includes Ailments from Hot Weather; Warmth; Warmth of Bed)

	PULS	BRY	NAT CAR	APIS	NAT M	SULPH	ACON	BELL	CARB V	LACH	LED	ANT C	GLON	IPEC	MERC	SIL	IOD	SEC
1	X	X			X					X								
4					X													
5	X		X							X								
7	**X**		X								X			X	X		**X**	**X**
8	X	X	X		X	X	X	X	X	X		X	X	X	X	X		
9	X	X		X		X												
10		X					X									X	X	
11											X							
14				X									X					
15		X					X	X										
18			X															
19	X				X				X		X	X	X					
20	X	X		X		X				X				X	X			
21	X	X		X	X	X		X										X
22	X	X		X			X		X		X							
25			X															
26	X	X	X			X		X	X			X				X		

Ailments from Hot/Warm Food

	CHAM	PHOS	PULS	BELL	BRY	AMBRA	ANAC	BAR C	CARB V	COFF	EUPHORB	IGN	KALI C	MERC	MEZ	NIT AC	NUX V	PH AC
7	X	**X**	**X**	X	X	X	X	X	X		X				X			X
8												X						
12	X			X														
14	X	X			X								X			X		
15	X													X			X	
19	X		X							X								
20			X															
22		X																

Ailments from Ice

	CARB V	PULS	ARS
8	X	X	X
17	X		
24		X	
26	X	X	X

Ailments from Ice Cream

	PULS	ARS	CARB V	ARG N	DULC	ELAPS	IPEC
1		X					
5	X						
8	X	X	X	X	X	X	X
10	X	X	X				
18	X						
19	X						
20	X	X					
21		X					
24	X						

Ailments from Injury

	ARN	ACON	LACH	RUTA	ART V	CALC PH	CAMPH	GLON	HYPER	IPEC	MEZ	MILL	SENEGA	STAPHYS	VER A
5	X														
6	X	X	X			X			X		X				
8	X	X	X												
10	X														
14	X	X					X								
17	X			X	X			X		X		X	X	X	X
19	X	X		X											
21	X														

Ailments from Injury, Skull/Head

	ARN	HYPER	CIC	NAT SUL	CON	HELL	HYOSC	MERC	OENANTH	OP	PETR	RHUS T	SULPH AC	ZINC
5		X		X									X	
8	X	X	X					X			X	X		
17					X									
19	X	X	X	X		X	X		X	X				X
21	X													

Ailments from Iron

	PULS	HEP	CHINA	ARN	ARS	BELL	FERR	IPEC	MERC	VER A
1	X									
8	X	X	X	X	X	X		X	X	X
10	X	X	X							
11	X	X								
28							X			

Ailments from Labour- See also Ailments from Exertion, Physical

	ARN	CAUL	SEC	KALI CAR	KREO	LIL T	LYC	SEP
1	X							
4						X		
6			X		X			
8	X		X					
14		X		X				
21							X	X
27		X						

Ailments from Laxatives

	CASC	COLLIN	HYDRAST	NUX V
5	X	X	X	
22				X

Ailments from Lead- See also Lead Poisoning

	ALUM	OP	PLAT	BELL	PLUM	NUX V	ARS	CAUST	POD	ALUMEN	CARB S	COLOC	CUPR	GLON	HEP	KALI IOD	MERC	STRAM	SULPH	SULPH AC
3								X												
6	X	X	X	X	X	X									X			X		
8	X	X	X	X		X	X		X	X										
10		X	X	X		X	X						X	X			X			
11	X	X			X											X				
12	X	X	X	X					X											X
13	X	X	X																X	
17											X									
24												X								
26	X							X												
27					X															
28					X															

Ailments from Lemonade

	SEL	CYCL
8	X	
13	X	X
17	X	

Ailments from Light- See also Photophobia

	BELL	NUX V	ACON	BRY	GLON	PHOS	SIL	SPIG
9	X							
10			X					
14	X			X	X	X	X	
19		**X**						
20								X

Ailments from Manipulation (Chiropractic or Osteopathic)

	RUTA
27	X

Ailments from Meat

	FERR	PULS	RUTA	COLCH	CARB V	CAUST	SIL	SULPH	CALC	KALI CAR	LEPT	MERC	NUX V	RUMEX	SEP
1			X		X								X		
5	X													X	
7	X	X		X	X					X					
8	X	X	X			X	X	X	X		X	X			X
10		X													
13			X	**X**		X	X	X							

Ailments from Meat, Smoked

	CALC	SIL	CAUST
7	X	X	X
8	X		
13	X	X	

Ailments from Meat, Spoiled

	CARB V	BRY	CHINA	KREO	PULS
15	X	X	X	X	X
17	X				

Ailments from Meat, Uncooked

	BRY	LYC	PULS	RUTA
13	**X**	X	X	X

Ailments from Medicines

	NUX V	BELL	NAT M	PHOS	PULS	TAB
5	X	X				
6	X					
7	X					
9	X			X		X
10	X				X	
14	X					
15			X			
18	X					

Ailments from Melons

	ZINC	ARS
8	X	
22	X	X

Ailments from Mercury

	HEP	NIT AC	AUR	CHINA	ASAF	CARB V	IOD	KALI IOD	LACH	STAPHYS	BELL	SIL	SULPH	DULC	MERC	MERC C	PH AC
2	X	X	X	X					X								
4	**X**							X	X								
6	X	X	X	X	X	X	X			X	X		X				
7	X	X															
8	**X**	X		X		X					X		X	X			
10	X	X	X	X		X	X			X	X		X				
11		X	X				X	X	X								
12			X														
15		X	X									X			X		
17	X	X	X	X	X	X	X	X	X	X							X
24	X				X							X					
25	X	X	X		X			X		X		X		X			X
28	X																
29[1]																X	
29[2]																X	
29[3]															X		

29[1] Datta S, et al. Comparitive efficacy of pre-feeding, post-feeding and combined pre and post-feeding of two microdoses of a potentised homeopathic drug, mercurius solubilis, in ameliorating genotoxic effects produced by mercuric chloride in mice. Evid Based Comp Alt Med, 2004, Dec, 1, 3, 291-300.
29[2] Cal JC. Chronobiological Approach of Protective Effect of Mercurius Corrosivus against Mercury induced Nephrotoxicity. Alternative Health Practitioner, Vol 3. No 3, Fall/Winter, 1997, 99-102.
29[3] Beringhs-Bueno, A, et al. Mercury Intoxication: High Dilution as Mercury's Chelating Agent. Int J High Dil Res, 2006, Vol 5, No 16.

Ailments from Milk

	AETHUSA	CALC	CARB V	CHINA	SEP	NAT CAR	SULPH	NIT AC	BROM	BRY	MAG CAR	ARS	NUX V	CON	LYC	ZINC	AMBRA	CHAM	CUPR	MAG M	PHOS	SULPH AC
1		X	X		X	X														X		
5	X	X		X	X	X			X		X		X					X		X		
6	X				X																	
7		**X**	X	**X**	**X**	X	**X**	**X**		X		X	X	**X**	X		X	X	X		X	X
8	X	X	X	X	X	X	X	X	X	X	X	X	X	X	X	X	X		X		X	X
9	X		X								X											
10	X	X				X	X				X											
11		X		X																X		
13		**X**	X	**X**	**X**	X	X	**X**	X	X		**X**	**X**	**X**	X	**X**	X	X	X		X	X
14					X		X															
15			X	X						X												
17	X					X										X						
18								X			X											
19	X							X	X													
20												X										
21	X																					
22			X																			
24	X								X													
26		X	X	X			X			X					X							

Ailments from Morphine/Painkillers- See also Ailments from Narcotics; Ailments from Opiates

	CHAM	IPEC	NUX V	AVENA	BELL	GELS
3	X			X	X	X
5	X					
6	X	X	X			
16	X					
17		X				
20			X			

Ailments from Mosquito Bites- See also Bites and Stings

	LED	CALAD	PSOR
19	X	X	X
24	X		

Ailments from Moulds

	BLATTA	SULPH
19	X	
27		X

Ailments from Mushrooms

	ABSINTH	ACON	ATROP	COFF	NIT S D	NUX V	PULS
8		X		X	X	X	X
9	X						
17	X						
23			X				

Ailments from Noise- See also Hyperaesthesia, Hearing

	BELL	COFF	SIL	NUX V	BRY	CHINA	COCCUL	LAC C	LAC D	NAT M	SANG	SPIG	SULPH	THER
19	X	X	X	**X**	X	X	X	X	X		X		X	
20	X		X									X		
21														X
22		X												
27										X				

Ailments from Narcotics- See also Ailments from Morphine/Painkillers; Ailments from Opiates

	CHAM	COFF	LACH	NUX V	MERC	PULS	SULPH	BELL	OP	ACET AC	ARS	CARB V	GRAPH	HYOSC	IPEC	LYC	SEP
2										X							
6	X	X	X	X	X	X	X					X					
8	X	X	X	X	X	X	X	X	X	X	X	X	X	X	X	X	X
13	**X**	**X**	**X**	X	X	X		**X**	**X**				X	X	X	X	X
16	X																
22		X		X													
26			X				X				X						

Ailments from Odours

	COFF	NUX V	IGN	SANG	SEP	SULPH
19	X	**X**	X	X	X	X
22	X					

Ailments from Onions

	LYC	THUJA	PULS	ALUMEN
1		X		
5	X			
7	X	X		X
13	X	X	X	
18	X			
21			X	

Ailments from Opiates- See also Ailments from Morphine/Painkillers; Ailments from Narcotics

	NUX V	IPEC	BELL	MERC	VER A	CARB V	CHAM
1	X	X					
6	X	X	X	X	X	X	X
8	X	X	X	X			
15	X						
17					X		
20	X						

Ailments from Overeating (Includes Ailments from Over-Indulgence)

	NUX V	ANT C	PULS	CHINA	CHAM	IPEC
4	X		X	X		
9	X					
14		X	X			
15	X	X	X	X	X	X
18	X					
19		X				
20	X					
21	X					
22	X	X				

Ailments from Over-lifting- See also Ailments from Exertion, Physical

	RHUS T	CALC	ARN	BRY	CARB V	COCCUL	FORMICA	GRAPH	LYC	MILL	RUTA	BOV	CALC PH	CON	KALM	MUR AC	NAT CAR	NUX V	OLEAND	PH AC	PHOS	SIL	VAL
2						X	X																
7	**X**	**X**	X	X	X	X	X	X	X	X		X		X	X		X	X		X		X	
8				X																			
13	X	X							X							X			X				X
14	X																						
15	X																						
16			X																				
17	X				X			X		X	X		X								X		
27											X												

Ailments from Oysters- See also Ailments from Oysters; Ailments from Shellfish; Allergy, Seafood

	LYC	BROM	SULPH AC	LACH
7	**X**	X	X	
8	X	X	X	X
13	X	X		
18	X			
19	X			

Ailments from Pastry- See also Ailments from Farinaceous Foods

	PULS	CARB V	ARS	IPEC	LYC	BRY	ANT C	CALC	CYCL	KALI BIC	KALI C	SULPH	VER A
1	X	X		X									
6	X			X									
7	**X**		X		X								
8	X	X	X	X	X	X				X	X	X	X
9	X												
12	X												
13	**X**	X	X					X					
14	X												
15	X	X			X	X			X				
18	X												
19							X	X					
24	X												

Ailments from Pepper

	CINA	ARS	CHINA	NUX V
8	X	X	X	X
13	X			

Ailments from Pork

	PULS	CARB V	IPEC	SEP	CYCL	COLCH	NAT M	ANT C	NAT C	THUJA	ACON L	ARS	DROS	NAT ARS
1			X											X
2											X			
5	X		X		X									
6	X													
7	**X**	**X**	X	**X**	**X**	X	X		X	X				
8	**X**	X	X	X		X	X						X	
9		X												
13	**X**	**X**	X	**X**	X	X	X	X	X	X				
15	X	X										X		
19	X							X						

Ailments from Potatoes

	ALUMEN	SEP	VER A	ALUM	AMM C	MAG C
1	X					
5	X					
7	X	X	X			X
8	X	X	X		X	
10				X		
13	X	X	X			
22				X		

Ailments from Pregnancy- See also Cramp, Calves, Pregnancy From; Dyspepsia, of Pregnancy; Dysuria, Pregnancy From; Hair, Falling of, Pregnancy During or After; Headache, Pregnancy, During; Heartburn, Pregnancy, During; Incontinence, Urinary; Insomnia, Pregnancy, During; Menses, Pregnancy, Continue Through; Morning Sickness; Oedema, Pregnancy During; Pain, Back, Pregnancy During; Pregnancy, Albuminuria From; Pregnancy, Bladder Disorders From; Pregnancy, Breasts Painful From; Pregnancy, Constipation From; Pregnancy, Diarrhoea From; Pregnancy, Diseases Of; Pregnancy, Dysuria From; Pregnancy, Indigestion From; Pregnancy, Pruritis From; Pregnancy, Oedema From; Pregnancy, Toothache From; Pregnancy, Urine, Retention/Suppression Of/From; Ptyalism, Pregnancy From; Pyrosis; Varicose Veins, Pregnancy, From

	SEP	BELL	NUX V	PULS	VER A	ACON	ALUM	LYC	NAT M	PLAT
6	X									
7		X	X							
8	X		X	X	X		X	X		
10		X	X	X		X				X
13	X				X		X			
17									X	
19	X								X	
21	X							X		
25				X						
26		X			X	X				X

Ailments from Radiation (Includes Radiotherapy)

	PHOS	RAD BR	ARN	CAD IOD	CAD S	CALC FL	PANAX	RUTA	X-RAY
1	X				X				
3	X			X					
17			X						
19	X	X				X			
27		X							
28									X
29[1]								X	
29[2]							X		

29[1] Khuda-Buksh AR, et al. Alterations of Cytogenic Effects by Oral Administration of a Homoeopathic Drug, Ruta Graveolens, in Mice exposed to Sub-Lethal X- Irradiation. Berlin Journal on Research in Homoeopathy, 1991, 1, 264-274.

29[2] Khuda-Bukhsh AR et al. Assessment of Cytogenetic Damage in X-irradiated mice and its Alteration by oral administration of a Potentised Homeopathic Drug, Ginseng D200. Berlin Journal on Research in Homoeopathy, 1991, 1, 254-263.

Ailments from Reading

	NAT M	ARN	RUTA	CALC	SIL	ARG N	CINA	CON	EUPHR	HEP	KALI C	NUX V	ONOS	PHOS	PULS	COCCUL
1			X													
5	X		X		X											
6	X	X		X											X	
8						X										
9					X				X							
11													X			
12		X														
13	**X**	X	X	**X**	**X**	X	X	X	X	X	X	X		X	X	**X**
14			X													
19	X															
21											X					
24	X	X		X			X	X		X			X			
26												X		X		

Ailments from Rhubarb

	PULS	CHAM	COLOC	MERC	NUX V
8	X	X	X	X	X
15	X				
26	X	X	X	X	

Ailments from Salt (Includes Ailments from Salted Food)

	CARB V	ARS	DROS	NAT M	SEL	PHOS	NIT S D	ALUM	COCA	IPEC	LYC	MAG M	MERC	NUX V	PULS
1				X				X				X			
6	X														
7	X		X	X	X	**X**			X						
8	X	X	X	X			**X**				X		X	X	X
10	X	X													
13	X		X		X					X					
15	X	X													
17					X	X									
26	X	X													

Ailments from Sauerkraut

	BRY	PETR	CALC	CHINA	LYC	PHOS	PULS	SEP
7	X	X	X	X	X	X	X	X
13		X						
26	X							

Ailments from Sausages

	BRY	ARS	BELL	ACET AC	CARB V	PH AC	PULS	RHUS T
2				X				
7	X	X	X					
8	X	X	X			X		X
15	X				X		X	

Ailments from Shellfish- See also Ailments from Oysters; Allergy, Seafood

	ANT C	ARS	CARB V	COP	DULC	TEREB
1		X		X		X
14	X					
15	X		X		X	

Ailments from Shock, Electric

	PHOS	ELECTR	MORPH
1		X	
17	X		X
20	X		
21	X		

Ailments from Sleep, Loss Of

	COCCUL	COLCH
2	X	
4	X	X

Ailments from Smoke

	SPIG	BROM	EUPHR	IGN	SEP
7	X		X		X
19	X	X		X	

Ailments from Spicy Foods

	NUX V	ARS	CHINA	SULPH
7	**X**			X
9	X			
10	X			
15			X	
18	X			
22		X		

Ailments from Spoiled Food- See also Food Poisoning; Ailments from Meat, Spoiled; Ailments from Fish, Spoiled

	ARS	CARB V	CARB A	PYROG
1		X	X	
5	X			X
10	X			
11	X			
14	X			
17		X		

Ailments from Stimulants (Wine, Coffee, Tea etc)

	NUX V
3	X
6	X
10	X
12	X
24	X

Ailments from Strawberries

	BRY	SEP	FERR	OX AC
8	X	X	X	
13		X		X
26	X			

Ailments from Sugar (Includes Sweet foods)

	ARG N	IGN	CHAM	MERC	ZINC	CAUST	IPEC	SEL	ACON	GRAPH	NAT C	SULPH	THUJA	ANT T	BAD	CALC	CROT T	CYCL	FL AC	IRIS V	MEDO	NIT AC	OX AC	SEP	SPONG	TROMB
1	X																					X				
4																				X						
5	X					X	X																			
6						X	X																			
7		**X**	X	X	**X**			X					X													
8	X	X	X	X	X	X	X		X	X	X	X				X	X		X					X	X	X
10	X			X																						
13		X	X	X				X	X		X	X	X	X				X					X			
14	X																									
15		X	X																							
17	X							X							X						X					
18	X																									
19	X				X					X																
27	X																									

Ailments from Sun- See also Hydroa; Photophobia; Sunstroke (Includes Ailments from Sunlight)

	GLON	BELL	LACH	NAT C	ACON	AGAR M	GELS	CAMPH	NAT M	NUX V	SANG	SEL	ANT C	PULS	BRY	SOL	BAR C	CACT	CARB V	EUPHR	MUR AC	VAL	VER V
1																X							
2												X						X					
4									X														
6			X	X	X	X		X	X								X						
7	**X**	**X**	**X**	**X**		X	X	X		X			**X**	**X**	X				X	X		X	
9	X	X					X		X														
10	X	X			X												X						
11	X									X	X												
13	X	X	X	X	X	X		X		X		X	X	X	X					X		X	
14	X	X	X			X		X															
15		X			X										X								X
17				X		X	X			X	X	X						X			X		X
18																					X		
19	X	X	X	X	X		X		X		X	X	X	X		X			X				
21	X																						
22							X				X												
25	X																						
28																X							

Ailments from Surgery

	ARN	STAPHYS	HYPER	PHOS	STRONT C	ACON	CALEND	CARB V	CAUST	CHINA	OP	BELLIS	GELS	MILL	PYROG	VER A
2			X													
4	**X**		X			X										
5		X							X		X	X				
10	X	X														
12	X															
13														X		
14	X				X			X								X
16		X		X	X		X									
17	X	X														
18	X	X		X						X				X	X	
19	**X**	**X**	X	**X**	**X**	X	X	X	X	X	X	**X**	X		X	
21	X	X	X	X				X	X							
22							X									
24	X		X			X				X	X		X			X
28	X	X														
29[1]	X															
29[2]	X															
29[3]	X	X														

29[1] Wolf M., et al. Efficacy of Arnica in Varicose Vein Surgery; Results of a randomized, double-blind, placebo-controlled pilot trial. Forsch Komplementarmed Klass Naturheilkd, 2003, Oct, 10, 5, 242-7.
29[2] Karow JH, et al. Efficacy of Arnica montana D4 for healing of wounds after Hallux valgus surgery compared to diclofenac. J Altern Complement Med. 2008 Jan-Feb;14(1):17-25.
29[3] Alecu, A, et al. Effect of the homeopathic remedies Arnica montana and Staphisagria on the time of healing of surgical wounds. Cultura Homeopática, 2007, 20, Jul- Sept, 19-21.

Ailments from Surgery, Dental

	ARN	HYPER	PHOS	RUTA	CALC	CALEND	CHAM	HECLA	IPEC	LED	STAPHYS	SYMPH
1	X		X		X				X			
6	X											
14	X		X									
16	X	X						X				
18	X											
19	X	X										
21	X	X	X	X						X	X	
22		X		X		E	X					
28	X											
29*												X

E- External
29* Mazzocchi A, Montanaro F. Observational study of the use of Symphytum 5CH in the management of pain and swelling after dental implant surgery. Homeopathy. 2012 Oct;101 (4):211-6.

Ailments from Surgery, Eye

	ACON	ARN	BRY	IGN	RHUS T	THUJA	ASAR	CROC	STRONT C	HYPER	LED	SENEGA	SENNA
1		X	X	X	X	X	X	X	X		X		X
4	**X**	**X**	X	X	X	X	X	X	X			X	
10	**X**		X	X	X	X							
19		X								X			
24	X												

Ailments from Tea

	CHINA	THUJA	COFF	FERR	SEL	NUX V	IGN	VER A	DIOSC	LACH	LOB I
1					X						
2	**X**	**X**				**X**			X		X
4	X										
6	X		X				X	X		X	
7	X	X	X	X	X						
8	X	X	X	X	X		X	X		X	
10	X		X				X				
11	X										
12		X		X							
13	X	X		X	X			X			
15	X					X	X				
17	X				X				X		X
21			X			X					
25						X					
26	X			X							

Ailments from Teething

	CHAM	CALC	BELL	IGN	ACON	POD	AETHUS	CALC PH	CIC	COFF	IPEC	MAG M	SULPH	NUX V
6	X	X	X	X	X									
7	X	X	X	X	X		X		X		X			
8	X	X								X	X		X	
10	X	X	X	X	X					X			X	
11	X	X	X		X		X	X				X		
12	X		X			X								
13	**X**	**X**	X	**X**		X	X	X		X	X	X	X	**X**
14	X					X		X	X			X		
15	X	X	X		X									X
17	X	X		X					X					
18	X													
21	X													
22						X								
24			X											

Ailments from Tobacco (Smoking or Smoke)- See also Tobacco Heart

	NUX V	IGN	GELS	STAPHYS	PULS	ARS	SPONG	COCCUL	CLEM	IPEC	PHOS	TAB	ARG N	CHINA	MERC	SEP	SPIG	THUJA	NAT M	ACON	ANT C	CHAM	EUPHR	LACH	LOB I	VER A	PLANTAG	
1		X	X		X	X			X				X															
2			X	X																								
4	X		X																									
5	X	X		X	X	X	X	X		X	X	X		X		X	X	X							X			
6	X	X				X		X					X	X	X							X				X		
7	**X**	**X**	X	**X**	**X**	X	**X**		X	X	X	X			X			X	X	X	X		X	X	X		**X**	
8	X	X		X	X	X	X	X	X	X	X			X	X	X			X		X	X	X	X		X	X	
9	X	X	X									X																
10	X	X			X	X																X						
11	X												X		X													
12	X																											
13	**X**	**X**	X	**X**	X		**X**	**X**	X	X	X					X		X	**X**	X	X		X	X				
14		X																										
15	X								X	X																		
17	X	X	X	X		X	X				X	X	X			X		X							X	X		
18		X																										
19	X																											
21	X	X										X																
22		X	X					X												X								
26	X				X									X														

Ailments from Turnips

	PULS	BRY
7	X	X
13	X	

Ailments from Turpentine

	CAMPH	NUX V	PHOS
2		X	
6	X		X

Ailments from Vaccination (AKA Vaccinosis)

	THUJA	SIL	SULPH	MALAND	VARIOL	ACON	APIS	ARN	BELL	KALI MUR	MERC	VACCIN	ANT T	HEP	CALEND	CHLORAL	CROT H	ECHIN	GRAPH	LAC C	MAG PH	MEZ	LED	SKOOK	VER V	NOSODE*
1	X			X								X	X													
2	**X**	**X**	**X**	**X**	X	**X**	**X**			X	**X**	**X**					X	X	X	X		X		X		
3	X	X						X			X			X												
5								X	X						X								X			
6	X	X																								
7	X	X	X				X																			
8	X	X	X							X				X												
9	X	X			X																					
10	X	X	X	X			X	X																		
11		X																								
15						X			X																X	
16	X	X	X		X											X					X					
17	X	X	X			X			X	X			X									X				
19		X																								
21	X	X																								
23	X			X																						
25	X				X																					
28																										X

*A remedy made from the vaccine

Ailments from Veal

	IPEC	NIT	CALC	CAUST	KALI NIT	SEP	ARS	ZINC
8	X	X	X	X		X		
13	**X**	**X**	X	X	X	X	X	X
15	X							
17					X			
22	X							

Ailments from Vegetables

	ARS	BRY	NAT CAR	CARB V	HELL	HYDRAST	MAG C	VER A	ALUM	CHINA	CIST	CUPR	LEPT	LYC	PULS	SEP	SULPH
7		X	X	X	X	X											
8	X	X	X			X	X		X				X	X		X	
13	X	X	X		X			X			X	X					
14	X																
15	X	X		X						X					X		X
24							X	X									

Ailments from Vegetables, Spoiled

	CARB A	CARB V	VER A																									
7	X	**X**	X																									
17	X																											

Ailments from Vinegar

	ARS	ANT C	ACON	CAUST	NUX V	SEP	SULPH	ALUM	ASAR	BELL	BOR	CALC	CARB V	FERR	HEP	IGN	LACH	NAT ARS	NAT M	PH AC	PULS	STAPHYS	THUJA					
1								X										X										
8	X		X		X				X							X					X							
13	X	**X**		X	X	X	X			X	X			X			X		X	X		X	X					
19		X																										
26	X		X	X		X	X					X	X		X													

Ailments from Warm Food or Drink

	CHAM	PHOS	PULS	BELL	MERC	AMBRA	ANAC	ARS	BAR C	BRY	CALC	CARB V	CHINA	COFF	DROS	HELL	KALI C	LACH	MERC I F	MEZ	NUX V	PH AC	PHYTO	SIL	STANN			
1		X																										
8	X		X								X								X		X			X				
9		X						X																				
10	X	X																										
12	X			X																								
13	**X**	X	X	X	**X**	X	X		X	X		X			X	X	X	X		X		X	X		X			
15	X												X															
19	X		X											X														

Ailments from Water (Bathing, Drinking or Working In)

	CALC	RHUS T	SULPH	ANT C	AMM C	DULC	SEP	PULS	SARS	BELL	CANTH	CARB V	CHAM	CLEM	MERC	NIT AC	NUX V	SPIG	CHINA	ARAN D	LYC	NUX M	PHOS	RHOD	STRONT C	URT U		
1				X																								
7	**X**	**X**	**X**	**X**	**X**		**X**		X	X	X	X	X	**X**	X	X		X		X	X				X			
8	X	X	X	X	X	X	X	X	X	X	X	X	X		X	X	X	X	X			X	X	X				
9	X			X		X											X							X				
10	X	X	X			X																						
12		X																										
13	**X**	X	**X**	**X**	**X**		**X**	**X**	**X**	X	X	X	X	**X**	X	X		X	**X**	X	X	X			X			
14	X																											
17		X															X						X					
20																										X		
21			X																							X		
24	X																											
26	X	X	X			X		X																				

Ailments from Wine

	NUX V	ZINC	ANT C	CARB V	OP	ARN	ARS	COFF	NAT CAR	PULS	SEL	CALC	IGN	LACH	LYC	NAT M	RAN B	SABAD	SIL	SULPH	ACON	GELS	GLON	NUX M	RHOD	THUJA	CHINA
1		X	X								X																
5		X											X					X									
6	X				X								X								X						
7	**X**	**X**	X	X	**X**	X	X	**X**	X	X	X	X		X	**X**	X	**X**	X	**X**	X	X		X	X		X	**X**
8	X	X	X		X	X	X	X	X	X	X	X		X		X				X			X		X		
10	X	X																									
12	X																										
13	X	X	X	X	**X**	X	**X**	**X**	X	X	X	**X**	X	X	**X**	X	**X**	X	**X**					X	X	X	
14				X																							
15	X									X												X					
16	X																										
17									X																		
18		X																									
19		X	X																	X		X					
21			X																								
22				X		X																					
24		X																									
26	**X**			X																							

Ailments from Writing

	NAT M	CALC	KALI C	RUTA	SIL	ZINC	ASAF	CINA	COCCUL	LYC	NUX V	OLEAND	RHOD	SEP	CANN S
6	X														
7	**X**	**X**	**X**	X	**X**	**X**	X	X	X	X	X	X	X	X	
13	**X**	**X**	**X**	X	X	X	X	X	X	X	X	X	X	X	**X**
14				X											
19	X														

Ailments from X-rays

	RAD BR	FL AC	PHOS	X-RAY
3	X	X	X	X
16	X			
28	X			

Airsickness, On Descent- See also Motion Sickness

	BOR
1	X
18	X
28	X

Albuminuria

	APIS	ARS	CANTH	TEREB	MERC C	HELON	HELL	PHOS	KALI CHL	LACH	PH AC	LYC	CALC AR	PLUM	AM BENZ	COLCH	NIT AC	GLON	ACON	AUR	DIG	SEC						
1	**X**	X	X	X	X	X	X	X	X	X	X	X		X		X		X			X							
2				X		X	X		X	X		X	X		X							X						
3	**X**		X			X	X				X																	
4	X	X	X	X	**X**			**X**	X	X				**X**				X	X		X							
5											X																	
6	X	X	X	X	X	X				X		X				X	X			X		X						
7	**X**	**X**	X	X	**X**	X	**X**	X		X	X	X	**X**	X	X	X	X	**X**		X		X						
8	X	X	X	X	X	X	X	X		X	X		X	X	X	X	X	X		X	X	X						
9	X	X	X		X				X								X											
10	X	X		X	X		X	X	X	X			X			X			X									
11	X	X			X				X					X	X													
12		X		X		X					X	X							X									
14	X	X						X	X																			
15	X	X	X				X	X			X								X									
17													X															
18			X																									
19		X																			X							
23				X		X						X			X		X											
24			X	X																X								

Alcoholism- See also Cirrhosis, Liver (AKA Dipsomania)

	NUX V	LACH	ARS	SULPH AC	SULPH	RAN B	ASAR	CAPS	OP	ANT T	CHINA	HYOSC	AVENA	PHOS	SEL	ZINC	AGAR M	APOMOR	STRAM	CANN I	STROPH	CALC	CARB V	CIMICI	KALI BIC	LED	NUX M	
1	X	X	X	X		X	X	X	X		X	X	X			X			X	X				X				
2	**X**	X	X			X	X			**X**	X		X		X	**X**		X			**X**							
3	X			X																								
4	**X**	X	X	**X**		X		X	**X**	X		**X**	X	X			X		X	**X**	X	X		X				
5	X	X	X	X		X	X	X	X			X		X			X								X			
6	X	X	X	X	X					X	X			X	X		X						X		X		X	
7	**X**	**X**	**X**	X	X	**X**	X		**X**	X	**X**	X		X	**X**	X	X		X			X	X			X	X	
8	X	X	X	X	X	X	X		X	X	X	X		X	X				X	X		X	X	X		X	X	
9	X	X		X			X	X					X					X										
10		X	X																									
14	X		X	X				X																				
16				X	X		X														X							
17	X		X	X		X																						
18		X																								X		
19																		X										
21	X	X			X			X					X			X									X			
22		X																										
25																		X										
26	X	**X**	X		**X**																							
28				X																								
29[1]			X																									
29[2]					X																							
29[3]	X				X																							
29[4]	X																											

29[1] Gopinadhan S, et al. A Pilot Study on the Effect of Arsenicum album in Alcohol Dependants. CCRH Quarterly Bull., 1994, 16, 1&2, 10-15.

29[2] Milewska G, et al. Homoeopathic Treatment of Alcohol Withdrawal. Brit Hom J, October 1993, 82, 249-251.

29[3] Rogers J. Homoeopathy and the Treatment of Alcohol Related Problems. Complement Ther Nurs Midwifery, 1997, Feb, 3, 1, 21-28.

29[4] Sukul NC, et al. Strychnos nux vomica extract and its ultra high dilution reduce voluntary ethanol intake in rats. J Altern Complement Med, 2001, Apr, 7, 2, 187-193.

Allergic Rhinitis- See Hay Fever

Allergy- See also Ailments from, Foods etc (Includes Urticaria from food)

	HIST	APIS	ARS	PULS	NAT M	NUX V	EUPHR	ALL C	ARS IOD	LYC	SABAD	ACON	ARG N	CALC	LACH	RHUS T	SANG	SIL	SULPH									
1													X															
3					X								X															
5	X	X	X	X	X	X	X	X	X		X			X	X		X	X										
9												X																
10				X												X												
14												X																
17			X					X																				
18	X	X	X		X				X	X				X														
19		X	X	X		X	**X**			X	X				X		X	X										
20			X			X	X	X			X					X			X									
21		X																										
22		X																										
27				X																								
28	X																											
29[1]				X	X	X			X	X									X									
29[2]	X	X																										
29[3]	X																											
29[4]	X																											
29[5]	X																											
29[6]	X																											
29[7]	X																											
29[8]	X																											
29[9]	X																											
29[10]	X																											
29[11]	X																											

29[1] Colin P. Homeopathy and respiratory allergies: a series of 147 cases. Homeopathy, 2006, 95, 68-72.

29[2] Poitevin B, et al. In Vitro Immunological Degranulation of Human Basophils is Modulated by Lung Histamine and Apis mellifica. Br J Clin Pharmacol, 1988, 25, 439-444.

29[3] Sainte-Laudy J, et al. Improvement of flow cytometric analysis of basophil activation inhibition by high histamine dilutions. A novel basophil specific marker: CD 203c. Homeopathy, 2006, 95, 3-8.

29[4] Sainte-Laudy J, et al. Analysis of Immunosuppressive activity of serial dilutions of Histamine on Human Basophil Activation by Flow Cytometry. Inflammation Res, 1996, 45, Supplement 1, S33-S34.

29[5] Sainte-Laudy J, Belon P. Inhibition of basophil activation by histamine: a sensitive and reproducible model for the study of the biological activity of high dilutions. Homeopathy. 2009 Oct;98(4):186-97.

29[6] Chirumbolo S, et al. Inhibition of CD203c membrane up-regulation in human basophils by high dilutions of histamine: a controlled replication study. Inflamm Res. 2009 November; 58(11): 755–764.

29[7] Belon P, et al. Histamine Dilutions Modulate Basophil Activation. Inflammation Research, 2004, May, 53, 5, 181-8.

29[8] Belon P, et al. Inhibition of Human Basophil Degranulation by Successive Histamine Dilutions. Inflammation Research, 1999, 48, Supplement 1, 17-18.

29[9] Sainte-Laudy J, et al. Application of Flow Cytometry to the Analysis of the Immunosuppressive effect of Histamine Dilutions on Human Basophil Activation: Effect of Cimetidine. Inflammation Res, 1997, 46, Supplement 1, S27-S28

29[10] Sainte-Laudy J, et al. Confirmation of biological effects of high dilutions. Effects of submolecular concentrations of histamine and 1-, 3- and 4-methylhistamines on human basophil activation. Inflammation Res. 2008;57 Suppl 1:S27-8.
29[11] Sainte-Laudy J, et al. Inhibition of human basophil activation by high dilutions of histamine. Agents Actions, 1999, 38, C245-7.

Allergy, Dust

	BLATTA
5	X
18	X

Allergy, Eggs

	FERR	SULPH	TUB	NAT M
1	X	X	X	X
3	X			

Allergy, Flowers

	SANG	SABAD
1	X	
17	X	X
19	X	

Allergy, Fruit

	ARS	PULS
4		X
10	X	

Allergy, Hair Dyes

	SULPH	TUB
1	X	X

Allergy, Meat

	SULPH	TUB	NAT M
1	X	X	X

Allergy, Milk

	SULPH	TUB	AETHUSA	CALC	NAT M	SEP	URT U
1	**X**	**X**			X		X
4				X		X	
19		X					
21			X				

Allergy, Sardines

	SULPH	TUB
1	**X**	**X**

Allergy, Shellfish

	ARS	TEREB
4	**X**	X

Alopecia- See Hair, Falling Of

Alopecia Areata (Includes Porrigo Decalvans)

	PHOS	ALOE	ARS	SEP	VINCA	BACILL	FL AC	GRAPH	HEP	MEZ	NAT M	PETR	SULPH	THUJA	TUB
3						X								X	X
6	X	X	X		X										
8	**X**	X	X	X	X		X	X	X	X	X	X	X		
10	X														
12				X											

Altitude Sickness

	COCA	ARS	ARG N	MEDO
1		X		
2	X			
5	X	X	X	X
8	X	X		
14	X			
18	X			
28	X			
29*	X			

29* Shackleton MF, et al. The Effect of Homeopathic Coca on High Altitude Mountain Sickness. Complementary Health Practice Review, 6, 1, Fall, 2000, 45- 55.

Alzheimer's Disease

	ALUM	ARS	BAR C	BELL	CANN I	HYOSC	OP	PHOS	STRAM																			
9			X	X	X		X		X																			
27	X	X				X		X																				

Amaurosis

	BELL	PLUM	PHOS	NAT M	SULPH	HEP	CAUST	CALC	PULS	SIL	GELS	ZINC	AUR	CON	MERC	ARS	AUR M	CHINA	DIG	ELAPS	HYOSC	MENY	SEP	STRAM	ACON	NUX V	TAB	
2	**X**	**X**	**X**		X	**X**	X		X		X						X		X	X	X	X			**X**	**X**	**X**	
4	X																											
6	X		X			X	X				X					X												
7	**X**	X	**X**	X	**X**			**X**	**X**	X				**X**	X	X	X	X		X		X		X				
8	X	X		X		X	X					X																
13	**X**	X	X	X	X		X	X	X	X	**X**	X	**X**	X					X		X		X	X				
17		X																										
24		X		X		X						X																
26			X	X	**X**			X		X			X		**X**			X					X					

Amblyopia

	PHOS	RUTA	CHINA	NAT M	SIL	NUX V	CALC	DROS	OP	PULS	SULPH	ZINC	PH AC	SANTON	ACON	ARN	BELL	CAUST	CINA	CROT H	HYOSC	LACH	PLUM	SEP	THUJA			
2	**X**	**X**	**X**			**X**		X				X	**X**	**X**						X		X						
4	X																											
7	**X**		**X**	X	X			X	X	X			X															
8	X	X	X	X	X		X		X	X	X	X					X	X	X	X	X	X	X	X	X			
12																X												
23		X				X								X	X													
24	X	X		X	X	X	X		X	X	X	X			X	X			X		X		X	X	X			
26	X	X	X	X	X		X	X			X						X	X										

Amblyopia Amaurotica

	AUR	PHOS	SIL	SULPH																								
8	**X**	**X**	**X**	**X**																								

Amenorrhoea

	PULS	SEP	ACON	SULPH	CALC	FERR	BRY	KALI CAR	LYC	SENEC	GRAPH	NAT M	BELL	DULC	LACH	PLAT	COCCUL	IGN	CON	APIS	GLON	PHOS	CYCL	GELS	NUX M	SIL	VER A	ZINC
1	X	X	X	X		X		X	X	X				X			X			X			X		X			
2	X	X		**X**			X	X		X	X					X											X	
3	X		X			X										X	X					X						
4	**X**	**X**	X	X	**X**	**X**	X		X	**X**	X		X	X	X					X	X	X		X			X	
6	X	X	X	X	X		X	X	X	X	X	X	X		X	X	X		X	X		X	X					
7	**X**	**X**	X	X	X	X	X	X	X	X	X	X	X	X	X	X	X	X	X	X			**X**	X	X	X		X
8	X	X	X	X	X	X	X	X	X	X	X	X	X	X	X	X	X	X	X	X	X	X	X	X	X	X	X	X
9	X	X	X	X	X	X	X					X	X					X										
11				X											X			X			X							X
13	**X**	**X**	X	**X**	X	X	**X**	**X**	**X**		**X**	**X**	X	**X**	X	X	X		**X**		X	X		**X**	**X**	**X**	**X**	**X**
14	X	X				X		X	X	X																		
19										X																		
18															X													
21		X	X		X	X			X			X		X				X										
23	X	X	X		X			X		X	X										X							
25	X	X	X	X	X	X	X					X	X					X										
26	X	X	X	X	X		X	X	X		X		X	X		X			X							X		
29^	X	X			X							X																

29* Cardigno P. Homeopathy for the treatment of menstrual irregularities: a case series. Homeopathy. 2009 Apr;98 (2):97-106.

Amoebiasis

	CALC AC	CINA	IPEC	MERC	NUX V	SANTON	SULPH	TEUCR	URT U
9	X	X				X	X	X	X
17			X	X	X				

Amyotonia- See also Fatigue; Myasthenia

	CAUST	COCCUL	GELS	LYCOP
1	X	X	X	
4				X
14	X			

Anaemia- See also Hydraemia

	CHINA	FERR	NAT M	ARS	CALC PH	PULS	FERR PH	PHOS	CALC	KALI CAR	PIC AC	AC ET AC	PH AC	ALET	HELON	PLUM	SULPH	CYCL	FERR AC	GRAPH	SIL	IGN	MERC	NUX V	SEP	STROPH
1	X	X	X	X		X	X	X	X			X		X		X			X			X		X	X	
2	**X**	X	**X**	**X**	**X**	**X**			**X**	X	**X**	X		X	X	**X**	X	X			**X**		X			X
3	X	X	**X**								X	X	X			X			X					X	X	
4	**X**	**X**	**X**		X	**X**	**X**	X	**X**	**X**		X		**X**	X			X	X	X			X			
5	**X**	X	X		X		X	X		X			X					X		X	X					
6	X	X	X	X					X						X					X		X				
7	**X**	**X**	**X**	**X**	X	X		**X**	**X**	X			X		X	X	**X**	X			X	X		X	X	
8	**X**	X	X	X		X		X	X	X			X		**X**		X			X	X	X	X	X	X	
9	X	X	X	X	X	X	X	X	X			X														
10	X	X	X	X	X			X		X	X					X										X
11	**X**	**X**	**X**		X	X	X	X		X			X	X				X		X						
12	X	X		X		X							X											X		
13	**X**	X		**X**		X							X				X					X	X		X	
14	X	X	X	X	X		X	X			X	X		X					**X**		X					
16			X		X		X																			
17	X	X	X	X	X	X	X	X			X		X				X			X			X			X
18	X	X		X						X																
19	X	X	X																							
21	X	X	X		X		X				X					X										
23	X	X	X		X	X					X			X	X			X	X							X
24		X					X																			
25	X	X	X	X	X	X	X	X	X																	
28		X																								

Anaemia, Cerebral

	FERR	ARS	NUX V	PHOS	ZINC	CHINA	ARN	CON	KALI PH	LACH	SIL
1	X	X	X	X	X	X					
4	**X**	X	**X**	**X**	**X**	X					
6	X	X	X	X		X	X	X		X	X
7					X			X			
8									X	X	
10									X		
14	X	X									
17	X						X				X

Anaemia, Haemolytic

	ARS	CROT H	KALI PH
7			X
10	X		
21		X	

Anaemia, Hypochromic Microcytic- See Green Sickness

Anaemia, Pernicious

	ARS	PIC AC	CHINA	CROT H	CUPR	FERR ARS	VER A	ANTIPYR	CALC	CAMPH	CANTH	CARB V	CURARE	FERR	HELON	HYDRAST	KALI C	KALI PH	MERC	NAT M	NUX V	PHOS	PLUM	SULPH	THYROID
1		X																							
2		X																							
3	X		X	X																					
4	**X**	X																							
6	X		X		X		X		X			X		X	X	X	X			X	X			X	
7																		X							
8	X			X			X			X	X		X												
9	X																								
10	X																								
11	X	X				X		X														X			X
12	**X**				X														X				X		
14		X																							
17	X																								
23	X	X				X																			
25	X																								

Anaemia, Retina

	CHINA	CHIN S	FERR PH
1	X		X
7		X	
8		X	
14	X		

Anaemia, Spinal Cord

	NUX V	KALI PH	PHOS	AGAR M	ARS	CALC	CHINA	CIMICI	FERR	GELS	GRAPH	IGN	LYC	PH AC	SEC	STRY PH
6	X		X		X	X	X	X	X	X		X		X	X	
7	X	X	X													
8	X	X		X							X		X			
14																X

Anaesthesia (Includes Sense, Vanishing of)

	ANAC	OP	PHOS	PLUM	ARS	LYC	OLEAND	STRAM	ACON	ALCOHOL	BELL	CAMPH	CIC	GELS	HYOSC	LACH	PH AC	ZINC										
6		X	X			X	X	X		X			X	X	X		X											
7	X	X	X	X		X		X				X		X				X										
8	X		X	X	X		X			X																		
12	X				X																							
13	X	X	X	X	X	X	X	X	X		X	X	X		X	X	X	X										
17									X							X												
19				X																								
23											X																	
27		X																										

Anaesthesia, Skin

	PLUM	ANAC	CAMPH	CAPS	KALI IOD	PHOS	ZINC																					
7	X	X	X	X	X	X	X																					
8	X																											

Anasarca- See also Oedema

	ARS	HELL	APIS	ADONIS	APOCY	DIG	TEREB	CRAT	DULC	LYC	RHUS T	ACET AC	BAR C	CONVAL	ELATAR	FRAG	HELON	HEP	LACH	MERC	STROPH	SULPH	URT U	VER A				
2																X								X				
3			X		X																							
4	X	X		X		X	X							X														
6	X	X				X			X	X									X	X								
8	X	X	X				X				X		X				X	X										
10	X						X	X			X																	
11	X																											
12	X	X																										
17				X																								
19					X																							
23	X		X	X	X	X		X				X			X						X		X					
26		X	X						X	X												X						

Ancylostomiasis- See Worms, Hook

Aneurism

	BAR C	LYC	BAR M	CACT	KALI IOD	SPONG	CARB V	LACH	SPIG	ACON	CALC	CARB A	CALC FL	ARN	ARS	DIG	PLUM	VER V	ARS IOD	BELL	FERR PH	FL AC	GUAIAC	LITH C	LYCOP	RAN S	SULPH
1	X	X										X															
2	**X**	**X**	X	X	**X**	X		X				X	X				X		**X**				X	X	X	X	
3	**X**	X										X															
7		X	X	**X**		X	X	X	**X**	X	X					X				X	X	X				X	X
8	X	**X**	**X**	X	X	X	**X**	**X**	X	X	X			X	X	X	X	X		X	X		X				X
10	X								X						X												
12	X	X								X				X			X										
14	X												**X**														
15	X									X				X													
17	X	X	X	X	X	X					X	X						X	X					X	X		
19				X				X																			
21	X	X			X																						
23		X	X		X								X			X		X				X					
24	X																										
26							X		X						X												
27			X			X	X				X																

Aneurism, Aorta

	SPONG	LYC	BAR M	CALC	CARB V	ARS	BAR C	BRY	CACT	CALEND	DIG	GALL AC	GRAPH	LACH	NAT M	PULS	RAN S	RHUS T	SEC	SPIG	SULPH
4			X																		
6	X				X			X				X									
7				X													X		X	X	
8	**X**	X		X	X	X			X		X		X	X	X	X		X			X
10			X																		
14		X																			
17	X	X					X														
21		X																			
24			X																		
27	X									X											

Aneurism, Carotid Artery

	LYC	CALC	CUPR	LACH
6	X			
7	X			X
17	X			
27		X	X	

Aneurism, Mesenteric Artery

	SEC	BAR M
6	X	
27	X	X

Angina Catarrhalis- See Pain, Throat
Angina Faucium- See Pain, Throat
Angina Follicularis- See Pain, Throat
Angina Granulosa- See Pain, Throat
Angina Ludovici

	ANTHRAC	LACH	ACON	BRY	HEP	IOD	KREO	MERC CY	SIL	TAR C
6	X	X	X			X				
8	X	X		X	X		X	X	X	X

Angina Pectoris

	CACT	ARS	SPIG	AMYL N	GLON	LATRO M	ARN	NAJA	SPONG	ACON	CRAT	TAB	CUPR	OXAL AC	VER A	MAG PH	LACH	AUR	CIMICI	HYDR AC	LIL TIG	CUPR AC	DIG	NUX V	AUR M	PHOS
1	X	X	X	X	X			X		X	X					X	X	X	X							
2	**X**		**X**	**X**	X	X		**X**	X		**X**	X	**X**	X	X			X		**X**	**X**	X	X		X	
3	X	X		X	X	**X**					**X**					**X**			X			X				
4	X	X	**X**	**X**	**X**	X	X			X	**X**	X	X			X		X	**X**		X			X		
5							X									X										
6	X	X	X	X	X		X	X	X	X		X	X	X	X		X			X			X	X	X	X
7	**X**		**X**	**X**			**X**	X	**X**	X		X	X	**X**	X	X	X	**X**					X	X	**X**	**X**
8	X	X	X	X	X	X	X	X	X	X		X	X	X	X	X	X	X	X	X		X	X	X		X
9	X	X	X			X		X						X												
10		X				X	**X**		X																**X**	
11	X	X	X	X	X	X	X	X	X	X	X	X	X			X				X		X		X		
12	X	X		X						X										X		X	X			
13		X												X	X		X						X			
14	**X**		X	X	**X**		**X**	X				X		X							X	X				
15	X	**X**	X							X									X							
16	X	X	X	X	X	X	X	X	X	X		X			X	X	X	X				X				
17	X	X	X	X	X	**X**		X	X	**X**	X	X	X	X	X		X		X	X	X			X	X	X
19	X	X	X		X	X	X	X	X	X	X	X		X			X	X			X		X	X		X
21	X		X		X	X		X													X					
23	X			X	X	X			X		X								X	X	X					
25	X																									
26		**X**							**X**				X		**X**											
27	X	X					X						X													
28											X															

Angular Stomatitis

	ARUM T	ANT C	CONDUR	GRAPH	NAT M	NIT AC	SIL	LYC	ZINC	AILANTH	HELL	HEP	KREO	LAC C	PETR	SEP
1	X	X	X					X	X			X	X			
5		X														
6		X					X									
7	X		X	X	X		X	X	X		X					X
10			X		X											
12										X						
14	X	X	X	X		X										
17	X													X		
19	X				X	X										
21	X														X	
27				X		X	X									

Anisocoria

	ABSINTH	PLUM	SULPH
14	X		
24		X	X

Ankylosing Spondylitis

	AESC	RHUS T	PHOS	AUR	BELLIS	BRY	KALI C	NUX V	APIS	ARG	ARN	CALC	CALC FL	CON	DULC	KALM	NAT M	RAD BR	SEP	SULPH
11	**X**	**X**	X		**X**	**X**	**X**	**X**			X	X							X	X
18		X							X				X		X			X		
19	X		X	**X**																
27	X	X								X				X		X	X			

Anorexia- See also Appetite, Decreased

	NAT M	SIL	ARS	NUX V	SULPH	ARG N	BRY	FERR	LYC	RHUS T	ANT C	IGN	IPEC	ARN	CHINA	COCCUL	MERC	SEP	CARB V	MUR AC	PHOS	CALC	CHAM	CYCL	HEP	HYDRAST	PULS	
1				X	X						X										X							
3				X					X	X		X																
4										X											X							
5	X	X	X					X				X		X				X		X								
7	**X**	X	**X**	**X**	**X**	**X**	**X**	**X**	**X**	**X**		X	X	**X**	**X**	**X**	**X**	**X**	X	X		**X**	**X**	**X**	**X**	**X**	**X**	
8	X	X	X	X	X	X	X	X	X	X	X	X	X	X	X	X	X	X		X		X		X	X	X	X	
9	X	X																										
10	X		X		X		X						X		X													
11			X																									
12											X						X											
13																					X							
14		X	X	X	X	X					X		X			X			X									
15				X			X																X					
18	X	X						X	X																			
25	**X**	X				X																						
26					X														X									
28	X																											

Anosmia- See also Smell, Sense of, Diseases Of

	PULS	NAT M	KALI BIC	SIL	CALC	ANAC	HEP	PHOS	MAG M	SEP	AMM M	PLUM	SANG	ALUM	CUPR	HYOSC	IOD	AUR	BELL	CAUST	CYCL	ELAPS	MEZ	TEUCR	MERC	MERC C		
1	X	X			X				X					X	X		X	X				X	X			X		
2											**X**		**X**															
4	X								X																			
6	X	X	X	X							X				X		X		X		X	X						
7		X	X	**X**		X	**X**	**X**		X	X	**X**	X		X	X	X	X		X						**X**		
8	X	X	X	X	X		X			X	X	X	X	X		X		X	X	X	X		X	X				
10	X					X																		X				
11	X	X	X			X	X		X					X							X							
12	**X**		X		X					X															**X**			
13		**X**		**X**		**X**	X	X	X	X		X	X			X												
14	X	X	X																									
15	X		X		X			X																				
17	X	X	X	X	X	X	X	X	X	X		X	X	X		X	X		X	X			X	X	X			
18	X																											
20		X																										
21		X			X																							
22		X																										
24	X	X	X	X				X							X							X						
25	X																											
26	X																											

Anthrax

	ANTHRAC	LACH	ARS	APIS	BELL	SIL	CAMPH	CARB V	KREO	RHUS T	TAR C
6	X	X									
7	**X**	**X**	X			**X**	X	X	X		
8	X	X	X	X	X	X	X	X	X	X	X
10	X										
12	X	X		X	X						
21	X										
24	X	X	X	X	X					X	X
26			X								

Anuria- See also Urine, Retention of; Urine, Scanty

	ACON	APIS	ARN	ARS	BELL	CARB V	URIN	VER V
24		X		X	X			X
27	X		X			X	X	

Anus, Diseases Of

	IGN	AESC	ALUMEN	ALUM	GAMBOG	GRAPH	ALOE	LACT V	NIT AC	NUX V	PAEONIA	SIN A
2	**X**	**X**	**X**	**X**	**X**	**X**	X	X			X	X
8	X											
9									X	X		

Anus, Dryness

	ALUM	NAT M	ALOE	MAG M	MUR AC	NUX M	RAT
5	X	X	X	X	X	X	X
7		X					
17	X						

Anxiety See also Delirium; Stress (This rubric combines Agitation [Mental]; Anguish; Distress; Excitability; Fright; Hysteria; Irritability; Nervousness; Stage Fright)

	ACON	IGN	GELS	ARS	PHOS	PULS	CALC	NUX V	MOSCH	ARG N	BELL	COFF	PLAT	AUR	LYC	ASAF	CHAM	NAT M	COCCUL	NUX M	SEP	HYOSC	LACH	VAL	IOD	RHUS T	VER A	KALI C
1	X	**X**	X	X		X	X	X	X	X	X	X	X	X		X		X	X	X	X	X	X	X	X		X	
2		**X**																										
3										X																		
4	X	**X**	**X**		X	**X**		X	X		**X**		**X**			**X**			X	X	X			**X**				
5	X	**X**	X	X	X	X	X	X	X	X			X	X	X	X	X	X		X	X	X	X	X	X	X	X	X
6	X	X	X	X	X	X	X	X	X		X	X	X	X	X	X	X		X	X	X	X	X	X	X	X	X	X
7	**X**	X	X	**X**	**X**	X	**X**	**X**	X	**X**	**X**	**X**	X	**X**	X	X	**X**	X	**X**	X	X	X	X	X	**X**	X	X	X
8	**X**	X	X	**X**	X	**X**	X	X	X		**X**	X	X	X	X	X	X	X	X	X	X	X	X	X	X	X	**X**	X
9	X	X	X	X	X	X	X	X	X	X	X	X	X	X		X		X			X	X	X			X	X	X
10	X	**X**		X		X	X	X		X	X	X	X					X	X		X	X	X		X	X	X	
11	X	X	X	X	X	X			X	X			X		X	X			X	X	X	X		X	X			
12	X	X	X	X	X	X		X	X		X	X	X	X		X			X	X		X						
13	**X**	X	X	**X**	**X**	**X**	**X**	**X**	**X**		**X**	**X**	**X**	**X**	**X**	**X**	**X**		**X**	**X**	**X**	X	X	**X**	X	**X**	**X**	X
14	X	X		X	X		X			X							X	X	X									
15	X	X	X	X		X	X	X			X	X	X	X			X				X							
16		X	X	X	X		X			X		X		X	X		X	X										
17	X	X	X	X	X			X	**X**	X		X		X	X	X		X	X	X		X	X		X	X	X	
18	X	X	X	X	X	X	X	X	X	X		X		X	X		X	X		X			X		X			X
19	X	X	X	X	X	X	X	X		X					X										X	X		X
20	X				X						X															X		
21	X	X	X	X	X	X	X		X	X			X		X			X					X	X				X
22	X	X	X	X	X												X											
23		X	X					X	X							X												
24	X	X	X	X							X																X	
25	X	X	X	X	X	X	X											**X**										X
26	X	X		X	X	X		X	X		X	X	X	X	X		X		X	X	X	X		X		X	X	
27	X		X	X	X		X			X		X											X					X
28	X									X							X											
29[1]	X																											
29[2]										X																		
29[3]			X																									
29[4]			X																									
29[5]			X																									

29[1] Alibeu JP, et al. Aconite in Post-Operative Pain and Agitation in Children. Pediatrie, 1990, 45, 7-8, 465-6.

29[2] Stanton H.E. Test and Anxiety- A Five Drop Solution. Education News, 1981, 17, 6, 12-15.

29[3] Bellavite P, et al. Homeopathic Doses of Gelsemium sempervirens Improve the Behavior of Mice in Response to Novel Environments. Evid Based Complement Alternat Med. 2009 Sep 14. [Epub ahead of print]

29[4] Venard C, et al. Comparative Analysis of Gelsemine and Gelsemium sempervirens Activity on Neurosteroid Allopregnanolone Formation in the Spinal Cord and Limbic System. Evid Based Complement Alternat Med. 2009 Jul 23. [Epub ahead of print]

29[5] Magnani P, et al. Dose-effect study of Gelsemium sempervirens in high dilutions on anxiety-related responses in mice. Psychopharmacology (Berl). 2010 Jul;210 (4):533-45.

Aorta, Aneurism- See Aneurism, Aorta

Aorta, Diseases Of

	LYC	CRAT
11		X
14	X	

Aortic Insufficiency

	OX AC	LITH C	SPONG
4	X		
8		X	
17	X		X

Aortic Regurgitation

	ADONIS	AUR	AUR M N	CACT	CONVAL	CRAT	DIG	STROPH
1	X							
17		X	X					
23	X			X	X	X	X	X

Aortic Valve, Insufficiency

	SPONG	ADONIS	ARS I	AUR M	CAFF	OX AC	VISC A
8	X						
11					X		X
14			X	X			
17	X	X				X	

Aortic Valve Stenosis

	ARS I	ASPIDO	AUR	HYDROC	LAURO
7				X	
8					X
14	X	X	X		

Aortitis

	ARS I	ADONIS	AUR	BAR M	ADRENAL	ANT ARS	AUR IOD	CACT	CARB V	EUC AL	PLUM IOD	SPONG	TAB
1		X	X										
2									X	X			
4	X			X									
5			X			X		X				X	X
10	X												
14	X												
17		X	X		X		X				X		
23		X											
24	X			X									

Aphasia- See also Speech, Disorders Of

	KALI BR	LYC	CAUST	GELS	NUX V	STRAM	ANAC	BOTHR	HYOSC	ARN	COCCUL	CON	GLON	GRAPH	HEP	LACH	MERC	NAT M	NIT AC
2	**X**	**X**				**X**							X						
6	X	X	X	X	X	X	X		X		X	X	X	X	X		X	X	
7	X	X	X	X	X	X	X		X		X	X	X	X	X	X	X	X	**X**
8	X	X																	
9	X		X	X		X	X	X		X									
13		X	X		**X**				X	X	X	X		X	X	X	X	X	X
14			X					X											
17					X			X											
21				X					X							X			
25	X	X		X			X	X		X									

Aphonia- See also Speech, Disorders Of

	CAUST	PHOS	CARB V	ARUM T	GELS	ANT C	ARG M	BELL	HEP	LACH	RHUS T	SPONG	OX AC	SULPH	IGN	BAR C	STRAM	ARG N	MERC	RUMEX	ARN	NUX M	PLAT	SENEGA	ALUMEN	IPEC		
1	X	X				X			X	X		X	X			X	X								X	X		
2	**X**		X		**X**		X								**X**					X								
3	X	X		**X**	X	X				X	X																	
4	**X**	**X**			X									X						**X**		X	X	X		**X**		
5	X	X	X	X							X							X			X							
6	X	X	**X**	X	X	X	X	X		X	X			X	X		X					X	X					
7	**X**	X		X	X	X	**X**			X	X	X		X	X		X	X	X	X		X		X	**X**			
8	X	X	X	X	X	X	X	X		X	X	X	X	X	X	X	X	X	X	X		X	X	X				
9	X	X	X	X			X	X	X	X			X				X	X			X							
10	X				X																							
11	X				X		X		X				X											X				
12	**X**	**X**	X					X	X			X				X			X		X							
13	**X**	**X**	X			X		X	X	X	X	X		X		X			**X**				X					
14	X		X					X		X			X			X										X		
15		X						X						X														
16	X																											
17	X	X	X	X		X	X		X		X	X	X				X	X		X				X	X	X		
18																					X							
19				X	X	X							X															
21		X					X				X	X			X	X					X							
22		X																										
23		X	X												X							X			X			
24	X	**X**		X																								
25	X								X			X							X									
26	X	X				X		X	X					X									X					
27	X																											
28	X																											

Aphthae- See also Stomacace (Includes Canker)

	BOR	MERC	ARS	NIT AC	SULPH AC	MUR AC	SULPH	BAPT	NAT M	CARB V	HELL	HYDRAST	MERC C	BRY	STAPHYS	CALC	KALI BIC	LACH	THUJA	CAPS	NUX V
1			X	X	X	X		X			X	X					X	X			
2	**X**	X	**X**		X	**X**			**X**		X		**X**	X						**X**	
3	X	X			X		X	X													
4	**X**	X	X	X	X	X					X	X									
5	X		X	X	X	X			X				X		X						
6		X		X	X		X		X			X				X		X	X		X
7	**X**	**X**	**X**	**X**	**X**	**X**	**X**	**X**	X	X	X		**X**	X	X	X	X	X		X	
8	X	**X**	X	X	**X**	**X**	**X**	X	X	X	X	X	X	X	X	X	X	X	X	X	X
9	X			X																	
10		X	X	X			X			X											
11			X	X																	
12		X																			
13	**X**	**X**	**X**	X	**X**		**X**	X		X	X			X	X				X		**X**
14	X		X	X																	
15		**X**	X	X			X	X		X		X									
17						X							X	X					X		
18	X				X							X									
19	X		X																		
21	X	X	X	X																	
23	X																				
24																	X				
26		**X**	X	X	X	X	X		X	X					X	X					
27	X																				
28		X		X																	
29*	**X**	X	X	X	X																

29* Mousavi F, et al. Homeopathic treatment of minor aphthous ulcer: a randomized, placebo-controlled clinical trial. Homeopathy. 2009 Jul;98(3):137-41.

Apnoea- See also Asphyxia, Dyspnoea

	CUPR	DIG	LATRO M	OP
6		X		
8	X			X
19			X	

Apoplexy- See Stroke

Appendicitis- See also Pain, Appendix

	BELL	BRY	LACH	RHUS T	IRIS T	PLUM	ARS	DIOSC	ECHIN	IGN	ACON	COLOC	LYC	MERC	FERR PH	KALI MUR	BAPT	COLCH	CROT H	MERC C	SULPH	THUJA
1	X	X	X	X	X	X	X	X		X		X	X	X	X	X					X	
2			X	X	**X**	X		X	X					X			X	X	X	X		
3	X	X	X		**X**	X		X	X	X		X					**X**				X	
4	**X**	X	**X**	**X**		X	**X**	**X**	X	X	X	X		X	X	X				X		
7	X		X	X		X							X	X				X	X			X
8											X								X			
9	X	X	X	X			X					X										
10	X	X	X	X		X	X	X	X	X				X								X
12	X	X																		X		
14	X	X		X	X					X			X									
16	X	X	X	X	X	X	X	X	X		X		X		X	X	X	X				
19	X	**X**									X											
21	X	X	X		X						X											
24	X	X	X	X		X	X	X	X	X		X	X		X	X					X	X

Appendix, Ruptured

	LACH
16	X
21	X

Appetite, Decreased- See also Anorexia (Includes Food, Aversion to)

	NUX V	ANT C	ARS	PULS	SULPH	CALC	CHINA	IGN	MERC	BRY	LYC	BELL	CARB V	PHOS	RHUS T	IRIS V	SEP	NAT M										
1	X		X			X	X	X	X								X											
2	X																											
3	X							X																				
4			X					X	X	X				X	X													
5		X	X				X																					
6	X	X	X	X	X	X	X	X	X	X		X	X	X	X		X	X										
7											X																	
8	X		X								X				X													
9	X	X	X									X				X												
10	X	X		X	X	X	X		X	X	X		X															
11						X			X																			
12		X				X	X							X														
13	X	**X**	X	X	X	X	X	X	X	X	**X**	X	X	X	**X**	X	X	**X**										
14	X	X	X	X	X	X							X					X										
15	X	X		X	X		X	X	X	X		X		X		X	X											
17	X			X																								
20					X																							
21	X							X			X																	
22																X												
24				X	X																							
25	X	X	X	X								X																
26	X	X		X	X	X	X			X			X															

Appetite, Increased

	IOD	CALC	SULPH	CINA	LYC	NAT M	CHINA	PETR	NUX V	PHOS	SEP	HYOSC	ZINC	ARS	MERC	VER A	ABROT	ANT C	IGN	PH AC	PSOR	RHUS T	SEC	STAPHYS	URAN N	AUR	GRAPH
1	X	X	X	X	X		X	X	X			X	X	X		X	X		X	X	X	X			X		
3	X	X										X								X							
4	**X**	X	X	X	X	X		**X**		X																	
5	X	X		X	X	X	X	X	X	X	X		X				X	X	X	X	X		X	X	X	X	
6	X	X	X	X		X	X		X	X	X	X	X		X	X		X				X					
7	**X**	**X**	X	**X**	X	X	**X**	X	**X**	X	X	X		**X**	X					X		X	X	X		X	**X**
8							X																				
9	X	X	X	X		X							X				X							X			
10	X		X			X				X				X			X				X				X		
11	X			X	X																				X		
12							X																				
13	**X**	X	**X**	**X**	**X**	**X**	X	**X**	**X**	X	**X**	**X**	X		**X**	**X**		X	X			X	X	X		**X**	X
14	X	X	X																								
15		X	X		X						X																X
17			X						X	X																	
18						X												X	X								
19	X							X						X													
21	X		X	X	X	X		X													X						
24	X																						X				
25	X																										
26		X	X	X	X		X				X				X	X											
27				X																							
28		X																									

Aqueous Humor, Opacity Of

	COLOC	EUPHORB	EUPHR	GELS	KALI IOD	MERC
7	X	X		X	X	X
8			X			

Arachnitis

	CHLF
2	X
8	X

Ardor Urinae- See also Dysuria

	OCIMUM	PIX	POP T	RHAMN F	RHEUM	SCUT
2		X	X	X	X	X
8	X					

Arrhythmia

	DIG	ARS	SPIG	CACT	LACH	NAJA	ARN	CRAT	VER A	CARB V	NAT M	AUR	KALI C	PH AC	LAURO	CONVAL	GELS	LYCOP	MUR AC	NUX V	TAB	VER V	NIT AC
1	X		X	X		X				X							X		X				
2																					X		
4	X	**X**	X					X								X			X			X	
5	X							X								X							
6	X	X	X	X	X		X		X	X	X	X	X	X	X		X		X	X	X	X	X
7	**X**	X	X	X	X	X	X		X	X	X		X		X		X	X			X	X	X
8	X	X	X				X		X	**X**	**X**		X	X	X	X	X	X	X	X	X	X	**X**
9						X		X															
10	X	X		X	X		X	X		X		X	X	X									
11	X							X								X		X					
12	X	X	X											X						X			
13	X	X									**X**		X	X	**X**								
14	X		X	X	X	X	X		X	X		X											
15	X	X												X									
17	X	X	X	X		X	X	X	X			X	X		X				X		X		X
18																						X	
19	**X**	**X**	**X**	X	**X**	**X**	X				**X**	X				X	X	X		X			
21	X		X	X	X	X																	
24	X	X							X			X						X		X			
25								X															
26	X			X					X														
27	X				X																		
28	X																						

Arteries, Diseases Of

	BAR C	STROPH	VANAD	PHOS	ARS	AUR M	BELLIS	CALC HP	EQUISET	LOB I	VER V
2				**X**		X		X			
4			X								
8											X
10	X										
18		X			X						
19		X									
27	X		X				X		X	X	

Arteriosclerosis

	BAR M	PLUM	AUR M	CRAT	ARS IOD	BAR C	STROPH	AUR	PHOS	PLUM IOD	NAT IOD	GLON	ADRENAL	BAR IOD	KALI IOD	ARN	CACT	SPIG	STRONT I	ERGOTIN
1	**X**	X	X		X		X	X					X			X		X		X
2										X										
3	X		X				X													
4	**X**	**X**	**X**	**X**	X		**X**				**X**	X	**X**	X	X	X			X	**X**
5	X				X	X		X	X	X	X			X			X			
9		X				X		X				X								
10	X	X	X	**X**			X	X	X											
11	X			X	X	X	X			X	X	X			X		X			
12									X											
14	X	X	X	X								X				X		X		
16	X			X		X														
17	X	X	X	X	X	X	X	X	X	X	X	X	X		X		X	X	X	
18		X	X		X	X			X	X				X						
21					X	X			X											
23					X					X										
24	X	**X**		**X**							X		X	X	X				X	
27			X					X												

Arteriosclerosis, Cerebral

	ARN	AUR M	BAR C	BELL	CANN I	OP	STRAM	STRY PH
1	X	X						
9	X		X	X	X	X	X	
10	X	X						
14	**X**							X

Arteriosclerosis, Senile

	STROPH	BAR M	BAR C	HAM
1	X	X		
10	X	X		
12				X
17			X	
24	X			

Arteritis

	CUPR AR	CUPR	PLUM	SEC
5	X			X
18		X	X	

Arthritis- See also Rheumatism; Polyarthritis; Pain by location for all of the following entries

	BRY	RHUS T	CAUST	COLCH	SULPH	GUAIAC	LED	ACON	BENZ AC	KALI BIC	KALI CAR	MANG	RHOD	SABIN	THUJA	ANT C	APIS	BERB V	CALC	MEDO	NAT SUL	SEP	ARN	BELL	DULC	PH AC	PULS	STAPHYS
1	X				X		X				X	X					X	X	X									
2			X																									
3				X											X						X							
4													X															
5	X	X	X	X			X		X	X				X		X	X			X	X				**X**			
6			X															X								X		
7	X		X					X				X										X						
8	X	X	X	X	X	X	X	X	X	X	X	X	X	X		X	X	X	X		X	X	X	X		X	X	X
9	X	X		X					X											X		X					X	X
10	X																											
11	X	X																										
12	X	X		X									X															
13	**X**	**X**	**X**	**X**	**X**	**X**	**X**	X		X	**X**	**X**	**X**	**X**	**X**	X			X			X	X	**X**	X	**X**	**X**	**X**
14			X																									
16		X			X	X																						
18			X		X						X				X				X		X							
19	**X**	**X**	X	X		X	X	X	X	X							X	X		X			**X**	X	X			
23				X		X		X		X				X	X	X				X								
24	X	X		X					X																			
25	X	**X**																										
27		X																										
29[1]	X																											
29[2]		X																										

29[1] Labrecque G, et al. Effect of Bryonia on Experimental Arthritis in Rats. Berlin J of Res in Hom, 1, 3, 1991, 169, Congress Report Poster.

29[2] Patel DR, et al.Toxicodendron pubescens retains its anti-arthritic efficacy at 1M, 10M and CM homeopathic dilutions. Homeopathy. 2012 Jul;101 (3):165-70.

Arthritis, Ankle

	LED	ABROT	CAUST	LITH C
5	X			X
19		X	X	
27	X			

Arthritis, Elbow

	EUP PERF	GRAT	MAG SUL	NAT PH
1	X			
3				X
13		X	X	

Arthritis, Foot

	CAUST	CHINA	PHOS
19	X		
26		X	X

Arthritis, Fingers

	ANT C	COLCH	RHOD	CAUST	ACT SP	ARAN D	BRY	CALC	CARB A	CAULO	CLEM	COLOC	EUP PERF	GRAT	GUAIAC	HEP	LYC	MANG	NICCOL	NIT AC	OX AC	PETR	PHYT	RHUS T	SARS	SEP	STELL AQ
1								X					X														
5	X	X	X		X	X				X		X			X								X				
13	X		X				X		X		X			X		X	X	X	X	X	X	X		X	X	X	X
14	X																										
19				**X**																							
24		X																									

Arthritis, Hand And Wrist

	HEP	SABIN	BELL	CALC	CALC HP	COCCUL	HYPER	KALI BIC	LYC	PHOS
1				X						
3							X			X
13	**X**	**X**	X			X		X	X	
25					X					

Arthritis, Hip

	RUTA	ABROT	AUR	CALC FL	CAUST	DROS	HECLA	KALI CAR	KALI IOD	SEC	TUB RES
5	X					X	X		X	X	X
19		X			X						
25	X		X	X							
27								X			

Arthritis, Joints, Small

	LED	ACT SP	LAC AC	RHOD
7			X	
12	X			X
14		X		
27	X			

Arthritis, Knee

	BRY	CALC FL	KALI CAR	PULS	RUTA	ABROT	ANGUS	BENZ AC	CALC	CAUST	CHEL	CHINA	CIMEX	COLCH	CON	HECLA	LED	PULS N	RAD BR	RHUS T	TUB
1									X												
2																		X			
3				X	X																
5	X	X	X	X	X		X	X			X		X			X			X	X	X
13												X			X						
14		X																			
19						X				X											
24														X							
25	X																				
27			X														X				

Arthritis, Lumbar- See Lumbago

Arthritis, Psoriatic

	SULPH	AUR	CALC	GRAPH	RHUS T	THYROID
19	**X**	X	X	X	X	X

Arthritis, Shoulder

	SANG	CAUST	GUAIAC	IRIS V	LOB I	LYC	MERC C	PALLAD	SULPH
3	X								
13	X		X	X	X	X	X	X	X
19		X							

Arthritis, Wrist- See Arthritis, Hand And Wrist

Ascarides- See Worms, Round

Ascites- See also Oedema, Abdomen

	ARS	APOC	APIS	HELL	COLCH	DIG	LYC	CHINA	BRY	MERC	SULPH	SENEC	DULC	PRUN S	TEREB	KALI C	LED	ACET AC	ADONIS	CANTH	FL AC	LACH	AGNUS
1	X	X	X	X	X	X	X						X		X							X	
2		X										X		X			X						X
3	X	X			X	X									X								
4		X	X	X																			
6	X	X	X	X	X	X	X	X	X	X	X	X				X				X	X	X	
7	**X**	X	**X**	X	X	X	**X**	X	X	X	X		X		X	X				X	X		
8	X	X	X	X	X	X	X	X	X	X	X	X	X	X			X						
9	X	X	X			X			X														
10	X														X								
11	X	X	X	X		X	X	X				X		X				X	X				
12	X	X						X															
13	**X**		X	X	**X**	**X**	X	**X**	X	**X**	**X**		X	X		**X**	**X**			X			**X**
15	X		X	X																			
17					X														X				
18	X																						
19	X	X			X	X	X			X								X				X	
23		X	X	X															X		X		
24	X	X	X	X	X		X		X	X	X	X											
26	X		X					X	X		X												

Asphyxia- See also Apnoea, Dyspnoea

	ANT T	ARS	CUPR	LACH	OP	CARB V	CARB S	CHINA	IPEC	SAMB	ACON	BELL	CAMPH	HEP	IGN	LAURO	PULS	VER A
1	X				X		X	X										
7	**X**	X		X	X		X	X	X	X		X	X	X		X	X	
8		X	X	X	X	X		X			X	X	X		X	X		X
10	X						X								X			
12		X		X							X							
13	X	X	X	X	X	X		X		X	X	X			X	X	X	X
14	X					X			X									
15		X		X					X					X			X	
16	X																	
17	X				X		X						X					
18			X							X								
19			X															
22	X																	
26	X	X	X			X			X	X				X				X

Asphyxia Neonatorum

	ANT T	LAURO	CHINA	OP	CAMPH	ACON	BELL	ARN	LACH	CARB V	CARB S	CHLF	COLCH	SINAP														
1			X																									
2	X	X																										
3	**X**	X	X	X					X	X																		
7	**X**	X		X	**X**	X	X	X																				
8	**X**	X	X	X	X	X	X																					
9	X																											
17	X	X		X	X		X	X			X	X	X	X														
26	X		X			X			X																			
28	X																											

Asthenopia

	ART V	CINA	CON	JAB	RUTA	NAT M	PHOS	ALUM	LACH	ONOS	KALM	AGAR M	AMMC	APIS	ARG N	ARN	ASAR	CINNAB	CROC	EUPHR	GELS	LIL TIG	LITH C	MANG	RHOD	SENEG	SEP	SULPH
1	X	X	X																									
2		X		X					X				X									X		X	X			
3	X				X			X		X										X								
4	X	X	X		X	**X**	X	X				X			X						X						X	
6				X																								
7			X				**X**		X		**X**					X		X	X									**X**
8	X	X	X	X	X	X	X	X	X	X	X	X	X	X	X	X	X	X	X	X	X	X	X	X	X	X	X	
17										X													X					
23					X	X								X			X									X		
24				X																								

Asthma (Includes Miller's Asthma) (Note that only the main remedies are used from 17)

	ARS	IPEC	ANT T	NUX V	NAT SUL	SULPH	KALI C	CUPR	CARB V	LACH	LOB I	ACON	PULS	CALC	LYC	PHOS	BLATTA	MEDO	THUJA	GRIND	IGN	KALI BIC	SAMB	ARS IOD	MOSCH	BROM		
1	X	X	X	X	X	X	X	X	X	X	X	X	X		X	X	X	X	X	X	X	X	X	X	X	X		
2	**X**	**X**	**X**	X	**X**	**X**	**X**	**X**	X	X	**X**	X			X	X	X	X	X	X		X	X			X		
3	X	X		X	X		X	X	X		X	X					X	X	X	X	X							
4	**X**	**X**	**X**	X	**X**		X		X		X				X		X			X		**X**			X	X		
5	X	X	X	X	X		X	X	X	X	X						X	X		X	X		X	X	X			
6	X	X	X	X	X	X	X	X	X	X	X		X						X					X		X		
7	**X**	**X**	X	X	X	**X**	**X**	X	X	X	**X**	X	**X**	X		X					X		X		X	X		
8	**X**	X	X	X	X	**X**	X	**X**	X	X	X	X	X	X	X	X			X	X	X	X	X	X	X	X		
9	X	X	X	X	X	X	X			X		X				**X**		X		X						X		
10	**X**	X	X	X	X	X	X		X								X	X	X			X						
11	**X**	**X**	X	X	**X**	X	X		X		X	X					X		X	X		X	X					
12	X	X	X	X	X	X		X			X	X							X					X				
13	X	X	X	X	X			X		X		X	X	X	X	X					X		X		X			
14	X	X	X					X	X	X		**X**		X	X													
15	X	X	X	X		X						X										X						
16	X	X												X					X									
17	X	X	X	X	X	X	X	X	X	X	X	X	X	X	X	X	X	X	X	X	X	X	X	X	X	X		
18	X	X	X		X	X	X	X		X			X	X	X		X	X	X					X				
19	**X**	**X**	X	X	**X**	X	**X**	**X**	X	**X**	**X**		**X**	X	**X**	**X**	X	X			X	**X**	**X**		X	X		
20	X	X											X															
21	X	X	X	X	X		X	X	X	X		X	X			X					X		X	X	X			
22	X	X		X					X																			
23					X						X						X			X								
24	X											X																
25	X	X		X		X	X									**X**		X										
26	X	**X**	X	X		**X**	X	X	X	X	X	X	X	X	X	X					X				X			
27	X	X	X		X	X	X	X			X				X			X										
28	X							X									X											
29[1]	X					X			X	X			X	X	X			X	X		X							
29[2]	**X**		X	X									X	X														
29[3]	X	X	X																	X								
29[4]				X		X								X	X													
29[5]									X	X														**X**				
29[6]	X		X							X				**X**		X						X						

29[1] Castellsague API. Evolution of 26 Cases of Bronchial Asthma With Homoeopathic Treatment. Brit Hom J, 1992, 81, 168-172.
29[2] Mohan GR. Efficacy of homeopathy in childhood asthmas. Homeopathic Links, Summer 2007, Vol 20, 104-107.
29[3] Riveron-Garrote M, et al. Clinical Trial of Asthma. Boletin Mexicano, 1998, 31, 54-61.
29[4] Castellsague API, Sturza CM. Retrospective Study in Asthma. Revista Homeopatica AMBH, 1998, 37, 5-21.
29[5] Van Wassenhoven M. Clinical verification in homeopathy and allergic conditions. Homeopathy. 2013 Jan;102 (1):54-8.
29[6] Shafei HF, et al. Individualized homeopathy in a group of Egyptian asthmatic children. Homeopathy, 2012 Oct;101(4):224-30.

Asthma, Cardiac

	DIG	ASPIDO	SPONG	ACON	ADONIS	ARN	BAR C	BAR M	CRAT	GRIND	LYC	NAJA	SUMBUL
1	X			X			X	X	X			X	
5					X				X				
7	X		X			X				X			
8	X									X			
9			X										X
11											X		
14	X	**X**		X			X	X			X		
17		X			X								X
19	X		X			X						X	
23		X											

Asthma, Senile

	CARB V	BAR M	ALUMEN	AMM C	ANT T	ARS	BAR C	KALI C
8	X							
10	X	X	X		X			X
12						X		
14	X	X						
16							X	
17				X				

Astigmatism

	LIL T	GELS	PHYSO
2	X	X	X
3	X		
4		X	
6	X		
7	X	X	X
8		X	X
9	X		X

Atelactesis

	ANT T	HYOSC	LAURO	STRY PH	SULPH
2					X
17	X	X	X	X	

Atheroma (Includes Blood Vessels, Fatty Degeneration of)

	LACH	BAR M	PHOS	VANAD	CRAT	CALC	GRAPH	LAC AC	PLUM	SIL
2	X			X						
4	X									
6			X							
7	X					X	X	X	X	X
8	X		X			X	X	X	X	X
10		X	X							
14		X			X					
16				X						
24		X			**X**					
27	X			X						

Atherosclerosis

	BAR C	GLON	PHOS	VANAD	ALL S	AMM IOD	ARS	ARS IOD	AUR IOD	BAR IOD	BENZ AC	CALC	CALC FL	KALI IOD	LYC	NAT IOD	NAT SUL	PLUM IOD	PLUM	POLYG A	RHUS T	SKOOK	SIL	STRONT I	SULPH	THUJA	X RAY
11	X	X		X	X	X		X						X		X		X		X				X			
16											X											X					X
18	X		X				X		X	X		X	X		X		X		X				X		X	X	
19																					X						
21	X	X	X	X																							

Athetosis

	LATH	STRYCHN
2	X	X
17	X	X

Atony- See Weakness

Atrial Flutter

	DIG	CALC	CHINA	CIMICI	LIL T	NAT M	NUX V	RHUS T
17	X	X	X	X	X	X	X	X
19	X							

Atrophic Pharyngitis

	SABAL	AESC	ALUM	CIST	COCCUS	HYDRAST	KALI BIC	MEZ	NAT M	SABAD
2	X	X	X	X	X	X	X			
8	X								X	X
17								X		

Atrophy

	PLUM	IOD	ARS	BAR C	PIC AC	NAT M	CALC SIL	CETRAR	CHINA	GRAPH	HYPER	KALI PH	PETR	PLUM IOD	PHOS	SABAL	SEC	SEL	SIL									
1															X													
2	X	**X**	**X**	X		**X**	X	X				X		X		X												
4	X										X																	
6	X				X												X		X									
10	X				X								X															
11		X																										
13									X	X								X										
14			X																									
19				X																								
24	X	X																										

Atrophy, Breast (Includes Emaciation, Breasts)

	IOD	CON	CHIM	KREO	NIT AC	NUX M	SABAL	KALI IOD	ONOS	ARS	BAR C	DULC	FRAG	LAC D	SARS													
1	X		X	X		X	X		X			X																
2			X				X		X																			
6	X			X																								
7	X	X			X	X		X																				
8	X	X	X		X	X							X	X	X													
10	X			X																								
13	X	X			X			X		X																		
14	X																											
18	X																											
19											X																	
21	X						X																					

Atrophy, Glands

	IOD	KALI IOD	BAR C																									
1		X																										
8	X	X																										
10	X																											
19			X																									

Atrophy, Liver

	PHOS	ACON	BELL	BRY	CALC	CROT H	DIG	IPEC	LEPT	LYC	ARS	AUR ARS	AUR	CHINA	HYDRAST	MERC	PH AC	SULPH AC
1	X											X			X			
4	X						X											
6	X	X	X	X		X		X	X									
7																X		
8	X	X	X	X	X	X	X	X	X		X			X			X	X
9	X																	
10	X																	
11										X								
19	**X**				X					X			X					
23	X																	

Atrophy, Muscles

	PLUM	PHOS	ARG N	CALC	CUPR	ARN	ARS	CAUST	GELS	THALLIUM	AGAR M	BAR C	BAR IOD	CIMEX	COCCUL	DULC	HEP	IGN	KALI BIC	KALI PH	LACH	MUR AC	PHYSO	SEL	STRY PH	SULPH	VER V	ZINC
1	**X**	X	X		X	X				X		X	X							X		X		X	X			
3	**X**	X	X		X	X		X	X		X			X	X	X		X	X								X	X
4		X															X											
6	X		X	X	X		X	X													X					X		
7	X	X		X			X																					
8				X																								
9	X								X																			
11	X																											
17										X																		
23	X																						X					

Atrophy, Muscular, Progressive

	PHOS	PLUM	PHYSO	ACON	ARG N	ARN	ARS	BAR C	BELL	CARB S	CAUST	CUPR	GELS	HYOSC	MERC	NUX V	RHUS T	SEC	SULPH
2	**X**	**X**	X							X									
8	X	X	X	X	X	X	X	X	X		X	X	X	X	X	X	X	X	X

Atrophy, Nipples

	SARS	NUX M
3	X	X
8	X	

Atrophy, Optic Disc

	CARB S
1	X
14	X

Atrophy, Optic Nerve

	NUX V	PHOS	ARS	CARB S	ARG N	IOD	OL JEC A	SANTIN	STRY N	TAB
1	X	X	X	X						
3				X						
4					X					
7	X	X								
8	X									
9			X			X	X			X
11		X							X	
17		X								
23								X		
24	X									

Atrophy, Pancreas

	PHOS
4	X
8	X

Atrophy, Testicles

	CAPS	IOD	KALI IOD	AUR	CARB A	SABAL	RHOD	STAPHYS	ZINC	AGNUS	APIS	ARN	AVENA	BAR C	BUFO	CAUST	CHIM	CON	LYSS	SIL	SULPH
1	X	X	X	X	X	X	X				X	X	X					X		X	X
2						X															
4							X														
7	X	X	X	X	X			X											X		
8	X		X	X	X			X	X						X		X				
11						X															
13	X	X	X						X	X						X					
19														X							
21		X																			

Atrophy, Tongue

	MUR AC
7	X
11	X
13	X
17	X

Attention Deficit (Hyperactivity) Disorder (Note that the entries from 7 are for Attention, Cannot Fix, and from Distraction)

	CALC	SIL	LYC	STRAM	HYOSC	AGAR M	ARS	BAR C	BELL	CAUST	LACH	MERC	NAT M	NUX V	PHOS	PULS	SEP	STAPHYS	CINA
1	X	X		X		X		X					X						
7	X	X																	
29[1]	**X**	X	X	X	X	X	X	X	X	X	X	X	X	X	X	X	X	X	
29[2]				**X**	**X**														**X**
29[3]	X	X	**X**				X		X	X	X	X		X	X	X	X	X	
29[3]	X	X	X									X		X					

29[1] Frei H, et al. Treatment for Hyperactive Children: Homeopathy and Methylphenidate compared in a Family Setting. Brit Hom J, 2001, 90, 183-188.
29[2] Lamont J. Homoeopathic Treatment of Attention Deficit Hyperactivity Disorder. Brit Hom J, 1997, 86, 196-200.
29[3] Frei H, et al. Randomised controlled trials of homeopathy in hyperactive children: treatment procedure leads to an unconventiona study design. Experience with open-label homeopathic treatment preceding the Swiss ADHD placebo controlled, randomised, double-blind, cross-over trial. Homeopathy. 2007 Jan;96(1):35-41.
29[3] Frei H, et al. Homeopathic treatment of children with attention deficit hyperactivity disorder: a randomised, double blind, placebo controlled crossover trial. Eur J Pediatr. 2005 Dec, 164, 12, 758-67.

Autism

	ARN	ARS	CARC	CHAM	HYOSC	NAT M	SECRETIN	SIL	STRAM
21				X	X			X	
29[1]							X		
29[2]	X	X	X			X			X

29[1] Robinson TW. Homoeopathic Secretin in Austism- A Pilot Study. Brit Hom J, 2001, 90, 86-91.
29[2] de Menezes Fonseca GRM, et al. Effect of homeopathic medication on the cognitive and motor performance of autistic children (Pilot study). Int J High Dilution Res 2008; 7 (23); 63-71.

Azospermia- See also Impotence

	CON	DAMIAN	CHIN S	IOD	STRYCH
1	X	X	X	X	X
3	X	X			

Balanitis (Includes Inflammation, Glans Penis)

	MERC	THUJA	NIT AC	RHUS T	APIS	ARS	CANTH	CINNAB	COR R	DIG	HEDEOM	MERC C	NAT CAR	SARS	SEP	SULPH	CALEND	KALI MUR
2	**X**	X									X			X			**X**	
3											X							
4										X								
5	X		X					X										
6	X		X															
7					X				X	X		X	X					**X**
8	X	X	X						X						X	X		
9	X																	
11		X																
12	X																	
13		X	X	X		X	X					X	X	X	X			
14	X	X		X														
21	X																	
27				X	X	X	X	X								X		

Balanorrhoea

	THUJA	MERC	NIT AC	SEP	SULPH	AMM M	CHINA	CINNAB	COR R	FL AC	JAC CAR	JAC G	MEZ	NUX V	PH AC	PULS
2	X										X					
7															X	
8	X	X	X	X	X		X					X	X	X		X
26	X	X	X	X	X	E		X	X	X						

E- External

Barber's Itch (AKA Pseudofolliculitis barbae) (Includes Mentagra)

	RHUS T	SULPH IO	GRAPH	CALC	LYC	TELL	THUJA	ANT T	CIC	LACH	LITH C	MEZ	NAT SUL	PHYTO	SULPH	NAT M
1	**X**	X	X		X	X			X	X	X				X	
2		X	X			X					X			X		
3	X	X	X	X						X		X				
7					X								X			**X**
8			X				X		X				X	X	X	
10							**X**									
12				X	X			**B**								
14	**X**	**X**	X													
19						X										
26				X								X				

B- Both Internal and External

Bartholinitis

	HEP	MERC	BELL	HYDRAST	KREO	MEDO	PYROG
5	X	X		X	X	X	X
21	X	X	X				

Basal Cell Carcinoma (AKA Rodent Ulcer)

	ARS	BELL	CIC	HEP	HYDROC	HYDRAST	MERC	NIT AC	SIL	STAPHYS	SULPH	URAN N	AUR	CALO	CINNAB	CONDUR	CURARE	FERR PIC	JUG C	KALI BIC	MERC N	MILL	PHYTO	THUJA
2																X		X	X			X	X	
6	X	X	X	X	X	X	X	X	X	X	X	X												
8	X	X	X	X	X	X	X	X	X	X	X	X	X	X	X		X			X	X			X

Basedow's Disease- See Exophthalmic Goitre

Bedsores

	ARN	SULPH AC	CARB V	LACH	SULPH	FL AC	CALEND	CHINA	PAEONIA	ARG N	CAMPH	HAM	HYDRAST	MUR AC	PETR	PLUM	PULS	ANTHRAC	ARS	BAPT	CHLOR	CROT H	HIPPOZ	HYPER	PH AC	PYROG	VAL	ZINC
1	X			X			E		X	X												X						
2	X			X	X	X			X		X				X						X		X			X	X	
3	X			X						X										X								
4	X		X											X														
7	X	X	X			X					X	X	X		X	X		**X**										
8	X	X	X					X				X				X	X		X						X			X
9	X			X	X	X	X																					
10						X		X																				
11	X													X														
13	X	X	X					X									X											
14	X	X	X		X		E		X																			
15													X															
16																								B				
24		X		X	X																							
25	X																											
26		E																										

B- Both Internal and External E- External

Bedsores, Prophylactic

	ARN
14	X
16	X

Bedwetting- See Enuresis, Nocturnal

Bell's Palsy (AKA Facial Palsy; Bell's Paralysis)

	CAUST	ACON	GELS	RHUS T	CAD S	DULC	PHOS	AGAR M	AMM PH	ARN	ARS	COCCUL	FL AC	GRAPH	IGN	KALI CHL	KALI IOD	NAT M	NUX V	OP	PLAT	PLUM	SENEG	SULPH
5	X	X		X		X																		
8		X		X																				
9	X		X	X					X	X			X		X							X		X
11	X	X	X	X		X	X				X			X		X	X						X	
14	X	X	X		X															X				
17	X																							
19	X	X	X		X		X	X				X						X	X		X			
21	X	X																						

Bell's Palsy, Left Side

	CAD S	CAUST	SENEG
11		X	X
14	X		

Benign Prostatic Hypertrophy- See Prostate, Benign Hypertrophy

Beri Beri

	ARS	LATH	RHUS T	ACON	ARS I	ELAT	GELS	LACH	PHOS	TUB
2		X	X							
12	X			X	X		X	X	X	
17	X	X	X			X				X

Bile, Deficiency Of- See Liver, Torpidity

Bile, Excessive Production Of

	POD	BELL	BRY	CHAM	IPEC	MERC	MERC C	NAT SUL	NIT AC	NUX V	PHOS	PULS	SULPH	VER A
7	X	X	X	X	X	X		X		X	X	X	X	X
10	X						X		X					
24	X													

Bipolar Disorder- See Mania; Manic Depression

Birthmark- See Naevi

Bites, Animals, Effects Of

	ECHIN	LED	ACET AC	AMM C	ARS	BELL	CAUST	CIST
1			X					X
2	X							
3		X	X					
5	E							
7				X	X	X	X	
10		X						
11	X							
19		X						

E- External

Bites, Dogs, Effects Of

	LACH	LYSSIN	CANTH	BELL	ECHIN	HYPER	LED
1	**X**	X	X			X	
2	X				X		
3	X	X					X
7	X	X					
10		X	**X**	X			
19		X					

Bites, Snakes Effects Of (Includes Bites, Animals, Poisonous)

	BELL	CEDRON	LACH	SENEGA	ARS	ECHIN	EUPH PO	EUPH PR	CAMPH	GYMNEM	OX AC	SELA
1	X	X		X			X	X			X	
2		X		X		X			X	X		
3		E					X					
7	X				X				X			
8	X		X	X	X							
10	X		X		X							
13				X								
15	X				X							
16		X	X				X	X		X		X
17		X		X								
19			X			X						
22			X			X					X	
23								X				X

E- External

Bites and Stings, Effects Of

	LED	APIS	HYPER	ARN	LACH	URT U	ARS	ECHIN	SENEG	TAR C	ACET AC	BELL	CALAD	CALEND	CANTH	GRIND	NAT M	SULPH AC	HYDR AC	MOSCH
1						X				X										
2	**X**				**X**			X	X		X					X			**X**	**X**
3						**X**					X									
5	E							X												
6																	X			
7	X	X	X	X								X	X				X			
8	X	X	X	X														X		
11	X	X	X		X		X	X								X				
12	E	X																		
13	X			X	X		X		X			X	X					X		
14	X	X					X													
17									X											
18			E																	
19	**X**	**X**	X							X										
20		X				X														
21				X	X					X				E	X					
22						X									X					
24	X																			
25			X	X										E						
28	X	X																		

E- External

Bites and Stings, Effects Of, Bees or Wasps

	APIS	LED	ARN	URT U	LACH	NAT M	CALEND	HYPER	MERC	SANIC
1	X	X		X						X
2				X						
3	X	X		X						
5	X									
7			X		X	X				
8	X		X							
9	X									
10	X	X	X			X				
14	X									
19		X								
20		**X**								
21		X								
22	X	X	X				X	X		
25	X									
26	**X**				X				X	

Bites and Stings, Effects Of, Hornets

	APIS	LED	ARN	CALEND	HYPER
1	X				X
21	X	X			
22	X	X	X	X	

Bites and Stings, Effects Of, Insects

	APIS	LED	CAMPH	CEDRON	HYPER	ACON	URT U	ACET AC	ARN	BELL	BERB V	CANTH	CROT H	ECHIN	EUPH PR	MERC	NAT M	NAT PH	TAR C
1				X	X										X		X		
2			X		X														
3	B	X		X															
4		X																	
5	X	X			X														
7	X		X					X											
8	X	X				X			X	X	X		X			X		X	
9	X	X																	
10	B																		
12			E																
14	X	X				X													
15	X	X	X			X													
17				X															
18	X											X							X
19		X					**X**							X					
24		X																	

B- Both Internal and External E- External

Bites and Stings, Effects Of, Jellyfish

	URT U	APIS	CHIRO	LED
19	**X**	X		
28			X	X

Bites and Stings, Effects Of, Leeches

	LACH
1	X
7	X

Bites and Stings, Effects Of, Mosquitoes

	LED	CALAD	APIS	NAT M	PSOR	STAPHYS
3	X					
4	X					
5	X					
7	X	X		X		
8	X					
9	X					
10	X					
16						X
19	X	X			X	
24	X					
25			X			
28	X					

Bites and Stings, Effects Of, Scorpions

	APIS	CROT H	LED	CARB AC	ECHIN	GUACO	LACH	OX AC
1		X						
2			X					
3	X		X					
5	X							
9	X							
10	X							
14	X							
16						X		
22		X		X	X		X	X

Bites and Stings, Effects Of, Spiders

	LACH	CROT H	ECHIN	OX AC	SELA
16					X
19	X				
22	X	X	X	X	

Bites and Stings, Effects Of, Wasps

	APIS	ARN	CALEND	CANTH	LED	MERC	HYPER	LACH
1		E	X	X		X		
3	X	E		X				
5	X							
9	X							
10	X							
21	X				X			
22	X	X	X		X		X	
26	**X**					X		X

E- External

Black Eye

	LED	ARN	HAM	ERIGER	SYMPH
1	X				
2	X	**X**	**X**	X	
28					X

Blackheads- See Comedo

Bladder, Diseases Of

	BERB V	CANTH	BENZ AC	CAUST	DULC	NUX V	APIS	BAROSMA	ELAT	EUCAL	GADUS	GEUM	LIL T	LYC	MUREX	PULS	ROSA C	SARS	SEP
2	**X**	**X**	**X**	**X**	**X**	**X**	X	X	X	X	X	X					X	X	
5													X		X				
9	X	X												X		X			X

Bladder Hernia- See Hernia

Blennorrhoea

	HEP	PULS	CARB V	EUPHR	LYC	MERC	THUJA
6			X				
7	X	X				X	X
8	X	X		X	X	X	X
26	X	X	X	X	X		

Blennorrhoea, Glans Penis

	CANN S	LYC	MERC	NAT M	NUX V	SEP	SULPH	THUJA	ALUM	CAUST	COR R	DIG	JAC CAR	LACH	MEZ	NAT CAR
13	**X**	**X**	**X**	**X**	**X**	**X**	**X**	**X**	X	X	X	X	X	X	X	X

Blepharitis

	GRAPH	HEP	EUPHR	PULS	RHUS T	NAT M	SULPH	PETR	STAPHYS	ACON	CALC	MERC	THUJA	APIS	ARG N	ARS	BELL	SEP	DIG	ANT C	CAUST	CON	KALI C	MERC C	PH AC	PSOR	SPIG
1	X	X	X	X	X			X	X		X											X		X			
2	X	X	X																								
3	X	X						X																			
4	**X**		X									X			X				X								
6	**B**	X	X	X	X	X	X	X	X	X	X		X	X	X	X	X	X	X		X	X	X	X	X	X	
7	**X**		X		**X**	X	X	**X**	**X**			**X**	X	**X**	**X**					**X**			X			X	X
8	X	**X**	X	X	**X**	X	X	X	X	**X**	X	**X**	X	X		X	**X**	X	X	X	X				X		X
9	X		X	X													X										
12		X			X					X				X			X					X					
13		**X**	X	X	X	**X**	**X**		X	**X**	X	X	**X**			**X**	X	**X**	X	X	**X**	X	X		X	X	**X**
14	X	X		X				X												X				X			
15			B			X				X	X				X	X		X			X						
17																								X			
19							X																				
21	X	X		X	X		X																				
23		X	X			X																					
24	**B**	X	X	X	X	X	X						X					X	X				X		X	X	
26		X										X															
27	X	X		X					X		X			X	X	X											

B- Both Internal and External

Blepharoadenitis

	SANG	DIG	PETR	PULS
2			X	
7	X			
8	X	X		X

Blepharospasm

	BELL	PHYSO	PULS	AGAR M	CHAM	MERC	NAT M	NUX V	CODEIN
2		X	**X**	X	X				**X**
6	X								
7		X							
8	X				X	X	X	X	
9		X		X					
17	X		X			X	X	X	

Blindness

	GELS	PHOS	SULPH	ACON	BELL	STRAM	LYC	NAT M	ARG N	BOTHR	CIC	KALI BIC	NUX V	PULS	SIL	ARS	CAUST	CHINA	DIG	FERR	GRAPH	MERC	PHYSO					
1	X	X	X	X			X			X	X	X			X		X	X		X	X	X						
2					**X**					X																		
3	X	X	X	X			**X**			X					X					X			X					
4	X					X		X				X																
5		X					X						X	X		X					X							
6	X	X			X	X			X									X	X				X					
7	X		**X**		**X**	X		**X**	X							X	X		X									
8	X	X	X	X	X	X	X	X	X		X		X	X	X	X	X		X	X	X	X						
9												X																
10														X														
11	X																											
12		X											X															
13		X		X		X		X			X		X	X	X							X						
14										X	X							X										
17	X																											
22												X																
24	X		X	X					X														X					
27		X																										

Blindness, Colour

	CINA	PHOS	AGAR M	BENZIN	CARB S	ACT SP	ANHAL	ARS	BELL	CAMPH	CAPS	CON	DIG	GRAT	HYOSC	ONOS	SANTON	STRAM	STRONT	TABAC								
1	X	**<u>X</u>**	X		X	X	X	X	X	X	X	X	X	X	X			X	X									
2				X												X				X								
3		X	X																									
8	**X**																											
9				X													X											
14					X																							
24	X																											

Blindness, Night- See also Nyctalopia

	LYC	CHINA	HYOSC	BELL	PHYSO	VER A	RAN B	STRAM	HELL	PULS	ACON	AGAR M	ANAC	ARG N	CAD	CALC SU	CARB S	CHEL	MEPH	MERC	NUX V	PETROS	PHOS	STRYCH	SULPH			
1	**<u>X</u>**	X	X		**<u>X</u>**		X																					
2			X	**X**		X	X		X												X	X		X				
3	**X**	X	X	X	X	X	X		X		X	X					X						X					
5	X				X																							
6	X	X	X	X		X	X	X		X				X											X			
7	**X**	**X**	X																									
8	X	X											X															
13			**X**	**X**		**X**		X		X					X			X	X	X								
14		X			X											X												
17								X																				

Blindness, One-Sided

	APOC
1	X
6	X

Blisters

	CANTH	NAT M	ANT C	ARS	RHUS T	CAUST	AMM M	BELL	DULC	MERC	RAN B	SULPH
13	X		**X**	**X**	**X**	X	**X**	**X**	**X**	**X**	**X**	**X**
14	**X**	X										
21	X	X	X	X	X							
22						X						
26		X										

Blood Poisoning- See also Sepsis; Septicaemia

	PYROG	ECHIN	GUNPOW	AILANTH	ANTHRAC	APIS	ARN	ARS	BAPT	CARB V	CROT H	GELS	HYOSC	IGN	LACH	TRAC D
1			X													
2		X														X
4													X			
6				X		X				X		X				
16		X	X													
21	X		X				X		X					X	X	
22	**X**	X														
23	X	X			X			X			X					
28	X															

Body/Skin Odour, Offensive- See also Perspiration, Offensive

	PSOR	MERC	HEP	RHEUM	CALC	NUX V	SIL	SULPH	ARS	BRY	COLCH	NIT AC	SEP															
1								X																				
2	X	X																										
3												X																
5	X	X	X	X		X			X	X	X	X	X															
6	X		X	X				X		X	X																	
8	X							X																				
9	X					X	X																					
10	X		X	X	X				X																			
14		X	X																									
15				X																								
18													X															
20		X																										
21	X	X			X		X																					
24																												
25		X			X	X	X																					

Boils (Includes Furuncle)

	HEP	BELL	SIL	SULPH	ARN	LYC	LACH	MERC	ARS	PH AC	CALC	LED	PHYTO	ANTHRAC	NIT AC	PHOS	PSOR	TAR C	THUJA	APIS	CALC SUL	NUX V	SEC	BELLIS	ECHIN			
1	X	X	X	X			X		X		X	X						**X**			X		X					
2	**X**	**X**	**X**	**X**	**X**		X			X		X	X	X			X				X		X	X				
3	X	X		X	X	X	X				X							**X**	X						X			
4	X	**X**	**X**	**X**	X	X			X	X			X				X				X			X	X			
5	X		X		X														X									
6	X	X	X	X	X	X	X	X	X		X				X	X				X		X	X					
7	**X**	X	X	**X**	**X**	**X**	X	**X**	X	X	X	X	X	X	X	X	**X**			X	X	X	X					
8	X	X	X	**X**	X	**X**	X	X	X	X	X	X	X	**X**	X	X	X		X	X		X	X					
9	X	X	X	X				X					X					X										
10	X	X	X	X	X			X	X	X																		
11	X	X		X	X							X	X					X						X	X			
12	X	X	X	X				X							X	X												
13	X	**X**	X	X	**X**	X	X	X		**X**	X	X			**X**	**X**			**X**	X			X					
14	X	X	X				X		X	X				X					X	X								
15	X	X		X	X	X		X																X				
16	X	X	X		X	X			X	X	X			X							X	X						
19	X	X		X	X		X				X	X				X			X		X							
20	X	**X**	X																									
21	X	X	X						X					X														
22	X																											
23	X		X	X	X																				X			
24	X	X	X		X	X	X	X							X					X		X		X	X			
25	X	X	X	X													X	X										
26	X		X	X	**X**	X																X						
27													X															

Boils, Arm

	SIL	PETR	AMM C	CALC	HYDRAST	LYC	MAG M	MEZ	NIT	PH AC	ZINC
7	X										
8	X	**X**	X	X	X	X	X	X	X	X	X

Boils, Axilla

	LYC	PH AC	BORAX	CARB A	CAUST	FL AC	HEP	MERC	MUR AC	NIT	SIL	SULPH AC
3				X								
7							X	X			X	
8	**X**	**X**	X		X	X			X	X		X

Boils, Ear (Includes Boils, Ear, Around)

	MERC	PIC AC	CALC PIC	SIL	SULPH	CON	PHYTO	BELL	BORAX	BRY	HEP	MORBIL
1		X									X	X
2		X										
3	X		X					X				
7					X	X	X					
8	X	X		X	X	X	X		X			
13				X	X					X		
14			X									
17	X	X	X	X								
27	X											

Boils, Face

	MEZ	ANT C	ALUM	AMM C	ARN	BAR C	BELL	CALC	CALC PH	CARB V	CHINA	CINA	HEP	LAURO	LED	MUR AC	NAT C	NAT M	NIT AC	SIL	SULPH
2									X												
7	X	X											X								X
8	X																				
13	X	X	X	X	X	X	X	X		X	X	X		X	X	X	X	X	X	X	

Boils, Finger

	LACH	CALC	IRIS V	SIL
7	X			
8	X	X	X	X

Boils, Gums- See also Epulis (AKA Gum boils)

	MERC	SIL	BELL	HEP	BOR	ACON	LYC	NUX V	PHOS	SULPH	ARN	CALC FL	CARB A	CARB V	GUNPOW	KALI IOD	KALI MUR	NAT M	PETR	PULS	SANIC
1	X	X																			
2	**X**																				X
3	X	X	X		X								X								
5					X																
6	X	X		X							X										
7	X	X					X	X	X					X		X	X	X	X		
8							X														
10	X	X	X	X		X															
12	**X**		X	X		X			X	X											
14	X	X	X		X							X									
15	X		X	X				X		X										X	
21		X													X						
25		X																			

Boils, Nates

	HEP	LYC	ACON	AGAR M	AUR	BOV	GRAPH	NIT AC	OLEAND	PH AC
7	X	X								
8	X	X	X	X	X	X	X	X	X	X

Boils, Neck

	HEP	KALI IOD	AMM C	CALC	CHINA	COLOC	GRAPH	IOD	MAG	NAT M	PETR	PSOR	SEP	SIL	SULPH
7	X	X		X							X	X		X	X
8	X	X	X		X	X		X	X	X			X		
13	X						X								

Boils, Nose

	CARB A	ALUM	AMM C	SIL	APIS	CAD SUL	MAG	MAG M	MUREX	TUB
1						X				
3										X
7	X									
8	X	X	X	X	X		X		X	
13	X	X	X	X				X		

Boils, Prophylaxis

	SULPH	ARN
12	X	
16		X
24	X	
25	X	

Boils, Scalp

	KALI C	HEP	LED	MEZ	ARS	AUR	BAR C	BELL	CALC	HELL	KALI BIC	MAG M	MERC	MUR AC	NAT C	NIT AC	NUX V	PETR	PSOR	PULS	RHUS T	RUTA	SEP	SIL	SULPH
7	X	X		X							X				X				X						X
8	X		X				X	X	X			X		X		X					X				
13	X	X	X	X	X					X			X				X	X		X		X	X	X	
21						X																			

Boils, Slow to Heal

	SIL	HEP
20	X	X
21	X	

Boils, Thigh

	LACH	NIT AC	SIL	HYOSC	IGN	PETR	ALUM	AUR	CALC	CLEM	COCCUL	LYC	MAG	NUX V	PH AC	PHOS	SEP
7	X	X	X														
8	X	X	X	**X**	**X**	**X**	X	X	X	X	X	X	X	X	X	X	X

Bone, Brittle- See Osteogenesis Imperfecta

Bone, Curvature Of- See also Pott's Disease; Rickets

	CALC	SIL	SULPH	ASAF	PULS	BELL	MERC	LYC	PHOS	CALC PH	HEP	NIT AC	RHUS T	STAPHYS	AMM C	ARN	IOD	PH AC	PLUM	RUTA	SEP
1	X	X																			
3		X																			
4		**X**																			
6	X																				
7	**X**	X	**X**				X		X												
8	**X**	X	**X**	X	X	X	X	X	X		X	X	X	X		X					X
10				X	X	X															
13	**X**	**X**	X	**X**	**X**	X	**X**	X	X	X	X	X	X	X	X		X	X	X	X	
14	X									X											
15	X																				
24		X																			
26	X	X	X	X	X	X		X													

Bone, Diseases Of

	SIL	AUR	CALC	FL AC	MEZ	CALC PH	PHOS	PH AC	SULPH	ASAF	CALC FL	HECLA	MERC	RUTA	OL JEC	PHYTO	STILL	SYMPH	NIT AC	THERID	BELL	CIST	GUAIAC	HEP	PULS	STAPHYS	STRONT C
1		X		X							X	X															
2		**X**	**X**	**X**	**X**		**X**			X	X	**X**		**X**	X	**X**	**X**			X		X	X			X	X
4	X	X	X	X	X	X	X	X	X	X	X	X	X	X			X	X	X								X
6	X								X						X												
7	**X**		**X**	**X**	X	**X**	X	X	X		**X**		X		X	X			X	X				X			
8	X	X	X		X		X	X	X	X		X	X	X	X	X	X		X	X	X	X	X	X	X	X	
9	X		X		X	X								X				X									
10	X	**X**	X	**X**	X		X	X	X	**X**			**X**					**X**			X				X		
12	X	X						X																			
16	X																										
18						X																					
24						X																					

Bone Inflammation- See Osteitis

Bone Pain- See Pain, Bone

Borborygmi (Includes Stomach, Rumbling)

	LYC	PH AC	PULS	PHOS	VER A	BISM	CROT H	POD	SULPH	THUJA	JATR	CHAM	GAMBOG	MUR AC	SIL
2	**X**										**X**				
4		X													
6	X	X	X	X							X	X			
7			X	X	X		X	X	X	X	X		X	X	
8	X	X		X		X			X						
9	X		X												
10	X	X	X	X		X						X			
11		X	X				X						X		X
12	X				X										
13					X	X			X	X				X	X
14	X						X	X							
15			X	X	X							X		X	
18	X							X	X	X			X		
19	X	X					X	X		X					
22	X														
24	X					X									X
27					X										
28	X														

Bowel, Atony/Torpor- See also Paralysis, Intestines (Includes Bowel, Congestion)

	OP	ALUM	BRY	HYDRAST	COLLIN	NUX V	CUPR AC	GRAPH	PLUM	POD	SEL	SEP
5			X	X	X	X				X		X
9	X	X										
12	X			X					X			
15	X					X	X					
17											X	
18	X	X	X									
21	X											
22			X									
24	X	X			X			X				
28				X								

Bowel Obstruction- See Bowel Atony; Ileus; Obstruction, Intestines; Paralysis, Intestines

Bradycardia

	DIG	OP	GELS	KALM	CUPR	APOC	NAJA	VER V	BERB V	ARS IOD	CAMPH	LAURO	VER A	ABIES C	APIS	CROT H	HELL	MYRICA	PLUM
1	X		X	X			X	X		X	X		X					X	
3										X		X							
4	X			X	X	X	X	X										X	
5			X				X							X					
6	X	X	X	X	X				X	X			X		X	X	X		X
7	X	X	**X**	X		X			**X**			X				X	X		
8	X	X	X	X	**X**	X		X	X		X	X	X				X	X	X
9	X	X	X	X		X								X					
10	X			X	X														
11	X	X	X																
12											X		X						
14	X	X	X				X			X									
15															X				
16		X																	
17	X	X	X	X	X	X	X	X	X		X	X		X	X	X			
18								X											
19	X			X															
21	X																		
24	X	X																	X
25	X	X																	
27	X				X														

Bradypnoea

	CAMPH	OP	DIG	HYDR AC	SPONG	CAPS	GELS	HELL	HYOSC	IPEC	MERC C	NUX V	BELL	CACT	LAURO
1	X														
4	X														
6		X	X					X							
7	X	X	X	X	X	X	X		X		X	X			
8		X	X	X	X					X					
13	X	X		X	X	X		X	X	X	X	X	**X**	**X**	**X**
17							X								

Brain, Diseases Of

	BRY	BELL	OP	PHOS	CUPR	NUX V	GELS	HELL	HYOSC	ARN	BAR C	CUPR AR
2	**X**	**X**	**X**	**X**		**X**	**X**			**X**	**X**	**X**
6				X								
7	X				X	X	X	X				
8	X	X	X		X				X			
9	X				X			X				
12		X	X	X					X			

Breasts, Diseases Of

	CIMICI	CON	PHYTO	AUR S	BELL	BROM	CARB V	COM	HELL	HELON	HEP	HYPER	IOD	LEPID	OL AN	ONOS	ORIGAN	PARAF	PHELL AQ	PULS	TRIFOL P	SULPH	ZINC
2	**X**	**X**	**X**	X				X	X	X	X	X	X	X	X	X	X	X	X			X	X
12					X															X			
20							X																
24						X																	
29*																					X		

29* Parvu E. Trifolium pratense for Breast Disease: A Case Series. Homeopathy, 2004, 93, 45-50.

Breast Lumps- See Tumor, Breast

Breath, Offensive- See Halitosis

Breathing, Stertorous

	OP	AMM C	BELL	CAMPH	CHLOR	GLON	HYOSC	NUX V	PULS	STANN
6	X									
7	X	X	X	X	X	X	X	X	X	X
8	X	X	X	X	X	X	X	X	X	X
12	X									
26	X									

Bright's Disease- See also Nephritis

	APIS	PHOS	ARS	MERC C	TEREB	COLCH	CANTH	NIT AC	PLUM	KALI CHL	DIG	GLON	LYC	PH AC	ACON	APOC	BRACH	CHEL	HELL	HEP	KALI IOD	KALM	SULPH	AUR M				
1	X	X	X	X	X	X	X	X	X	X	X		X		X	X			X									
2	**X**			X				X	X		X	X	X				X				X	X	X					
3	X			X	X	X	X	X		**X**						X			X									
4	**X**	**X**	X	X					X	**X**					X					X				X				
6		X																										
7	X	X	**X**	**X**	**X**	X	X	X	**X**		X	**X**	**X**	**X**			X	X		X	X	X	X	**X**				
8	X	X	X	X	X	X	X	X	X		X	X		X			X	X	X	X	X	X						
9	X			X		X																						
10	X	X				X																						
11					X																							
12	X	X	X	X	X	X	X	X						X	X	X		X					X					
14	X	X	X		X		X			X																		
17			X																									
24		X																										

Bronchiectasis (Note that only the main remedies from 17 have been used here)

	HEP	ANT T	PHOS	CALC	IPEC	KALI BIC	LYC	STANN	MERC	ACON	AMM M	BACILL	BRY	CAUST	DROS	KALI CAR	KALI SUL	KREO	PULS	SENEG	CON							
3																				X								
6	X						X	X			X																	
7	X	X	X	X				X																				
8	X					X					X				X													
11		X	X	**X**			X		**X**			X				X	X	X			**X**							
17	X	X	X	X	X	X	X	X	X	X		X	X	X	X	X	X	X	X	X								
19					X																							
21	X	X	X		X	X				X			X	X					X									

Bronchiolitis (Note that only the main remedies from 17 have been used here)

	IPEC	CARB V	ACON	ANT T	BELL	CALC SUL	DULC	FERR PH	KALI CAR	KAOLIN	PH AC	SENEG	SOLAN	TEREB	TUB													
14	X		X			X		X	X	X	X				X													
17	X	X			X		X							X														
19	X																											
20	X																											
21		X		X																								
27												X	X															

Bronchitis (Note that only the main remedies from 17 have been used here)

	ACON	ANT T	BRY	IPEC	PHOS	HEP	PULS	BELL	MERC	KALI BIC	SPONG	ARS	CARB V	CAUST	LYC	SULPH	CALC	IOD	DROS	FERR PH	KALI CAR	LACH	SENEG	NUX V				
8	**X**	X	X	X	X	X	**X**	X	**X**		X	X	X	X	X	X	X	X	X			X	X	**X**				
9	X	X	X		X	X		X		X	X									X	X							
10	X		X					X	X							X												
11									X																			
12	X	X	X	X	X		X	X		X	X							X					X					
13	X		X		X	X			X	X	X	X	X	X	X		X	X	X			X		X				
14	X	X	X	X			X			X																		
15				X																								
16	X	X	X	X	X	X	X					X	X															
17	X	X	X	X	X	X	X	X	X	X	X	X	X	X	X	X	X	X	X	X	X	X	X	X				
18		X	X														X											
19		X	X	X	X		X		X			X		X	X	X					X		X					
20				X																								
21	X	X		X	X	X	X	X		X			X	X														
22																				X								
23							X				X							X		X								
24					X	X																						
25	X	X	X		X	X		X		X																		
26	**X**	X	X	X	X	X		X	**X**		X	X	X	X	X	X	X		X		X	X						
27		X		**X**											X	X												

Bronchitis, Acute

	ACON	ANT T	BRY	IPEC	BELL	FERR PH	MERC	HEP	KALI BIC	PHOS	PULS	RUM	ARS	HYOSC	STICTA	CACT	CALC	CARB V	CAUST	CON	GELS	SULPH						
1	X	X	X	X	X		X	X		X		X		X	X		X											
2	**X**	**X**	**X**	**X**		X	**X**	**X**	**X**	**X**	**X**	**X**	**X**	**X**	X	X		**X**	**X**	**X**		**X**						
3	X	X		X		X			X																			
4	**X**	**X**		X	**X**	X															X							
5	X	X	X	X	X	X	X	X		X																		
6			X		X		X																					
7	X	**X**	X	X	X	X	X	**X**	X	X	X	X	X	X		X	**X**	X	X	X	**X**							
8	**X**	X	**X**	X	**X**	X	X	X	X	**X**	X	X	X	X	X	**X**	X	X	X	X	X	X						
10	X		X		X	X	X															X						
12	X	X	X	X					X	X																		
14		X	X	X							X																	
15	X	X	X	X				X	X	X	X		X															
18	X	X	X	X	X	X	X	X			X	X			X													
19									X																			

Bronchitis, Chronic (Note that only the main remedies from 17 have been used here)

	CARB V	KALI BIC	ANT T	ARS	HEP	SENEGA	SULPH	STANN	PHOS	AMM C	IPEC	SIL	NIT AC	PULS	CALC	HYDRAST	LYC	ANT IOD	CACT	DROS	ARS IOD	CAUST	COP	KALI CAR	LACH	NUX V	VER A
1	X	X	X	X		X				X				X				X		X		X					
3	X								X	X				X				X		X							
4	X	X	**X**	X	X	X	**X**		X		X			X				X						X	X	X	X
5		X	X		X	X		X			X	X				X											X
6									X				X		X		X								X		
7	X	X		X	X	X	X	X	X	X		**X**	X		X	X	**X**		X	X		X	X	X	X	X	
8	X	X	X	X	X	X	X	X	X	X		X	X		X	X	X		X	X		X	X	X		X	X
10	X		X		X				X					X													
11	X	**X**	X	X	X	X	X	**X**		**X**	**X**	X	X	X	X		X				X						
12	X	X	X	X			X		X	X		X	X						X								
14	X		X				X											X			X						
15	X	X		X	X		X	X	X		X		X	X	X	X			X	X					X		
17	X	X		X	X	X	X	X		X	X	X	X	X	X		X	X	X		X		X			X	X
18	X	X	X	X		X		X			X	X				X						X		X			
23	X	X			X	X	X	X				X									X		X				
26	X		X	X	X						X																

Bronchorrhoea

	BERB A	COP	FERR IOD	AMM C	ARS	BACILL	CHINA	EUCAL	GRIND	STANN	TEUC S
2	X		X								X
8		X	X	X	X		X		X		
23	X	X				X		X		X	

Bruising (Includes Contusions; Ecchymoses; Haematomas)

	ARN	LED	HAM	RUTA	SULPH AC	BELLIS	CON	HYPER	PHOS	CARB V	LACH	PULS	RHUS T	BRY	HEP	SYMPH	BAD	IOD
2	**X**	X	X	**X**	X		**X**	**X**	X								X	
3	X																	
4	X									X								
5	X																	
6	X								X	X								
7	**X**	X	X	**X**	X		X	X	**X**	X	X	X			X	X	X	X
8	**X**	X	X	X	X		X	X	X		X	X	X	X	X	X	X	X
9	B	X	X			X	X	X					X			X		
10	B	X	E	X		X			X	X			X					X
11	X		X		X				X	X								
12	X		X															
13	X			X	X		X			X		X	X	X	X			
14	**X**																	
15	E					E												
16	X				X													
17	X	X																
18	X	X	X								X							
19	**X**	**X**	X	X	X	**X**	X		X		X	X		**X**	X			
20	**X**	X																
21	X		X	X		X		X										
22	X	X						X										
23	X	X		X			X									X		
24	**X**				X	X					X		X	X				
25	B	X	X			X												
26	**B**			**X**														
27	X																	
28	X																	
29*	X																	

B- Both Internal and External E- External

29* Seeley BM, et al. Effect of homeopathic Arnica montana on bruising in face-lifts: results of a randomised, double-blind, placebo-controlled clinical trial. Archives of Facial and Plastic Surgery, 2006, Jan-Feb, 8, 1, 54-9.

Bruising, Bone

	RUTA	SYMPH
2	**X**	
3	X	
14	X	
24	X	
25	X	X
26	X	X
28	X	

Bruising, Cartilage

	RUTA
3	X
14	X

Bruising, Eye (AKA Black Eye)

	LED	ARN	HAM	SYMPH	RUTA	TAMUS
9	X	**B**	E	X	X	
14	X	X				
15		X				X
18	X		X			
21	E	X			X	
22	X					
24	X					
25	X	**B**	E	X		

B- Both External and Internal E- External

Bruising, Glands

	CON	ARN
24	X	
26	X	X

Bruising, Tendons

	RUTA	RHUS T
3	X	
14	X	
18		X
24	X	

Bruxism

	CINA	BELL	HYOSC	ZINC	ARS	STRAM	ACON	APIS	CALC	IGN	POD	VER A	ASAF	BRY	CAUST	CHAM	CIC	COFF	KALI BR	MERC	PHYTO	PLUM	SANTON	SQUILL	BUFO
1	X		X																						
3	X	X				X							X												
4	X	X		X																					
5	X		X							X	X					X			X		X				
6	X	X	X	X	X		X	X						X										X	
7		**X**	**X**	X			X		X	X			X		X					X		X			
9	X											X							X						
10	X								X									X							
11	X	X												X			X						X		
13	X	X	**X**		**X**	**X**	X	X	X	X	X	**X**			X	X	X	X		X		X			
14		X									X														
15		X	X					X																	
18	X																								
19			X																						**X**
21	X			X	X																X		X		
24						X																		X	
25	X																								
27	X																								

Bubo

	CARB A	BAD	HEP	NIT AC	KALI IOD	MERC	MERC I F	AUR	BUFO	LACH	MERC C	SIL	SULPH	ARS IOD	CINNAB	MERC I R	PHYTO	SYPH	CALEND
2	**X**	X	X	**X**	**X**	**X**			X	X					X			X	**X**
3	X						X				X								
4	X		X								X					X			
6	X	X	X	X	X	X	X	X		X	X	X	X		X	X			
7	X	X	X	**X**	X	**X**	X	X	X	X		X	X	X			X	X	
8	X	X	X	X	X		X	X	X			X	X	X			X		
16		X																	
23		X																	

Buerger's Disease (AKA Thromboangiitis Obliterans)

	ARS	CARB V	ECHIN	EUPHORB	LACH	SEC	SULPH AC	TAB
8								X
11	X	X	X	X	X	X	X	

Bulimia- See also Appetite, Increased

	CALC	IOD	IPEC	NAT M	NUX V	ABIES C	ALL S	ANAC	ANT C	BRASS	CALC IOD	CAPS	CARB V	CIMICI	FERR	FERR SU	GELS	LYC	NAT C	NUX M	PETR	PHOS	PLAT	PULS	STAPHYS	THUJA		
2										X						X												
5	X		X		X	X	X	X	X			X		X			X		X	X	X		X		X	X		
8	X	X			X						X											X						
14			X																									
18		X		X																								
21	X			X											X													
23													X											X				
24																		X										

Bunion

	BENZ AC	SIL	HECLA	AGAR M	HYPER	NIT AC	VER V	RHOD	ARN	CALC	CARB V	KALI MUR	KALI IOD	ANT C	LAPPA	FERR PIC	GRAPH	HEP	PULS	RAN B	RUTA	SEP	SULPH	THUJA				
1																							X					
2	**X**	**X**		X	X		**X**	**X**				X	**X**		X													
6									X	X																		
7					X					X		X																
9	X	X	**X**	X		X					X																	
10																			X									
11						X								X		X	X			X		X		X				
12							**<u>E</u>**		E									X			E							
14	**<u>X</u>**							X																				
19		X			X																							
25		X	**<u>X</u>**	X		X					X																	

E- External

Burns

	CANTH	CAUST	URT U	ARS	CALEND	ACON	HEP	ARN	CARB V	STRAM	HYPER	KREO	KALI BIC	RHUS T	HAM	PETR	PHOS	SEC	SULPH	APIS	BELL	CARB AC	LACH					
1	B	X	B	X						X	B					X	X											
2	**X**	X	**X**		X		**X**		X	X			**X**		**X**	X						X						
3	**X**	X	E	X	E	X	X			X			X				X											
5	X			X	E									X						X	X							
6	X	X	X	X		X		X	X			X											X					
7	**X**	**X**	X	**X**	X		X		X	X					X			X				X	X					
8	X	X	X	X	X	X	X	X	X	X		X		X	X				X				X					
9	X	X	B	X	B			X			X						X	X	X									
10	B	X				X	X																					
12	E		E	X		X			X			E						X										
13		**X**		**X**					X	X		X		X					X									
14	B	X																										
15	X	X				X																						
16	E																											
18	X			X								X	X							X	X							
19	**X**	X	**X**	**X**	**B**	X	X						X		E	X		X		**X**	X	X						
20	X		X		E						X						X											
21	X	X	X		E		X	X			E		X															
22	X	X	B		E			X			E																	
23	X		X											X														
24	**B**		X	X	X	X		X	X	X		X		X		X												
25	X		B					X			E								X									
26	B	X																										
28	X	X																										

B- Both Internal and External E- External

Bursitis- See also Housemaid's Knee

	STICTA	SIL	RUTA	APIS	ARN	BELL	BRY	IOD	PULS	RHUS T	SULPH	ANT C	ARS	BENZ AC	GRAPH	HEP	KALI IOD	ACON	AGAR M	CAUST	COCCUL	FRAG	KALM	LED	PHYTO	SANG	SANIC	
1	X	X			X			X																				
2			X																									
6	X	X		X	X	X			X		X	X	X									X						
7	X	**X**									X																	
8	X	X		X				X	X		X	X	X		X	X												
12		X	**B**	B	B	E	B	B		B					X	X	X	X	B					B				
14	X	X			X									X							X							
19	X		X				X			X										X			X		X	X	X	
21	X		X	X		X	X		X	X							X											
28														X														

B- Both Internal and External

Cachexia- See Emaciation

Calcification (of various parts)- See also Ossification, Arteries

	CALC FL	CALC	SIL	CALC PH	CAUST	HECLA	KALI NIT	MAG CAR	MAG M	MAG SUL	NAT CAR	NAT M	SULPH IO
1		X		X									
5	X	X	X			X	X	X	X	X	X	X	X
19	X		X		X								
28	X												

Calculi- See Lithiasis

Calculi, Biliary (AKA Cholelithiasis)

	BERB V	CHEL	CALC	CHINA	CARD M	CHION	HYDRAST	NUX V	CHOLEST	DIOSC	LYC	BELL	LACH	POD	CHLF	ARS	HEP	LITH C	NAT S	SEP	SULPH	TER	FEL
1	X	**X**	X	X	X	X	X		X				X						X				
2	X	X	X		X			X	X		X		X	X	X			X					X
3	X	X	X		X	X	X		X	X													
4	X	**X**	X	X		**X**	**X**			**X**													
5	X	X					X		**X**											X			
6	X	X	X	X	X	X		X				X	X	X	X	X	X				X	X	
7	**X**	X	**X**	**X**	X			X			**X**	**X**	X	X	X	X	X	X				X	
8	X	X	X	X	X	X		X		X		X	X	X	X	X	X			X	X	X	
9	X	X									X												
11	**X**	**X**	**X**		**X**	X	X	X	X	X													**X**
12	X		X									X											
14	X	X		X																			
15								X						X									
16		**X**	X	X	X	X					X							X					
18			X								X												
19		X		X	X			X		X									X	X	X		
21	**X**			X																			
23	X	X	X	X	X		X			X													
24	X			**X**								X											
27	X		X				X		X		X								X				

Calculi, Biliary, Prevention Of

	CHINA	CHEL
12	X	
14		X
16	X	

Calculi, Bladder (AKA Vesical Calculi)

	SARS	BERB V	CALC	LYC	CANTH	NUX V	BENZ AC	GELS	NUX M	PULS	SEP	STPAHYS
3					X	X						
7	X	X	X	X	X	X	X		X	X	X	
9	X	X		X				X				
10		X										
11	X	X	X	X	X		X				X	X
13	**X**								X			
15						X				X		
18			X									
21	X		X	X								X
24	X											
25								X				

Calculi, Renal- See also See Colic, Renal; Oxaluria; Phosphaturia; Uric Acid, Deposits of/Excess

	LYC	BERB V	SARS	CALC	CANTH	NUX V	PARIERA	TAB	CALC REN	LITH C	PHOS	SEP	URT U	BELL	CANN I	BENZ AC	COCCUS	DIOSC	IPOMOEIA	OCIMUM	PULS	ASPARAG	OX AC	PH AC	TEREB
1	X	X	X	X			X						X	X				X		X					X
2						X			X											X					
3	X	X	X				X							X	X		X	X	X	X	X				
4		**X**			**X**							X													
5		X	X				X		**X**			X	X			X					X				X
6	X	X	X	X		X		X	X	X	X				X				X		X	X			
7	**X**		**X**			X		X			X	X						X	X						
8	X	X	X		X							X							X						
9	X	X	X										X												
10		X																							
11	X		X	X	X		X			X	X					X									
12	X	X			X	X									X					X			X	X	
13			**X**																						
14	X	X					X						X				X								X
16	X	X	X	X					X	X	X		X									X	X	X	
17								X																	
18	X	X	X	**X**			X			X		X				X									
19				X	X			X						**X**			X	X							
21	X	X			X	X		X																	
23	X	X	X		X				X																
24	**X**	X	X	X		X		X		X	X			X			X					X	X	X	
26	**X**		X												**X**						X				
27		X		X		X	X									X									
28	X																								
29*		X																							

29* Jyothilakshmi V, et al. Preliminary investigation on ultra high diluted B. vulgaris in experimental urolithiasis. Homeopathy, 2013 Jul;102 (3):172-8.

Calculi, Renal, Left Side

	BERB V	BENZ AC	HYDRANG	PERIERA																								
19	**X**	X	X	X																								
28	X																											

Calculi, Renal, Right Side

	LYC	NUX V	OCIMUM	SARS																								
19	**X**	**X**	X	X																								

Calluses

	ANT C	GRAPH	SEP	CALC	LYC	PHOS	RAN B	SIL	SULPH	ARS	ASAF	CARB V	CHINA	CLEM	DULC	GASTEIN	HEP	JUG C	KALI BIC	LACH	MERC	PETR	RHUS T	TAR H	THUJA			
2	X															X								X				
7	X	X		X																								
8	X	X	X	X	X	X	X	X	X	X	X	X	X	X	X		X	X	X	X	X	X	X					
10	X																											
13	X	X	**X**			X	X	X																				
14	X				X				X																X			
21	X																											

Cancer- See also Scirrhus (AKA Carcinoma)

	HYDRAST	ARS	CON	PHYTO	CONDUR	PHOS	LYC	SIL	THUJA	ARS IOD	AST R	CARB A	CARC	KALI CY	NIT AC	SEP	APIS	AUR ARS	CALEND	CARB AC	CIST	CLEM	KALI ARS	BAPT	KREO			
1	X	X	X	X	X	X		X							X	X	X	X	X			X			X			
2	**X**	**X**	**X**	**X**	**X**	**X**	**X**	**X**	**X**	**X**	**X**	X		**X**		**X**		X			X	X	X	**X**	**X**			
3													**X**															
4						X														X								
7	X	**X**	**X**	**X**	X	X	**X**	**X**	X	X	X	**X**		X	**X**		X		X	X	X	X	X					
8	X	X	X	X	X	X	X	X	X	X		X		X	X	X	X	X	X	X	X		X					
9	X										X																	
12		**X**																										
15	X	X	X		X																			X				
16	X																											
17	X																											
19													X															
23	X		X						X																			
24	**X**																											
29[1]	X			X									X															
29[2]							X																					

29[1] Maliekal TP. Homoeopathic Medicines Successful in Tumour Reduction. CCRH Quarterly Bull, 18, 1&2, 1986, 12-14.

29[2] Samadder A, et al. The Potentized Homeopathic Drug, Lycopodium clavatum (5C and 15C) Has Anti-cancer Effect on HeLa Cells In Vitro. J Acupunct Meridioan Stud, 2013 Aug;6(4):180-7.

Cancer, Bladder

	CROT H	TARAX
24	X	
14		X

Cancer, Bone- See also Enchondroma; Osteosarcoma

	CON	PHOS	AUR IOD	AUR	HECLA	SIL	SYMPH
1	X		X				
2		**X**					X
3					X		
8	X						
10	X						
12				X			
16						X	

Cancer, Bone, Pelvic

	EUPHORB
1	X
6	X

Cancer, Brain- See Tumor, Brain

Cancer, Breast

	CON	CARB A	AST R	HYDRAST	PHYTO	ARS	SIL	APIS	BELL	BROM	CHIM	CLEM	SULPH	GRAPH	LACH	LAPIS	SEP	LYC	NIT AC	THUJA	HEP	BAD	CALC	CALC O T	PHOS			
1	X	X	X	X	X						X		X			X												
2		X								X	X			X								X						
3	X														X													
4	**<u>X</u>**	**X**		X	X				**X**	X			X			X												
5	X																			X								
6	X	X	X	X	X	X	X	X	X	X	X	X	X	X	X	X	X	X	X	X	X	X	X	X	X			
7	**X**	X	X	X	X	X	X	X		X	X	X					X		X			X			X			
8	**X**	X	**X**	**X**	X	X	X	X	X	X	X	X	X	X		X	X	X	X	X	X							
10	X		X	X		X	X	X	X	X		X		X	X	X	X	X					X	X	X			
12	X																											
13	**X**	X	X		X	**X**	**X**	X	**X**			X	**X**	X	X		X	X	X		**X**		X	X				
14	X		X		X	X					X				X													
23	X	X	X	X	B																							
24		X		X				X				X																
26						X	X																					
29*	X				X															X								

B- Both Internal and External

29* Frenkel M, et al. Cytotoxic effects of ultra-diluted remedies on breast cancer cells. International Journal of Oncology, 2010, 36: 395-403.

Cancer, Cervix

	CARB A	KREO	CALTHA	IOD	SEC
1		X			
4	X				
14		X			
23			X	X	X
24	X				

Cancer, Connective Tissue- See Sarcoma; Cancer, Scirrhus Form

Cancer, Eyelid

	CONDUR
7	X
19	X

Cancer, Face

	CON	AUR ARS	ARS	CALC	CARB A	BRY	KALI MUR	LAPIS	SIL	SULPH
1		X								
7	X				X			X		
8	X						X			
14		X								
26	X		X	X		X			X	X

Cancer, Glands

	AUR M	CARB A	HOANG	HYDRAST
1			X	
8	X	X		
12				B

B- Both Internal and External

Cancer, Larynx

	ARS	THUJA	CON	HYDRAST	KALI BIC	LAPIS	NIT AC	PHYTO	SANG
8	X	X		X		X	X		X
14	X	X	X		X			X	

Cancer, Lips

	CON	COND	HYDRAST	ARS	SIL	LYC	SEP	SULPH	AUR ARS	AUR	CLEM	STAPHYS	TAB	ANT M	BELL	BRY	CALC	CARB V	CIC	CIST C	DULC	KALI MUR	KREO	LACH	PHOS	PHYTO
1	**X**	X	B		X		X	X	X		X	X	X					X			X				X	
2			**X**			**X**							X	X												
3	X		X																							
7	**X**	**X**		X		X	X			X		X							X	X						X
8	X	X		X	X			X			X				X											
10	X	X		X	X	X	X			X												X	X	X		
14	X	X	X						X																	
23	X			X	X			X								X	X									

B- Both Internal and External

Cancer, Liver

	CHOLEST	HYDRAST	ARS	CHEL	BELL	CARB A	CON	LYC	PHOS	SEP	SIL	BRY	LOB E	LACH	LOB L	MUR AC	NIT AC	ORNITHO
1	X								X							X		
2	X																	
6		X	X		X	X	X	X		X	X							
8		X	X		X	X		X		X	X							
11	**X**	**X**	**X**	**X**			X		X			X		X			X	
12		X		X									X		X			X
14	X																	
23	X																	

Cancer, Liver, Prophylaxis

	CHEL	CARC	LYC
29[1]		X	
29[2]	X		
29[3]	X		
29[4]			X

29[1] Biswas SJ, et al. Efficacy of the potentised homeopathic drug, Carcinosin 200, fed alone and in combination with another drug, Chelidonium 200, in amelioration of p-dimethylaminazobenzene-induced hepatocarcinogenesis in mice. J Alt Comp. Med, 11, 5, 2005, 839-845.
29[2] Biswas SJ, et al. Effect of Homeopathic Drug, Chelidonium, in Amelioration of p-DAB Induced Hepatocarcinogenesis in Mice. Complement Altern Med, 2002, April 10, 2:4.
29[3] Biswas SJ, Evaluation of protective potentials of a potentized homeopathic drug, Chelidonium majus, during azo dye induced hepatocarcinogenesis in mice. Indian J Exp Biol. 2004 Jul;42(7):698-714.
29[4] Pathak S, Protective potentials of a potentised homeopathic drug, Lycopodium 30, in ameliorating azo dye induced hepatocarcinogenesis in mice. Mol Cell Biochem, 2006, Apr, 285, 1-2, 121-31.

Cancer, Lungs

	ANT T	ARS	CALAD	HYDRAST	LOB I	MILL	MORGAN	PHOS	SIL
14						X		X	X
23		X							
27	X		X	X	X		X		

Cancer, Mouth

	ARS	AST R	AUR M	CARB A	CIST	HEP	KALI MUR	PHOS
3								X
7		X	X	X	X			
8	X					X	X	

Cancer, Nose

	AUR	CALC	ARS	SULPH	EUPHR	SEP	ALUM	AUR M	CARB A	CONDUR	NAT M	PHYTO	SIL
1											X		
2					**X**								
7	X	X	X				X					X	
8	X												
10	X									X			
13	**X**	X	X	X		**X**			X				
17	X	X						X					
26		X	X	X									X

Cancer, Oesophagus

	ARS	CONDUR	SPIG	AST R	CARB V	CARC	CIST	EUPHORB	HYDRAST	KREO	LACH	LYC	MERC	THUJA
3		X												
10			**X**											
14	X													
24	X	X		X	X	X	X	X	X	X	X	X	X	X

Cancer, Ovaries

	LACH	ALUMEN	ARS	CON	GRAPH	HYDRAST	KREO	LAPIS	PALLAD	PSOR	PULS
1		X				X			X		
4											X
7	X			X							
8			X		X		X	X		X	
14	X										

Cancer, Pancreas

	CALC ARS	PHOS	RHUS T	SIL
2	X			
8	X	X	X	X
23	X			

Cancer, Penis

	CON	ARS
1	X	X
14	X	

Cancer, Prostate Gland

	CROT H	CON	ARS	BAR C	CHIM	LYC	SABAL	SOLID	THUJA
1	X								
11		X		X	X	X		X	X
14	X	X	X						
24	X								
29*							X		

29* MacLaughlin BW, et al. Effects of homeopathic preparations on human prostate cancer growth in cellular and animal models. Integr Cancer Ther. 2006 Dec;5(4):362-72.

Cancer, Pylorus

	ACET AC	BISM	SPIG	ANANTH	ORNITHO
1					X
6		X			
8	X		X	X	
10	X	X	X		

Cancer, Rectum

	HYDRAST	SEP	ALUM	NIT AC	RUTA	ARS	SPIG	NAT SUL
1	X		X	X	X			
2		X					X	
8	X	X						
10	X	X				X	X	
14			X	X	X			
19								**X**
27	X	X	X	X	X	X		

Cancer, Scirrhus Form- See also Sarcoma; Scirrhus

	CON	CARB A	AST R	BELL	CARB V	CONDUR	HYDRAST	LAPIS	SIL	THUJA
7	X	X	X	X	X	X	X	X	X	X
8	X	X								
24	**X**	X								

Cancer, Skin- See also individual sites (Includes Cancroid)

	CALC	ARS	ANTHRAC	CALEND	CAUST	CONDUR	CON	LACH	LYC	NAT M	PHOS	SEP	SIL	SULPH	THUJA	VISC A
1										X						
14	X		X			X										
26	X	**X**			X		X	X	X		X	X	X	X		
28	X			X											X	X

Cancer, Stomach

	ARS	PHOS	CON	BISM	KREO	COND	HYDRAST	MEZ	CARB A	LYC	SEP	CARB V	LACH	ORNITHO	ARS IOD	BELL	SULPH	ACET AC	KALI BIC	NUX V	CARB AC	CAD S	CROT H	SIL	STAPHYS			
6	X	X	X	X	X	X	X	X	X	X	X	X	X		X	X												
7	**X**	**X**	**X**	**X**	X	**X**	X	X	**X**		X	X	X		X		X	X			**X**			X	X			
8	X	X	X	X	X			X			X	X			X	X	X		X	X			X					
10	X	X	X	X	X	X	X	X	X	X	X	X	X		X	X	X	X				X		X	X			
11	**X**	**X**	X	**X**	X	X	**X**	**X**	**X**				X	X		X		X	X									
13	**X**	X	X		X					**X**										X								
14	X	X												X														
19									X					X								X						
23	X					X	X							X							X							
24	X	X	X	X		X	X	X		X	X		X						X				X					
26		**X**			X					**X**	X	X					X			X								
28														X														

Cancer, Stomach and Intestines

	BISM	CONDUR	ACET AC	ARS	HYDRAST	PHOS	ACT S	ART V	CAD S	CARB V	CARB AC	CHEL	CON	CROT H	LACH	MAG PH	NIT AC	ORNITHO	PLAT M	PLUM	SEC	SULPH						
1	X	X		X	X	X				X		X					X	X				X						
2	X		X				X		X							X			X		X							
3						X																						
4		X																										
5	X																											
8	X	X	X	X	X			X			X		X	X	X													
19																				X								

Cancer, Testes

	CON	ARS	CARB A	BELL	PHOS	PHYTO	AUR	CROT H	SCIRR	SIL	SPONG	SULPH	THUJA															
1	X	X							X		X																	
6	X		X	X	X	X							X															
7	X		X			X																						
8	X	X	X	X	X		X			X		X																
14	X	X						X																				

Cancer, Tongue

	ARS	CON	HYDRAST	APIS	KALI CY	LACH	MUR AC	NIT AC	PHYTO	SIL	ALUMEN	AUR M	CARB A	SEP	SULPH	AUR	CARB V	CAUST	COND	CROT H	PHOS	SEMP						
1	X	X	X	X	X						X	X				X			X	X	X							
3					X											X												
6	X	X	X			X	X	X	X	X			X	X	X		X	X				X						
7	X	X	X	X		X	X	X	X	X		X	X															
8	X	X	X	X	X	X	X	X	X	X	X	X		X	X							X						
10	X	X	X			X	X	X	X	X	X		X	X	X		X	X	X									
14				X																X	X							
23					X																							

Cancer, Uterus

	HYDRAST	CARB A	KREO	ARS	IOD	GRAPH	PHOS	LYC	MUREX	SEP	CON	LAPIS	NIT AC	PHYTO	SIL	THUJA	LACH	CALC	CARB V	STAPHYS								
1	X		X									X																
2		X				X																						
3	X						X																					
4	X				X							X																
6	X	X	X	X	X	X	X	X	X	X	X		X	X	X	X	X	X	X	X								
7	X	X	X	**X**	X	X	**X**	**X**	**X**	X	**X**		X	X	X	X	**X**	X	X	X								
8	X	X	X	X	X	X	X	X	X	X			X	X	X	X			X	X								
10	X	X	X	X	X	X	X	X	X	X	X	X	X	X	X	X	X	X	X									
12	X											X																
13	**X**	**X**	**X**	**X**	X	**X**	X	X	X	**X**	**X**		X	X	X	X		X		X								
14		X	X	X								X					X											
19		X																										
24	X				X																							

Cancrum Oris (AKA Noma)

	MERC	ARS	BAPT	KALI CHL	MUR AC	NIT AC	ARS IOD	MERC C	DULC	HYDROC	KALI PH	LACH	SULPH AC															
1	X	X				X				X		X																
2	X			X			**X**	**X**			X		X															
8			X						X																			
12	**X**	X		B	X																							
15		X	X		X	X																						

B- Both Internal and External

Candidiasis

	CAND A	BOR	KALI MUR	MERC	NIT AC	SEP																						
5	X			X		X																						
27	X	X	X		X																							
28	X																											

Carbuncle

	ARS	ANTHRAC	SIL	LACH	TAR C	BELL	ARN	APIS	RHUS T	HEP	CARB V	BUFO	CALEND	ECHIN	NIT AC	SEC	SULPH	BOR	CARB AC	KREO	MYRIST	ACON	BRY	CROT H	KALI IOD	PHOS	THUJA	CALC CHL
1	**X**	X		X	X										X				X									
2	**X**	X	**X**	**X**	**X**	**X**	**X**	**X**		**X**	**X**	X	X	X		X			X	X				X				**X**
3	X	X	X	X	**X**	X	X		X	X			X						X		**X**							
4	**X**	**X**	**X**	**X**	**X**		X		**X**		X		E	B	X													
6	X	X	X	X	X	X	X	X	X	X	X	X			X	X				X						X		
7	X	X	X	X			X			X							X											
8	X	**X**	X	X	X	X			X	**X**	X	X			X	X	X			X				X	X			
9	X	X	X	X	X	X		X										X										
10	X		X	X			X		X	X													X			X		
12	**X**		X	X		X		X			X		E				X					X						
13	**X**		**X**			**X**						X				X												
14		X				X		X																			X	
16	X	X					X		X		X										X							
19	**X**	**X**	X				X					X					X								X		X	
23		X						X		X			X	X				X										
24	X	X	X	X	X		X	X	X		X			X								X						
25	X	X	X	X	X	X		X										E										
26	X		X	X					X														X					

B- Both Internal and External E- External

Cardialgia- See Heartburn

Cardiomegaly- See Heart, Dilatation; Hypertrophy, Heart

Cardiomyopathy- See Heart, Diseases of

Carditis- See Rheumatic Carditis

Caries

	ANGUST	ANTHROK	ARG	ARS S F	ASAF	AUR	AUR M	BUFO	CALC	CINNAB	FL AC	GUAIAC	HECLA	HIPPOZ	KALI IOD	NAT SIL	PLAT M	THER										
2	X	X	X	X			X	X	X	X		X		X	X	X	X	X										
23					X	X					X		X															

Caries, Bone

	ASAF	AUR	PHOS	FL AC	SIL	CALC	SULPH	NIT AC	LYC	MERC	MEZ	STAPHYS	ARG	CALC PH	ANGUST	HECLA	HEP	PH AC	CALC FL	CHINA	CIST	CON	CUPR	GUAIAC	PLAT M	RHUS T	RUTA	STRONT C
1	X		**X**									X		X														
3		X	X									X									X							X
4	X	**X**	X	**X**										X		X			**X**						X			X
6	X	X	X	X	X	X	X	X	X	X	X						X			X								
7	X	X	**X**	**X**	**X**	**X**	X	X	**X**	X	X		X	**X**	X		X	X					X	X				
8	X	X	X	X	X	**X**	X	X	X	X	X	X	X		X		X	X				X				X	X	
10		X	X	X	X	X	X																					
11		X																										
13	**X**	X	X		**X**	X	X	**X**	**X**	**X**	**X**	X	**X**					X		X	X	X	X	X		X	X	
14																			X									
17	X		X																									
23	X	X		X												X												
24	X				X										X										X			
26	X	X		X	X	X	X	X																				
27																X												

Caries, Bone, Cheek

	AUR
6	X
8	X

Caries, Bone, Cranial

	AUR	NIT AC	PH AC	SIL	ASAF	CALC	CALC PH	FL AC	HEP	PULS	STAPHYS
4	X										
6				X	X	X	X	X		X	
7	**X**	**X**	X	X					X		
8		X									
13	X	X	X								X
14	X										
24	X										

Caries, Bone, Ear (AKA Caries, Ossicles)

	NIT AC	AUR	SIL	ASAF	CALC	HEP	NAT M	THUJA
1		X	X					
6	X							
8	X	X	X	X	X	X	X	X
24	X							

Caries, Bone, Facial

	AUR	AUR M	HECLA
7	X	X	
11	X		
24			X

Caries, Bone, Jaw, Lower

	CIST	PHOS	CON	MERC	SIL
7	X	X	X	X	X
8	X				
24		X			

Caries, Bone, Long

	ANGUST	FL AC	STRONT C	ASAF
1	X	X	X	X
6	X			
7		X		
8	X			
24		X	X	

Caries, Bone, Mastoid

	NIT AC	AUR	CAPS	SIL	FL AC
1			X	X	
6	X	X	X		
7	X		**X**	**X**	
8	X	X	X	X	
11	X				
13	X	**X**		X	
14		X			
24	X	X			X

Caries, Bone, Nasal

	AUR	ASAF	CAD S	MERC	AUR ARS	AUR M N	CALC	CALC F	FL AC	HECLA	KALI IOD	NIT AC	PH AC	PHYTO	SIL	SULPH
1	X		X		X				X		X			X		
3	X	X														
6	X									X						
8		X		X		X	X	X				X	X		X	X
11	X															
14	X		X	X												
17		X														
24	X															

Caries, Bone, Tarsal

	PLAT	PLAT M
1	X	
4	X	
8		X

Caries, Bone, Temporal

	FL AC
6	X
8	X
24	X

Caries, Dental

	KREO	STAPHYS	CALC	MERC	SIL	CALC F	CALC PH	CARB V	PULS	ANT C	FL AC	PHOS	BELL	BRY	CHAM	MEZ	PLANTAG	RHUS T	SEP	TEREB	THUJA
1	X	X	X		X	**X**	X	X			X					X	X				X
2	**X**		**X**		**X**																
3																					X
4	X	X					X													X	
5	X	X	X		X	X	X	X			X								X		
6			X	X					X											X	X
7	X	**X**	X	**X**	X	X		X	X	**X**					X			X			
8		X	X	X	X					X			X	X				X			
9	X																				
10											X										
12	X	X		X	X					X		X	X								
13	X	X	X	X	X							X				X			X		
14	X	X	X			**X**	X	X				X					X				
15			X																		
17	X	X																			
19	X	X	X	X		X	X		X	X	X	X	X	X	X	X	X	X	X		
21	X			X																	
24		X	X						X											X	
25	X							X													
26		X	X	X	X				X					X	X						

Caries, Dental, Enamel

	CALC FL	FL AC	KREO
1	X		
4	X		
7	X		
14	X		
19		X	
21			X

Caries, Jaw

	SIL	CIST	PHOS	FL AC	HECLA
2	**X**				
3	X		X		
4		X	X		X
5				X	
8		X			

Caries, Ossicles- See Caries, Bone, Ear

Caries, Palate

	AUR	BELL	MERC
1	X		
4	X		
6		X	
7	X		
8	X		
11	X		
13	**X**		X
14	X		
17	X		
24	X		

Caries, Spine/Vertebra

	CALC	PH AC	PHOS	ANGUST	BAR C	BUFO	DROS	HEP	HIPPOZ	KALI IOD	SYPH
1		X					X		X	X	
2		X									X
3	X										
4	X	X	X					X			
7		X	X			X					
8				X	X						
24	**X**		X								

Caries, Tibia

	LACH	SIL	ASAF	FL AC	GIAUAC
1				X	
7	X	**X**			
8	X				
14	X				
24			X		X

Caries, Vertebra- See Caries, Spine/Vertebra

Carotid Artery, Aneurism- See Aneurism, Carotid Artery

Carpal Tunnel Syndrome

	RUTA	ACON	CALC PH	CAUST	HYPER	MAG PH	NAT M
19	X						
21		X				X	X
27	X		X	X	X		

Cartilage, Diseases Of

	ARG	AUR	RUTA	SYMPH																								
1	X	X																										
2	X																											
7	**X**																											
9			X	X																								
19	X																											

Catalepsy

	ACON	OP	CIC	MOSCH	STRAM	LACH	BELL	HYOSC	IGN	PLAT	AGAR M	CANN I	CHAM	VER A	CURAR	ART V	ARAN D	BRY	COFF	CUPR	FERR	GELS	IPEC	PH AC	PIPER M	SULPH	THUJA	
2	X	**X**	**X**	**X**	X	**X**			X			**X**			X	X	X				X				X		X	
6	X	X	X		X	X	X	X	X	X			X	X				X	X			X		X		X		
7			X			X			X	X	X					X					X		X				X	
8	X	X			X	**X**	X	**X**	**X**	X		X	X	X	X	X	X	X	X			X		X	X	X		
11				X																								
13	X	**X**	**X**	**X**	**X**		**X**	X	X	**X**			X	X						X			X					
17	**X**	**X**	X	**X**								**X**			**X**					X								
26	X				X		X	X					X	X														
29[1]											X																	
29[2]											X																	
29[3]											X																	

29[1] Sukul NC, et al. Prolonged cataleptogenic effects of potentized homoeopathic drugs. Psychopharmacology (Berl). 1986, 89, (3), 338-9.
29[2] Sukul NC, Haloperidol-induced Catalepsy in Mice and Rats suppressed by orally Pre-administered Potentised Agaricus. Brit Hom J, 84, 1, January 1995, 6-11.
29[3] Ghosh, S. Suppression of Alpha Adrenergic Induced Catalepsy in Mice by Potentised Agaricus muscarinus. Brit Hom J, July, 1997, 86, 139-141.

Cataract

	PHOS	CAUST	SIL	CALC	CON	CALC FL	NAT M	SULPH	CANN S	MAG C	LYC	EUPHR	BAR C	CINERAR	SEP	COLCH	BELL	CHEL	NAPHTHA	CALC PH	PULS	RUTA	SANTON	SEC	AMM C	MERC
1	X	X				X		X											X	X						X
2	**X**	X	**X**	**X**	**X**	X		X	X		X	**X**		X		**X**			X		X		X	X		
3	X	X					**X**	X						E	**X**	X				X						
4	X	X	X		X	X	X			X					X											
5	X	X												E					X							
6	X	X	X	X	X	X	X	X	X	X	X	X	X		X	X	X	X						X		
7	X	X	**X**	**X**					X		X		X					X								
8	**X**	**X**	**X**	X	X	X	**X**	X	X		X		X		**X**	X	X	X			X	X				
9	X	X	X	X	X	X	X			X				X					X				X			
12	X		X	X	X			X	X			X					X									
13	X	**X**	**X**	X	X		X		**X**	**X**	X	X	X				X	X			X	X			**X**	**X**
14	X	X		X		X		X											X							
16		X	X		X	X																X				
21	X		X	X																						
23	X				X								X	X												
24	X	X	X	X	X	X	X	X	X	X	X	X	X		X	X	X	X						X	X	
25	**X**	X				X	X			X				X						X			X			
26			X	X	X			X	X	X	X	X														
27				X		X														X						

E- External

Catarrh

	ARS	PULS	AMM BR	ARS IOD	HYDRAST	KALI MUR	MEDO	RUMEX
10	X	X			X			
11	X							
15		X						
17								X
21		X	X		X	X	X	
23		X	X	X		X	X	X
24	X			X				
27	X							

Catarrh, Bladder

	DULC	NUX V	PULS	BENZ AC	CALC	CARB V	COLOC	LYC	SULPH	APIS	CAUST	CHIM	CON
1	X												
7	X	X	X	X	X	X	X	X		X	X	X	X
8	X	X	X	X	X	X	X	X	X	X	X	X	X
13	X												
15	X	X	X		X				X				
23	X			X									
26	X	X	X			X	X	X	X				

Catarrh, Bronchial- See also Bronchorrhoea

	KALI BIC	ANT T	SULPH	NUX V	CHAM	IPEC	PHOS	PULS	NAT M	ARS	BRY	CARB V	CHINA	MERC	RUMEX	CALC	DROS	DULC	EUPHR	STICTA	ACON	HEP	RHUS T
1	X	X		X					X													X	
2	**X**	**X**	**X**		X	X	X	**X**	**X**			X			X		X	X		X			
3			X																				
4																			X	X		X	
5									X														
6	X	X	X	X	X	X	X	X	X	X	X	X	X		X	X	X		X	X		X	X
7	X	**X**	**X**	**X**	X	X	X	**X**	X	X	X	X	X	**X**	**X**	X	X	X	X	X	**X**	**X**	**X**
8		X	X	X	X	X	X	X		X		X	X	X						X			X
9	X	X									X				X								
10	X																		X				
11										X													
12	X			X	X	X		X		X	**X**			X	X			X			X		
13		X	X	X	X	X	X		X			X	X	X		X	X	X			X		
17	X												X			X							
23	X																	X					
24							X																
26			X	X	X	X	X	X		X	X	X	X	X		X	X		X		X		X

Catarrh, Ear- See also Deafness, Otitis media, Otorrhoea

	CHAM	HYDRAST	PULS	MERC DULC	AGRAPH	BAR M	FERR PH	GELS	HEP	KALI MUR	LACH	MEDO	MEZ	NAT SUL	TELL	VISC A
1		X	X	X					X				X			X
3				X												
4		X														
5					X							X				
6	X		X				X	X								
7	X					X									X	
8											X					
14		X								X						
24	X													X		
25			X													

Catarrh, Eustachian Tube

	MERC D	PULS	CALC	FERR PH	IOD	KALI MUR	PETR	AGRAPH	ARS	ARS IOD	AUR M	BAR C	CARB S	GELS	GLON	GRAPH	KALI SUL	LOB SYPH	MANG AC	MERC	MERC I F	NAT SAL	PHYTO	PSOR	SAL AC	SANG	SANG N	SIL
1		X																										
2	X																X	X					X				X	
5						X		X											X									
6	X	X	X	X	X							X																
7					X															X						X		X
8													X		X							X			X			
16																X												
17																					X							
18						X			X	X	X																	
19	X						X																	X				
24	X	X	X	X			X							X														
27	X																											

Catarrh, Eyes (Includes Discharge, Eyes)

	EUPHR	PULS	ARG N	MERC	HEP	SULPH	ACON	BELL	APIS	CHAM	DIG	GRAPH	RHUS T	SEP
6	X	X	X	X		X	X	X	X	X	X	X	X	X
7			X				**X**	**X**	X					
10		X	X	X						X				
12	X													
14	X	X	X	X	X									
18	X	X	X	X	X									
19					X	X						X		
21	X	X												
24	X	X		X							X		X	X
26						X								

Catarrh, Gastric

	HYDRAST	IPEC	KALI BIC
1	X		
8		X	X
23	X	X	X
24	X		

Catarrh, Intestines

	MERC	VER A	APIS	ARS	ARUNDO	BAD	BRY	CALC	CHAM	CHEL	CHINA	COLCH	COLOC	COP	COTO	DULC	EUCAL	FERR	IPEC	LYC	MAG C	SULPH	TEREB
7		X		X	X	X	X	X	X	X		X	X	X		X		X	X		X		
8	X	X	X								X									X		X	X
23															X		X						
24	X																						

Catarrh, Larynx

	CAUST	RUMEX	HEP	MANG	ALL C	ARG	ARS IOD	CALC IOD	CIST	COCCUS	COTYL	FERR PIC	GELS	ILLICIUM	KALI BIC	MEDO	MERC I R	SPONG										
7		**X**	X	X						X								X										
8	X		X	X	X		X	X				X					X											
9		X																										
17																X												
23	X								X		X		X	X	X													
24	X					X																						

Catarrh, Lungs- See also Lungs, Congestion

	ANT T	ARS	FERR PH	ACON	APIS	AUR M	CALC SUL	DIG	DULC	HEP	KALI BIC	KALI C	KALI SUL	LACT V	LYC	MERC	PHOS	PULS	SENEC	SIN N								
7	X	X	X	X	X	X		X	X	X	X	X	X	X	X		X	X	X	X								
9	X																											
11		X					X									X												
21	X																											
22	X																											
24			X																									

Catarrh, Mucous Membranes

	AMM M	KALI BIC	MERC	PULS	ANT T	BENZ AC	HEP	NAT M	AESC	AMM C	ARG N	BAD	BAR M	CALC	GELS	HYDRAST	IOD	OL JEC A	PETR	SENEC	SULPH	THUJA						
7	X	X	X	X	**X**	**X**	**X**	**X**		X	X	X	X	X	X			X		X	X							
8	X	X							X							X												
10			X														X											
17																			X									
18				X																		X						

Catarrh, Nasal- See also Coryza; Ozaena (Includes Nose, Blockage)

	KALI BIC	PULS	HEP	HYDRAST	SULPH	ELAPS	KALI IOD	LYC	NUX V	ARS	CALC	SEP	SIL	ARS IOD	AUR	BELL	NAT M	PHOS	PSOR
1			X		X		X						X						
3	X	X	X	X	X	**X**		X										X	
4	X		X	X			X			X									
5				X										X					
6	X	X	X	X	X	X	X	X	X	X	X	X	X			X	X	X	X
7	X	X	X	X	X	X	X	X			X	X	X	X	X		X	X	X
8	X	X	X	X	X	X	X	X	X	X	X	X	X	X	X	X	X	X	X
9		X							X	X					X	X			
10									X										
11							X												
12															X				
13		X							X	X						X			
14	X	X				X		X	X		X	X		X				X	
15												X							
16	X	X																	
17		X	X	X	X	X						X				X			X
18						X											X		
19	X		X	X	X			X					X		X				X
20	X																		
21	X	X	X	X	X						X			X			X		
23	X					X		X											
24	X																		
25	X	X					X		X	X									
26					X						X		X						

Catarrh, Ophthalmic- See Catarrh, Eyes

Catarrh, Post Nasal (Includes Post-Nasal Drip)

	HYDRAST	KALI BIC	LEM MIN	PSOR	SEP	SPIG	KALI CAR	NAT CAR	NAT M	PENTHOR	SANG N	THUJA
1			X								X	
2	X	X				X		X		X	X	X
4			X									
6						X			X			
8	X						X					
10	X											
14		X			X	X						
17			X	X	X		X	X		X		
19	X	X	X	X	X							X
20		X							X			
21	X			X								

Catarrh, Senile

	AMM C	BAR C	CALC	POTHOS
8	X	X		
13				X
17			X	

Catarrh, Sinuses, Frontal- See also Sinusitis, Frontal

	KALI IOD	SIL	CUPR	MERC	NUX V	LYC	CALC	CAMPH	KALI BIC	KALI MUR	MAG M	NAT M	SABAD	THUJA	VERBASC
2											X	X		X	
4	X			X	X			X	X						
6			X												
7	X	**X**	X	X	X	**X**	X			X					X
9													X		
18	X														
19		X													

Catarrh, Stomach- See Gastritis

Catarrh, Throat (Includes Catarrh, Trachea)

	ACON	CAUST	HEP	HYOSC	MERC	NAT M	NUX V	SULPH	SUMBUL
1			X						X
2									X
7					X	X	X	X	
8			X						
12	X								
13	X	X		X	X	X	X	X	
17				X					
24		X							

Catheter Fever

	CMPH AC	ACON	PETROS
2		X	X
3	X		
16	X		

Cellulitis

	RHUS T	APIS	LACH	GRAPH	SULPH	BELL	CANTH	HEP	LED	MERC	SIL	ARN	BUFO	CALEND	ECHIN	EUPHORB	NAT M	NIT AC	PHYTO	PYROG	STAPHYS	THUJA
2											X											
8	X		X																			
9	X																					
14	X	X							X													
17	X																					
18				X													X					X
19	X	X	X	X	**X**			X	X				X	X					X	X	X	
21	X	X	X			X				X												
23	X						X															
24	X	X	X	X	X	X	X	X		X	X	X			X	X		X				

Cellulitis, Orbital

	RHUS T	APIS	HEP	ACON	LACH	MERC	PHYTO	SIL
4	**X**	X	X					
6	**X**			X	X	X		X
8	X						X	
21	X	X	X					
24	X							

Cellulitis, Pelvic

	APIS	ACON	BELL	CHINA	FERR IOD	KALI IOD	MEDO	MERC I F	PYROG	RHUS T	SULPH	VER A
2							X					
8	X	X	X	X	X	X		X			X	X
16	X								X	X		

Cephalaetoma

	CALC FL	SIL	ARN	CALC	CHINA	MERC	RHUS T
7	X	X				X	
8	X	X	X	X	X		X

Cerebral Palsy- See Palsy

Cervicitis

	HYDRC	KREO	ACON	CIMICI	AESC	ANT T	BELL	CARB A	FERR PH	MAG PH	MERC	SULPH
1		X		X	X							
8						X					X	
9	X		X				X		X	X		X
14	X	X										
19								X				

Chalazion- See also Stye

	STAPHYS	GRAPH	THUJA	CALC	CON	SEP	BAR C	BAR IOD	KALI IOD	LACH	MERC	NIT AC	PULS	SIL	SULPH	ZINC
2	X															
5	X	X	X		X											
6	X	X	X	X	X	X										
8	X	X	X	X		X	X	X	X	X	X	X	X	X	X	X
14	X															

Chancre

	MERC	NIT AC	HEP	MERC I F	MERC I R	MERC C	ARS	CINNAB	COR R	THUJA	ARG N	AUR M	KALI BIC	KALI IOD	JAC CAR	LAC C	LACH	LYC	PH AC	SIL	APIS	BAD	CAUST	CON	MERC AC	PHYTO	SULPH
2	X	**X**		X		**X**		X	X		X	X			X	X	X		X		**X**				X		X
4	X	X	X	X	X													X									
6	X	X	X	X	X		X		X	X	X		X		X		X			X			X			X	X
7	**X**	**X**	X	X		X	X	X		X		X		X		X		X	X	X	X	X		X		X	
8	X	X	X		X	X	X	X	X	X		X	X	X	X		X	X	X	X		X	X	X			
12	X	X				X	X			X																	
13	**X**		X								X					X											
14	**X**				X									X													
23		X		X	X			X	X																X		
24			X										X														

Chemosis (Includes Chemosis, Conjunctiva)

	APIS	HEP	RHUS T	ACON	EUPHR	KALI IOD	ARG N	DULC	GUAREA	CON	KALI BIC	KALI IOD	IPEC	LACH	MERC C	NAT M	NIT AC	PHYTO	TER	VESPA
2									X											X
4			X																	
5		X																		
6	X	X	X				X													
7	**X**	X	X	**X**			X			X		X	X	X		X				
8	X	X	X	X		X		X			X						X	X	X	
11						X														
12															X					
16					X															
27	X				X															

Chest, Diseases Of

	ACON	ARN	CHEL	OX AC	SAMB	BROM	BRY	CALC	CUPR AC	LAURO	MENISP	MYRTUS
2	**X**	**X**	**X**	**X**	**X**						X	X
8	X					X	X	X	X			
17										X		

Cheyne Stokes Breathing

	ACON FE	OP	ANITIPYR	GRIND	KALI CY	PARTHEN	TUB	VANAD
2	X		X	X	X	X	X	X
8		X						
19		X						
23	X							

Chickenpox (Includes Varicella)

	ANT T	RHUS T	MERC	PULS	BELL	ACON	ANT C	SULPH	BRY	VARIOL	APIS	ARS	THUJA	CANTH	CARB V	HEP	HYOSC	MEZ	SEP	SIL
1	X		X						X	X										
2	**X**		**X**			X														
3	X	X	X						X	X										
5		X			X		X							X		X		X		
6	X	X	X	X	X	X	X										X			
7	X		X	X	X		X	**X**					X				X			
8	X	X	X	X	X	X	X	X				X	X	X	X				X	X
9		X																		
10	X		X	**X**	X	X		X												
11	X	X				X					X									
12		**X**	X		X	X														
13	**X**	X		**X**	X	X	**X**					X	X		X				X	X
14	X	X	X					X	X	**X**										
15	X		X		X	X					X									
16	X	X	X						X							X				
17	X																			
18	X	**X**	X															X		
19							X													
20	X	**X**	X	X	X		X					X								
21	X	X	X	X	X	X		X												
22	X	X		X			X	X												
25	X	**X**	X	X	X	X					X									
26	X			X				X												
28				X																

Chicken Pox, Prophylaxis

	PULS	RHUS T
10	X	
16		X

Chilblains

	AGAR M	PULS	PETR	SULPH	BELL	RHUS T	CARB V	NIT AC	NUX V	PHOS	ARS	CALC	TAMUS	ARN	CHAM	ZINC	CALEND	KALI CAR	LACH	LYC	CARB A	HEP
1	**X**	X	X	X		X		X				X										X
2	**X**	**X**	**X**	**X**		**X**	**X**	X		X		X	X			X	X	X	X			**X**
3	X	X	X					X														
5	X	X	X								X	X										
6	X	X	X	X	X	X	X	X	X	X	X			X		X		X	X			X
7	**X**	X	**X**	X	X		X	X	X	X				X	X	X			X	X	X	
8	X	X	X	X	X	X	X	X	X	X	X			X	X			X		X	X	
9	X	X	X	X	X		X		X			X					B					
10	**X**	X	X	X	X	X			X		X				X		E					
11																X						
12	X	X	**X**	X	X	**X**		X		X		X	E	X								
13	**X**	**X**	**X**	X	X	X	**X**	X	**X**	**X**	X				X	X				X	**X**	
14	X																					
15		X		X							X		E	E								
16	X	X																				
17	X				X	X																
21	X	X	X									X										
23	X	X																				
25	X	X		X	X		X		X			X	**E**				B					
26		X	X	X	X			X	X	**X**	X				X			X	X	X		
28							X															

B- Both Internal and External. E- External

Chloasma

	SEP	CAULO	LYC	SULPH	ANT C	ARG N	ARN	ARS	CALC	CAUST	GRAPH	KALI C	NAT C	NAT M	NIT AC	PETR	PHOS	PULS	SEC
2	X	X		X															
8	X		X	X	X				X	X	X	X	X		X	X	X	X	
11	X	X	X			X	X	X						X					X
14	X																		
17	X																		
21	X																		
28	X																		

Chlorosis- See also Anaemia (AKA Green Sickness or Hypochromic Microcytic Anaemia)

	CALC	PULS	FERR	NAT M	SEP	SULPH	ARS	CHINA	PHOS	PLUM	COCCUL	LYC	NUX V	ANT C	BELL	CALC PH	CYCL	ALUM	GRAPH	CON	PLAT	ALET	CUPR	HELON	IGN	IPEC	SABIN	
1	X	X	X	X	X	X	**X**	X	X		X	X	X	X											X			
6	X	X	X	X	X	X	X	X	X	X	X		X	X	X		X	X	X	X		X	X	X	X	X	X	
7	**X**	X	**X**	**X**	**X**	X	X	X	X	X	X	X	X	**X**		**X**	**X**	X	X		X		X	X		X	X	
8	X	X	X	X	X	X	X	X	X	X	X	X	X	X	X	X	X	X	X	X	X	X	X	X	X	X	X	
10	X	X		X		X	X	X	X			X			X	X												
12	X	X	X		X	X																						
13	**X**	**X**	**X**	X	X	**X**	X	X	X	X	**X**	**X**	X		**X**			X		**X**	**X**							
15	X	X			X		X	X								X												
17			X							X																		
23	X		X	X													X					X						
26	X	**X**		X	X	X			X	X									X									

Cholecystitis

	CHEL	CHINA	COLOC	DIOSC	BELL	BERB V	BRY	CALC	CARD M	HYDRAST	MAG PH	POD	CHION	CHOLEST	LYC	MAG M	NAT S	NUX V	PTELEA	TARAX								
1	X								X			X	X	X														
4					X																							
5	X	X	X			X	X		X	X	X	X			X	X	X	X	X	X								
6					X		X																					
7	X	X		X						X		X																
11	X			X		X		X	X	X			X	X				X										
17				X																								
19	X	X	X		X	X	X	X							X	X	X		X	X								
21	X	X	X	X							X																	
27								X																				
28			X								X																	

Cholelithiasis- See Calculi, Biliary

Cholera (Includes Asiatic Cholera and Cholera Morbus)

	CAMPH	ARS	VER A	CUPR	CARB V	SEC	IPEC	ACON	PH AC	HYDR AC	JATR	CHINA	CUPR AC	PHOS	POD	SULPH	DULC	TAB	ANT T	ELAT	LACH	CANTH	CHAM	CROT H	IRIS V	MERC	NUX V
1	X	X	X	X	X	X				X	X									X	X						
2	**X**	**X**	**X**	X	X	X	X	X	X	X	X						X	X	X	X				X			
3	**X**	X	X	X			X			X					X												
4	X	**X**	**X**	**X**	**X**	**X**	X	X		X	**X**				X	X					X			X			
5															X												
6	**X**	X	X	X	X	X	X	X	X	X	X	X	X	X		X		X			X	X	X	X	X	X	
7	**X**	**X**	**X**	**X**	**X**	**X**	**X**	**X**	X	X	**X**		X	X	**X**	**X**	X	X	**X**	**X**	**X**	X	X	X	X	X	X
8	X	X	X	X	X	X	X	X	X	X	X	X		X	X		X		X	X		X	X		X	X	X
10	**X**	X	X	X	X	X										X											
11	**X**	X	**X**	**X**	X	X	X	X	X	X		X	**X**					X									
12	**X**	**X**	X		X		X	**X**	X			X	**X**														
13	**X**	X	**X**	X	**X**	**X**	**X**	X	**X**		X			**X**			X										X
14	X	X	**X**	X	X	X									X												
15	**X**	**X**	**X**	**X**	X				X			X		X								X					
16	X	X	X		X	X							X												X		
17	X	X	X	X	X													X	X								
19	**X**	X																									
23	X	X	X	X			X						X	X													
26	X	X	**X**	X		X	**X**					X				**X**	X						X			X	X
29*	X	X		X								X															

29* Gaucher C, Homoeopathic Treatment of Cholera in Peru. Brit Hom J, 1992, 81, 18-21.

Cholera Infantum

	ARS	AETHUSA	IPEC	VER A	SEC	POD	ACON	ANT C	SULPH	TAB	CALC	CALC PH	CAMPH	CHINA	CUPR	FERR PH	KREO	LAURO	PHOS	CHAM	CROT T
1	X	X																			
2		**X**			X	X	**X**			X		X					X	X			
3		X																			
4	**X**						**X**				**X**					X					
6	X		X	**X**	X				X	X			X		X				X		
7	**X**	**X**	**X**	**X**	X	**X**	X	X	X	X	X	X	X	X	X	X	X	X	X	**X**	**X**
8	X	X	X	X	X	X	X	X	X	X	X	X	X	X	X	X	X	X	X	X	X
10																	X				
11												X									
13	X	X	X	X	X	X		X	X		X		X	X				X	X		X
14			X			X															
17	X	X								X											
23	X	X	X	X				X							X	X					
26	X		**X**	X	X			X	X					X						X	

Cholera, Prophylaxis

	VER A	CUPR AC	CAMPH	CUPR	SULPH	ARS
2		X				
10	X			X	X	
12		X	X			
16	X	X	X	X		X
26	**X**				X	

Cholerine

	VER A	CROT T	PH AC	CUPRARS	DIOSC	ARS	ASAR	EUPH C	IPEC	JATR	KALI PH	NUPH	NUX M	SULPH
2	**X**	X		**X**	**X**		X	X		X	X	X	X	
6	X		X						X					
10	X	X	X			X								X

Chordee

	CANN I	CANTH	CANN S	ACON	ARG N	CAMPH	MYGALE	TEREB	KALI BR	PULS	CAPS	MERC	NIT AC	PETROS	THUJA	KALI MUR
2	X	X				X	X	X	**X**							
4	X		X	X												
6	X				X			X			X			X		
7	X	**X**	X			X	X	X	X	**X**	X	X	X	X	X	**X**
8	X	X	X	X	X	X	X			X		X	X		X	
12		X		X	X											
23			X													

Chorditis

	PULS	BERB V	NUX V	SYPH
7	X	X		X
13	X		X	

Chorea- See also Huntington's Chorea (Includes St Vitus Dance)

	AGAR M	STRAM	CUPR	CAUST	HYOSC	IGN	BELL	MYGALE	ZINC	NUX V	CROC	SULPH	TAR H	CINA	MAG PH	CALC	NAT M	ARS	ASAF	COCCUL	LAURO	VER V	CIMICI	OP	SEP	CIC	PHOS	VISC
1	X	X	X	X	X	X		X	X	X					X			X			X							
2	**X**	**X**	X	X	X	**X**		X	X		X		X	X	X	X	X		X	X	X	**X**			X		X	X
3	X																		X									
4	**X**	**X**	**X**	**X**	X	X	**X**	**X**	**X**	X	X	X		X	X	**X**	X	**X**	X	X	X	X		X	X	X	X	
6	X	X	X	X	X	X	X	X	X	X	X	X	X	X		X	X			X	X	X	X	X	X		X	X
7	**X**	**X**	**X**	**X**	X	X	**X**	X	X	X	X	X	**X**	**X**	X	**X**	X		X	X	X			X		**X**	X	
8	X	X	X	X	X	X	X	X	X	X	X	X	X	X	X	X	X	X	X	X	X	X	X	X	X	X	X	
9	X	X	X	X	X			X	X				X		X													
10					X	X	X			X		X								X								
11	X																											
12	X	X	X		X	X	X		X			X		X				X					X					
13	**X**	**X**	**X**	X	**X**	X	**X**			X	**X**	X	X				X	X	X		X	X		**X**	**X**	**X**		
14	X	X	X	X		X			X	X													X					X
15		X	X																									
16	X							X																				
17	**X**	**X**	**X**	**X**	**X**	**X**	**X**	**X**	**X**	**X**	X	X	X	**X**	**X**	**X**	**X**	**X**	X	X		**X**	**X**	X	X	X	X	X
19	X			X																								
23	X				X			X			X		X		X								X					X
26		X	X	**X**		X	X			X	X	X		X														

Chorea, Left Sided

	CIMICI	RHOD	CUPR AC	CUPR	LACH	SPIG
1		X				
4	**X**					
6	X					
8		X				
17	X		X	X	X	X

Chorea, Right Sided

	TAR H	CAUST	ARS	COCCUL	IOD	MAG PH	PHYSO
1	X	X					
4	X						
6				X			
17	X	X	X		X	X	X

Choroiditis

	PRUN S	BELL	BRY	GELS	KALI IOD	ARS	AUR	MERC C	PHOS	PHYTO	SULPH	ASAF	CEDRON	COLOC	HEP	IPEC	MERC	NUX V	RHUS T	SPIG								
1	X				X		X	X	X	X					X													
2	**X**			X															X									
4				X																								
6	X	X	X	X	X	X	X	X	X	X	X	X		X	X	X	X	X		X								
7	X	X	X	X	X	X		X			X		X	X		X	X	X		X								
8	X	X	X		X		X			X	X	X							X									
21		X				X			X																			
23	X		X										X															

Chronic Obstructive Pulmonary Disease (AKA COPD)

	ANT T																											
19	X																											
28	X																											

Cicatrix- See also Keloid; Scars

	SIL	GRAPH	FL AC	CAUST	HYPER	KALI BIC	LACH	MERC	THIO	PHYTO	ALL C	ASAF	BAD	BOR	CALEND	CARB A	CROC	CROT H	HEP	IOD	NIT AC	PETR	PHOS	SULPH AC				
1																	X											
2	**X**		**X**	X					X	**X**																		
3					X																							
8	X	X	X		X	X	X	X			X	X	X	X	X	X		X	X	X				X				
13	X					X	X	X													X		X					
18		X		X																								
24		X																				X						
28									X																			

Circulation, Cerebral, Poor- See also Anaemia, Cerebral

	BAR C	CON	FERR	GLON	LYC	STERCUL																						
1						X																						
4		X	X																									
9	X																											
14				X																								
25	X				X																							

Circulation, Congestion Of

	ACON	PHOS	CARB V	BELL	CACT	FERR PH	PULS	SULPH	ARN	AUR	AUR M	CALC	FERR	GLON	IOD	MILL	NUX V	SANG	VER V
5	X	X							X	X			X	X	X			X	
7	**X**	**X**		**X**	**X**	**X**	**X**	**X**			X	X				X	X		X
10			X																
17			X																

Circulation, Peripheral, Poor- See also Acrocyanosis; Circulation, Poor; Cyanosis (Includes Extremities, Cold; Skin, Cold)

	CARB V	VER A	CAMPH	SEC	BELL	ARS	LACH	IPEC	SEP	CALC	CALC PH	NUX M	PULS	FERR	NAT M	OP	PLUM	SIL
1		X	X	X	X		X					X			X			
5	X		X	X					X									
6		X	X			X		X	X	X		X	X	X	X	X	X	
7	X	X	X	X	X	X	X	X	X	X	X	X	X	X	X	X	X	X
8					X		X											
9	X						X					X						X
10	X	X	X		X	X		X		X	X		X					
11	X	X			X		X				X							
12	X	X	X			X		X								X	X	
13		X	X	X	X	X		X	X	X		X						X
14	X	X	X	X		X	X			X				X	X			
15	X	X				X			X				X					
16	X																	
17		X		X	X			X										
18	X			X														
19					X				X									
21	X													X				
22											X							
24	X	X	X	X							X					X	X	
25	**X**						X						X					X
26		X																
28				X														

Circulation, Poor- See also Acrocyanosis; Circulation, Peripheral, Poor; Circulation, Poor; Cyanosis

	CARB V	CAMPH	LYC	DIG	SIL	CUPR	HAM	HYDRAST	LACH	SEC	VER A	RHUS T
1			X			X			X			
2					**X**							**X**
4	X			**X**								
5										X		
6	X	X						X				
8	X	X	X	X				X	X			
9	X		X				X					
10	X									X		
11	X	X				X					X	
12		X									X	
25	X				X		X					

Circulation, Portal, Poor- See also Obstruction, Portal Circulation

	NUX V	SULPH	AESC	SEP	ASAF	APOC	CARB V	CARD M	COLLINS	KALI MUR	LED	MERC C	POD	POLYPOR	VER A
4	X	X	X	X											
6	X														
7	X	X	X		X	X	X	X	X	X	X			X	
8	X	X										X			X
10	X														
15													X		
18		X		X											
19	X	X	X												
24			X	X											

Cirrhosis, Kidney

	GLON	ARS	AUR M	DIG	NIT AC	PHOS	PLUM
7	X	X	X	X	X	X	X
8	X						

Cirrhosis, Liver- See also Alcoholism

	PHOS	NUX V	LYC	CHINA	MERC	CARD M	AUR	IOD	LACH	NIT AC	ARS	CHEL	NAT M	MAG M	PLUM	ARG N	AUR M	BRY	LEPT	MUR AC	SEP	SULPH
1		X																				
2				X																		
3	X		**X**		X															X		
4	X	**X**	X																			
6	X		X	X	X	X	X	X	X	X		X	X	X	X	X			X		X	
7	**X**	X			X	X	**X**	**X**	X				X		X	**X**		X		X		X
8	**X**	X	X	X	X	X	**X**	**X**	X	X	X	X	X	X	X	X		X	X		X	
9		**X**											X									
10		**X**	X																			
11	X	X	**X**	**X**	X	**X**	X	X	X	X		**X**	X	X	X		X				X	
12	X		X		X		X			X												
14	X	X										X										
18	**X**			X					X		**X**						X	X	X			
19	X	X	X	X	X	X			X	X	X	X		X								X
21	X			X							X											
23	X					X				X												
27	X		X	X	X	X		X			X						X			X		X

Claudication, Intermittent- See also Cramp, Calves

	ARN	CALC	CUPR	VER A
9		X	X	X
18	X			

Claustrophobia

	ARG N	SULPH	GELS	PULS
21	X	**X**		X
25	X		X	

Clavus- See also Lichen; Scleroderma; Skin, Thick/Hard

	IGN	THUJA	KALI C	NUX V	PULS	AQUILEG	CHIN S	NICCOL	PLAT	PULS N
2	**X**	X	**X**	**X**	**X**	X		X		X
8	X	X					X		X	

Climacteric- See Menopause

Clubbing, Fingers

	LAURO																											
1	X																											
17	X																											
19	X																											

Coccydynia (Includes Coccygodynia)

	KALI BIC	SIL	CARB A	FL AC	HYPER	CIC	LACH	CAUST	CANTH	EUPHORB	PHOS	RUTA	BELL	CALC PH	KALI CAR	KREO	MERC	MUR AC	PH AC	PLAT	RHUS T	TAR H	THUJA	ZINC	APIS			
1	X									X																		
2	**X**	**X**	X	X	X	**X**		**X**		X	X					X			X			X	X					
3					X																							
4					X																							
5		X		X			X											X		X								
6		X	X	X		X	X	X			X	X	X	X	X	X	X	X	X	X	X	X	X	X				
7	X		X	X	X		X		X	X	X	X		X	X		X				X			X	**X**			
8		X	X	X	X		X	X	X	X	X	X	X	X	X	X	X	X	X	X	X	X	X	X	X			
9									X																			
10													X															
14						X	X		X			X																
17						X																						
18	X																											
19	X	X	X																									
21	X	X			X	X		X																				
23			X	X																								

Cold, Common- See also Catarrh, Nasal (Includes Coryza)

	NUX V	ARS	ACON	PULS	GELS	ALL C	MERC	EUPHR	BRY	BELL	CALC	CAMPH	HEP	DULC	NAT M	SULPH	FERR PH	KALI BIC	RHUS T	SABAD	CHAM	SIL	ARS I	LYC	PHOS	STICTA		
1												X																
2	**X**	**X**	**X**	**X**	X	**X**		**X**			**X**	X	**X**			**X**									X	X		
3				X		X	**X**		X		**X**		X			X	X		X									
4	**X**	**X**	**X**	**X**	**X**	**X**	X	**X**		X	X	**X**		**X**	**X**		X						X	X		X		
6	X	X			X		X				X																	
9	**X**	X	X		X	X		X	X											X								
10	X	X	X	X		X	X		X			X				X												
11	X	**X**			X	**X**	X	**X**			X	X	**X**		**X**			X		**X**	X		X	X		X		
12	X	X	**X**	X	X	X	X	X	X					X				X			X							
14	X	X	X	X	X		X	X	X		X			X				X				X	X	X	X			
15	X	X	X	X	X		X	X			X	**X**		X		X		X			X	X		X				
16	X	X	X		X	X		X	X	X		X			X	X	X			X					X			
17	X	X	X	X	X	X	X	X	X	X		X	X	X	**X**	X	X	X	X	**X**	X	X	X			X		
19	X			X		X													X	X		X						
20	X	X	X	X	X	X		X	X	X			X		X		X	X	X						X			
21	X		X	X	X	X	X	X	X	X			X	X	X		X											
22	X	X	X	X	X	X	X	X	X	X			X	X	X		X											
24	X	X		X	X		X			X																		
25	**X**	X	X	X	X	X	X		X																			
26			X	X			X		X	X	X			X		X			X		X	X						
27	X	X	X	X	X				X	X			X			X			X									

Cold, Common, Prophylaxis

	PSOR	BELL	BRY	CALC	CARB V	CHINA	CIST	COFF	DULC	LACH	LYC	MERC	NAT M	NIT AC	PULS	RHUS T	SABAD	SEP	SIL	SULPH	TUB	VER A						
16	X						X						X				X											
17	X																											
26		X	X	X	X	X		X	X	X	X	X		X	X	X		X	X	X		X						
27																					X							

Cold Sores- See also Herpes

	NAT M	RHUS T	CALC FL	DULC	HEP	ARS	CAPS	NIT AC	RAN B	SEMP	SEP	SULPH IO																
2			X																									
3			X									X																
4	X			X	X	X																						
10	X										X																	
14		X			X			X	X																			
18		X																										
20	X																											
21	X	X		X			X			X																		
28	X																											

Coeliac Disease

	MORG G	CALC	LYC	SIL																								
27	**X**	X	X	X																								

Colibaccilosis- See Infection, Urinary Tract, E Coli

Colic, Abdomen- See also Spasm, Abdomen (Includes Colic Infantile)

	COLOC	CHAM	NUX V	BELL	PLUM	MAG PH	DIOSC	CHINA	PULS	VER A	BRY	IPEC	ACON	CARB V	POD	COCCUL	IGN	OP	ALOE	CUPR	STANN	COFF	STAPHYS	SULPH	LYC	MAG C	RHEUM	
1	X	X	**X**	X	X	X	X	X	X	X			X	X		X		X		X	X	X	X		X	X		
2	**X**	**X**	**X**	**X**	X	X	X			**X**						**X**		**X**	X		**X**	X	X					
3	X	X	X	X	X	X	X	X	X			X					X		X	X	X		X					
4	**X**	**X**	X	X	X		**X**			X		X	X			**X**	X	X		X	X		X			X	X	
5	X	X	X					X						X									X			X		
6	X	X	X	X	X	X	X	X	X	X	X	X	X	X	X	X	X	X		X	X	X		X	X	X	X	
7	**X**	**X**	X	**X**	X	**X**	X	**X**	X	X	X	X	X	X	X	X	X	**X**	**X**	X	X	X	X	X	X	X	X	
8	**X**	X	**X**	**X**	X	X	X	X	**X**	X	X	X	X	X	X	X	X	X	X	X	X	X	X	X	X	X	X	
9	X		X	X	X	X		X	X		X			X	X				X									
10	**X**	**X**	X	X		X	X		X	X	X	X	X	X	X			X	X			X		X	X		X	
11		X			X		X		X									X		X							X	
12	X	X	X	X	X		X		X	X	X	X			X									X				
13	**X**		**X**	X	X		X	X	X	**X**		X	X	X	X				X	**X**		X		**X**				
14	X	X	X	X	X	X		X		X	X	X		X	X				X				X		X			
15	**X**	**X**	**X**	**X**			**X**	X	**X**				X			X	X					X					X	
16						X							X															
17	X				X													X										
18																	X											
19	X	X	X	X	X	X	X	X													X							
20	X																											
21	X				X	X					X				X		X											
22	X	X				X					X				X													
23		X			X	X																						
24	X	X	X	X	X	X	X	X	X	X	X	X	X	X		X	X		X	X	X		X	X	X	X		
25	X	X	X	X	X	X		X		X	X	X			X											X		
26	X	**X**	**X**	X			X	X	X	X	X	X	X	X		X	X					X	X	X	X		X	
28	X																											

Colic, Biliary- See also Calculi, Biliary, Gall Bladder

	BERB V	DIOSC	CHINA	CHEL	BELL	CALC	CHION	NUX V	CARD M	VER A	COLOC	NAT SUL	HYDRAST	LYC	MAG C	BRY	CHAM	CHOLEST	IRIS V	KALI CAR
1	X		X			X	X		X			X	X					X		
2	X		X				X							X						
3	X	X	X	X		X	X	X		X	X	X	X					X		
4									X											
6			**X**																	
7	**X**			X	**X**			X		**X**						X	X		X	X
8	X	X																		
9	**X**	X		X						X		X		X	X					
10					X	X														
11	X	X	X	X	X	X	X	X	X		X		X							
14			X				X													
18	X	X			**X**	X		X			X					X	X			
19			X	**X**				X	**X**		X	X		X					X	X
23		X																		
24	X	**X**	X		X															
25	X	X		X						X					**X**					

Colic, Lead- See Ailments from, Lead

Colic, Menstrual- See Dysmenorhoea

Colic, Ovarian- See also Ovaritis; Pain; Colic

	COLOC
1	X
4	X

Colic, Painters

	ALUM	OP	BELL	PLAT	CHAM	POD
10						X
13	X	X		X		
15	X	X	X			
24		X				
26	X		X	X	X	

Colic, Renal- See also Calculi, Renal; Infection, Urinary; Pain, Kidney (AKA Nephritic Colic)

	BERB V	SARS	LYC	CALC	PARIERA	DIOSC	OCIMUM	BELL	NUX V	TAB	CANTH	MAG PH	ARN	ARS	COLOC	NUX M	APIS	ARG N	COCCUS	EUP PUR	HYDRANG	SIL	THLASPI	URIC AC	ZINC			
1	**X**		X	X		X	X	X																				
2	X	X	X	X	X	X	X									X				X								
3	**X**	X	X	X	X	X	X	X	**X**	X	**X**	X						X	X	X			X	X				
4							X																					
5	X	X	X	X	X			X	X			X			X						X	X		X				
6	X	X	X			X			X	X	X		X	X								X			X			
7	**X**	**X**	**X**		**X**	X		**X**	X	X	X		X	X		X	X	X										
8	X	X	X	X	X	X	X	X	X	X	X		X	X		X	X	X	X	X		X		X	X			
9	X			X		X	X					X																
10		X						X						X														
11		X																										
13	X	X					X									X									X			
14		X	X		X																X							
16																							X					
18	X	X	X	**X**	X			X					X		X		X											
19	X	X	X						X						X						X							
23															X													
24	X		X		X					X									X									
25	X			X		X	X					**X**											X					

Colitis- See also Inflammation, Bowel

	SULPH	COLOC	MERC C	ALOE	LACH	LYC	NAT SUL	POD	STAPHYS																			
1	**X**				X																							
3		X	X																									
5		X		X		X	X	X	X																			
9			X																									
14	X		X		X																							
19	X			X		X	X	X	X																			
23		X																										

Collapse- See also Fainting

	CARB V	VER A	CAMPH	ARS	HYDR AC	ACON	MOSCH	CARB AC	ANT T	ARN	CHINA	CUPR	OP	CANTH	DIG	LAURO	STRONT C	AETHUSA	ANTHRAC	CANN I	COLCH	CROT H	GELS	HYOSC				
1	X	X	X		X																							
3	X	X	X	X	X							X					X											
5	X	X		X																								
6	**X**					X	X							X						X				X				
7	**X**	**X**	**X**	X			X	**X**			**X**			X										X				
8	X	X	X	X		X	X		X		X	X		X	X			X	X	X		X						
9	**X**	X	X					X		X	**X**		X		X	X							X					
10	**X**	X	X	X		X			X	X			X					X			X	X						
11	X		X																									
12	X	X		X		X																						
14	X	X	**X**	X								X																
15						X																						
16	X				X		X										X											
17	X	X			X		X		X	X											X							
18		X																										
19	X	X	X	X	X				X							X	X						X					
20		X																										
21	X							X					X															
22	X	X																										
23	X							X																				
24	X			X								X							X									
25	X	X		X						X			X		X	X												
26	X																											
27	X				X																							
28	X																											

Coma

	OP	BELL	ARN	ANT T	HELL	PHOS	ZINC	BAPT	BAR C	NUX M	PH AC	STRAM	VER A	CAMPH	CUPR	CAUST	LED	PLUM	SEC									
1	X		X	X	X	X	X	X	X									X										
3	X		X			X		X	X																			
6	X	X								X			X			X												
7	**X**	X			X							X			X													
8	X	X	X	X	X	X				X	X	X	X	X	X		X		X									
9	X	X																										
11	**X**		X	X	X		**X**	**X**			X			X														
12	X	X																										
13	**X**	X		X		X	**X**		**X**	**X**	**X**	**X**	**X**	X	X	**X**	**X**	**X**	**X**									
14	X																											
15		X																										
17	X	X	X	X	X	X	X	X	X	X	X	X	X	X	X	X	X	X	X									
19	X	X																										

Comedo (Includes Acne Punctata)

	SULPH	GRAPH	HEP	NIT AC	SEL	BELL	CARB V	ARS	CALC	EUGEN	SABIN	BRY	DIG	DROS	HYDRAST	NAT M	SABAD	SEP	SIL
2					**X**					X									
6	X		X			X	X	X	X										X
7	**X**	**X**	X	X		X	X	X	X	X	X	X			X	X		X	X
8	X	X	**X**	X	X	**X**	**X**		X	X	X	**X**	X	X	X	X	X	X	
10	X																		
13	**X**	X	X	X	X						X		X	X			X		
14				X															
19	X	X	X					X											
26	X	X		X	X														

Conception, Failure Of- See also Impotence; Sterility

	NAT CAR	AGNUS	ALET	AUR	AUR M N	BAR C	CAULO	KALI BR	PHOS	PITUIT	PLAT	SULPH	THUJA
1	X	X	X	X	X	X	X	X	X	X	X		X
8	X											X	

Concussion- See also Injury, Spinal Cord

	ARN	CIC	HYPER	BELL	HELL	NAT SUL	ACON	RHUS T	HYOSC	OP	SULPH AC	BRY	KALI PH	NAT M	PHOS	PULS	RUTA	SPIG	LED	CALC	COCCUL	CON	LACH	VER A	ZINC	BAD
1	X																									
2	X	X	X		X						X		X													
3	X	X			X			X				X	X		X					X						
7	**X**	**X**	**X**	X	X	**X**		X	X				X	X		X		X	X		X		X			**X**
8	X	X	X		X			X			X					X	X	X				X	X			
9	**B**	X	X	X		X	X			X				X	X		X							X		
10	B																									
12	X			X			X		X	X																
13	**X**	X		X				X			X	X		X		X		X	**X**		X	X				
14	**X**	X	X																							
15	X						X																			
16	X																									
17	X	X	X	X	X				X		X															
19	**X**	X	X		X	X	X		X	X															X	
24	X																									
25	**X**		X	X		X	X			X							E							X		
26	**X**	X		X				X				X			X					X					X	
28		X				X																				

B- Both Internal and External E- External

Condylomata- See also Warts

	NIT AC	THUJA	STAPHYS	SABIN	EUPHR	CINNAB	MERC	MERC N	NAT SUL	PH AC	AUR	AUR M	CALC	CAUST	CHAM	EUPHORB	KALI IOD	LYC	MEDO	MERC D	PHYTO	PIC AC	PLAT M	SANIC	SEP			
2	**X**	**X**	X	**X**	**X**		X	X	X	X		X					X			X		X	X	X	X			
3	X	X	X																									
6	X							X																				
8	X	X	X			X	X				X			X														
9	X	X		X					X										X									
13	X	**X**	X	X	X	X				X			X		X	X		X			X							

Conjunctivitis- See also Inflammation, Eye

	EUPHR	BELL	ACON	PULS	ARG N	APIS	HEP	SULPH	RHUS T	MERC	ARS	ARN	CALC	SEP	CHAM	FERR PH	KALI BIC	KALI IOD	MERC C	HAM	NUX V	ALUM	IGN	SIL	SPIG	STRAM		
1	X	X	X		X	X	X	X	X									X	**X**									
2	X																X											
3	X	X	X	X		X	X	X	X	X			X												X			
4	X	X	X	X	X		**X**	**X**	X	X	X		X			**X**												
5	X	X	X	X	X	X	X		X	X	X					X		X										
6	X		X	X	X		X	X		X	X				X		X	X		X	X					X		
7		**X**		X	**X**	X	X	**X**	**X**		**X**	**X**	**X**	**X**	X	**X**						X	X			X		
8	**X**	X	X	X	X	X	**X**	**X**	**X**	**X**	X	X	X	X	X						X	X	X	X	X			
9	X	X	X	X							X						X											
10	X	X	X	X		X				X	X				X				X									
12		X	X		X																							
13	X	X	X		X	X	X	X	**X**		X	X	X	X				X			X		**X**	**X**	**X**	**X**		
14	X	X		X	X	**X**	X	X											X									
15		X	X											X						X								
16	X																											
17		X					X		X			X				X												
18	X	X	X			X														X								
19	X	X	X	**X**	X	X	X	X		X														X				
20	X	X	X	X		X	X			X																		
21	X		X		X																							
23	X				X				X																			
24	X	X		X						X		X		X			X		X	X								
25		X						X			X																	
26			X																									
27	X	X	X	**X**	X	X		X	X	**X**	X	X	X	X	X		X	X			X	X						
28	X																											

Conjunctivitis, Catarrhal- See Catarrh, Eye
Conjunctivitis, Purulent- See Catarrh, Eyes

Constipation- See also Bowel, Atony; Weakness, Intestines

	NUX V	OP	BRY	PLUM	ALUM	LYC	NAT M	SULPH	HYDRAST	SEP	GRAPH	COLLIN	SIL	PLAT	MAG M	VER A	CALC	POD	ANAC	AESC	CAUST	LACH	NIT AC	PHOS	ANT C	PULS	KALI CAR	
1	X	X	X	**X**	X	X	X	X	X	X	X	X	X	X	X	X		X	X		X	X				X		
2	**X**	**X**	**X**	**X**	**X**	**X**	**X**	**X**	**X**		**X**	X	X	X	X	**X**			X	**X**	**X**		**X**	X	X			
3	X	X	X	X	X	X	X	X	X	X			X	X			X	X	X			X		X	X			
4	**X**	**X**	**X**	**X**	**X**	**X**	**X**	**X**	**X**		**X**	X	**X**	**X**	X	**X**		X	X					X				
5	X	X	X	X	X	X	X		X	X	X	X	X	X	X	X	X	X	X	X	X	X	X			X	X	
6	X	X	X	X	X	X	X	X	X	X	X	X	X	X	X	X	X	X	X	X	X	X	X	X	X	X	X	
7	**X**	**X**	**X**	**X**	X	**X**	**X**	X	X	**X**	**X**	**X**	**X**	**X**	**X**	X	X	X	**X**	**X**	**X**	**X**	X	**X**	X	X	X	
8	X	X	X	X	X	X	X	X	X	X	X	X	X	X	X	X	X	X	X	X	X	X	X	X	X	X	X	
9	X	X	X	X	X	X	X	X	X	X		X	X	X	X	X	X		X						X			
10	**X**	**X**	**X**	**X**	**X**	**X**	**X**	**X**	X	X	**X**			**X**	X	X	X				X	X		X	X	X		
11	X	X	X	X	**X**	X	X	X	X	X		X	X	X	**X**	X	X		X	X						X		
12	X	X	X	X	X	X	X	X	X	X		X				X		X		X			X					
13	**X**	**X**	**X**	**X**	X	**X**	**X**	**X**		X	**X**		**X**	**X**	X	**X**	**X**	X	X		X	**X**	X	X	X	X	**X**	
14	X	X	X	X	X	X	X	**X**		X	X	X	X		X						X		X			X		
15	X	X	X	X		X	X	X	X	X			X	X			X	X					X			X		
16	X		X			X			X																			
17	X	X	X	X	X		X		X	X							X	X									X	
18		X	X	X	X	X	X		X	X	X	X	X		X		X				X						X	
19	X	X		X	X	X		X		X	X									X							X	
20	X	X	X																									
21	X	X	X	X	X	X	X	X		X	X	X	X				X			X			X					
22	X		X		X		X	X			X	X	X															
23	X	X	X		X		X	X	X	X	X	X	X	X	X					X		X			X			
24	X	X	X	X		X		X	X	X	X	X						X						X				
25	X	X	X	X	X		X	X		X		X		X		X												
26	**X**	X	**X**	X	X	X	X	X		X	X			X	X	X	X					X		X	X		X	
27		X		X								X																
28		X			X				X																			

Constipation, Diarrhoea, Alternating

	ANT C	NUX V	POD	SULPH	BRY	CARD M	COLLIN	LACH	CHEL	NIT AC	ARG N	CON	PULS	IOD	ABROT	ANT T	CALC	HYDRAST	LYC	NAT M	NAT SUL	PHOS	RHUS T	OP				
1			X			X	X	X	X						X								X					
3	X	**X**	X																									
4				X																								
5	X						X			X							X				X							
6			X			X				X		X										X						
7	X	X		X	X	X		X	**X**	**X**	X	X	X					X		X	X			**X**				
8	X	X		X	X			X						X		X			X			X						
9															X													
10		X		X																								
11	X	X	X	X		X	X		X									X										
12	X																											
13	X	X			X			X			X			**X**		X				X			X					
14						X							X															
15	X	X	X		X								X															
19	X	X																	X									
21	X			X							X																	
22				X																								
24	X		X									X																
26																	X											
28			X																									

Constipation, Senile

	ALUM	ALOE	ASAF	CALC PH	CAUST	COLLIN	GRAPH	HYDRAST	MEZ	NAT M	OP	PHYTO	PLAT	PLUM	POD	SEP												
8		X										X																
9											X																	
10				X																								
11	X		X			X	X	X	X	X			X	X	X	X												
18	X				X																							

Contracture, Fingers- See also Dupuytren's Contracture

	CAUST	LYC	CALC	COCCUL	MERC	NAT CAR	SEC	GRAPH																				
7	X		X	X	X	X	X																					
13	X	**X**	X	X	X	X	X	**X**																				
14		X																										
17	X																											
28	X																											

Contracture, Muscles (Includes Contracture, Limbs)

	CAUST	GUAIAC	NAT M	LACH	AMM M	BAR C	COLOC	GRAPH	LYC	NUX V	PLUM	RHUS T	SEP	SULPH
1	X													
3	X													
6	X	X	X	X										
7	X	X	X	X										
8	X		X	X	X	X	X	X	X	X	X	X	X	X
11	X	X												
13	X	X	X	X	X	X	X	X	X	X	X	X	X	X
17	X													
19		X	X											
27	X													
28	X													

Contracture, Tendon, Achilles

	CALC	CANN S	CARB A	EUPHR	GRAPH	KALI C
7	X	X	X			X
13				X	X	

Contracture, Tendons (Includes Tendons Shortening of)

	CAUST	GUAIAC	MEZ	CIMEX	KALI IOD	LACH	NAT M	SIL	TELL	AETHUSA	AMM M	LYC	NAT C	NAT PH	PHOS	PULS	SEP	ZINC
1	X			X		X												
2	X		X															
3	X																	
4	X	X																
5		X																
7	**X**		X	X	X													
8	X	X			X													
10	X							X										
12	X																	
13	X		X			X	X	X		X	X		X		X	X	X	X
14									X			X						
17	X								X									
19		X					X							X				
28	X																	

Convalescence– See Recuperation, Failure of

Convulsions

	BELL	CUPR	CIC	HYOSC	OP	NUX V	CHAM	CINA	IGN	STRAM	VER V	ACON	HYDR AC	AETHUSA	CALC	GELS	IPEC	ZINC	CAMPH	CAUST	OENANTH	AGAR M	COCCUL	COFF	GLON	SULPH	APIS	BUFO
1	**X**	X	X	X	X	X	X	X		X	X			X	X	X			X				X		X			
2	**X**	X	X	X		**X**	X	X	X		X	X	X	**X**		X	X		X	X	X		X	X	X			
3	X	X	X	X	X	X	X	X	X	X	X	X		X								X		X				
4		X	X					X		X	X	X			X						X							
5	X																											
6	X	X	X	X	X	X		X	X	X	X				X	X	X	X					X		X		X	
7	**X**	**X**	**X**	**X**	**X**	**X**	X	X	X	**X**	X	X	X	X	**X**		X	X	X	**X**	X	X	X	X	X		**X**	X
8	X	X	**X**	X	X	X	X	X	**X**	X	X		X	X	X	X	X	X	X	X		X	X	X			X	
9	X	X	X	X		X	X			X				X		X		X							X			
10	X	X	X	X	X	X	X	X	X	X	X	X		X			X	X	X					X				
11	**X**	**X**	**X**	X	X		**X**	**X**	X	X			X	X		X		X	X		**X**						X	
12	X	X	X	X	X		X	X	X		X	X	X			X												
13		X		X	X	X			X								X											
14	X	X	X	X	X	X	X	X	X		X	X	X				X		X			X						X
15	X	X	X	X	X	X	X			X	X	X				X												
16	X	X	X	X	X		X	X	X	X		X					X			X				X				X
17	X	X	**X**	X	X	X	X	X	X	X	X		X		X				X	X	X	X	X				X	X
18	X	X																										
19	X		X	X	X	X		X		X					**X**			X		X	X	X						X
20		X																										
21	X				X		X		X			X													X		X	
23	X		X	X				X			X			X							X				X			
24					X	X				X			X									X						
25	X															X												
26	X	X	X	X		X	X		X			X			X		X			X			X	X				
27	X		X										X					X										
28																												X

Convulsions, Arm

	BELL	CHAM	COCCUL	OP	STRAM	IOD	BRY	CAMPH	CAUST	IGN	IPEC	PLUM	SABAD	SQUILLA														
6	X																											
7	X		X		X						X																	
9					X																							
10	X	X	X																									
13	**X**	**X**	X	**X**		**X**	X	X	X	X		X	X	X														
15	X			X																								
16		X																										

Convulsions, Extremities

	CUPR	IGN	OP	KALI BR
6		X	X	X
10	X	X		
15			X	
26	X			

Convulsions, Eyes, Muscles Of

	BELL	IGN	CUPR	CANTH	COCCUL	HYOSC	SPIG
13	**X**	**X**	**X**	X	X	X	X
15	X	X					

Convulsions, Face

	BELL	CHAM	DIG	IGN	LAURO	OP	STRAM	IPEC	AGAR M	BROM	CALC	CANTH	CIC	CUPR	GLON	HYDR AC	HYOSC	LACH	LYC	MEPH	NAT CAR	OENANTH	PHOS	RAN B	SULPH	ZINC
1					X																					
6	X																									
7	X	X		X	X	X	X						X	X	X		X									X
8			X						X	X						X		X		X		X		X		
12	X																									
13	X	**X**	X			X	X	**X**			X	X							X		X		X		X	
15	X			X																						

Convulsions, Febrile

	BELL	ACON	AETHUSA	HYOSC	OP	STRAM	ZINC SUL
8				X			
19	X				X	X	
21	X	X	X				X

Convulsions, Feet

	CUPR	NUX V
7	X	X
8	X	

Convulsions, Legs

	CHAM	BELL	COCCUL
10	X		X
12		X	
16	X		

Convulsions, Limbs

	BELL	CHAM	CIC	CINA	HYOSC	IGN
10		X	X		X	
12	X					
15	X	X				X
16				X		
24	X					

Convulsions, Mouth

	BELL	CUPR	ART V	CANTH	HYOSC	IGN	OENANTH	OP
6	X							
7	X	X	X	X	X			
8		X					X	X
15	X					X		

Convulsions, Puerperal

	BELL	HYOSC	COFF	GELS	HYDR AC	IGN	CIC	KALI BR	ACON	AMYL N	ANT C	ARG N	CANTH	COCCUL	CUPR	GLON	HELL	KALI CAR	LACH	MERC C	NUX M	OENANTH	OP	PHOS	PLAT	STRAM	VER A	VER V
7	**X**	**X**	X	X	X	X	**X**	**X**			X	X	X	X	X	X	X	X	X	X	X	X	X	X	X	X	X	X
8			X						X																			
9										X																		
17	X	X		X	X	X																						

Convulsions, Right Side

	ART V	BELL	CAUST	NUX V
6	X			
17			X	X
19	X	X		

Convulsions, Tongue

	LYC	CHAM	ARG N	COCCUL	CON	HYOSC	RUTA
7	X		X	X	X		
10						X	
13	**X**	**X**					X

Convulsions, Uraemic

	CUPR AR	CUPR	HYDR AC	MOSCH	JAB	KALI BR	LONICER	OENANTH	PLUM	TEREB	VER V
2			X								
7	X	X	X	X		X			X	X	
8		X	X					X			
14	X										
17				X							
23	X	X			X		X				
24											X

Copper Poisoning (Includes Colic, Copper, From)

	BELL	HEP	ARS	CUPR	NUX V	VER A
6	X	X			X	
24	X					
26		X	X			X
28				X		

Cor Pulmonale

	ANT T	ARS	ANT ARS	APIS	ASPIDO	CASSIA S	LACH	LOB I	NAT ARS	NAT SUL	SPONG
11	X	X	X	X		X				X	
17	X	X			X		X	X	X		X

Cornea, Diseases Of

	ARS	CALC	EUPHR	SIL
8	X	X	X	X
19				X
24	X			
26		X	X	

Cornea, Inflammation- See Keratitis, Cornea

Cornea, Opacity Of (Includes Obscuration)

	CALC	CANN S	NIT AC	CALC FL	ARG N	MAG CAR	CHEL	CROT T	SULPH	ZINC SUL	APIS	EUPHR	PULS	SACCH	ZINC	PHOS	SENEG	CAD S	CALC SUL	CAUST	CHINA	HEP	KALI BIC	NAPHTH	SIL			
1				**X**	X	X											X		X					X	X			
2		X		X		X		X		X				X				X				X	X					
4	**X**	X	**X**	X											X													
6	**X**	X	X		X		X	X	X		X	X	X			X						X	X		X			
7	**X**			X	**X**	X	X	X	X		X									X								
8	**X**	**X**	X				X		X	**X**		X	X		X	**X**				X	X							
13	X	**X**	X		X	**X**	X	X	X		X	X	X	X	X		**X**	X			X							
14																			X					X				
23		X	X							X				X														

Cornea, Specks On

	EUPHR	CALC	HEP	NIT AC	SIL	SULPH	CANN S	ARS	AUR	BELL	APIS	CADM	CAUST	CHEL	CON	HYDRAST	KALI BIC	LYC	NUX V	RUTA	SENEGA	SEP	SPIG					
8	X	**X**	X	X	**X**	**X**	X	X					X			X	X				X		X					
13	**X**	X	**X**	**X**	X	X	X	X	**X**	**X**	X	X		X	X			X	X	X		X						

Cornea, Spots (Includes Cornea, Maculae)

	AUR	CALC	CON	EUPHR	NIT AC	APIS	ARS	CAD	CANN S	SIL	SULPH	BELL	HEP															
6						X																						
7	X	**X**	**X**	X	X		X		X	X	X																	
8								X																				
13	**X**	X	X	**X**	**X**	X	X	X	X	X	X	**X**	**X**															

Cornea, Ulceration Of- See Ulceration, Cornea

Corneitis- See Inflammation, Cornea

Corns (AKA Clavus)

	ANT C	SULPH	LYC	NIT AC	PH AC	THUJA	CALC	NAT M	ARN	FERR PIC	IGN	NAT C	RAN S	RHUS T	SEP	SIL	BRY	RAN B	PETR	PHOS								
1	X	X				**E**		X		**X**	X							X										
2	X	X	X	**X**	X			X	X	X	X	X	X					X										
3	X			X	X	X																						
7	X	X	X	X	X		X	X	X			X	X	X	X			X										
8	X	X	X	X	X	X	X	X		X	X	X	X		X	X			X									
9				X		X										X												
10	X	X	X		X				B					X			X			X								
12		X					X		E																			
13	**X**	X	**X**	X	**X**		**X**	**X**			X	X	X	X	X	X	X		**X**	**X**								
14	X	X	X			X																						
15									E																			
21	X																											
26	X	X	X	X			X							X	X	X	X											

B- Both External and Internal E-External

Coronary Insufficiency- See also Arteriosclerosis

	CHOLEST	ACON	ARN	ARS	AUR M	CACT	DIG	KALI CAR	KALM	LACH	NAJA	OX AC	PHOS	RHUS T	SPIG	SPONG	STROPH	SULPH										
3	X																											
16	X																											
17		X																										
18					X																							
19			X	X		X	X	X	X	X	X	X	X	X	X	X	X	X										

Coronary Thrombosis

	BOTHR	ARN	CACT	LACH	LIL T	MERC	SEC	SPIG	ASPIDO	DIG	KALI C	KALM	LYC	MEDO	NAJA	OX AC	PHUS	RHUS T	SPONG	STROPH	SULPH	SUMBUL						
1		X			X	X	X		X				X	X														
3	X			X		X	X	X														X						
14	**X**	X	X	X	X																							
19		X	X					X		X	X	X			X	X	X	X	X	X	X							
28	X																											

Coryza (AKA Rhinorrhoea)

	ALL C	ARS	EUPHR	PULS	ACON	NAT M	NUX V	GELS	KALI BIC	KALI IOD	SABAD	ARS IOD	DULC	HEP	MERC	ARUM T	BRY	SIL	AMM C	CAMPH	LACH	CALC	IPEC	KALI CAR	SANG	BROM	SULPH	
1	X	X	X	X	X	X		X		X	X	X	X	X		X	X		X				X	X		X		
2	X								X		X						X	X				X						
3	X	**X**	X		X										X	X	X											
4	X	**X**	X	X	X	X	X	X	X	**X**	X	X	X		**X**					X	X				X			
5	X	X	X	X	X		X		X	X	X	X	X	X		X		X	X	X			X					
6	X	X	X		X		X		X	X				X		X		X	X	X	X	X						
7	X	X	X	X	X	X	**X**	X	X	X	X	X	X	X	X	X	X	X		X	X	X	X	X	X	X	X	
8	X	X	X	X	X	X	X	X	X	X	X	X	**X**	X	**X**	X	X	X	X	X	X	X		X	X	X	X	
9	X	X	X	X	X	X	X	X			X					X	X						X					
10	X	X		X	X	X		X							X												X	
11	**X**	**X**	X			**X**	X	X	X	X	**X**	X		**X**		X			**X**	X		X	X	X		**X**		
12	X	X	X	X	X		X	X					X		X		X						X		X			
13	X	**X**	X	**X**	X	X	X	X	X	X	X		X	X	**X**		X	**X**	**X**		**X**	X	X	X	X	X	**X**	
14	X	X	X	X		X		X	X	X		X				X	X		X									
15		X	X	X				X	X						X			X				X					X	
16			X	X					X		X	X																
17	X	X	X	X		X	X			X	X	X	X	X		X	X	X	X	X	X	X	X	X	X	X		
18	X	X	X	X	X	X	X		X	X	X	X	X	X							X				X		X	
19	**X**	**X**	X	X		X	X			X	X	X				X	X		X						X	X	X	
20	X	X	X	X	X	X	X	X						X														
21	X			X			X						X					X										
22	X	X	X	X	X	X		X	X				X	X	X													
23	X				X					X		X	X							X	X				X	X		
24	X	X	X	X	X	X		X	X			X				X		X		X	X	X		X			X	
25	X	X	X				X								X									X				
26		X	X	X										X	X		X						X					
27																								X				
28	X																											

Coryza, Dry

	AMM C	NAT M	NUX V	PHOS	PSOR	SAMB C	SULPH	BRY	CARB A	KALI CAR	LYC	ACON	CAUST	CHINA	NIT AC	SIL	SPONG	STANN	STICTA	AMM M	CALC	CAPS	GRAPH	IPEC	PLAT	SULPH AC	THUJA	
2						X																						
7		X	X	X		X	X		X	X		X	X	X	X	X	X		X									
8	X	X	X	X	X	X	X	X	X	X	X	X	X		X	X	X	X		X	X	X	X	X	X	X	X	
13	**X**	**X**	**X**	**X**	X	X	X	**X**	**X**	**X**	**X**	X	X	X	X	X	X	X		**X**	**X**	**X**	**X**	**X**	**X**	**X**	**X**	
14	X						X				X								X									
17	X	X	X		X			X						X				X										
18																			X									
19					X																							
24				X																								

Cough (Note here that only the main remedies are used from 2)

	DROS	HEP	PHOS	BRY	PULS	SULPH	AMBRA	BELL	CAUST	ACON	RUMEX	SPONG	ARS	NUX V	CARB V	CHAM	IPEC	ALL C	ANT T	RHUS T	SIL	CALC	EUPHR	HYOSC	IGN	KALI CAR	NAT M	NIT AC
1	X	X	X				X				X							X	X				X			X	X	
2	**X**	**X**	**X**	**X**	**X**	**X**	**X**	**X**	**X**	**X**	**X**	**X**		**X**	**X**		**X**		**X**		**X**	**X**		**X**		**X**	**X**	**X**
3		X		X			X	X	X	X	X		X	X	X	X		X		X		X	X					
4	X				X		X											X			X				X		X	X
5					X		X		X	X									X									
6	X	X	X	X	X	X	X	X	X		X	X	X	X	X	X	X	X		X	X		X		X	X		X
7	**X**	**X**	**X**	**X**	X	**X**	X	X	**X**	X	**X**	**X**	**X**	X	X	X	X	X	**X**	X	X		X	**X**	X	X	**X**	**X**
8	X	X	X	X	X	X	X	X	X	X	X	X	X	X	X	X	X	X	X	X	X	X	X	X	X	X	X	X
9	X	X		X			X				X						X	X	X	X			X	X	X			X
10	X		X	X		X			X							X				X		X						
11																		X										
12		X	X	X	X	X		X	X			X	X		X	X	X		X			X						X
13	X	X	**X**			**X**		X		X			X	**X**	X	**X**				X	**X**					X	X	
14	X	X		X				X															X					
15	X	X	X	X	X			X		X		X	X	X	X	X	X					X		X	X			
17	X	X	X		X	X	X	X	X	X	X	X	X	X	X		X	X	X	X	X	X	X	X	X	X	X	X
18				X						X										X								
19	X	X	**X**	**X**	**X**	X	X	X	X	**X**	**X**	**X**	X	X		X	X	X	X	X	X	X	X	X	X	**X**	X	
20					X								X															
22			X		X							X																
23	X			X			X	X																	X			
25			X			X																						
26		X	X	X	X	X				X				X	X	X	X							X				
27	X	X				X			X		X	X	X									X						

Cough, Bloody- See Haemoptysis

Cough, Cardiac

	NAJA	HYDR AC	LAURO	LACH	SPONG	DIG	AUR M	CAPS	CARB V	FERR M	KALI CAR	OX AC
1	X	**X**			X	X	X					X
3	X	**X**	X			X		X				
6			X									
7	X			X	X					X		
8		X										
17	X		X	X	X				X		X	
19	X		X	X								

Cough, Dry (Includes Cough, Hacking)

	BRY	ACON	BELL	PHOS	SPONG	NUX V	SULPH	RHUS T	ARS	HYOSC	CHAM	KALI CAR	RUMEX	CAUST	CON	SANG	PULS	CALC	DROS	HEP	IOD	BROM	EUPHR	STICTA	IPEC	MANG	LYC	OP
1	X	X	X		X		X	X		X			X	X		X			X		X					X		
3	X		X																									
4	X		X	X	X	X	X	X		X		X	X	X	X	**X**		X			X		X	X				X
5	X	X		X	X					X		X	X	X		X						X		X				
6		X	X	X	X	X	X	X	X	X	X	X	X			X	X	X		X	X		X	X	X	X	X	X
7	**X**	**X**	X	**X**	**X**	X	**X**	X	**X**	**X**	X	X	**X**	X	X	X		X			X	X		X		X		X
8	X	X	X	X	X	**X**	X	X	X	X	X			X	X	X	X	X	X	X	X	X				X	X	X
9	X	X	X																									
10	X	X	X	X		X	X				X						X		X	X			X		X		X	
11						X									X													
12	X	X	X	X	X		X			X					X							X						
13	**X**	**X**	**X**	**X**	X	X	X	X	X	**X**	**X**	**X**		X	**X**		X	**X**	**X**	**X**	**X**	X	X		**X**	**X**	X	X
14	X	X	X	X	X	X		X	X		X			X	X		X											
15	X		X	X	X	X	X		X	X	X				X			X		X			X		X			
16								X				X																
17	X	X	X	X	X	X	X	X	X	X	X	X	X	X			X	X	X	X	X	X		X		X	X	X
18	X	X	X	X	X				X			X	X				X		X					X				
19	X	X	X	X	X	X	X	X					X			X						X			X		X	
20	X	X		X		X		X					X						X				X					
21	X	X	X	X	X	X			X		X	X	X	X										X				
22	X	X	X	X	X	X			X				X							X			X					
24	X	X		X	X	X	X		X			X				X	X											
25	X	X	X	X	X						X																	
26	X	X	X	X		X	X	X	X	X	X	X		X	X										X			
27	X	X	X		X	X	X	X																				
28	X																											

Cough, Loose- See also Bronchorrhoea (Includes Cough, Catarrhal)

	ANT T	IPEC	HEP	PULS	KALI BIC	DULC	PHOS	STANN	LYC	SENEG	ARS	CAUST	CALC	SIL	SULPH	CARB V	COCCUS	MERC	SEP	AMM C	CHAM	KALI SUL	NAT S	EUPHR	SQUILLA	HYDRAST	BRY
1	X	X	X	X	X		X					X					X		X	X			X				
3									**X**		X		X			X				X						X	
4	X	X	X		X	X		X	**X**	X	X																
5	X	X	X	X	X	X	X	X		X	X	X					X							X		X	
6	X			X	X	X	X			X			X								X				X		
7	**X**	X	**X**	**X**		X			X			X	X	X					X		X				**X**	X	
8	**X**		X	**X**		X	X	X	X	X	X	X	X	X	X	X	X	**X**	X		X			X			**X**
9	X	X																				X					
10	X	X	X	X	X	X	X	X						X	X						X		X				
11	X	X	X		X			X						X	X			X		X		X	X				
12	X	X	X	X	X		X	X			X				X	X		X									X
13	X			**X**			**X**	**X**	X	**X**	X	X	**X**	**X**	**X**	X	X	X	**X**	X			X	**X**			X
14	X	X	X	X	X	X								X			X					X	X				
15	X	X		X	X	X	X						X			X		X			X				X	X	
16	X																										
17	X	X		X		X	X			X	X	X					X		X	X		X	X	X	X		
18	X	X	X	X	X			X		X		X					X					X				X	
19	X		X	X	X	X		X								X						X					
20	X	X	X																					X			
21	X	X	X		X																						
22		X	X		X																						
24	X					X			X		X									X					X		
25	X	X			X										X												
26	X	X	X	X		X	X	X	X			X	X	X	X	X		X	X		X						X
27									X	X																	
28	X																										

Cough, Senile

	ALUMEN	AMM C	ANT T	CON	HYDRAST	HYOSC	KREO	NAPHTHA	NUX V	SENEG
8	X	X	X	X	X		X	X	X	X
12						X				

Cough, Spasmodic

	DROS	IPEC	BELL	CUPR	COR R	HYOSC	CARB V	AMBRA	BRY	NUX V	CINA	BAD	KALI CAR	CON	ALL C	IGN	PULS	RUMEX	BROM	MOSCH	NAT M							
1				X																								
4						X																						
5	X	X		X	X						X				X													
6		X	X	X	X	X				X		X	X					X										
7	X	**X**	**X**	**X**	X	**X**	X	X	**X**	**X**	X	X	X	X	X	X		X	**X**	**X**	**X**							
8	X	X	**X**	X	X	X	**X**	X	**X**	X	X	X	X	X		X	X	X	X	X	X							
9					X			X																				
10	X				X																							
11					X																							
12	X	X	X			X									X													
13	**X**	**X**	**X**	X	X	**X**	**X**	**X**	**X**	X	**X**	X	X	**X**	X	X	X		X	X	X							
14		X					X																					
15	X	X	X			X	X		X	X				X		X	X											
17	X	X	X	X	X	X	X	X	X	X	X	X					X	X	X		X							
18	X	X	X	X	X							X	X		X													
19								X																				
20	X	X							X				X															
22			X				X											X										
23	X			X																								
25	X																											
26	X	X	X	X		X	X	X		X	X			X		X	X			X								

Coxalgia

	RHUS T	CALC	BRY	BELL	CAUST	COLOC	MERC	PULS	PHOS	STRAM	SULPH	ARS	FERR	KALI CAR	SIL	CHAM	HEP	LED	LYC	SEP	AUR	NUX V						
3			X							X				X		X												
4					X																							
5	X												X															
6	X	X		X		X	X		X	X	X	X		X	X		X	X	X									
7	X	X			X	X	X	X	X	X		X		X	X			X	X	X	X							
8	**X**	**X**	X	**X**	X	**X**	X	X	X	X	X	X	X		X		X	X	X	X	**X**	X						
13	**X**	**X**	X	**X**	X	**X**	**X**	**X**	X		X	**X**	X			**X**	**X**			X		**X**						
14		X	X					X		X	X		X		X													
15			X	X												X												
19					X																							
24	X			X										X														
25	**X**		X																									
26	X	X			X	X	X	X	X		X																	

Coxalgia, Left Side

	CAUST	BELL	CHAM	KALI BIC	NAT SUL	STRAM	SULPH
5	X				X	X	
7			X	X			
8							X
9		X					
19	X						

Coxalgia, Right Side

	HELON	HYDRAST	KALI BIC	KALI CAR	LIMUL	LED	MUREX
5				X	X	X	X
7	X	X	X				

Crack, Anus- See also Rhagades

	NIT AC	GRAPH	AGNUS	ALL C	ALUM	PAEONIA	RAT	SARS
5	X				X	X	X	X
8	X							
13		X	X	X				
14	X	X						
19	X							

Crack, Mouth, Corners Of- See Also Angular Stomatitis

	ARUM T	ANT C	GRAPH	NIT AC	AMM C	CINNAB	CONDUR	MERC	MEZ	ZINC
3	X		X	X						
6	X									
8		X					X			X
13	X	X			X	X		X	X	
14			X							
19				X						

Cracking, Lips- See also Rhagades

	NAT M	BRY	ARUM T	GRAPH	ARS	IGN	CARB V	NIT AC	PULS	SULPH	CROC	MERC	VER A	BELL	BOV	CALC	CAPS	CARB A	CHAM	COLCH	LACH	MUR AC	PH AC	SEP	AMM CAR	AMM M	ARN
1	X	X	X																					X			
2				X									X														
3	X		X																								
6		X			X		X		X	X				X						X	X						
7	X	X	X	X	X	X	X			X	X	X				X		X	X								
8		X				X			X						X												
9	X			X																							
10	X																										
11																							X				
13	**X**	**X**	X	X	**X**	**X**	X	X	X	X	**X**	**X**	**X**	X	X	X	X	X	X	X	X		X		**X**	**X**	**X**
14		X						X																			
15																						X					
17	X	X																				X		X			
18	X																										
19			X	X				X																			
20	X																										
21	X																X										
26		X			X	X	X																				

Cracking, Skin (Includes Heels, Cracked)

	PETR	GRAPH	SULPH	NIT AC	SIL	CALC	CALC FL	HEP	LACH	SEP	NAT M	CONDUR	ALUM	ARS	CIST	FL AC	NAT CAR	PULS	SARS
1	X								X						X				
2	X										**X**	**X**							
3	X																		
5	X	X					X			X			X	X		X	X		
6		X																	
7		X																	
8	X	**X**	X	X	X	X		X	X	X			X				X	X	
9	X	X																	
10		X																	
14	X	X	X	X	X		X	X							X				X
18	X																		
19	**X**	**X**	X	X	X	X	X	X		X		X				X		X	X
20		X												X					
21	X	X	X			X													
24	X								X										
25	X		X		X						X								
27	X			X															
28		X																	

Cracking, Sound/Sensation Of, Hip

	CAMPH	COCCUL	CROC
7	X		X
19		X	

Cracking, Sound/Sensation Of, Jaw

	RHUS T	AMM C	MENY	ARUM T	CALC	CARB A	GRANAT	NIT AC	THUJA
1	X			X			X	X	
5			X						
8		X				X			
13	X	X	X						X
14	X								
21	X								
24					X				

Cracking, Sound/Sensation Of, Joints

	BENZ AC	LED	CAPS	ANGUST	COCCUL	NIT AC	CALC FL	ACON	CAUST	FERR	KALI BIC	NAT M	THUJA	ZINC	CALC	CAMPH	NAT SUL	RHUS T
1	X			X			X											X
2		X					X						X	**X**				
3								X										X
4	X																	
5	X	X							X									
7			X		X	X				X						X	X	
8	X		X	X	X	X		X		X	X	X	X	X	X		X	
9									X									
11		X																
13	X	**X**	**X**	X	X	**X**		X		X	X	X	X		X	X		
14					X						X							
19			X	X					X			X						
24							X											
27	X																	

Cracking, Sound/Sensation Of, Knee

	COCCUL	BENZ AC	CAUST	PULS	LED	WILDBAD	ANGUST	CALC	CAMPH	CHAM	CON	IGN	NAT SUL	SEP	SULPH
1	X														
2	**X**					X									
3						X									
5		X													
6													X		
7	X			X	X			X	X		X			X	X
8		X													
9				X											
11					X										
13	X									X		X			
14	X		X				X								
19			X												
21		X	X												
25				X											

Cracking, Sound/Sensation Of, Neck

	CHAM	BRY	NAT CAR	SULPH
8	**X**		X	X
27		X		

Cracks, Fingertips

	PETR	SIL	GRAPH	NAT M	ARS	RHUS T
1	X	X		X	X	X
5	X					
9			X	X		
10	X					
14	X	X	X			
19	**X**		X			
21		X				
25		X				
28	X					

Cracks, Nipples- See also Fissures, Nipples

	SULPH	GRAPH	PHYTO	CAST EQ	CAUST	RAT	SEP	SIL	ARN	CALC	CHAM	LYC	AGAR M	AUR S	CALEND	COLCH	FL AC	IGN	MERC C									
1		X	X	X		X																						
5			X	E		X	X	X					X															
6	X	X																										
7	X	**X**	**X**	X	**X**	X		X				X			X		X		X									
8				X	X		X																					
9	X		X																									
13	**X**	X		X	X		X		X																			
14	X	X	X											X														
15	X	X							E		X																	
21	X	X						X		X																		
24	X	X																										
25			X																									
26	X									X	X	X				X		X										

E- External

Cradle Cap- See also Crusta Lactea (Includes Milk Crust)

	CALC	HEP	LYC	SEP	ARS	CALC PH	CARB V	CIC	DULC	GRAPH	HYDRAST	MEZ	NAT M	OLEAND	PETR	PSOR	SIL	STAPHYS	STILLING	VINCA	VIOL T							
8	X	X	X	X	X	X	X			X	X		X		X	X	X	X	X									
11	X	X	X	X					X			X								X	X							
19								X						X														

Cramps

	CUPR	NUX V	VER A	CAMPH	MAG PH	CALC	CHAM	COLOC	GELS	SEC	BELL	CUPR AR	HYOSC	ARN	ARS	CUPR AC	GRAPH	MENYANT	PLUM	RHUS T	SULPH	VIB OP	AGAR M	COLCH				
1	X			X	X	X			**X**	X		X								**X**								
2	**X**	**X**	X		X		X			X				**X**				X				X	**X**	**X**				
3			X					X													X							
4	**X**											X				X												
5	**X**									X																		
6		X		X														X										
7	**X**	X	**X**	**X**				X	X				X			X	X		X									
8	X	X	X	X	X	X	X	X	X	X	X		X	X	X	X	X	X	X	X	X	X	X	X				
9	X	X	X		X	X	X	X	X			X									X							
10	X																											
11					X																							
12	X		X												X													
13						**X**				X	X		X		X		X		X									
14	X										X		X															
15		X	X																									
17	X	X	X	X																								
19		X																										
20	X																											
21		X	X	X		X	X							X														
22	X	X																										
23					X		X	X				X										X						
24											X																	
27	X																											
28	X																											
29*	X																											

29* Hariveau E, et al. A study of the effectiveness of ultra low doses of copper in the treatment of hemodialysis related muscle cramps. Ultra Low Doses, Ed- C Doutremepuich, Taylor & Francis, London, 1991.

Cramp, Abdomen- See also Colic, Abdomen

	CUPR	NUX V	CUPR AR	MAG PH	CHAM	PULS	VER A	ARS	COLOC	LACH	COCCUL	IGN	KALI CAR	CHINA	DIOSC	GRAPH	MAG M	VIB OP	CALC	HYOSC	SEP	SPONG	STANN
1		X	X		X						X	X	X										
3																		X					
5	X			X			X																
6	X						X	X	X	X					X	X		X					
7	X	X		X				X	X	X					X		X	X				**X**	
8						X				X				X			X						
9			**X**																				
10		X		X	X	X			X							X				X			
11	X																						
13	**X**	**X**			**X**	**X**	**X**	X		X	**X**	**X**	**X**	X		X	X		**X**	**X**	**X**	X	**X**
14	X			X									X										
15	X						X																
18	X																						
19															X								X
21						X			X					X					X				
22			X		X			X															
24	X			X																			
25		X	X																				
26											X	X									X		

Cramp, Achilles Tendon

	CAUST
6	X
7	X

Cramp, Arms

	BELL	GELS	PH AC
4	X	X	
10			X

Cramp, Back

	BELL	EUPHR	ANAC	BRY	CHINA	CON	EUPHORB	IGN	OP	PHYSO	RHUS T	SEP	STRYCHN	VIOL T
1										X				
4	X													
8			X											
10								X	X		X			
13	X	**X**		X	X	X	X					X		X
19													X	

Cramp, Bladder

	CARB V	NUX V	PARIERA
7	X	X	
19			X

Cramp, Buttocks (Includes Cramp, Gluteals)

	BELL	CUPR	GRAPH
6	X		
13			X
19		X	
24	X		

Cramp, Calves- See also Pregnancy, Cramp, Calves, From

	CUPR	VER A	CALC	NUX V	CHAM	ANAC	ARS	CAMPH	SEC	COLOC	FERR	SULPH	FERR M	GRAPH	CON	CUPR AR	SIL	CUPR AC	NIT AC	SEP
1	X			X														X		
3	X										X									
4	X																			
6							X	X	X											
7	**X**	X	X	X	**X**				X		X	X	X	X	X		X	**X**		
8	X			X	X	X	X		X		X	X	X	X	X		X		X	X
9	X	X	X																	
10	X	X																		
11	X							X								X				
13	X	X	**X**	**X**	**X**	**X**	**X**	**X**	**X**	X	X	X	X	**X**	X		X		**X**	**X**
14	X	X	X			X				X						X				
17				X			X									X				
18	X																			
19	X		**X**			X														
21		X						X												
24										X										
25		X																		
26	X	X			X					X		X								
28	X																			

Cramp, Calves, Pregnancy From– See Pregnancy, Cramp, Calves, From

Cramp, Chest

	CUPR	COCCUL	CUPR AC	VER A
1		X	X	
6				X
10	X			
17	X			

Cramp, Extremities

	VER A	CUPR	CIC	STANN	THYROID
1	X				
9		X		X	
10	X	X			
14	X				X
17			X		
22	X				

Cramp, Face

	COCCUL	MAG PH	NIT AC	OL AN	RHUS T	STRYCHN
7		X				
13			X	X	X	
19	X					X

Cramp, Feet

	CUPR	SEC	CALC	CAUST	BERB V	COLCH	FERR	LAC C	NAT CAR	POD	STRAM	VER A	BELL	SULPH
1		X												
2		**X**												
3		X			X	X	X		X					
6			X											
7	**X**		X	**X**		X	X		X			X	**X**	
8										X				
9										X				
10	X	X										X		
11	X													
13		X		X	X			X			X			**X**
14								X						
15											X			
19	X		**X**											
21	X													
25	X													
27			X											

Cramp, Fingers

	CUPR	KALI CAR	MAG PH	SEC	SIL	STANN	AMBRA	CUPR AR	DIOSC	NAT M	VER A	ZINC PH
1			X									X
6	X	X										
7	X					X		X		X	X	
10	X	X										
14	X		X	X			X		X			
19	X											
21	X											
26				X	**X**	X						

Cramp, Forearms

	GELS
1	X
14	X

Cramp, Hands

	KALI CAR	BELL	AGAR M	AMBRA	CUPR	EUPH C	GRAPH	MAG PH	NAT M	NAT PH	STRAM	VER A
1										X		
6	X					X						
7	X	**X**	X				X		X			
10	X											X
14				X				X				
15											X	
19					X							

Cramp, Hip

	COLOC	PH AC	SEP
7			X
13	**X**	X	
14	X		

Cramp, Jaw (Masseter muscle)

	COCCUL	CUPR	RHUS T	STRYCHN
9	X			
14		X		
19	X			X
21			X	

Cramp, Knee

	CALC	CANN S	CAUST	COLOC	NIT	PAEONIA	PETR	PHOS	SULPH
7	X								
13	**X**	**X**	X		X	X	X	X	X
14				X					

Cramp, Legs

	CUPR	SEC	CUPR AR	CALC	CHAM	COLOC	NUX V	VER A	SULPH	GELS	JATR	LATH	MAG PH	PLUM	VIB OP	KALI MUR
1													X	X		
3		X	X												X	
4	X															
6		X		X												
7	**X**			X	**X**	X			**X**	X	X				X	**X**
9	X		**X**													
10		X					X					X				
13	X	X				X		X			X					
14	X															
15	X			X		X	X	X	X							
17												X				
18		X											X			
19	X															
21	X				X											
24														X		
25	X		**X**		X		X	X		X						
27				X												

Cramp, Legs, Nocturnal

	CUPR AR	CHAM	NUX V
25	**X**	X	X

Cramp, Limbs

	PHYSO	VER A	HYOSC	CALC	CHAM	COCCUL	COLOC	CUPR AC	CUPR	EUP PER	IRIS V	MAG PH	NUX V	PLUM	ROBIN	SULPH	TAB	VIB OP
1	X																	
5												X						
6		X															X	
7		X	X					X	X	X					X			
8											X			X				X
10	X	X	X	X	X	X	X						X			X		
11	X																	

Cramp, Neck

	ARN	ASAR	BAR C	CIC	NIT AC	SQUILLA	STRYCHN
7			X				
8					X		
13	X	X				X	
14				X			
19							X

Cramp, Palms

	CUPR	SCROPH
1	X	
2		X
3		X
14	X	

Cramp, Sole

	CUPR	AMM C	CALC	PHOS	SULPH	ANGUST	BERB V	CALAD	CARB V	CHEL	COFF	EUGENIA	FERR	HEP	NUX V	PETR	PLUM	SEC	SEL	SIL	STAPHYS
13		**X**	**X**	**X**	**X**	X	X	X	X	X	X	X	X	X		X	X	X	X	X	X
14	X																				
17															X						
19	X																				

Cramp, Stomach- See also Colic, Abdomen

	NUX V	CARB V	CUPR	BISM	CAUST	CHAM	LYC	NAT M	ANT C	CALC	CARB A	CHINA	COCCUL	COFF T	COLOC	GRAPH	HYOSC	ARS	BELL	HELON	MAG CAR	NAT CAR	NIT AC	PHOS	PLUM	SEP	VER A
1	X	X																									
2																X											
4		X																									
5					X																						
6	X		X					X									X										
7	**X**	**X**		X	X		**X**	X	X	X				X	**X**			X	X	X		X		X		X	X
8												X															
10			X			X												X									
11				X							X																
12																									X		
13	**X**	**X**	X	**X**	**X**	**X**	X	**X**	**X**	**X**	**X**	**X**	**X**	**X**		**X**	**X**		X		X	X	X	X	X	X	X
15	X					X							X							X							
18							X																X				
19	X		X	X											X						X						
24			X																								

Cramp, Rectum

	PHOS	LYC	ARG N	CALC	CAUST	FERR	KREO	NUX V	SANIC
2									X
6	X								
7	X	X			X	X	X		
8			X						
13	X	X		X					
19								X	

Cramp, Soles

	NUX V	SULPH
10		X
21	X	

Cramp, Thighs

	HYOSC	CHAM	RHUS T	SEP	ASAR	CANN S	AGAR M	ARG M	IPEC	PETR	SULPH
6			X								
7	X			X			X	X			X
13	**X**		X	X	**X**	**X**			X	X	
21		X									
25		X									

Cramp, Toes

	CALC	CUPR	LYC	FERR	CAUST	HEP	HYOSC	NUX V	AMM C	BAR C	BAR M	CARB A	CROT H	CUPR AR	DIOSC	GELS	GAMBOG	NICCOL	OL AN	PLAT	SEC	SIL	SULPH
5								X															
6		X																					
7	X	X	X	X	X	X							X	X									
8				X																			
10		X																					
13	**X**		**X**	X	X	X	X	X	X	X	X	X				X	X	X	X	X	X	X	X
14							X								X								
17			X																				
19	**X**																						
21		X																					

Cramp, Tongue

	LYC	RUTA	BORAX	PIPER N
2	X	X		
3	X	X		X
13			X	

Cramp, Uterus

	COCCUL	MAG M	BELL	NUX V	SEP	CAUST	CON	IGN	PULS	AMBRA	AMM C	CACT	CAUL	CHAM	CIMICI	DIOSC	GELS	GRAPH	HYOSC	KALI IOD	LACH	NAT M	ONOSM	PIPER N	PLAT	STANN	VIB P	
1	X	X		X		X	X	X										X							X		X	
2													X										X	X				
6											X																	
7	X		X	X					X								X		X									
8		X							X						X					X								
9					X																							
10	X				X																							
13	X	**X**		X	X	X	**X**	**X**														X				X		
19	X		X							X		X		X														
25			X																		X							
27																X												

Cramp, Vagina

	IGN	HAM	SIL	BELL	COCCUL	KREO	MERC	NUX V	PLAT	PLUM	SEP
2	**X**	**X**	**X**							X	
7						X					X
8	X			X	X		X	X	X		

Cramp, Writers (AKA Spasmus Scriptorum)

	GELS	MAG PH	ARG	SIL	SULPH AC	BELL	CAUST	CUPR	CYCL	FERR IOD	NUX V	RUTA	SEC	STANN	STAPHYS	ZINC	ZINC PH
1	X	X			X			X		X							X
2	X	X		X					X	X							
3	X	X	X														X
6	X			X		X	X				X	X	X	X	X	X	
8	**X**			X		X	X		X		X	X	X	X	X	X	
9	X	X			X												
14		X	X														
17			X		X												
18		X															
21	X							X									
25	X																

Craving, Acids

	VER A	ARS	SEP	ANT T	ANT C	BRY	CARB V	KALI BIC	MYRICA	POD	SEC	STRAM	ALUM	CIST	HEP	KALI CAR	PHOS	PULS	ARN	CHAM	CHEL	CHINA	CON	IGN	LACH	MAG C	SULPH
1	X			X			X	X	X	X			X	X										X			
4			X						X												X						
5	X	X	X	X	X						X																
6						X			X																		
7	X	X	X		X	X	X			X	X				X	X	X	X		X			X		X		X
8	X	X		X	X			X		X	X		X	X	X	X	X		X			X				X	
9	X							X																			
10	X	X																X			X						
11									X																		
13	**X**	X	X	X	X	X	X	X		X	X		X	X	X	X	X	X	X	X		X	X	X	X	X	X
15	X	X				X																					
17				X			X																				
18			X																								
21			X																								

Craving, Alcohol- See also Alcoholism; Craving, Beer; Craving, Whisky; Craving, Wine (Includes Craving, Brandy, Spirits)

	SULPH	ARS	SEL	NUX V	PULS	STAPHYS	SULPH AC	LACH	ARN	CHINA	HEP	SEP	ASAR	CAPS	CROT H	OP	AMM C	CALC	COCA	CUPR	IOD	LYC	MOSCH	PHOS	SPIG
1	X		X	X	X		X	X				X							X		X			X	
4	X																								
6			X				X		X																
7	X	**X**	**X**	**X**		X	X	**X**			X	X	**X**	**X**	**X**	**X**					X	X		X	X
8	X	X	X	X	X	X	X	X	X	X	X	X	X	X	X	X	X	X	X	X		X			X
9				X																					
13	X	X			X	X			X								X			X					
14	X																								
15		X			X					X													**X**		
17			X																						
26	X	X				X				X	X							X							

Craving, Apples

	ALOE	ANT T	GUAIAC
8	X	X	X
13	X		
17		X	

Craving, Bacon

	CALC PH	MEZ	TUB
1	X		
8	X		
10			X
19		X	

Craving, Beer

	KALI BIC	NUX V	ACON	COCCUL	SULPH	BRY	PULS	CAUST	LACH	PETR	PH AC	STRONT	PHELL	ALOE	GRAPH	MERC	NAT C	OP	SABAD	SPIG	ZINC
1	X			X																	
5	X																				
6		X																			
7	X	**X**	**X**	X	**X**	X		X	X	X		X					X			X	X
8	X	X	X	X	X	X	X	X	X	X	X	X	X	X	X	X		X	X		X
11	X																				
13	X	X	X	**X**	X	X	**X**	X	X	X	X	X	**X**	X		X	X	X	X	X	
15		X			X		X				X				X						
18	X																				
19			X			X															

Craving, Brandy

	ARS	HEP	LACH	SULPH	CUBEB	IGN	NUX V	OP	SEL	SEP
13	X	X	X	X	X		X	X	X	X
15						X				
26	X	X	X	X						

Craving, Bread- See Craving, Farinaceous Foods

Craving, Bread and Butter

	MAG C	FERR	MERC	PULS
8	X		X	X
13	X	X		

Craving, Butter

	MERC	PULS	IGN
8		X	
10	X		
13	X		
15		X	X

Craving, Cake

	PLUM	CORNUS	CHINA	NIT AC	NUX V																							
8	X	X	X	X	X																							
13	X																											

Craving, Cheese

	IGN	ARG N	CIST	NAT M																								
1			X																									
7			X																									
8	X	X																										
11		X																										
13	X																											
15	X																											
27				X																								

Craving, Chocolate

	LYC	LYSSIN																										
9	X																											
13		X																										
25	X																											
27	X																											

Craving, Cloves

	ALUMEN	ALUM	ALUM O	CHLOR																								
7	X			X																								
8			X																									
13		X																										

Craving, Coffee

	ANGUST	CARB V	ARS	AUR	NUX M	BRY	CHAM	CHINA	CON	NUX V	SEL	ARG M	CAPS	COLCH	LACH	AGARICIN	ALUM	BOV	CALC PH	COFF	GRAN	LOB I	MEZ	MOSCH	PH AC			
1	**X**	X																										
4																X												
5				X	X																							
6	X						X								X													
7		X	X	X	X	X			X		X												X					
8	X	X	X	X	X	X		X	X	X	X	X	X	X	X				X	X	X	X		X	X			
9										X																		
10			X							X																		
11	X																											
13	X	X	X	X	X	X	X	X	X		X	X	X	X			X	X										
15							X																					
17		X																										
20								X																				
24	X																											

Craving, Cucumbers

	ANT C	VER A																										
8	X	X																										
13	X	X																										
15	X	X																										

Craving, Drink, Cold (Includes Craving, Cold Milk; Craving, Cold Water)

	PHOS	VER A	BRY	ARS	DULC	RHUS T	ACON	CHINA	MERC	CHAM	ANT T	CAUST	COCCUL	PH AC	SULPH	THUJA	ANGUST	BOV	OLEAND	SABAD								
1													X															
5	X		X			X		X		X																		
7	**X**	**X**	**X**	**X**	X	X	X	X	X		X	X		X		X												
8	X	X	X	X	X	X		X	X	X	X	X	X	X	X	X	X	X	X	X								
9	X		X																									
10	X	X		X	X																							
11	X	X																										
13	X	**X**	X	X	X	X		X	**X**	X		X	X	X	X	X	**X**	**X**	**X**	**X**								
14			X																									
15		X		X						X																		
16	X																											
17	X	X				X	X				X																	
18	X		X	X		X	X																					
19	X			X			X								X													
20	X		X				X	X																				
21	X	X			X																							
22	X	X			X				X																			
25			X																									

Craving, Drinks, Hot

	SPIG	CHEL	CASC	HEP	LYC
1	X				
10					X
13		X	X		
17	X	X			
21	X			X	

Craving, Drinks, Warm

	CHEL	LYC
5	X	
17	X	
18	X	
19	X	X

Craving, Drugs- See Drugs, Addiction to

Craving, Eggs

	CALC	OL AN	NAT PH	PULS
1	X			
4	X			
5	X		X	
7	**X**			
8	X	X		X
9	X			
10	X			
11	X			
13	X	X		
14	X			
19	X			
21	X			
24	X			
25	X			

Craving, Fish

	NIT AC	NAT M	PHOS	CYCL	NAT PH	PULS	VER A
5		X	X		X		
6	X						
7	**X**	X		X		X	X
17			X				

Craving, Food, Farinaceous

	NAT M	FERR	PULS	ARS	MERC	PLUM	SABAD	STRONT C	AMM C	AUR	CALC	CINA	COLOC	CORNUS	GRAT	IGN	MAG CAR	OL AN	STAPHYS
5	X	X			X		X												
7	X	X			X						X	X	X	X			X		
8	X	X	X	X		X		X	X						X			X	X
13	X		X	X		X	X	X		X									
15			X													X			

Craving, Food, Fatty

	NIT AC	NUX V	MEZ	SULPH	HEP	MEDO	SANIC	TUB
1	X		X					
5	X	X						X
6	X							
7	**X**	X	X		X			
8	X	X						
10				X			X	
13	X	X	X					
15	X	X						
17	X							
19			X	X		X		
21		X		X				

Craving, Food, Hot

	LYC	SABAD	CALC	CHEL
1	X			
5		X		
7	X	X		
17	X			X
21			X	

Craving, Food, Seasoned- See Craving, Spicy Foods

Craving, Food, Smoked

	CAUST
8	X
13	X
26	X

Craving, Food, Sour- See also Craving, Vinegar

	HEP	ANT C	ANT T	SEP	ARS	AUR M	CHINA	CON	DIG	MEDO	SULPH	VER A	ACON	BOR	BRY	CALC	CARB A	CHAM	CHEL	CORNUS	EUP PUR	PHELL	PLUM	POD	POLYPOR	PULS	SQUILLA	
1			X							X																		
5				X																								
6						X	X				X					X												
8	X	X	X		X			X	X											X	X				X	X		
10	X	X		X		X		X											X									
11				X																								
13	X		X						X			X		X	X		X	X				X	X				X	
15																								X				
17		X																										
19										X																		
24	X																											
26	X				X		X				X	X	X															

Craving, Food, Spicy

	HEP	CHINA	FL AC	NUX M	SULPH	LAC C	MEPH	NUX V	PHOS	PULS	SANG	SEL
1										X	X	
5		X		X				X	X			X
6					X							
7	X					X						
8	X	X	X				X					
13	X		X									
14				X								
19					X							

Craving, Food, Starchy

	ALUM	NIT AC	PULS	CALC PH	LYC
1	X				
4				X	
5	X				
7	X				X
8	X	X			
9			X		
13	X	X			
25			X		

Craving, Food, Warm

	CHEL	ANGUST	CUPR	CYCL	FERR	LYC
8	X	X	X	X	X	
11						X
13	X	X	X	X	X	
17	X					
18	X					

Craving, Food or Drink, Bitter

	NAT M	DIG	ACON
5	X		
7	X		
8	X	X	X
13	X	X	
26	X	X	

Craving, Food or Drink, Cold

	PHOS	VER A	SIL	CUPR	THUJA	AGAR M	ANT T	CALC	CHAM	CROT H	EUP PERF	NAT SUL	PULS
1	X	X				X				X		X	
4	X												
5	X												X
7			X				X						
8	X	X	X	X	X			X					
9	X	X											
11	X	**X**											
13		X	X	X	X								
15									X				
19	X										X		

Craving, Fruit

	VER A	IGN	MAG C	PH AC	SULPH AC	ANT T	ALOE	ALUMEN	ALUM	CHINA	PULS	CIST	CUBEB	HEP	MAG M
5			X						X						
7	**X**	X	X	X	X	X		X							
8	X	X	X	X	X	X	X	X		X	X	X	X	X	
13	X	X	X	X	X		X		X	X					
15	X	X									X				
17						X									
19															X

Craving, Fruit, Green

	MEDO
1	X
5	X

Craving, Ham

	MEZ	CALC PH	NIT AC	NUX V	TUB
1	X	X			
5	X				X
7	X				
8			X	X	
13	X				

Craving, Herring

	NIT AC	VER A
8	X	X
13	X	X
15	X	X
26	X	X

Craving, Ice

	MEDO	PHOS	NAT SUL
1	X		X
10		X	
11		X	
19	X		
21			

Craving, Ice Cream

	PHOS	EUP PERF	CALC	LYC	RHUS T	SULPH
1			X			
8	X	X			X	
11	X					
17	X					
19	X	X				X
21	X					
27				X		

Craving, Indigestible/Abnormal Articles (AKA Pica) (Includes Craving, Chalk; Craving, Charcoal; Craving, Clay; Craving, Dirt etc)

	CALC	NIT AC	ALUM	CIC	NUX V	CALC PH	TAR H	BRY	CHAM	CHINA	CINA	CON	LAC FEL	MERC	SANG	SIL
1	X	X	X	X			X			X			X	X	X	
4	X															
5	X	X	X			X										X
6	X		X		X											
7	X	**X**	X	X	X		X									
8		X		X	X							X				
9	X		X	X							X					
11	X		X													
13		X	X	**X**	X			X								
14	X															
15		X							X							
17		X														
21	X															
23			X													
24						X										
26		X			X											

Craving, Lemonade

	BELL	PULS	CYCL	NIT AC	SABIN	SEC	EUP PURP	JATR
4		X						
5			X					
7	X	X		X				X
8	X		X	X	X	X	X	
11	X	X						
13	X				X	X		
19	X							

Craving, Meat

	MAG CAR	ABIES C	SULPH	HELL	KREO	MENY	ALL S	CALC PH	CANTH	IOD	LIL T	MERC	PHYTO	SANIC	TRIFOL P	TUB
1	X	X					X			X			X			
5	X				X											
7	X		X		X											
8	X	X	X	X		X			X						X	
10														X		
11																X
13	X		X	X		X						X				
16		X						X			X					

Craving, Meat, Salted- See Craving, Salt

Craving, Meat, Smoked- See also Craving, Food, Smoked

	CAUST	CALC PH	TUB	KREO	PHYTO
1		X			X
5	X	X	X		
7	X			X	
8	X				
10			X		

Craving, Milk

	CHEL	RHUS T	BRY	MERC	PH AC	APIS	ARS	CALC	SIL	STAPHYS	SULPH	AUR	BAPT	NUX V	PHELL	PHOS	SABAD	STRONT	TUB	CARB V	LACH	MEZ	NAT M	THLASPI
1		X																				X		X
4											X													
5	X	X	X	X												X			X					
7			X	X	X		X	X	X	X				X				X					X	
8	X	X	X	X	X	X	X	X	X	X	X	X	X	X	X	X	X			X	X			
10						X																		
11		X																	X					
13	X	X	X	X	X		X	X	X	X	X	X	X		X		X	X						
15					X																			
17						X																		
19	X																							
20	X																							

Craving, Milk, Cold

	PH AC	RHUS T	PHELL	SABAD	STAPHYS
8	X	X	X	X	X
11	X	X			

Craving, Mustard

	ARS	COCCUL	COLCH	HEP	LAC CAN
5	X	X	X	X	
7					X

Craving, Onions

	ALL C	CUBEB
1	X	
7	X	
8	X	X
13		X

Craving, Oranges

	CUBEB	MEDO
1		X
13	X	

Craving, Oysters

	LACH	RHUS T	LYC	NAT M	APIS	BRY	CALC	BROM
4	X							
5	X	X	X	X		X	X	
7	X	X	X	X		X	X	
8	X	X	X	X	X			X
13	X	X			X			

Craving, Pastry- See also Craving, Farinaceous Foods

	PLUM	SEP
5		X
13	X	

Craving, Pickles

	ANT C	HEP	SEP	ABIES C	CHEL	LACH	ARS	HAM	STAPHYS	SULPH	SULPH IO	VER A
1		X		X								
4			X		X							
5	X	X	X			X					X	X
7	X					X		X		X		
8	X			X			X					
10					X							
13		X							X			
21			X									

Craving, Pork

	CROT H	TUB
7	X	
5		X

Craving, Potatoes

	CALC PH	OL AN
4	X	
7	X	
8	X	X

Craving, Potatoes, Raw

	CALC
5	X
7	X
13	X

Craving, Rice, Dry

	ALUM
1	X
7	X
13	X

Craving, Salt (Includes Craving, Meat, Salted)

	NAT M	CALC	CARB V	PHOS	VER A	CALC PH	NIT AC	CAUST	CON	ARG N	THUJA	ALOE	COR R	MEDO	MEPH	MERC I F	SANIC	FERR IOD	LAC C	MANC	SEL	SEP	TAR H	TUB
1	X		X		X	X	X							X										
4	X		X			X																		
5	X			X	X	X	X	X	X	X		X					X						X	X
6	X					X					X													
7	X	X	X	X	X	X	X	X	X			X							X	X				
8	X	X	X	X	X	X	X	X	X		X		X		X	X					X			
9	X																							
10	X	X		X					X	X							X							
11	X	X																						
13	X	X	X		X		X	X	X		X		X		X	X								
14		X																						
16	X																							
17	X	X	X	X	X		X	X		X				X										
18	X																							
19				X														X						
21	X			X						X												X		
22	X																							
25	X																							
26		X	X		X																			
27	X																							

Craving, Sardines

	CYCL	FERR IOD	VER A
1	X		
8			X
19		X	

Craving, Stimulants

	NUX V	CAPS	CARB AC	COCA	HEP	NAJA	STAPHYS
1	X			X			
9	X						
12					X		
14	X	X	X				X
17						X	

Craving, Sugar (Includes Craving, Sweets)

	LYC	ARG N	SULPH	CALC	CHINA	KALI CAR	IPEC	AMM C	CARB V	MAG M	RHUS T	SABAD	RHEUM	SEP	ARG	BRY	CINA	MEDO	MERC	NAT C	NAT M	TUB						
1	X	X	X						X					X				X										
4	X	X	X			X														X								
5	X	X			X	X	X	X		X	X	X	X			X	X				X	X						
6	X	X	X																									
7	X	**X**	**X**	X		X	X		X	X	X					X												
8	X	X	X	X	X	X	X	X	X	X	X	X	X		X				X	X								
9	X	X																										
10	X	X	X	X	X																	X						
11	X	X		X								X					X											
13	X		X	X	X	X	X	X	X	X	X	X	X		X				X		X							
14		X		X																								
15	X	X	X																									
17	X	X	X											X				X										
18	X																											
19	X		X	X																								
20					X																							
21	X	X	X	X										X														
22	X																											
25	X	X																										
26	X				X	X	X	X																				
27		X																										
28		X																										

Craving, Tea

	ALUM	AGARICIN	CHINA	HEP																								
1	X																											
4		X																										
5	X																											
6			X																									
13	X			X																								

Craving, Tobacco

	DAPHNE	STAPHYS	NUX V	TAB	CALAD	CAMPH	EUGEN	IGN	THERID	ARS	CALC PH	CHINA	PHOS	PLUM	SPIG	TAR H	AGARICIN	ALUMEN	ASAR	CAPS	CARB AC	COCA	NAT PH	PLANT	QERC G S	SASSAF	SULPH AC
1				X	X																	X					
2			**X**			**X**				**X**	**X**	**X**	**X**	**X**	**X**									X			
3			X			X																					
4																	X										
5		X		X	X																					X	
6								X																			
7	X			**X**												**X**		X									
8	X	X					X		X																		
9			X																X	X					X		X
13	X	X					X		X																		
14		X																			X						
19																							X				
28	X				X			X																			

Craving, Vegetables

	MAG C	MAG M	ALUMEN	ALUM	CHAM
7		X			
8	X		X		
13	X			X	
15					X
19		X			

Craving, Vinegar- See also Craving, Acids, Craving, Food, Sour

	ARN	SEP	HEP	CHEL	APIS	ARS	KALI PH	SULPH FL
1	X	X	X					
4				X				
5	X	X	X	X	X	X	X	X
8	X	X	X					
13	X							
18		X						

Craving, Whisky

	ARS	LACH	SEL	SPIG	ACON	ARN	CALC	CHINA	CUBEB	FL AC	HEP	NUX V	OP	PULS	STAPHYS	SULPH	THERID
5	X	X															
8			X	X	X	X	X	X	X	X	X	X	X	X	X	X	X
13	**X**	**X**	**X**	**X**	X	X	X	X	X	X	X	X	X	X	X	X	X

Craving, Wine

	CALC	BRY	HEP	LACH	ACON	CIC	STAPHYS	SEP	PHOS	SULPH	ARG	CHEL	CHINA	CUBEB	FL AC	MERC	SPIGEL	THERID	AETHUSA	IGN	MEZ
5									X												
7	X	X	X	X		X		X	**X**										X		X
8	X	X	X	X	X	X	X	X		X	X	X	X	X	X	X	X	X			
10	X																				
13	X	X	X	X	X	X	X	X		**X**	X	X	X	X	X	X	X	X			
15																				X	
26	X	X	X	X	X		X														

Crepitus- See Cracking, Sound Of

Cretinism- See also Development, Delayed

	LAPIS	THYROID	BAR C	CALC PH	NAT C
2	X			X	
7	X				
8	X				
9					X
12		X			
23		X	X		

Crohn's Disease- See Enteritis

Croup

	ACON	SPONG	HEP	KALI BIC	BELL	IOD	BROM	ANT T	SAMB	PHOS	SANG	LACH	IPEC	KALI MUR	GELS	ACET AC	ARS	BRY	CUPR	FERR PH	KAOLIN	AMM C	CAUST	CHAM	DROS	LYC	RUMEX	STRAM
1	X	X	X	X	X			X	X		X	X																X
2	**X**	**X**	**X**		**X**	**X**	**X**	**X**	**X**	X	X			X		X	X		**X**	X	X			X				
3	X	X	X						X																			
4	**X**	**X**	**X**	X		**X**	**X**	X			**X**	X		**X**	X			X		X	**X**							
5	X	X							X																			
6	X	X	X	X	X	X	X	X		X	X	X	X			X	X		X	X	X	X	X			X		X
7	**X**	**X**	**X**	X	X	X	**X**	**X**	X	X	X	X		X	X	**X**	X	X					X	X			X	X
8	X	X	X	X	X	X	X	X	X	X	X	X	X	X		X	X	X	X		X	X	X	X	X	X	X	X
9	X	X																										
10	**X**	X	X	X	X	X				X																		
11	**X**		X	X	**X**		X	X			X		X	**X**	X			**X**		**X**			X		X		X	
12	**X**	**X**	X			X	X																					
13	X	**X**	**X**	X	X	X	X	X	**X**	**X**	X													X	X			
14	X	X	X	X	X			X					X		X													
15	X	X	X	X				X					X		X				X									
17	X	X	X	X		X	X		X	X		X		X		X						X				X		X
18	X	X																										
19	**X**	**X**	**X**	X	X	X	X		X	X		X	X														X	
20	**X**	**X**	**X**									X													X			
21	X	X	X																									
22	**X**	X	X	X											X													
23	X	X	X	X		X	X		X													X						
24	X	X	X																									
25	X																											
26	**X**	**X**	X		X				X	X			X				X									X		
27		X	X		X	X		X																				
28		X																										

Crusta Lactea- See also Cradle Cap

	VIOL T	ARS	CALC	SULPH	RHUS T	LYC	DULC	MEZ	BELL	CIC	HEP	MERC	SARS	BAR C	CROT T	GRAPH	IRIS V	NAT M	OLEAND	PHOS	PSOR	SEP	VINCA					
2	X		X				X	X									X				X		X					
4	X							**X**											X									
6	X	X	X	X	X	X			X	X					X													
8	X	X	X	X	X	X	X	X			X	X	X	X	X	X	X	X	X	X	X	X	X					
10	X	X		X	X	X			X	X	X																	
12	X																											
13	**X**	**X**	**X**	**X**	X	X	**X**		X	X	X	**X**	**X**	X		X		X		X		X						
23	X																											
26		X	X	X	X																							

Crusta Serpiginosa- See also Ringworm

	SULPH	ARS	CALC	DULC	PSOR	RHUS T
2	X				X	
26	X	X	X	X		X

Cuts- See Wounds, Incisional

Cyanosis (Note that only the main remedies from 17 are used here)

	CUPR	CARB V	DIG	LAURO	VER A	LACH	ARS	CAMPH	ANT T	OP	SAMB	IPEC	HYDR AC	SEC	RHUS T	PULS	ACON	AMM C	CALC	CUPR AC	SPONG	SULPH	CINA
1	X			X																			
2	X		X	X		X									**X**								
3			X																X			X	
4	**X**	**X**	X					X		X		X											
5	X	X		X					X			X	X							X			
6	X	X	X	X	X	X	X	X	X	X	X	X	X	X	X	X	X	X					
7	**X**	**X**	**X**	**X**	X	**X**	X	**X**	**X**	X	X		X	X	X	X				X	X		X
8	X	X	X		X	X	X	**X**	X	X	X	X		X	**X**	X	X	X				X	
9	X	X				X	X			X													
10		X	X		X	X		X		X									X		X		
11		X	X		X	X	X							X						X			
12	X				X																		
13	**X**	X	X	X	**X**	**X**	**X**	X		**X**	**X**	X	X	X		X	X		X		X	X	**X**
14	X	X	X		X		X	X				X	X										
16		X																					
17	X	X	X	X	X	X	X	X	X	X	X		X		X			X		X	X		
18	X	X			X				X		X			X		X							
19	X	X		X			X		X		X	X	X					X					X
23				X																			
26			X								X	X					X		X			X	
27	X			X		X			X														
28														X									

Cynanche Cellularis

	ANTHRAC	AUR M N
2	X	
8	X	X

Cystalgia

	ACON	CANTH	BERB V	ARS	NUX V	PULS	TEREB	BELL	CAUST	COP	EQUISET	LYC	THUJA															
1										X																		
4											X																	
6	X	X	X	X	X			X				X																
7	X	X	X	X	X	X	X		X	X	X	X																
8		X	X																									
10							X	X																				
11			X										X															
13	X	X	X	X		X																						
14	X						X						X															
15	X																											
19		X	X	X	X	X		X																				
20						X			X		X	X																
21		X								X			X															
24	X	X					X		X																			
26				X	X																							

Cystitis

	CANTH	ACON	APIS	TEREB	BERB V	EQUISET	NUX V	DULC	PULS	SARS	CHIM	SEP	BELL	MERC	UVA	DIG	ARS	CANN S	CAUST	LYC	EUP PUR	NIT AC	SABAL	SULPH				
1	X	X	X	X	X	X		X							X								X					
2		X		X		X					X	X						X		X	X		X					
3	X		X		X	X					X								X									
4	X			X		X	X					X				X												
5	X			X	X	X				X	X	X			X						X		X					
6	X	X		X	X		X	X	X	X	X	X	X	X	X		X		X	X		X		X				
7	**X**	**X**	**X**	**X**	X	X	X	X	**X**	**X**	X	**X**	**X**	X		X	X	X	X	**X**	X	X		X				
8	X	X	X	X	X	X	X	X	X	X	X	X	X	X	X	X	X	X	X	X	X	X		X				
9	X				X	X	X	X								X						X	X					
10	X												**X**															
12	X	X	X					X	X		X		X					X			X							
13	**X**		X													**X**												
14	X																											
15	X	X					X	X	X							X								X				
18	X			X													X											
19	X	X	X		X	X	X	X		X		X			X		X	X	X	X		X						
20	X	X	X		X		X		X	X				X														
21	X	X	X	X	X		X	X	X	X			X				X		X					X				
22	X	X					X							X														
23	X	X	X	X		X									X			X					X					
24														X														
25	X																											
26	**X**	**X**							X																			
27	X		X							X	X				X													
28	X																											
29*														X														

29* Kawakami AP, et al. In vitro growth of uropathogenic Escherichia coli isolated from a snow leopard treated with homeopathic and isopathic remedies: a pilot study. Int J High Dilution Res 2009; 8(27): 41-44.

Cystitis, Interstitial

	AUR M	GLON	LYSS
4	X		
17		X	
19			X

Cystitis, Traumatic (AKA Honeymoon Cystitis)

	STAPHYS	MEDO
18	X	
19		X
21	X	

Cystospasm- See Spasm, Bladder

Cysts

	BAR C	CALC	APIS	GRAPH	HEP	SIL	ACON	AGAR M	BOV	BROM	CALC SUL	IOD	KALI CAR	NIT AC	PHOS	RUTA	SABIN	SPONG	STAPHYS	SULPH
2	X								X		X								X	
7	**X**	**X**	X		X					X										
8						X														
9	X	X		X											X	X				
13	X	X		X	X	X	X	X					X	X			X	X		X
14			X									X								

Cysts, Eyelid

	CALC FL	NIT AC	CALAD	KALI IOD	STAPHYS	THUJA
1	X	X	X		X	X
2				X		
3	X	X				
4	X					

Cysts, Ganglion (Includes Ganglion, Wrist)

	RUTA	BENZ AC	SIL	BAR C	CALC	GRAPH	PH AC	PHOS	PLUM	AMM C	ARN	ARUM T	BELL	BOV	CALC FL	CARB V	CAUST	CON	FERR MA	IOD	MEZ	NAT M	PHYTO	RHUS T	STICTA	SULPH	THUJA	ZINC
1	X	X	X																									
2	**X**	**X**	X				X		X					X					X							X	X	
3	**X**	X																										
4	X																											
7	X	X																							X			
8	**X**	**X**	X	X	X						X	X	X			X	X	X		X		X		X				
9	X	X		X	X	X		X																				
12		X																			X		X					
13			X				X	X	X	X																		X
14															X													
21	X	X																										
24	X																											
28	X	X				X																						

Cysts, Genital, Female

	SABIN
7	X
8	X

Cysts, Hydatid, Uterus

	CANTH	ACON	ARS	BELL	CALC	CHINA	FERR	GRAPH	HYOSC	LYC	MERC	NAT CAR	PULS	SABIN	SEC	SEP	SIL	SULPH
8	X	X	X	X	X	X	X	X	X	X	X	X	X	X	X	X	X	X
9	X																	

Cysts, Meibomian Glands

	HEP	MERC	SIL
8		X	
27	X		X

Cysts, Ovaries

	COLOC	APIS	IOD	BUFO	KALI BR	LYC	PLAT	PULS	THUJA	BOV	CANTH	CARB A	LACH	OOPHOR	PRUN S	RHOD
1				X										X		
2																X
4		X														
5	X	X											X			
7	X	X	X	X	X		X					X				
8	X	X	X		X		X		X	X	X				X	
14	X					X										
18						X										
19									X							
21	X		X													
28								X								
29*								X								

29* Sanchez-Resendiz J, et al. Polycystic Ovary Syndrome. Boletin Mexicano de Homeopatica, 1997, 30, 11-15.

Cysts, Ovary, Left

	LACH	USTIL
7	**X**	
19		X
21	X	

Cysts, Ovary, Right

	APIS	ARS
7	X	X
21	X	

Cysts, Sebaceous

	BAR C	CALC	CON	GRAPH	STAPHYS	HEP	KALI BR	NIT AC	SIL	SULPH	THUJA
2					X		X				
5		X	X	X							X
8	X		X		X				X		
21	X			X		X					
26		X						X		X	

Cysts, Sebaceous, Scalp

	BAR C	CON	PHYTO	BELL	NIT AC	SIL	THUJA	CALC	CAUST	CLEM	GRAPH	KAI CAR	PH AC	RHUS T	SULPH	HEP	BENZ AC	KALI BIC	KALI IOD	LOB I	SEP
2	**X**	**X**	**X**		X						X	X	X	X		**X**	X		X	X	
3							X														
6	X		X	X		X	X	X	X	X					X						X
7	**X**	X		X	X	X					X	X									
8	X	X	X	X	X	X	X	X	X	X			X	X	X			X			
21	X																				

Cysts, Synovial

	SIL	BENZ AC	CALC	CAUST	KALI IOD	RUTA	STICTA
5	X	X	X	X	X	X	X
8	X						

Cysts, Tarsal

	FERR PH	FERR PY	GRAPH	KALI IOD
2	X	X		X
8			X	

Cysts, Vagina

	SIL
1	X
8	X
14	X

Dacryoadenitis- See Inflammation, Lachrymal Glands

Dacryocanaliculitis

	PETR	SIL	ARG N	BELL	CALC	GRAPH	KALI IOD	PULS																				
1	X					X																						
6			X	X			X																					
7	X	X			X																							
19		X						X																				

Dacryocystitis

	PULS	SIL	HEP	MERC	NAT M	PETR	APIS	ACON	ARG N	ARUM T	BELL	CALC	CALEND	CIMICI	CINNAB	CON	EUPHR	GRAPH	HYDRAST	KALI IOD	SANG	STRAM	STILLI	SULPH				
6	**X**	X	X				**X**																					
7	X			X		X												X										
8	X	X	X	X	X	X		X	X	X	X	X	X	X	X	X	X		X	X	X	X	X	X				
17		X			X																							

Dandruff

	ARS	NAT M	SEP	PHOS	SULPH	THUJA	CALC	GRAPH	LYC	STAPHYS	MEZ	OLEAND	CANTH	AMM M	BRY	FL AC	KALI MUR	KALI SUL	PSOR	SANIC								
1	X	X	X	X	X	X		X			X			X		X			X	X								
2	**X**		**X**	X														X		X								
3	X	X			X	X	X		X																			
7	X	**X**	X	**X**	**X**	**X**	X	X	X	X	X	X	**X**	X	X		X		X									
8	X	X	X	X	X	X	X	X		X			X		X		X	X										
9	X	X	X	X	X	X	X		X																			
13	X			X		X	X	X		**X**	X	X																
14	X			X		X																						
21	X	X	X		X			X				X				X												
25	X	X	X		X		X		**X**																			
28			X																									

Deafness (Includes Catarrhal Deafness; Hardness of Hearing; Hearing, Impaired)

	PHOS	PULS	GRAPH	HEP	CALC	IOD	NIT AC	SAL AC	SULPH	ARN	CAUST	MERC	BELL	MERC D	ARS	BAR C	CARB V	CHENO	GELS	PETR	SIL	CHINA	CON	ELAPS	KALI MUR	LACH	LYC	PH AC
1	X	X	X	X		X		X			X			X		X		X			X				X			
2			X								X			X			X	X	X	X		X		X				
3	X	X		X	X		X			X			X	X		X	X		X					X	**X**	X		
4		X	X			X		X						X				X							**X**			
5	X						X	X															X					
6	X	X	X		X	X	X		X	X	X	X	X		X		X		X	X	X		X	X		X		X
7	X		X	X			X		X		X	X		X					X			X		X			X	
8	**X**	X	X	X	**X**	X	X	X	X	X	X	X	X		X	X	X		X	X	X	X	X	X		X	X	X
9	X	X	X			X		X					X	X				X				X						
10		X		X	X				X	X		X			X		X									X		X
11							X									X												
12	X	X		X		X			X			X			X					X	X	X						X
13	X	X	X	X	X	X	X		X	X	X	X	X	X	X	X	X			X	X	X	X	X		X	X	X
14		X	X	X	X	X					X							X							X			
15	X	X		X	X		X		X	X		X	X		X	X			X			X				X		X
16	X																											
17	X	X	X	X	X	X	X	X	X	X	X	X	X	X	X	X	X			X	X		X		X	X	X	X
18								X																				
19								X																				
21	X		X					X		X	X							X	X			X					X	
22																									X			
24	X	X	X		X	X	X		X	X		X	X			X		X	X	X	X		X	X				
25	X	X	X			X		X										X										
26	X	X	X	X	X		X		X	X	X	X	X		X		X			X	X		X				X	
27		X		X	X				X					X													X	
28								X																				

Deafness, Senile

	PHOS	MERC D	CARB A	CHENO	CIC	GRAPH	IOD	KALI PH	PULS	SAL AC
6		X								
8					X			X		
9	X									
24		X								
25	**X**		X	X		X	X		X	X

Decubitus- See Bedsores

Dehydration- See Ailments from Fluid, Loss Of

Delirium

	BELL	HYOSC	STRAM	OP	ARS	BRY	BAPT	LACH	RHUS T	PHOS	VER A	AGAR M	GELS	CIMICI	PH AC	VER V	ACON	PLUM	AILANTH	APIS	ARN	CANTH	CHINA	NUX V				
1	X	X	X	X	X		X	X	X			X				X		X	X			X	X					
2																							X	**X**				
3	**X**	**X**	**X**						X			X				X			X									
4	**X**	**X**	**X**		X	X	X	X	X	**X**	**X**	X		X														
5	X	X	X	X		X		X		X	X			X	X													
6	X	X	X	X	X	X	X	X	X	X	X	X	X	X	X	X		X		X	X	X		X				
7	**X**	**X**	**X**							X			X											X				
8	**X**	X	X	**X**	X	X	X	X	X	X	X	X	X	X	X		X	X	X	X	X	X	X					
9	X	X	X	X									X		X													
10	X	X			X	X			X								X											
11	X	X	X	X	X	X	X	X			X	X		X	X						X	X						
12	X	X	X	X				X								X												
13	**X**	**X**	**X**	**X**	**X**	**X**		X	**X**	X	X	X					**X**	**X**			X	X	**X**	X				
14	X				X		X													X								
15	X	X		X	X	X	X		X	X			X	X	X	X			X									
16		X	X													X												
17	X	X									X		X								X							
18	X						X																					
19	X					X													X									
20	X																			X								
21	X	X	X	X	X	X		X									X			X								
22	X																											
23	X						X																					
24	X				X		X											X										
25	X												X															
26	X	X	X	X		X		X									X											
27	X			X																								

Delirium Tremens

	HYOSC	STRAM	BELL	NUX V	AGAR M	ARS	CIMICI	CANN I	OP	CAPS	RAN B	DIG	CALC	KALI BR	LACH	ANT T	BISM	COFF	CROT H	GELS	ARN	NAT M	ACON	CYPRIP	IGN	LOL T	NUX M
1		X		X			X																				
2	**X**	**X**	X		X	X	X	X		X	X	X	X		X	**X**	X		X					X		X	
4	**X**	X	X	X	X		X		**X**	X													X				
6	X	X	X	**X**	X	X	X	X	X			X	X	X				X	X	X			X		X		
7	X		**X**	X	**X**	**X**		X			**X**	X		X	X	X	X	X	X		**X**	**X**			X		**X**
8	X	X	X	X	X	X	X	X	X	X	X	X	X	X	X		X	X		X	X	X					
11	X	X	X		X		X	X	X	X																	
14								X																			
15	X					X	X		X			X				X				X							
16															X												
17											X															X	
19	X	X		X																							
21	X	X	X			X																					
23				X	X					X	X			X										X			
26		X	X	X		X			X	X			X														

Dementia

	ANAC	NUX V	BELL	CUPR	PHOS	MERC	OP	PIC AC	AGAR M	AUR	CALC	CALC PH	CROT H	HYOSC	IGN	LACH	LIL TIG	NAT M	PLAT	SIL
1		X				X									X					
2													X				X			
4	**X**							X				X								
6		X	X	X	X					X						X		X		X
8	X	X	X	X	X	X	X		X		X	X	X							
9	X	X					X			X										
10					X															
11	X		X	X	X			X	X					X			X		X	
14	X																			
23								X												
26		X	X	X		X	X				X			X	X	X		X	X	X

Dementia, Senile

	BAR C	ANAC	AUR IOD	CROT H	PHOS	AMBRA	CON	GLON	LYC	SEC
7				X						
8	X	X		X			X			X
11	X	X	X		X	X		X		
21	X		X		X				X	

Dengue Fever

	EUP PERF	RHUS T	ACON	BRY	GELS	ARS	BAPT	BELL	NUX V
1	**X**	X		X					
2	**X**	**X**	**X**		**X**				
3	X		X	X					
7	X	X	X	X					
8	X	X	X	X		X		X	X
11	X	X	X	X	X	X	X	X	X
12	X				X	X	X		
23	X	X							
28	X								

Dental Caries- See Caries, Dental
Dentition, Delayed- See Development, Dental, Delayed
Dentition, Diseases of- See Teething
Depression (Includes Depression, Post-natal; Grief; Melancholy; Sadness; Weeping)

	AUR	IGN	NAT M	SEP	PULS	LYC	PLAT	GRAPH	ARS	ACON	CALC	PH AC	CIMICI	NUX V	PHOS	LACH	PSOR	ARG N	CAUST	ANAC	HELL	KALI PH	PLUM	STANN
1	X	X	X	X	X	X	X	X		X		X	X	X	X	X	X	X	X	X	X	X	X	X
2	**X**	**X**	**X**				**X**		**X**												**X**		**X**	
3	X	X	X	X	X	X		X				X					X			X				X
4	**X**	**X**	**X**	X	X	X	X		**X**	X		**X**	**X**	X		X		X		**X**		X		X
5	X	X	X	X	X	X	X	X	X		X	X	X	X	X	X	X	X	X	X		X		X
6	X	X	X	X	X	X	X	X	X	X	X		X	X	X	X		X	X		X		X	
7	**X**	**X**	**X**	X	**X**	**X**	**X**	**X**	X	X	**X**	X		**X**	**X**	**X**	**X**	X	**X**	X	**X**	**X**	X	X
8	X	X	X	X	X	X	X	X	X	X	X	X	X	X	X	X	X	X	X	X	X	X		X
9	X	X	X	X	X	X	X				X		X				X	X	X		X			X
10	X	X		X	X	X		X		X	X			X			X		X	X			X	
11	X	X	X	X		X							X			X		X				X		
12	X	X	X		X		X		X	X										X				
13	**X**	**X**	**X**	X	**X**	**X**	**X**	**X**	**X**	X	**X**	**X**		X	X	**X**	X		**X**	X	**X**		**X**	X
14	X	X	X	X	X	X		X		X		X		X	X			X	X		X	X		
15		X		X	X		X	X		X	X			X	X									
16		X		X								X										X		
17	X	X	X	X	X												X	X					X	
18	X		X	X		X		X	X			X	X		X	**X**	X			X		X		
19				X	X					X	X		X											X
21	X	X	X	X	X	X		X	X			X		X										
22			X		X										X									
23	X	X							X				X					X				X		
24	X					X																	X	X
25	**X**		X	X	X	X	X				X		X		X			X						
26	X	X	X	X	X	X	X	X	X	X	X	X	X	X		X			X		X			
27	X	X	X	X	X		X			X	X						X							
28	X			X																				

Dermatitis- See also Dermatitis, Atopic; Eczema; Psoriasis (Includes Eruptions)

	RHUS T	DULC	SULPH	CANTH	KALI MUR	PETR	PSOR	ACON	AGAR M	APIS	ARS	BAR M	BELL	BRY	CALC	CHAM	CUPR	GRAPH	HEP	LYC	RAN B	SARS
1	X	X		X	X	X	X			X	X									X	X	X
2			X				X							X			X					
3	X		X							X								X				
5		X																				
7	X	X		X	X		X	X				X			X	X			X			
8	X			X	X	X							X									
9			X						X													
13	X	X	X			X		X	X		X	X	X	X	X	X	X	X	X	X	X	X

Dermatitis, Atopic- See also Dermatitis; Eczema

	SULPH	ARS	GRAPH	PULS	AILANTH	ANAC	APIS	BRY	CALC	CALEND	CHLOR	DULC	LYC	NAT PH	NAT M	NAT SUL	PSOR	RHUS T	SEP	SIL	THUJA	URT U
3	X	X			X		X				X	X		X		X						X
20	X		X			X		X		X								X	X			
29[1]	X			X					X				X				X			X		
29[2]	X	X	X	X											X						X	
29[3]	X																					

29[1] Itamura R, Hosoya R. Homeopathic Treatment of Japanese patients with intractable Atopic Dermatitis. Homeopathy, 2003, 92, 108-114.

29[2] Mohan GR, Anandhi KS. Efficacy of homeopathic drugs in dermatitis of atopic diathesis. Homoeopathic Links, 2003, Winter, 16, 4, 257-260.

29[3] Eizayaga JE, Eizayaga JI. Prospective observational study of 42 patients with atopic dermatitis treated with homeopathic medicines. Homeopathy. 2012 Jan;101 (1):21-7.

Descemetitis

	KALI BIC	CON	MERC D
2	X		
7	X		X
8	X	X	

Desquamation, Skin- See Skin Peeling

Development, Dental, Delayed (Includes Delayed Dentition)

	CALC	CALC PH	CALC FL	FL AC	SIL	ZINC	CALC AC	CALC IOD	FERR	MAG CAR	NAT M	PHOS	PHYTO	RHEUM	SULPH	TUB												
1	X	X	X													X												
3														X														
4		**X**													X													
5	X	X	X		X																							
6	X	X						X																				
7	X	**X**		X		X			X	X			X															
8		X				X																						
9							X																					
10	X	X																										
11	X																											
12	X																											
14	X	X																										
15	X																											
16											X	X																
19	X	X		X	X																							
22		X																										
25	X																											

Development, Mental, Delayed

	BAR C	CALC	NAT M	AGAR M	BAR M	BUFO	CALC PH	HELL	SIL	TUB	PH AC	AMBRA	BRY	CALEND	CAUST	KALI BR	MEDO	NAT CAR	SEP	STRAM	SYPH	THUJA	THYROID	XERO				
1	X	X	X	X	X	X			X	X				X	X						X	X		X				
3	**X**	X	X	X					X	X																		
4													X															
5	X			X		X		X			X	X				X				X								
8							X																					
9	X						X	X										X										
10	X		X																									
11	X																											
17	X				X																							
18											X																	
19	X		X																									
21	X	X															X		X									
24	X																						X					
27	X	X																										
28	X																											

Development, Physical, Delayed (Includes Puberty, Delayed)

	BAR C	CALC	CALC PH	SIL	SULPH	THYROXIN	NAT M	BAR M	PHOS	PULS	SABAL	SEP	TUB
1	X	X	X		X			X					X
3	X	X	X	X	X								X
4	**X**												
6	X		X										
8	X	X	X	X	X				X	X		X	
9	X	X	X	X	X		X			X	X	X	
10	X	X	X	X									
11	X												
12			X										
13		X	X	X	X								
14		X			X								
16							X		X				
17	X							X					
19		X					X						
21	X	X		X									
22			X										
25	X	X		X							X		
26		X		X	X								
29[1]						X							
29[2]						X							
29[3]						X							
29[4]						X							
29[5]						X							
29[6]						X							

29[1] Graunke H, et al. Treatment of lowland frogs from the spawn stage with homeopathically prepared thyroxin (10(-30)). Scientific World Journal. 2007 Oct 22;7:1697-702.

29[2] Endler, PC, et al. Effects of Highly Diluted Succussed Thyroxine on Metamorphosis on Highland Frogs. Berlin J on Res in Hom, June 1991,1, 3, 151-160.

29[3] Endler PC et al. Pretreatment with Thyroxine 10^{-8} Enhances a Curative Effect of Homeopathically prepared Thyroxine 10^{-13} on Lowland Frogs. Forschende Komplementarmedizin Und Klassiche Naturheikunde, 2003, 10, 137-42.

29[4] Lingg G, et al. Treatment of highland frogs from the two-legged stage with homeopathically prepared thyroxin (10-11 - 10-21). Scientific World Journal. 2008 Apr 20;8:446-50.

29[5] Welles SU, et al. Pretreatment with thyroxin 10(-8) and the effect of homeopathically prepared thyroxin 10(-30) on highland frogs--a multi-researcher study. Forsch Komplementmed. 2007 Dec;14 (6):353-7.

29[6] Harrer B. Replication of an experiment on extremely diluted thyroxine and highland amphibians. Homeopathy. 2013 Jan;102(1):25-30.

Development, Physical, Breasts, Delayed

	SABAL	CALC PH	LECITHIN	LYC
3	X	X	X	
4	X			
9	X			
14				X
19	X			
25	X			

Development, Walking, Delayed

	SIL	CALC	SULPH	ALUM	BELL	CALC PH	CHINA	CINA	FERR	LYC	NAT C	NAT M	PINUS S	PULS
4						X								
8	X	X	X		X		X	X	X	X			X	X
10	X			X										
19												X		
26	X	X	X								X			

Diabetes (Undifferentiated) See also Diabetes Insipidus; Diabetes Mellitis

	PH AC	URAN N	LAC AC	PHOS	ARS	NAT SUL	SYZIGIUM	ACET AC	PLUM	ARG	NAT M	NUX V	ARG N	ARS BR	LYC	CALC	CARB AC	HELON	SULPH	CANTH	CURARE	MOSCH	ARN	INSULIN	SQUILLA	OP	RAT
1	X	X	X	X	X		**<u>X</u>**	X	X	X	X	X	X	X						X		X	X				X
2	**X**		X			**X**	X	X		X	X		X	X		X	X	X	X		X	X	**X**		**X**		X
3	X	X	X	X	X	**X**	X	X	X	X			X	X	X			X		X	X				X		
4	**X**	**<u>X</u>**	X	**X**	X	X	X	X		X							X							**X**			
5				X		X		X				X						X									
6	X	X	X	X	X	X	X		X	X	X	X			X		X	X	X	X	X	X				X	X
7		X	**X**					**X**	X		X	X			X	X	X		X		X						
8		X		X	X																						
9		X		X								X		X													
10	X	X	X	X	X	X			**X**	X	X				X									X			
11	X	X	X	X		X																		X			
12	**X**	**X**			X		**X**		X			X								X							
13	X			X							X														X		
14	X		X		X	X	X	X		X				X			X										
15	X				X							X				X											
16				X							X		X			X			X								
17	X	X							X									X				X				X	
18																X											
19			X																								
21	X	X											X										X			X	
23	X	X	X				X	X						X													
26	X				X				X	X					X				X								
27						X									X												
28		X																									

Diabetes Insipidus- See also Diabetes

	PH AC	SQUILLA	URAN N	ACET AC	ARG	BELL	CAUST	LYC	EUP PUR	MUREX	LAC AC	APIS	ARS	CANTH	DIG	HELON	KALI NIT	LAC D	NAT M	RHUS T	SPIG	FERR M	RHUS A	SYZIG				
2		X	**X**														X											
4	X	X			X		X	X																				
6	X					X						X																
7	X			X		X	X	X						X		X		X	X	X	X							
8	X	X		X		X	X			X	X		X			X	X	X	X	X	X							
10	X	X			X							X																
11	**X**	X	X	**X**	**X**			X	**X**	**X**	**X**				X							**X**	**X**					
12	**X**		**X**						X				X	X	X									**X**				

Diabetes Mellitis- See also Diabetes

	URAN N	PLUM	PH AC	BOV	LYC	OP	TEREB	ACET AC	ARG	CODEIN	HEP	KALI MUR	KALI PH	LACH	LAC AC	LAC D	LYCOP	NAT SUL	PHOS	PIC AC	POD	SIL	SULPH AC	HELON				
2	**X**					X																						
4		**X**																										
7	**X**	**X**	**X**	**X**	**X**		X	X	X	X	X	X	X	X	X	X	X		X	X	X	X	X	**X**				
8	X	X	X	X	X	X	X	X	X		X	X	X	X	X	X	X	X	X	X	X		X					
21	X		X							X								X				X						

Diaphragm, Diseases Of

	ACON	APIS	ASAF	BELL	BRY	CACT	CHAM	CIC	CIMICI	COLCH	CUPR	DIG	MEZ	NUX V	OP	RAN B	RHUS T	STANN	STRAM	SULPH	TAB							
8	X	X		X	X	X	X	X	X	X	X	X		X		X	X		X	X	X							
13			X										X		X			X										

Diarrhoea (Note that only main remedies used from 2 and 8)

	ARS	POD	CHAM	SULPH	VER A	PHOS	CHINA	COLOC	PULS	PH AC	IPEC	CALC	RHEUM	ALOE	IRIS V	DULC	ANT C	ARG N	BRY	NUX V	ACON	CROT T	MERC	MERC C	BAPT	RHUS T	GELS
1	X	X	X	X	X	X	X	X	X	X	X		X	X	X	X	X	X	X	X	X	X		X	X	X	
2	**X**	**X**	**X**	**X**	**X**		**X**		**X**	**X**	**X**		**X**	**X**	**X**	**X**	**X**			**X**		**X**		**X**			
3	X		X	X	X	X		X	X	X	**X**	X	X	X	X	X	X		X	X	X		X		X		X
4	**<u>X</u>**	**X**		X	**<u>X</u>**	**X**	**X**	X	X	X	X	**X**	**X**	**X**	X	X		**X**	X		X	**X**	X	**X**		X	X
5	X	X	X		X		X	X	X	X	X	X	X	X	X	X	X	X	X	X	X	X		X		X	X
6	X	X	X	X	X	X	X	X	X	X	X	X	X		X	X	X	X	X	X	X	X	X			X	X
7	**X**	**X**	**X**	**X**	**X**	X	**X**	X	X	X	**X**	X	**X**	**X**	**X**	**X**	**X**	**X**	**X**	X	X	**X**	**X**	**X**	**X**	X	X
8	**X**	**X**	**X**	X	X	X	X	X	**X**	X	X	X	X		**X**	**X**	X	X	X	X	X	X	**X**		X	X	X
9	X	X	X	X	X		X			X	X	X		X	X		X	X				X		X			X
10	X	X	X	X	X	X	X	X	X	X	X	**X**	X	X		X	X	X	X		X	X	X		X	X	X
11	X	X	**X**	X	X	X	X	X	X	X	X	X	**X**	X				X		X	**X**	X	X	X	X	X	X
12	**X**	**X**	X	X	**X**	**X**	**X**	**X**	X	**X**	X	X			X	X	**X**		X		X		X	X	X		
13	X	X	**X**	**X**	**X**	**X**	**X**	**X**	**X**	**X**	**X**	**X**	**X**	X	X	X	**X**	X	**X**	**X**	X	X	**X**	**X**		**X**	
14	X	X	X		X	X		X				X						X						X	X	X	
15	**X**	X	**X**	X	**X**	X	X	X	X	X	**X**		X		**X**	X							**X**				
16		X									X																
17	X					X	X			X								X									X
18	X	X	X	X	X	X	X	X	X	X	X		X	X	X		X	X				X			X		X
19	**X**	**X**	X	**X**	**X**	**X**	X	X	X	X		X	X	**X**		X	X	X	X	X	X	X	X	X	X	X	X
20	X	**X**			X	X													X								
21	X	X	X	X	X	X	X	X	X	X				X	X	X		X	X	X	X			X	X		
22	X	X	X		X			X												X	X						X
23	X	X	X	X	X	X	X	X	X	X	X	X	X	X	X	X	X	X	X		X	X			X		
24	X		X	X		X	X	X	X			X		X											X	X	X
25	X	X	X	X	X	X	X	X	X	X	X	X		X	X				X								
26	X		**X**	**X**	X	X	X	X	**X**	X	X	X	X			X	X		X	X			X			X	
27				X				X																			
28	X			X																							
29[1]	**X**	**X**	X	**X**		X			X			X															
29[2]	**X**	**X**	X	X								X															
29[3]	X																										

29[1] Jacobs J, et al. Treatment of Acute Childhood Diarrhoea with Homoeopathic Medicine. Paed, May, 1994,93, 5, 719-725.

29[2] Jacobs J, et al. Acute Childhood Diarrhoea- a Replication. J Alt and Comp Med, 2000, 6, 131-139.

29[3] Kayne S, et al. The Use of Arsenicum album to Complement Conventional treatment of Neonatal Diarrhoea (Scours) in Calves. Brit Hom J, 83, 4, Oct 1994, 202-204.

Diarrhoea, Senile

	ANT C	CARB V	CHINA	COFF T	GAMBOG	HYOSC	NIT AC	PH AC	PHOS	SULPH
8		X		X	X	X				
10	X	X	X							X
12	X						X	X	X	

Digestion, Diseases Of

	LYC	CARB V	NUX V	PULS	SULPH	ANT C	BRY	CHINA	NUX M	ARS	CALC	CALC PH	CHAM	CHEL	CYCL	DIOSC	FERR	GRAPH	HEP	IGN	KALI BIC	NAT CAR	SANIC	SIL	URAN N			
2																							X					
4																			X									
5	X	X				X								X				X			X							
6		X			X		X		X											X								
8	X	X	X	X	**X**	X	X	X	**X**	X	X	X	X	X	X	X	X	X	X		X	X	X	X	X			
9	X	X	X	X				X		X						X	X							X				
10																									X			
12				X		X																						
15			X										X															
17	X		X				X																					
18	X							X							X					X								
19	X	X																				X						
24					X							X																
25				X							X																	

Digestion, Slow- See also Lientaria; Weakness, Digestion

	CHINA	CALC	NUX V	CARB V	PULS	ANT C	LYC	OP	AESC	ALET	ARN	BRY	CALC PH	CUPR	EUCAL	GRAPH	HEP	IGN	MERC C	NAT SUL	NUPHAR	PHOS	PSOR	SANIC	SIL	TAR H		
6	X		X					X										X				X						
7	X		X				X	X											X		X				X	X		
8	X	X			X	X			X	X		X				X				X			X	X				
9		X																										
10				X																								
14	X			X																								
15			X		X	X																						
17															X													
18							X																					
21				X																								
22													X															
25		X																										
26	X	X	X		X						X						X											
29*														X														

29* Santini R, et al. Effects of low dose treatment with cuprum 4CH on neostigmine digestive action in female mice. Drug Develop Res1991;24: 231-233.

Digestive System, Congestion Of

	BERB V	CALC	CHINA	HYDRAST	IGN	IRIS V	JUG R	NAT M	PHOS	SOLID																		
5	X		X	X		X	X			X																		
6		X			X			X	X																			

Dilation, Ventricle, Cardiac, Right- See Heart, Dilatation, Ventricle, Right

Diphtheria

	MERC CY	LACH	APIS	KALI BIC	PHYTO	LYC	LAC C	ARS	BROM	NIT AC	MUR AC	MERC I R	ARUM T	BAPT	DIPHTHER	KALI MUR	KALI PER	AMM C	CARB AC	GELS	IGN	RHUS T	AILANTH	BELL	CANTH	CROT H	NAJA	NAT ARS
1	X	X	X	X	X	X	X		X	X	X		X		X				X	X				X	X	X	X	
2	**X**	**X**	X	X	**X**	**X**	X	**X**	X		**X**	**X**	X	X		X	X		X	**X**	X	X	X		X	X		X
3	X	X	X		X	X							X		X			X			X		X					
4	**X**	**X**	**X**	**X**		**X**	X	**X**	X	**X**	**X**				**X**	**X**	**X**		X			X			X			
6	X	X	X	X	X	X	X	X	X	X	X	X	X	X		X	X	X	X	X	X	X	X	X	X		X	
7	X	**X**	**X**	**X**	**X**	X	**X**	**X**	**X**	X	X	X	**X**	**X**		X	X			X	**X**	**X**				X	X	**X**
8	X	X	X	X	X	X	X	X	X	X	X	X	X	X		X	X	X	X		X	X	X	X	X	X	X	X
9												X			X													
10	X	X	X	X		X									X						X	X				X		
11	**X**	**X**		**X**	**X**				X									X	X				X					
12	**X**	X		X		X		X		X	X			X			X	X						X				
14	X	X		X	X		X					X						X		X				X				
15			X	X				X		X	X			X														
16		X	X		X	X		X							X		X											
17	X	X	X	X		X	X		X	X		X				X		X		X							X	
19					X		**X**																					
21	X																											
23	X	X	X	X	X	X	X	X	X			X	X	X	X	x			X				X		X			X
26			**X**		X																							

Diphtheria, Prophylaxis

	DIPHTHER	APIS	BAPT	LAC C	MERC CY	MUR AC
10	X					
15			X			X
16	X	X		X	X	
28	X					

Diplopia

	GELS	BELL	HYOSC	AUR	PLUM	VER V	NAT M	NIT AC	CAUST	CYCL	STRAM	CIC	DIG	AGAR M	ARG N	CON	LYC	OLEAND	SENEG	SPONG	STROPH
1	X		X	X	X	X			X		X								X		
2					X	X				X										X	X
3					X	X					X								X		
4	X	X																			
5	X	X								X											
6	X	X	X		X	X						X			X					X	
7	**X**	X	X	X	X		**X**	**X**			X		X		X	X					
8	X	X	X	X	X	X	X	X	X	X	X	X	X	X	X		X	X	X		
9	X																				
10	X	X		X																	X
11	X	X	X					X		X											
12	X		X																		
13	X	X	**X**	X			X	X		X	X	**X**	X	X		X	X	X		X	
14	X		X	X	X	X															
15	X	X				X															
17	X	X					X	X	X				X			X		X			X
18	X					X															
19	X								X												
24	X		X		X		X							X							
25	X																				
26									X			X					X				

Diplopia, Horizontal

	AUR	CAUST	LYC
19	X		
26	X	X	X

Discharge, Ear, From- See Otorrhoea

Discoloration, Face, Blue- See also Circulation, Cyanosis (Includes Spots)

	ARG N	NAT M	OP	CACT	CAMPH	CHLOR	CIC	CROT H	CUPR	DIG	HYDR AC	HYOSC	IPEC	KALI IOD	PHYTO	PULS	SAMB	SPONG	TAB	VER A
6										X										
7	X	X	X		X	X	X	X	X		X			X	X	X	X	X	X	X
13		X	X																	
15	X			X								X	X							

Discoloration, Face, Green (Includes Spots)

	ARS	CARB V	VER A	ARN	FERR IOD	CON	LACH	SEP	SULPH
5				X		X	X	X	
7	X	X	X		X				X
13	X	X	X						

Discoloration, Face, Yellow (Includes Spots)

	SEP	LYC	ARS	CHEL	NUX V	CHINA	IOD	ARN	FERR	HEP	LACH	MERC	NAT M	ARG N	BRY	CALC	CANTH	CAUST	MAG M	PLUM
1	X																			
6	X	X	X		X	X	X	X	X				X							
7	X	**X**	X	**X**	X	**X**			X	X	X	**X**	X	**X**	X	**X**	X	X	X	X
8	X	X		X			X	X			X									
10	X									X										
12	X																			
13	**X**	**X**	**X**		**X**	X	**X**	X	X	X	X	**X**	X		**X**	X	**X**	**X**	**X**	**X**
14	X		X	X																
17	X																			
19				X																
21	X																			
24	X													X						
26	**X**	X			X															
28	X																			

Discoloration, Skin- See all Discoloration entries also Erythema; Jaundice; Liver Spots; Vitiligo

Discoloration, Skin, Black (Includes Spots)

	ARS	CROT H	SULPH AC	ARG N	ARS IOD	AETHUSA	CARB V	FERR	LACH	PHELL	PLUM	RHUS T	SEC	VIP
1	X		X		X	X			X					
3	X				X									
5	X	X	X	X			X				X		X	X
7	X	X	X					X						
8		X								X				
13	X	X		X								X		

Discoloration, Skin, Blue- See also Circulation, Cyanosis (Includes Spots)

	ARS	LACH	VER A	CARB V	OP	DIG	IRIS V	LED	MANG	NUV M	NUX V	PHOS	SEC	SULPH	SULPH AC
1	X						X								
3	X	X					X								
5	X	X	X	X	X	X					X	X	X		
7	X	X							X	X					
8								X	X	X				X	X
13	X	X	**X**	X	**X**	**X**		X			X	X	X	X	X
14	X	X	X	X											

Discoloration, Skin, Brown- See also Skin, Discoloration, Copper; Skin, Discoloration, Yellow (Includes Spots)

	SEP	THUJA	NIT AC	IOD	PHOS	PLUM	SULPH	ARS	CARB A	CON	HYOSC	LYC	PETR	ARS I	BELL	NAT M	MERC
1				X													
5	X	X	X	X	X	X			X	X						X	
6		X	X						X				X				
7	X	X	X	X		X	X	X	X	X	X			X	X		
8	X			X	X						X		X	X		X	
9	X							X									
12					X												
13	**X**	X	**X**		X	X	**X**	X		X	X	X	X				**X**
14		X										X					
15															X		
17	X																
21						X											
24							X										
25	X																
26												X					

Discoloration, Skin, Copper- See also Discoloration, Skin, Brown

	NIT AC	CARB A	KREO	LACH	MEZ	RHUS T	ARG N	ARS	BELL	CARB V	COR R	MERC D	RUTA
5	X	X	X	X	X	X							
6	X	X											
7	X	X					X				X		
13	X		X	X	X	X		X		X			X
14												X	
15									X				

Discoloration, Skin, Green (Includes Spots)

	ARN	CON	CARB V	LACH	SEP	SULPH	VER A	ZINC
3		X						
5	X	X		X	X			
7						X		
13	X		X				X	
17								X

Discoloration, Skin, Grey

	LYC	ARS	BOR	BRY	BUFO	CANTH	CARB V	CHEL	CHINA	CROC	IGN	IPEC	KREO	LACH	MERC	NUX V	SAMB	SEP	SIL
7					X			X											
13	X	X	X	X		X	X		X	X	X	X	X	X	X	X	X	X	X
15	X																		

Discoloration, Skin, Purple- See also Discoloration, Skin, Blue (Includes Spots)

	LACH	APIS	CROT H	FERR	RHUS T	VER A
1	X					
3	X					
5	X					
6			X			
7		X		X		
13	X					X
14	X				X	

Discoloration, Skin, White- See also Vitiligo (Includes Spots)

	ARS	BERB V	CALC	SEP	SIL	ALUM	APIS	AUR	CLEM	FL AC	KALI CAR	MERC	NAT CAR	PHOS	PIPER M
5	X	X	X	X	X	X	X	X		X	X	X	X	X	
7		X	X												
8	X			X	X										X
13									X						

Discoloration, Skin, Yellow (Includes Spots)

	MERC	PLUM	BRY	CHINA	DIG	NIT AC	CROT H	PHOS	RHUS T	SEP	IOD	NUX V	ARS	CALC	CARB V	CAUST	CHAM	CHEL	FERR	HEP	MEZ	MYRICA	PULS	SIL	SULPH	THUJA	CON	SEC
5									X												X							
6	X	X	X	X			X		X						X								X					
7	**X**	**X**	X		X	**X**	X					X	X	X				X	X	X		X		X	X	X		
10										X						X												
13	**X**	**X**	X	**X**	**X**	X		X	X	X	**X**	**X**	X	X	X	X	X		X	X	X		X	X	X	X	**X**	**X**
14					X	X	X	X			X							X				X						
15	X		X														X											
16				X																								
19										X																		
21		X						X																				

Dislocation

	ARN	RUTA	RHUS T	AGNUS	BRY	FORMICA	CALC	LYC	NAT CAR	NAT M	PETR	PHOS	AMM C	BELL	CARB A	CALC FL	IGN	MERC	NIT AC	NUX V	PULS	SULPH
2		X		X		X																
7	X	X	**X**	X	X	X	**X**	**X**	**X**	**X**	**X**	**X**	X	X	X		X	X	X	X		X
8																					X	
9	X	X	X																			
10	X																					
20	**X**																					
21		X																				
24	X		X																			
26	X		X		X																	
27		X														X						

Dislocation, Easy- See also Jaw, Dislocation, Easy; Sprain, Easy; Weakness, Ligaments

	RHUS T	CARB A	PHOS	NAT CAR	CALC	NUX V	RUTA	LYC	ACON	AGNUS	ARN	BELL	BOV	BRY	CANN S	CALC FL	HEP	MAG P A	NAT M	NIT AC	PETR	PULS	SULPH	TEUCR
2																		X						
7	X	X	X	**X**	X	X	X	X												X	X		X	
8																						X		
9		X																						
13	X	X	X	X	X	X	X	X		X	X	X	X	X	X		X		X					X
14									X															
24	X		X																					
28																X								

Dislocation, Easy, Hip

	CALC	RHUS T	SULPH	BELL	COLOC	BRY	CAUST	CHINA	LYC	MERC	PULS	ZINC
3	**X**	X	**X**	X								
13	X	**X**	X	**X**	X	X	X	X	X	X	X	X

Dislocation, Easy, Jaw

	PETR	RHUS T	STAPHYS
2	**X**		X
3	X		
24		X	

Distension, Abdomen– See also Flatulence (Includes Bloating; Meteorism; Tympany)

	LYC	CARB V	CHINA	BELL	NUX V	PULS	ARG N	ARS	BRY	CHAM	COLOC	SULPH	CALC	COCCUL	VER A	COLCH	OP	ACON	LACH	NUX M	KALI CAR	MERC	PH AC	IGN	PHOS	RHUS T	SEP	SIL
1	X	X	X	X		X	X		X	X			X	X		X	X	X	X							X		X
2	**X**	**X**	X			**X**								X			X											
3	X	X			X	X		X				X	X								X							
4	X	X	X	X	X			X	X			X	X	X	X					**X**	X		X					
5		X					X																					
6	X	X	X	X	X			X	X	X	X	X	X	X	X	X	X	X	X		X	X	X	X	X	X	X	
7	**X**	**X**	**X**		X	X	X	X	X	X	**X**	X	X	X		**X**	X		X	X	X	X		X	X		X	X
8	X	X	**X**	X	X	**X**	X	X	X	X	X	**X**	X	X	X	X	X	X	X	X	X	X	X	X	X	X	X	
9	X	X	X		X	X		X							X			X										
10	X	X	X	X	X	X	X	X		X		X	X	X		X			X			X	X		X	X	X	
11	X	X		X		X	X	X					X			X						X	X					X
12	X			X	X			X	X		X	X																
13	X	**X**	X	X	X	X		X	X	X	**X**	X	X	X	X	X	**X**	X	X	X	X	X	X	X	X	X	X	X
14	X	X	X	X	X		X													X								X
15			X	X	X	X		X	X	X	X							X				X		X				
16			X														X											
17							X														X							
18	X		X									X								X								
19	X	X	X				X			X				X		X												
20	X	X			X																							
21	X		X	X			X		X	X	X							X	X					X			X	
22	X	X			X					X	X																	
23							X																					
24	X	X	X	X		X	X			X	X		X		X		X	X	X	X								X
25									X						X													
26	X	X	X	X	X	X		X	X		X	X		X	X								X		X	X		
27	X		X	X											X													
28	X	X																										

Diuresis– See Urination, Profuse

Diverticulitis

	LYC	NUX V	BELL	CHAM	COLOC	DIOSC	IRIS V	PULS	THUJA	VER A
11						X		X	X	
27	**X**	**X**	X	X	X		X			X

Dizzyness- See Vertigo

Drowsiness- See Stupor

Drugs, Addiction To

	ARS	NUX V	ABSINTH	ACON	ARG N	ASAR	AVENA	BRY	CAPS	CHAM	HYOSC	LACH	RHUS T
5					X								
9		X				X			X				
21	X		X	X							X	X	
29*	X	X					X	X		X			X

29* Rai Y. Treatment of Drug Dependants with Homoeopathy. CCRH Quarterly Bull, 1994, 16, 3&4, 25-28.

Duodenum, Ailments Of

	ARS	BERB V	POD	RHEUM	RICIN
2	**X**	X	**X**	X	X

Dupuytren's Contracture- See also Contracture, Fingers

	GELS	CALC FL	CAUST	LAPPA	THIO
2	**X**			X	
3			X		
21	X	X			X
28		X			

Dysentery

	MERC C	SULPH	ALOE	ARS	COLOC	MERC	NUX V	ACON	IPEC	COLCH	BELL	CANTH	TROMB	RHUS T	BAPT	CAPS	NIT AC	ARN	CARB V	PULS	KALI BIC	PHOS	DIOSC	FERR PH	STAPHYS	DULC
1	**X**	X	X		X		X			X			X													
2	**X**	**X**	**X**		**X**	X	**X**	X	X	X	X	X	X	**X**	X	X	**X**	X	X				X	X	X	X
3	X	X	X	X	X	X	X	X	X			X	X		X						X	X		X		
4	**X**	**X**	X	**X**	X			**X**		X	X	**X**												X		
5			X	X																		X				
6		X	X	X	X	X	X	X	X	X	X	X	X	X	X	X	X		X	X	X		X	X	X	
7	**X**	**X**	**X**	**X**	**X**	**X**	**X**	X		**X**	**X**	**X**	**X**	**X**	X	**X**	X	**X**	X	X	**X**	**X**	X			X
8	X	X	X	X	X	X	X	X	X	X	X	X	X	X	X	X	X	X	X	X	X	X	X	X	X	X
9	X		X						X				X													
10	X	X	X	X	X	X	X	X			X			X												
11	X	X	X	X	X	**X**	X		X	X	X	X	X			X		X		X	X			X		
12	X	X	X	X	X	X	X	X	X	X	X			X	X		X		X			X	X			
13	**X**	**X**	X	X	**X**	**X**	X	**X**	**X**	**X**	X	**X**	X	X		**X**	X		X		X				X	
14	**X**	X	X			**X**	X		X					X	X			X		X						X
15	**X**			**X**			X	X	**X**						**X**		X			X		X	X			
18	X																	X								X
19																		X							X	
23	X	X	X	X	X		X	X	X				X		X	X										
24	X	X		X	X	X		X				X				X			X							
26	**X**	X		X	X	X		**X**	X	X	X			X						X					X	

Dysentery, Amoebic

	IPEC	ALOE	COLOC	EMETINE	MERC C	MERC	THUJA
1							X
3	X	X	X		X		
9	X						
11	X						
14	X			X			
17	X					X	

Dyslexia- See also Aphasia

	LYC	CON	STRAM	COLCH	GRAPH	LACH	MEPH	NUX V
1		X			X		X	
6	X		X					
8	X	X	X	X		X		X
10	X							
14	X							
21	X							

Dysmenorrhoea- See also Pain, Ovaries; Premenstrual Syndrome (AKA Menstrual Colic)

	PULS	MAG PH	CHAM	BELL	VIB OP	SEP	COCCUL	COLOC	NUX V	CIMICI	CAULO	GELS	SULPH	XANTHO	IGN	CALC	LACH	VER A	CUPR	GRAPH	MAG CAR	PLAT	CACT	PHOS	CYCL	SABIN	SEC	BROM
1	X	**X**	X		X	X		X	X		X		X	X				X	X		X	X		X		X	X	
2	X	**X**	X		**X**	X	**X**	X			X	**X**		**X**	X			X		X		X	**X**			X		X
3		X	X		X	X	X	X					X	X			X				X							
4	**X**	**X**	X	**X**	**X**	X	**X**	**X**		**X**	**X**	**X**		**X**	X							X						
5	X		X	X		X										X				X							X	
6	X		X	X	X	X	X	X	X	X	X		X	X		X	X		X	X	X	X	X	X	X			X
7	**X**	**X**	**X**	**X**	**X**	**X**	**X**	**X**	X		**X**	**X**	**X**	X	X	X	X	**X**		**X**	X	X	X	**X**	X	X	X	**X**
8	**X**		**X**	**X**	X	X	X		**X**				X	X	X	X	X	X	**X**	**X**	X	X		X	X		X	
9	X	X	X	X	X	X				X		X	X															
10	X	X	X	X		X	**X**		X	X	X	X	X			X	X	X				X						
13	X												X			X				X	X			X				
14	X	X		X	X	X			X	X								X	X						X	X		
15	X		X	X		X	X		X	X		X			X	X							X	X				
16	X	X		X	X			X	X	X						X			X									
18	X	X	X		X	X		X	X	X	X				X		X	X			X				X	X	X	X
19					X		X																					
20	X	X	**X**	X				X		X	X																	
21	X	X	X	X	X				X	X		X											X					
23	X	X			X			X				X		X											X			X
24																	X											
25	X	X	X	X	X					X		X	X															
26	**X**		X	X		X	**X**		X		X				**X**				**X**									
27	**X**	X		X		**X**		X	X		X				X		X									X		
28								X																				

Dysmenorrhoea, Membranous

	BOR	CHAM	KALI BIC	USTIL	VIB OP	ACET AC	BROM	BRY	CALC	CANTH	COLLIN	CYCL	GRAPH	GUAIA	LAC C	MAG PH	MILL	PHYTO	RHUS T
4	X			X	X									X		X			
7		X	X					X	X						X				X
8	X	X	X	X	X	X	X			X	X		X				X	X	
18												X							

Dyspareunia

	NAT M	THUJA	FERR	PLAT	SEP	SPIRA	STAPHYS	STROPH
2	X	X	X			X		X
18	X							
21	X	X		X	X		X	

Dyspepsia- See also Hyperacidity; Indigestion

	NUX V	CARB V	PULS	ARS	LYC	SULPH	KALI CAR	CALC	BRY	HYDRAST	ANAC	KALI BIC	SEP	ABIES N	ANT C	ARG N	NAT M	PHOS	CHINA	ROBIN	SANG	NUX M	LACH
1	X	X	X		X	X	X	X			X		X	X	X			X		X		X	
2	**X**	**X**	**X**	**X**	**X**		**X**	**X**	**X**	**X**	X	**X**	X	**X**	**X**	**X**	**X**		X	X	**X**	X	X
3	X	X	X	X	X		X				X	X		X		X			X	X			
4	**X**	**X**	X	X		**X**	X	X		X		X				X		X					
5	X	X	X					X	X	X	X		X	X									
6	X	X	X	X	X	X	X		X	X		X	X				X	X	X		X		X
7	**X**	**X**	**X**	**X**	X	X	X	**X**	**X**	**X**	X	**X**	X	X	X	X	X	**X**	X	X	X	X	**X**
8	**X**	**X**	X	X	X	**X**	X	X	X	X	X	X	X	X	X	X	X	X	X	X	X	X	X
9	X	X	X	X	X	X		X	X								X						
10	X	X	X	X		X		X	X	X	X				X	X			X				X
11																X							
12	**X**	X	X	X	X	X		X	X		X	X			X			X	X	X			
13																					X		
14	X	X	X	X	X										X								
15	X																						
17	X		X				X									X	X					X	
18					X		X						X							X			
23	X	X				X	X						X	X			X	X				X	
24			X	X						X													
25				X		X																	
28	X	X			X																		

Dyspepsia, Flatulent

	LYC	NUX M	NUX V	ARG N	CARB V	HEP	HYDRAST	SAL AC	ALET	ANAC	ANT C	CALC PH	CHINA	DIOSC	GRAPH	KALI CAR	LACH	MERC	PHOS	PULS	URAN N
1												X									
2								X													
3	X		X		X		X		X				X								
4			X																		
5		X																			
7	X	X		X		X	X										X		X	X	X
8	X			X		X		X		X											
12	X		X		X						X										
14		X																			
15																		X			
17		X																			
18															X	X					
24														X							

Dyspepsia, Nervous

	ANAC	ARG N	AUR M N	CARB AC	CUPR AR	GINSENG	HELON	KALI PH	NICCOL
2								X	
8		X							
10	X								
23			X	X	X	X	X		X

Dyspepsia, Senile

	CARB V	ABIES	ALL S	AMM C	ANT C	BAR C	CHINA	CIC	KALI CAR	NUX M	NUX V	VIP T
8	X		X	X	X	X	X	X	X	X	X	X
9		X										
10	X											
12	X											
14		X										

Dysphagia- See also Oesophagitis; Stricture, Oesophagus; Stenosis, Oesophagus

	BELL	LACH	BAR C	IGN	HYOSC	PHYTO	GELS	NIT AC	APIS	STRAM	HEP	MERC	RHUS T	ACON	CANTH	CIC	BRY	KALI CAR	CAUST	NUX V	ARS	IOD	LYC	MERC C	SIL
1	X	X		X	X	X	X	X	X	X	X		X	X		X		X	X			X	X	X	
4	X	X						X	X																
5	X																				X				
6	X	X	X	X	X	X	X	X	X	X		X	X	X	X	X		X	X		X		X		X
7	X	**X**	X	X	X	X	X	**X**	X	X	X	X	X		X	X	X	**X**	X	X	X	X	X		
8	**X**	**X**	X	X	X			X	X	X	**X**	**X**	**X**	X	X	X	**X**		X	**X**	X	X	X		X
9	X	X	X	X	X												X								
10					X						X			X			X								
11	X	X	X	X	X	X		X		X			X		X	X		X		X				X	
12	X																								
13	**X**	X		**X**	X		X		X	X	X	X	X	X	X	X	X	X	X	X	X	X	X		X
14	X	X	X			X			X		X				X				X					X	
15	X			X	X		X		X			X		X											
17	X	X	X		X	X	X	X		X			X	X	X			X		X		X		X	X
18	X	X				X																		X	
19		X	X	X			X																		
20	X	X				X																			
21		X		X		X	X	X		X															
22			X									X													
24	X					X	X									X									
25	X	X	X									X													
27	X		X								X														X

Dyspnoea (Includes Breathing, Oppressed; Breathlessness; Wheezing)

	ARS	IPEC	ANT T	CARB V	ACON	PHOS	NUX V	KALI CAR	LACH	APIS	CACT	SPONG	BRY	SULPH	CALC	AMM C	CUPR	GLON	IOD	SAMB	BELL	LOB I	LYC	NIT AC	PSOR	PULS	FERR	SENEG
1	X		X	X		X	X		X	X	X		X		X	X		X	X	X	X	X	X	X	X	X	X	X
2					X												X											
3	X		X			X	X				X					X												
4	**X**	X	X	X		X		X	X	X	X		X	X			X	X	X	X				X				
5	X	X	X	X	X	X	X	X	X			X				X	X			X		X	X	X	X			X
6	X	X	X	X	X	X		X	X	X	X		X	X	X	X	X	X	X		X	X	X		X	X	X	X
7	**X**	X	X	X		**X**	X	**X**	**X**	**X**	X	X		X	X		X	X	X		X	X	**X**	X	X		**X**	
8	**X**	**X**	X	X	X	X	X	X	**X**	**X**	X	X	X	X	X	X	X	X	X	X		**X**	X	X	X	X	X	X
9	X	X	X		X			X	X	X																	X	
10	X	X	X	X	X		X	X	X	X		X	X	X	X	X	X	X			X				X	X		
11	X	X	X		X		X			X	X		X	X	X	X		X			X	X		X				
12	X	X	X		X	X						X	X	X					X	X		X						
13	X	**X**	X	**X**	X	**X**	X	X	X		X	X	**X**	**X**	X	X	X		X	X	**X**		X	X	X	X	X	**X**
14	X	X		X	X	X	X				X		X		X								X					
15	X	X	X	X	X	X	X				X	X	X	X	X											X		
16		X	X																									
17	X		X	X	X	X	X	X	X	X	X	X	X	X	X	X	X	X	X	X	X	X	X	X	X	X	X	X
18	X	X	X	X		X		X	X	X										X								X
19	X	X	X	X	X	X		X	X		X	X			X	X			X	X		X				X	X	X
20			X	X																								
21	X	X		X	X		X				X	X				X		X							X			
22		X	X	X			X			X		X																
24	X						X			X		X		X							X			X				
25		X	X		X	X		X										X										
26	X	X		X	X	X	X	X	X				X	X	X		X			X	X		X			X		
27	X				X			X				X							X									

Dysuria (Includes Strangury)

	CANTH	PULS	NUX V	ACON	SARS	SULPH	TEREB	APIS	CAMPH	CANN S	BERB V	COP	ARS	BELL	STAPHYS	PARIERA	THUJA	CHIM	EQUISET	HEP	LYC	MERC	MERC C	CLEM	NAT M	NIT AC		
1	X	X	X	X	X	X	X	X	X	X		X		X	X	X	X	X		X		X		X	X	X		
2	**X**				X		**X**		**X**					**X**		X												
3	X		X				X				X	X	X	X	X		X		X									
4	**X**		X	X		X	X			X		**X**		X		X	X		X				X					
6	X	X	X	X		X	X	X		X	X	X	X	X	X	X		X		X	X				X	X		
7	**X**	X	X	X	**X**	X	**X**	X	X	**X**	X	X	X	X	X	X	X	X	X	X	X	X	**X**	X	X	X		
8	**X**	X	X	X	X	X	X	X	X	**X**	X	X	X	X	X	X	X	X	X	X	X	X	X	X	X	X		
9	X		X					X																				
10	X	X	X	X		X			X				X	X						X		X	X					
11	X	X			X			X		X	X	X						X					X					
12	X	X	X	X	X				X				X	X							X			X				
13	**X**	**X**	X		X	X	X		X	**X**	X	X	X		**X**	X	X			X	X	X	X	X	X	X		
14	X	X		X	X	X	X	X	X	X							X	X										
15	X	X		X		X																						
17	X								X																			
18	X		X		X	X							X		X	X			X									
19	X	X			X		X	X	X	X	X	X	X		X					X								
20	X	X	X	X	X			X			X											X			X			
21				X			X		X		X		X															
22				X				X			X								X									
23	X																	X	X									
24	X	X	X		X	X	X	X			X	X			X		X				X			X		X		
25	X							X																				
26	X	X	X	**X**		X				X											X	X						
27					X	X																						
28	X																											

Dysuria, Pregnancy From- See Pregnancy, Dysuria From

Ear, Disorders Of

	CALC	CAPS	SIL	ACON	BELL	FERR PH	GRAPH	HEP	HYDRAST	KALI MUR	NIT AC	SULPH	AUR	MERC D	PULS	ARS	CHIN S	COLCH	CROT T	MANCIN	MERC	MEZ	PETR					
2	**X**	**X**	X	**X**	**X**	**X**	**X**	**X**	**X**	**X**	**X**	**X**	X			**X**	**X**	**X**	**X**	**X**	**X**	**X**	**X**					
4	X	X	X	X	X	X	X	X	X	X	X	X	X	X	X													
9			X											X	X													
12		X																										
25	X																											

Earache- See Otalgia

Eardrum, Perforation Of- See Tympanic Membrane, Perforation Of

Ears, Dry- See Earwax, Deficiency Of

Earwax, Accumulation Of

	CON	LACH	CARB V	CAUST	HEP	PETR	CALC	ELAPS	MUR AC	SIL	GRAPH	KALI CAR	PSOR	PULS	SEL	THUJA
1	X															
2		X						X								
3	X															
4	X															
6	X					X			X							
7	X	X	X	X	X	X	X	X	X	X		X	X	X		
8	X	X	X	X	X	X	X			X	X				X	X
13	**X**				X					X					X	
14	X															
17	X	X	X	X	X		X	X				X	X	X		X
21				X												
24	X	X	X			X			X		X					
26	**X**															

Earwax, Deficiency Of

	CARB V	GRAPH	LACH	PETR	CALC	CARB A	CAUST	COLCH	LAC C	MUR AC	NIT AC	NUX V	SPONG	SULPH
6	X	X	X				X							
7	X			X								X		
8	X		X			X				X				
10	X		X											
12		X											X	X
13		**X**	X	X				X	X		X			
14		X												
26	X				X									

Eclampsia

	BELL	CUPR	VER V	CIC	IGN	CHAM	GELS	HYOSC	NUX M	OP	PHOS	PLAT	STRAM	ACON	AETHUSA	AMBRA	CHIN S	CHLOR	COFF	NUX V	OENANTH	PULS	SEC	CINA
2			X	X			X		X	X	X					X	X	X			X	X		
4		X									X													
6	X	X	X		X		X	X		X		X	X				X							
8		X	X						X						X	X								
13	X			X	X	X			X		X	X	**X**							X				**X**
17	X	X	X	X		X		X						X				X	X	X	X	X	X	
19	X	X		X																				
23					X										X									
26	**X**		X		X	X	X	X		X		X		X					X				X	

Ecthyma- See also Impetigo

	ANT T	MERC	RHUS T	ARS	JUG C	SIL	SULPH	ANT C	CIC	CROT T	KALI BIC	LYC	NIT AC	SEC	THUJA
2	**X**	**X**	**X**		X										
6	X	X		X			X	X	X		X	X	X	X	
7			X	X	X	X				X					
8	X	X	X	X	X	X	X	X	X	X	X		X	X	X
26	X	X	X	X		X	X					X			X

Ectropion

	APIS	ARG N	HAM	MERC	BELL	MERC C	NIT AC	RHUS T	SULPH	BOR	EUPHR	HEP	LYC
6	X	X	X			X		X					
7	X	X	X	X			X		X				X
8	X	X	X	X	X		X						
12				X					X		X		
14	X												
21										X			
24	X	X	X			X		X					
26				X	X							X	

Eczema- See also Dermatitis, Atopic

	GRAPH	SULPH	ARS	RHUS T	PETR	LYC	MEZ	PSOR	CALC	HEP	NAT M	CROT T	CIC	VIOL T	ANT C	MERC	SEP	CALC SUL	THUJA	DULC	OLEAND	ALUM	ANAC	HYSRAST	LED	BOV
1	X	X	X	X	X	X	X	X	X	X	X		X		X			X	X			X				X
2	**X**	**X**	**X**	X	X	**X**		X		**X**		X	**X**	**X**	**X**	X	**X**	X			**X**	X	X	X	X	**X**
3	X	X		X	X	X	X		X		X	X	X		X		X		X			X	X	X	X	X
4	**X**	X	**X**	X	X			X	X		X	**X**							X							
5	X		X	X	X	X	X				X			X	X					X			X	X		
6	X	X	X	X		X			X	X	X	X	X	X	X	X			X		X		X			
7	**X**	**X**	**X**	X	**X**	**X**	X	**X**	**X**	**X**	X	**X**		X	X	X	X	X	X	**X**	X		X	X	X	
8	X	X	X	X	X	X	X	X	X	X	X	X	X	X	X	X	X	X	X	X	X	X	X	X	X	X
9	X	X	X	X	X		X	X		X	X		X													
10	X	X	**X**	X	X	X	X	X	X	X	X					X	X		X	X		X				
11	X	X	X	X	X		X	X	X	X		X	X					X		X	X				X	
12		X	X	X		X			X	X		X		X		X										
14	X	X	X	X	X	X	X		X		X			X											X	
15	**X**	X		**X**												**X**	X			X				X	X	
16																						X				
17																		X								
18	X	X	X	X	X	X	X		X		X	X		X	X		X									
19	**X**	**X**	**X**	X	**X**	X	X	**X**	X	X	X		X			X	X	X	X	X	X					
21	X	X	X	X	X	X	X	X		X				X												
23	X				X			X			X	X	X	X				X			X		X	X		X
25	X	**X**	X	X	X		X	X																		
27	X	X	X		X	X	X	X		X			X		X							X				X
28	X																									
29*						X	**X**	X	X								X									

29* Van Wassenhoven M. Clinical verification in homeopathy and allergic conditions. Homeopathy. 2013 Jan;102 (1):54-8.

Eczema, Anus

	BERB V	GRAPH	NIT AC	PETR	SEP	STAPHYS
5	X	X		X		X
7			X			
14	X	X				
19					X	

Eczema, Back

	BOV	BROM	CALC	LYC	PSOR	PULS	SIL
7		X	X	X	X		X
8	X						
19						X	

Eczema Capitis- See also Eczema, Head

	GRAPH	KALI MUR	CIC	LYC	MEZ	SULPH
4		**X**				
8	X		X			X
14	X			X	X	

Eczema, Cheeks

	ANT C	CALC	LED
5	X	X	
14			X

Eczema, Chin

	CIC	GRAPH	BOR	RHUT T	SEP
5	X				
8	X	X	X	X	X
14		X			
27	X				

Eczema, Dry

	ARS	PETR	ALUM	SEP	CALC	GRAPH	PSOR	RHUS T
1			X				X	X
5	X	X	X	X				
8	X			X	X			
10		X	X		X		X	
14	X							
15						X		
18		X		X		X		
19	X	X			X	X		
25								X
27	X	X	X					

Eczema, Ear

	LYC	GRAPH	PETR	CALC	LACH	MERC	OLEAND	APIS	BAR C	HEP	KALI MUR	MERC	MEZ	NIT AC	RHUS T	SCROPH	STRONT N	SULPH	TELL	THUJA								
1	X												X						X									
2	X																X											
4			X								X																	
6	X	X	X	X			X		X	X		X		X	X			X										
8	X		X													X				X								
10		X		X	X	X		X																				
21	X																											
24		X																										
26		X	X		X	X	X																					

Eczema, Ear, Behind

	GRAPH	LYC	PETR	CALC	CAUST	OLEAND	SEP	BAR C	CARB A	CIC	HEP	KALI CAR	NIT AC	SIL	STAPHYS	SULPH	TUB											
1	X																											
5	X																											
6	X						X																					
8	X	X	X	X	X	X	X		X	X		X	X	X	X													
9	X																											
10	X		X														X											
12					X																							
14		X																										
18	X																											
19	X																											
21	X	X																										
24	X																											
25	X																											
26	X	X	X	X		X		X			X					X												
27		X	X																									

Eczema, Ear, In Front Of

	TEREB
6	X
24	X

Eczema, Extremities, Flexures Of

	GRAPH	MERC	SEP	SULPH	AMM C	BRY	LED	PSOR	RHUS T	NAT M	AETHUSA	BAR C	BERB V	CALC	LYC	MANG	PETR	SYPH	TUB
1					X	X													
6	X	X	X	X			X							X					
8	X	X	X	X	X	X	X												
10	X							X		X		X						X	X
14	X								X	X	X		X				X		
19		X	X	X				X	X						X	X			

Eczema, Eyelids

	GRAPH	BACIL	MEZ	NAT M	TELL
1			X		
6					X
14	X	X			
18	X			X	

Eczema, Face

	GRAPH	RHUS T	CALC	LYC	CROT T	HEP	ARS	CIC	SULPH	VINCA	VIOL T	BOR	CLEM	DULC	IRIS V	MERC	PSOR	SEP	STAPHYS
5										X	X								
6	X	X	X	X	X	X	X	X	X		X	X	X	X	X	X		X	X
7	**X**	X	X	X	**X**	**X**	X	X	X			X			X		X		
8	X	X	X	X	X	X	X	X	X	X	X		X	X		X	X	X	X
10	X	X	X	X															
14	X	X								X									
18	X																		
19	X																		

Eczema, Feet

	APIS	SULPH
10	X	
19		X

Eczema, Feet and Toes

	GRAPH	PETR
5	X	X
18	X	

Eczema, Fingers (Includes Eczema, Fingers, Between)

	BOR	MERC	NAT M	PETR	SEP	SULPH	AGAR M	ANAG	ARS	BERB V	BOV	CARB V	CIC	LYC	PULS	SEL	STILL
1									X								
5	X			X			X	X		X						X	X
10		X			X	X											
14	X																
15															X		
18			X								X						
19			X	X									X	X			
26		X			X	X						X					

Eczema, Forehead

	RHUS T	LED	MERC	NIT AC	PETR	SARS	SEP	SULPH
5	X			X	X	X		
8	X		X				X	X
14		X						

Eczema, Genitals

	GRAPH	RHUS T	NAT M	CROT T	SEP	LYC	ARG N	ARS	CALAD	CANTH	HEP	NIT AC	PETR	PH AC	SULPH	THUJA	ANT C
5				X													
6	X	X	X	X	X	X	X	X	X		X	X	X		X	X	
8	X	X	X	X	X	X	X	X	X		X	X	X		X	X	
9	X									X							
10		X	X			X								X			
14	X	X								X				X			
18	X																
19		X	X		X												
27																	X

Eczema, Hands (Includes Eczema, Hands, Backs of; Eczema, Palms)

	GRAPH	RHUS T	BERB V	PETR	ARS	LYC	MERC	SEP	SULPH	BOV
1	X				X					X
5			X							
8	X		X		X	X				
9		X								
10	X	X		X			X	X	X	
14	X		X	X						
19				X		X				
21	X	X								
25		X								
26							X	X	X	
27	X									X

Eczema, Head- See also Eczema Capitis

	GRAPH	MEZ
1		X
6	X	
19		X
24	X	

Eczema, Joints, Around

	GRAPH	SEP	NAT M	PSOR	AETHUSA	AMM C	BRY	CALC	LED	MANG AC	MERC	NAT PH	PH AC	SIL	SULPH
5	X	X								X		X		X	
6	X	X				X	X	X	X		X				X
10	X		X	X											
14			X		X										
15		X											X		
25				X											

Eczema, Legs

	GRAPH	MERC	ARS	CARB V	LACH	LYC	NAT M	RHUS T	SULPH	CALC	PETR	PSOR	PULS	SARS	SEP	SIL
6	X	X	X	X	X	X	X	X	X	X			X	X	X	X
8	X	X	X	X	X	X	X		X							
10		X						X								
14	X										X					
21												X				

Eczema, Lips

	GRAPH	ALUM	SEP	APIS	KALI CAR	PHOS
1	X					
10	X	X	X	X		
26	X	X	X		X	X

Eczema, Moist

	GRAPH	RHUS T	MEZ	DULC	CALC	HEP	MERC	NAT M	SULPH	CLEM	LYC	PSOR	SEP	ARS	CAUST	KALI BR	PETR	PHYTO	SIL	VINCA
1	X																			
5	X	X		X			X			X					X					
6	X	X			X	X														
7	X	X	X	X		X	X	X	X	X	X		X			X		X	X	X
8	X	X	X	X	X	X	X	X	X	X	X		X			X		X	X	X
9	X																			
10	X	X	X	X	X	X		X				X					X			
15							X							X	X					
18	X		X														X			
19		X						X	X		X	X	X							
25	X		X																	
26	X	X	X	X	X				X					X						
27	X											X								

Eczema, Mouth, Around

	GRAPH	LYC	ANT C	ARUM T	HEP	MANG	RHUS T	SEP	SIL
5	X		X						
8	X	X		X	X		X		X
19		X				X		X	

Eczema, Neck

	CALC	PULS
7	X	
19		X

Eczema, Nose

	GRAPH	SEP	ALUM	ANT C	APIS	CALC SUL	CAUST	CIST	KALI CAR	MANG	PHOS
8								X			
10	X	X	X		X		X				
14	X			X							
19		X				X				X	
24	X										
26	X	X	X						X		X

Eczema, Penis- See Eczema, Genitals

Eczema, Perineum

	PETR	NIT AC
6	X	
7	X	X

Eczema, Scalp

	MEZ	NAT M	CALC	GRAPH	LYC	KALI BIC	LAPPA	VINCA	ARS	BOR	BROM	CALC SUL	CIC	IRIS V	OLEAND	PSOR	RHUS T	SULPH
1		X				X												
5	X		X				X											
8			X	X	X		X	X	X	X	X			X				X
9	X			X														
10		X	X													X	X	
14	X				X	X		X										
18	X	X																
19		X			X							X	X		X			
21	X																	
25	X			X														
27	X																	

Eczema, Scrotum- See Eczema, Genitals

Eczema, Weeping- See Eczema, Moist

Eczema, Wrist

	RHUS T	JUG C
19		X
21	X	
25	X	

Effusion, Pleural

	BRY	ARS	SULPH	CANTH	IOD	APIS	APOC	ARN	HELL	KALI IOD	RAN B	SENEG	DIG	KALI CAR	ASC T	BELL	CHINA	COLCH	FERR PH	HEP	MERC	PHOS						
1			X	X	X																							
3		X				X	X																					
6									X																			
7	**X**	X	X	X																X								
8	X	X								X	X				X			X										
10	X	X	X																									
11	X	**X**	X	X	X	X	X					X	**X**	**X**					X		X							
12		X			X			X																				
16	X				X	X			X								X											
17	X	X	X	X	X	X		X		X	X	X	X	X	X	X	X	X	X	X	X	X						
18	X			X				X																				
19							X																					
23									X																			
24	X	X	**X**	X	X					X	X	X				X						X						
28	X																											

Effusion, Serous Membranes

	APIS	ARS	BRY	APOC	COLCH	HELL	JAB	KALI IOD	KALI MUR	KALI SUL	LYC	MERC	MERC C	NAT M	SAMB	SULPH	URT U											
7	**X**	**X**	**X**	X					X	X	X			X		X												
8		X			X			X																				
18	X		X																									
23						X	X								X		X											
24												X	X															

Ejaculation, Premature

	LYC	SEL	CON	ZINC	BERB V	PH AC	PHOS	SULPH	CALAD	CALC	CARB V	GELS	GRAPH	NAT CAR	NUX V	PLAT	BAR C											
7	**X**			X			X							X			**X**											
8					X																							
9	X	X	X			X						X			X													
11	X	X	X	X	X	X	X	X	X	X	X	X	X	X		X												
13	X	X	X	**X**	X		X	X	X		X					X												
14		X				X		X		X																		
17	X																											
19	X		X																									
21	X												X															
24		X																										
25	**X**														X													

Elephantiasis (Includes Elephantiasis arabum; Spargosis)

	HYDRC	MYRIST	ANAC	HYDRAST	ARS	CALO	ELAEIS	SIL	CANTH	CLEM	GRAPH	HAM	HIPPOZ	IOD	LYC	MERC C	MERC	NAT C	PHOS	SIL	STILLING	SULPH
1	X					X														X		
2		X	**X**	**X**	X		X	X					X								X	
7	X																					
8	X	X	X	X	X			X		X	X	X		X	X	X	X	X	X			X
9	X																					
12	X																					
23	X	X				X	X		X													

Emaciation- See also Anorexia; Marasmus (Includes Cachexia)

	IOD	ARS	NAT M	PLUM	PHOS	LYC	SULPH	CALC	CALC PH	BAR C	SIL	NIT AC	SEC	TUB	ARS IOD	PETR	ARG N	CHINA	FERR	OL JEC	PH AC	SARS	GRAPH
1	X		X	X	X			X	X		X	X	X	X			X					X	X
2	X			X			X													X			
3			X	X					X		X												
4	X	X	X		X	X	X	X	X	X					X	X							
5	X	X	X																				
6	X	X	X	X	X	X	X	X	X		X	X	X				X	X	X		X		X
7	**X**	**X**	**X**	X	**X**	**X**	**X**	X	**X**	X	**X**	**X**	X		X	X	X	**X**	**X**	X	**X**	**X**	X
8	X	X	X	X	X		X	X	X	X	X	X	X			X	X	X		X	X	X	X
9	X		X		X	X								X					X	X			
10	X	X	X	X	X	X	X	X	X	X	X		X	X		X	X	X					
11	X	X			X			X	X			X		X			X					X	
12		X			X			X							X				X		X		
13	**X**	**X**	**X**	X	X	**X**	**X**	**X**		**X**	X	**X**	**X**			**X**		**X**	**X**		**X**	**X**	**X**
14	X		X			X									X								
15		X		X	X		X	X															
16	X		X		X	X	X		X	X				X	X								
17	X	X		X		X						X	X	X	X	X				X			
18		X	X						X		X			X									
19	X	X		X		X				X										X			
21		X	X			X				X	X												
23				X																			
24	X	X	X				X								X								
25	X		X		X																		
26		X					X	X		X													
27	X			X																			

Emaciation, Breast- See Atrophy, Breasts

Emaciation, Feet

	AMBRA	ARS	CAUST
7		X	X
8	X		

Emaciation, Legs

	ABROT	ARG N	LATH
6		X	
9	X		
10	X		
11	X		
14		X	
16			X
17	X		

Emaciation, Limbs

	CALC	SULPH	ACET AC	BAR C	NAT M	PLUM
4	X					
7	X	X				
8			X		X	
10		X		X		
19						X

Emaciation, Muscles

	LACH	LATH
7	X	
19		X

Emaciation, Neck

	NAT M	CALC PH	SARS
7	X	X	
8	X	X	
10	X		
11			X
21	X		
27	X		

Emaciation, Senile

	BAR C	LYC	OP
7	X		
9		X	
16	X	X	X

Emaciation, Thighs

	NAT M	BAR M
6	X	
8		X
10	X	

Emaciation, Upper Body

	LYC	NAT M	NIT AC
4	X	X	
6	X		
8	X		X
10		X	
17	X		
24	X		

Embolism- See also Cerebral Anaemia; Circulation, Cerebral, Poor; Thrombosis

	ARN	ARS	CACT	COLCH	KALI MUR	ZINC PH	APIS	ARG N	BELL	CALC ARS	FERR PH	GELS	GLON	HEP	KALI IOD	LAURO	MERC	OP	SIL
1			X	X		X		X											
2					X					X									
3			X	X		X													
7		X			X		X												
16	X								X		X	X	X	X	X		X	X	X
17	X	X														X			

Embolism, Pulmonary

	ACON	ARN	ARS	AS[PODO	CARB V	CEANOTH	LAURO	VANAD	VER A
17		X	X	X	X	X	X	X	X
21	X								

Emphysema (Note that only the main remedies are used from 17)

	LOB I	AMM C	IPEC	ARS	HEP	ANT T	LACH	ANT ARS	BROM	CARB V	DIG	NAT M	BELL	CAMPH	NAPHTHA	PHOS	SENEG	CHLOR	CUPR	CURARE	GRIND	LYC
1				X											X						X	
2	**X**	X			X			X	X	X										X	X	
5	X		X					X			X						X					
6	X		X	X	X	X	X		X	X	X	X	X	X	X	X	X		X			X
7	**X**	**X**	X	X	**X**	**X**	**X**		X		X	X	X	X		X		X	X			
8	X	X	X	X	X	X	X		X	X	X	X	X	X	X		X	X	X	X		
10		**X**																				
11	**X**	**X**	**X**	X	X	**X**	X	X				X				X						X
14		X	X	X						X												
17	X	X	X	X	X	X	X	X	X	X	X	X	X	X		X	X	X				X
19																					X	
23	X							X							X					X		

Empyema (Note that only the main remedies are used from 17)

	HEP	CHINA	ARS	MERC	SIL	SULPH	CALC	CHIN A	LACH	APIS	ARS I	CALC SUL	CARB SUL	CARB A	CARB V	DIG	FERR	IOD	KALI CAR	LYC	NAT ARS	NIT AC	PHOS	SEP
2		X												X										
6	X																							
8	X	**X**	**X**	**X**	**X**	**X**	X	X	X	X						X	X	X		X				
17	X	X	X	X	X	X	X	X	X		X	X	X		X				X		X	X	X	X
21	X																							
23	X																							

Empyema, Lungs

	ARS	MERC	SIL	CHINA	HEP	KALI SUL	CALC SUL	CHIN ARS	KALI CAR	LACH	NAT ARS	PHOS	SULPH
7	X	X	X	X	X			X		X			X
11	**X**	**X**	**X**	X	X	**X**	**X**		X		X	X	

Encephalitis

	GELS	HELL	ACON	BELL	STRAM	BRY	HYOSC	MERC	PHOS	CAMPH	CUPR	ARS	BAPT	CANTH	OP	ZINC
1	X	X			X		X					X	X			
3	X															
8	X		X													
11	X							X	X			X		X		
13		**X**	**X**	**X**	X	**X**	**X**	X	X	**X**	**X**			X		
14	X												X			
15	X	X	X	X	X	X	X								X	X
16		X			X											
17		X	X	X		X		X	X	X	X				X	
19																X
21	X			X												

Encephaloma- See Tumor, Brain

Enchondroma- See also Cancer, Bone; Osteosarcoma

	SIL	CALC FL	CALC	CONCH
2	**X**			X
4		X		
7	X		X	
8	X			
24		X		

Endocarditis- See also Inflammation, Heart (Note here that only main remedies are used from 17)

	SPIG	AUR	ACON	ARS	KALM	NAJA	CACT	BRY	LACH	PHOS	KALI CAR	VER V	ADONIS	BISM	CALC	COLCH	CONV	MAGN GR
1	X		X		X	X			X									X
3		X																
4	X		X	X				X				X						
5						X												X
6	**X**	X									X	X		X				
7	X	X	**X**	**X**	X		X	X	X	X	X			X	X			
8	X	X	X	X	X	X	X		X	X	X	X	X	X		X	X	
10	X	X		X	X			X		X					X			
11													X					
14			X		X	X	X											
16							X											
17	X	X	X	X	X	X	X	X	X				X			X	X	
19	X	X		X	X	X	X		X	X	X							
23						X						X				X	X	X
26	X	X	X	X				X		X					X			

Endocarditis, Bacterial

	CACT	ARS IOD	CEANOTH	CRAT	LAURO	STAPHYL
1		X				
11				X		
14	X					
17	X		X		X	X

Endocarditis, Rheumatic

	BRY	KALM	PHOS	SPIG	SPONG	ACON	ADONIS	ARS IOD	AUR	AUR M	BELL	CACT	CHIN S	HYOSC	KALI NIT	LACH	PHYTO	PSOR	PULS	SUMBUL	VER V
7		X	X		X					X				X	X					X	
8			X		X				X								X				X
11							X														
17	X	X		X				X				X	X			X					
19																		X			
26	X			X		X					X								X		

Endocervicitis

	BELL	CALC	CALC PH	CALEND	HEP	HYDROC	LIL T	MERC I F	SIL
7							X		
8	X	X	X	X	X	X		X	X

Endometriosis

	SEP	APIS	CACT	CAUL	COCCUL	FOLLIC	HYDRAST	LACH	PALLAD
18							X		
19	X				X				
27		X	X	X				X	X
28						X			

Endometritis

	ARS	ALET	BELL	HYDRAST	BOR	LYC	NUX M	PHOS	POD	SANG	VISC
2	X	X									X
4			X								
5					X						
7				X		X					
8	X		X				X	X	X	X	
18				X							
23		X									

Enteralgia- See Pain, Abdomen
Enteric Fever- See Typhoid Fever
Enteritis

	ACON	COLOC	BRY	ARS	LACH	MERC	BELL	CHAM	RHUS T	BAPT	NUX V	SULPH	CHINA	IPEC	POD	ARG N	PULS	VER A	ALOE	ANT C	CALC	CARB V	CROT T	IRIS V	NIT AC	NUPH	PHOS	SEP
2	X																											
4							X																					
6	X	X	X	X	X	X		X	X	X	X	X	X	X	X	X	X	X	X	X	X	X	X	X	X	X	X	X
7	**X**		**X**		X	X	**X**	X	X																	X		
8	X	X	X	X	X		X	X	X	X	X	X	X	X	X		X	X		X				X				
9		X																										
11		X	**X**	**X**	**X**	**X**				**X**		**X**		X		X					X	X	X		X	X	X	X
13	**X**		X	X	X	X	X	X	X		**X**			X			**X**	**X**		X			X					
15										X																		
19		X		X		X		X			X		X		X				X					X	X			
23	X	X													X	X												
25		X																										
26	**X**	X	**X**		X		**X**		X			X									X	X					X	X
27				X		X							X						X									

Enterobiasis- See Worms, Pin
Entropion

	BOR	CALC	ACON	MERC	MERC C	NAT M	SULPH	SEP	ARG N	EUPHR	GRAPH	LYC	RHUS T	TELL
2	X										X			X
6		X	X		X	X		X						
7	X	X		X	X									
8	X	X	X	X		X	X		X			X		
12				X			X			X				
14	X													
21	X													
24		X	X		X	X	X	X					X	

Enuresis- See Incontinence, Urinary
Enuresis, Coughing/Sneezing- See Incontinence, Urinary, Coughing/Sneezing From

Enuresis, Nocturnal

	CAUST	BELL	SULPH	SEP	CINA	EQUISET	SIL	BENZ AC	CALC	KREO	AMM C	ARG N	ARS	CARB V	FERR	FERR PH	MERC	PULS	THUJA	ARN	CON	GRAPH	HEP	RHUS T
2												X												
6	X	X	X	X	X	X	X	X	X	X	X	X			X	X			X					
7	**X**	**X**	X	**X**	X	X	X	X	X	X	X	X	X	X	X		X	X	X	**X**		X	X	
8	**X**	**X**	X	**X**	X	X	X	X	**X**	X	X	X	X	X	X	X	X	X	X	X	X	X	X	**X**
9	X					X										X								
10	X	X	**X**	X			X		X					X			X	X						X
13	X	X	**X**	X	X		X		X	X	**X**		X	X			X	X	X	X	**X**	**X**	**X**	X
14	X	X						**X**		X														
16					X																			
23	X				X	X		X							X						X			
24				X			X																	
25		X				X							X			X								
27			X																					

Eosinophilia

	ARS	LACH
3		X
17	X	

Ephelis

	LYC	PHOS	ANT C	CALC	CAUST	GRAPH	HYOSC	KALI CAR	LAURO	MUR AC	NAT M	NIT AC	PETR	PULS	SEP	SULPH
2	X	X								X						
8	X	X	X	X	X	X	X	X	X		X	X	X	X	X	X

Epicondylitis, Lateral- See Tennis Elbow

Epidermolysis

	RAN B
1	**X**
3	X

Epididymitis

	PULS	HAM	GELS	RHOD	ACON	SPONG	ARN	AUR	BELL	CLEM	CON	IOD	MERC	PHYTO	RHUS T	AGNUS	BROM	CHINA	GRAPH	HYDROC	NIT AC	NUX V	TAR H	THUJA	TUSSIL	VIB OP		
2																										X		
4	X		X			X																						
7	X	X	X	X				X			X							X										
8	X	X	X	X	X	X	X	X	X	X	X		X	X	X	X	X				X	X	X	X	X			
9	X			X			X					X			X				X	X								
12	X	X	X		X					X		X	X	X														
21	X	X			X				X																			
23	X	X		X		X																						

Epiglottis, Diseases Of

	ALL C	CHLOR	HEP	LACH	WYETHIA																							
2					X																							
17	X	X	X	X																								

Epilepsy- See also Status Epilepticus (Note here that only the main remedies are used from 17)

	BELL	CUPR	CIC	IGN	HYOSC	BUFO	CALC	SIL	STRAM	CAUST	NUX V	AGAR M	KALI BR	OP	OENANTH	SULPH	ABSINTH	ARG N	ART V	HYDR AC	PLUM	COCCUL	LACH	ARS	GLON	STANN	CALC AC	AETHUSA
1	X	X	X	X	X	X	X			X	X	X	X		X	X	X	X	X		X				X	X		
2	**X**	X	**X**	**X**	X	**X**	**X**	**X**	**X**	X	X		X	**X**	**X**	X	X	X	X	X	**X**		X		X	X	X	X
3	X	X	X	X	X	X		X				X	X	X		X	X			**X**					X			
4	**X**	**X**	**X**		**X**	**X**	**X**	**X**	**X**	X	**X**	X			**X**	X		X	X	X	X					X		
5	X	X	X			X			X						X		X											
6	X	X	X	X	X	X	X	X	X	X	X	X	X	X	X	X		X	X		X	X	X	X	X	X	X	
7	X	**X**	**X**	X	X	**X**	X	**X**	X	**X**	**X**	X	**X**	X	X		X	**X**	**X**	X	X	X	X	X	X	X	X	X
8	**X**	X	X	X	X	X	X	X	X	X	X	X	X	X	X	X	X	X	X	X	X	X	X	X	X	X	X	X
9	X	X	X		X			X	X		X		X										X		X			X
10	X	X		**X**	X		**X**	X	X	**X**	X					X						X						
11	X	X	X	X	X	X	X	X	X	X	X	X	X		X		X	X	X	X		X	X					
12	X		X	X	X		X		X			X	X	X	X	X			X	X	X			X				
13	**X**	**X**	**X**	X	**X**	X	**X**	X	**X**	**X**	X	**X**		**X**		**X**		X			X	X	X	**X**	X	**X**		X
14	X	X	X	X	X	X			X			X					X											
15	X	X		X	X				X		X			X								X						
16		X		X		X	X			X										X								
17	**X**	**X**	**X**	**X**	**X**	**X**	**X**	**X**	**X**	**X**	**X**	**X**	**X**	X	**X**	**X**	**X**	**X**	**X**	**X**	X	**X**	**X**	**X**		X	**X**	
19																											X	
21	X	X	X	X	X									X											X			X
23	X		X	X		X						X	X		X		X	X	X	X							X	X
26	X	X		**X**			X	X		X				X		X							X	X				
27	X		X			X	X	X					X	X			X				X							
28	X				X	X	X																					
29*	X																					X						

29* Varshney JP. Clinical management of idiopathic epilepsy in dogs with homeopathic Belladonna 200C: a case series. Homeopathy. 2007 Jan; 96 (1):46-8.

Epilepsy (Petit Mal)

	CAUST	ABSINTH	ART V	BELL	HYOSC	ZINC CY	CINA	PHOS
2						X		X
4	**X**		X					
7	X	X		X	X		X	
8	X			X				
17	**X**	**X**	**X**	**X**		**X**		X
19	X	X	X		X		X	
27		X						
28					X			

Epiphora- See also Lachrymal Duct Blockage; Lachrymation Profuse/Frequent

	ALL C	**MERC P**	**SQUILLA**
2		X	X
8	X		

Episiotomy- See Wounds, Incisional

Epistaxis

	ARN	**PHOS**	**HAM**	**BRY**	**IPEC**	**CARB V**	**ACON**	**BELL**	**MILL**	**PULS**	**CROC**	**CHINA**	**ARS**	**CROT H**	**DROS**	**RHUS T**	**FERR PH**	**SEC**	**LACH**	**SULPH**	**ERIGER**	**MERC**	**NUX V**	**TRILL P**	**GRAPH**	**NIT AC**	**VIP**
1	X	X	X	X		X			X	X	X		X	X		X			X		X			X	X	X	X
2		**X**	**X**	**X**		**X**			**X**	X	**X**			X			**X**	X		**X**					**X**		X
3		X	E	X	X			X	X								X							X			**X**
4	X		X	X				X	X	X		X	X			X			X			X		X			
5		**X**		X					E			**X**			X						X						
6	X		X	X	X	X	X	X		X	X	X	X	X		X		X	X	X	X		X	X		X	
7	**X**	**X**	**X**	X	X	X	X	X	X	X	X	**X**	X	X		X	X	**X**	**X**	X	X	X	X		X	**X**	
8	X	X	X	X	X	X	X	X	X	X	X	X	X	X		X		X	X	X	X	X	X		X	X	
9	X	X									X																
10	X			X	X	X	X	X		X				X						X		X	X				
11	X	X		X	X	X		X						X													
12	X		X		X		X	X		X		X			X	X		X									
13	X	X		X	X	X	X	X	X	X	X	X	X		X	X		X	X	X		X	X			X	
14	X	X	X			X	X		X		X		X	X	X									X			
15	X	X	X			X	X				X	X			X												
17	X	X	X	X	X	X	X	X	**X**	X	X	X		X	X	X	X	X	X		X	X	X	X		X	X
18		X			X										X		X								X		
19	X		X		X				X						X												
20							X																				
21	X	X	X	X	X			X									X								X		X
22		X			X																						
23			X																		X						
24	X		X			X	X		X	X			**X**				X							X			
25	X		B	X			X	X		X			X				X										X
26	X	X	X	X	X	X	X	X		X	X	X	X		X	X		X		X		X	X				
28		X																									

E- External, B- Both Internal and External

Epithelioma

	CONDUR	CON	HYDRAST	ARS	CIC	KREO	ARS I	BELL	LAPIS	PHYTO	SEP	SIL	THUJA	LYC
2	X			X	X	X	X		X					**X**
4	X	X	**X**		X									
5													X	
7	X	X		X		X		X		X		X		
8	X	X	X	X		X	X	X	X	X	X	X	X	
10	X	X									X			
24	X	X	X		X									

Epithelioma, Eyelid

	APIS	HYDR AC	LACH	CALC OX	CON	HEP	KALI SUL	SEP
1					X			X
6	X	X	X					
8	X	X	X	X		X	X	

Epithelioma, Face

	KALI SUL	ARS
4	X	
8	X	X

Epithelioma, Lip

	ARS	KREO	ACET AC	ARG N	ARS IOD	AUR	BELL	CARB A	CHEL	CLEM	CON	AUR M N	HYDRAST	LACH	PULS	SEP	SIL	SULPH	THUJA	KALI SUL
1																X				
2	X	X																		
6	X	X	X	X	X	X	X	X	X	X	X	X	X	X	X		X	X	X	
8	X	X	X	X	X	X	X	X	X	X	X		X	X	X		X	X	X	X
10												X				X				

Epulis- See also Boils, Gums

	THUJA	CALC	CHAM	LAC C	NAT M	PLUM	BRY	GRAPH	HEP	MERC I F	SEP	SIL
1	**X**			X		X	X					
2	X	X		X		X						
6	X	X	X		X							
8	X	X	X		X			X	X	X	X	X

Erethism- See also Hyperaesthesia

	CHINA	AUR	CAMPH	CLEM	MUR AC	PASS	STRAM	STRY VAL
2		X						
10	X							
17	X				X			
23			X	X		X	X	X

Eructation, Gas (Includes Belching, Burping)

	CARB V	ANT C	NUX V	ARG N	PULS	CHINA	SULPH	LYC	CALC	IGN	SULPH AC	BRY	CARB A	KALI CAR	ARN	CHAM	SEP	ARS	PHOS	AMBRA	BELL	GRAPH	MERC	NUX M	LACH	ASAF	CAUST
1	X	X	X	X	X	X	X				X	X	X			X		X									
2	**X**			**X**			**X**						**X**			**X**								**X**			
3	X	X		X																						X	
4	X	X	X	X	X	X	X							X			X		X			X					
5	X	X	X	X	X	X		X		X	X			X	X		X			X		X		X	X	X	X
6	X	X	X		X	X	X	X	X		X	X	X	X	X	X	X	X	X		X		X		X	X	X
7	**X**	X	**X**	**X**	**X**	X	**X**	**X**	X	X	X	**X**	X	X	**X**	X	**X**		**X**	X	**X**	X	**X**	X	X		X
8	X	X	X		X	X	X	X	X	X	X		X		X		X	X	X	X		X	X		X		X
9	X	X			X		X																				
10	X	X		X	X	X	X		X	X		X	X		X	X					X		X				
11			X	X		X		X	X	X			X						X		X						
12		X	X		X				X			X															
13	X	X	X	X	X	X	X	X	X	X	X	X	X	X	X	X	X	X	**X**	**X**	X	**X**	X	X	X		X
14	X	X		X	X	X		X										X									
15	X	X	X		X					X	X	X						X				X	X				
17											X			X						X				X		X	
18		X	X	X										X												X	
19	X		X	X		X	X	X												X							
20						X																					
21	X		X	X	X	X		X		X																	
22	X	X	X							X																	
24	X			X					X		X			X													
25							X																				
26	X	X	X		X	X	X	X	X			X			X	X	X	X			X				X		
28	X							X																			

Eructation, Food (Includes Regurgitation/Reflux; Regurgitation via mouth or nose)

	NUX V	PHOS	BRY	CHAM	LYC	FERR	PULS	SULPH	BELL	CALC	CARB V	NAT M	CHINA	AETHUSA	LACH	MERC	POD	RHUS T	SARS
6		X																	
7	X	X	X		X	X					X		X		X				
8	X	X	X	X	X	X	X	X	X	X	X	X	X	X		X	X	X	X
10				X															
11	X	**X**	X	X	X	**X**	**X**	**X**		X	X	X	**X**		X	X			
13	X	X	**X**	X	X	X	X	X	X	X	X	X			X	X	X	**X**	**X**
15	X			X			X		X										
17					X				X					X					
18	X																		
19								X											
21		X																	
26	X		X							X		X		X			X		

Eruptions, Skin- See Dermatitis

Erysipelas (AKA St Anthony's Fire)

	RHUS T	BELL	APIS	GRAPH	LACH	ARS	CANTH	SULPH	EUPHORB	ACON	BOR	MERC	PULS	ARN	CUPR	HEP	SIL	VER V	CAMPH	CHINA	BRY	CHAM	CROT H
1	X	X	X	X	X	X	X	X		X	X					X	X						X
2	**X**	**X**	**X**	**X**	X	**X**	X		X		X				X	X		X	X	**X**		X	**X**
3	X			X																			
4	**X**	**X**	**X**	**X**	**X**	X	X	X	X	X				X				X					
5	X				X																		
6	X	X	X	X	X	X		X	X		X		X		X	X	X	X	X	X		X	
7	**X**	X	**X**	**X**	X	X	X	X	X			X	X	X	X		X		X	X		X	
8	X	X	X	X	X	X	X	X	X	X	X	X	X	X	X		X		X	X	X		X
10	X	**X**	X	X	X	X		X		X		X	X		X	X					X		
12	X	X	X		X	**X**	X	X		X			X	X				**X**			X		
13	**X**	**X**	X	**X**	X	X	**X**	X	X	**X**	X	**X**	X	X		X	X		**X**	X	X	**X**	X
14	X	X	X		X	X	X				X					X	X						
15	**X**	**X**	**X**							X		**X**	X					**X**					
16	X	X	X	X																			
21	X	X	X		X							X											
23	X	X	X	X	X		X		X		X			X									
24	X	X	X	X					X														
26	**X**	**X**	X	X	X	X		X							X						X		

Erysipelas Bullosum

	EUPHORB	KALI CAR	TEREB
2			X
7	X	X	

Erysipelas, Extremities

	HEP	ARN	BOR	CALC	GRAPH	PETR	PULS	RHUS T	ZINC
8	X		X	X	X	X	X	X	X
13	X	X							

Erysipelas, Face

	BELL	APIS	RHUS T	CANTH	CARB A	GRAPH	HEP	LACH	PULS	SEP	SULPH
8	X	X	X		X	X	X	X	X	X	X
10	**X**										
14				X							
26	X	X	X								

Erysipelas, Nose

	GRAPH	APIS	AUR M	CANTH	PLUM	RHUS T
7	X	X	X			X
8	X			X	X	

Erysipelas, Prophylaxis

	GRAPH
10	X
16	X

Erysipelas, Scalp

	APIS	BELL	CARB S	RHUS T	SIL
1			X		
8					X
26	X	X		X	

Erysipelas, Scrotum

	ARN	CANTH	CARB V	GRAPH	MERC	NAT M	PULS	RHUS T
8			X					
13	X	X		X	X	X	X	X

Erysipelas, Senile

	AMM C	LACH
10	X	
14		X

Erysipelas, Vesicular

	CANTH	EUPHR	URT U
2			X
8	X	X	

Erythema

	BELL	APIS	RHUS T	MERC	ACON	ARS	PULS	SULPH	CANTH	LACH	LYC	GRAPH	AGAR M	ANTIPYR	ARN	BRY	NUX V	URT U
2	**X**													X				X
5	X	X	X	X		X	X		X		X	X	X			X	X	
6	X		X	X	X			X	X	X	X							
7			**X**	**X**	**X**	**X**	X	X							X			X
8	**X**		X	**X**	**X**	**X**	X	X	X	X	X	X		X	X			X
10	X	X	X				X			X								
12	X	X			X	X										X	X	
13	**X**	X	**X**	**X**	X	X	X	X	X	X	X	**X**	X		X	X	X	
14	X																	
18		X											X					
21								X										
23														X				
28		X																
29*		X																

29* Bildet J, et al. The Effect of Dilutions of Apis mellifica and Apium virus on Ultra-violet light induced erythema in the Guinea pig. Ann Pharm Fr, 1989, 47, 1, 24-32.

Erythema, Ears, Behind

	GRAPH	PETR	MERC	OLEAND	SULPH
6	X	X			X
8	X	X	X	X	

Erythema, Face

	BELL	ACON	OP	NUX V	STRAM	CHAM	CUPR	GLON	PULS	RHUS T	SAMB	FERR	GRAT	ARG N	ARS	CACT	CANTH	CHINA	CIC	CROC	GUAIAC	LACH	LYC	NAT CAR	PHOS	SPIG
7	X	X	X	X	X	X	X	X	X	X	X	X	X	X	X		X	X	X	X	X	X	X	X	X	X
8	X		X	X						X																
9	X	X																								
10	X	X			X			X																		
12	X						X				X															
13	**X**	**X**	**X**	**X**	**X**	X	X	X	X	X	X	**X**	**X**	X	X	X	X	X	X	X	X	X	X	X	X	X
14	X		X																							
15	X	X				X			X							X										
16	X																									
19	X																									

Erythema, Hands

	ACON	ALL S	JUG C	PHOS
7			X	X
14	X			
26		X		

Erythema, Nose

	ALUM	PHOS	CHINA	SULPH	HEP	MERC C	BELL	CALC	MERC	RAN B
7	**X**	**X**	**X**	**X**	X	X				
13	**X**	**X**	X	X	X	X	**X**	**X**	**X**	**X**

Erythema Nodosum

	LED	RHUS T	APIS	LACH	ARN	JUG C	RHUS V	SULPH AC	SULPH	ACON	ALL C	BRY	CON	KALI BIC	KALI BR	KALI IOD	LYC	MEZ	NUX V	PHYTO	PTEL	OP	SANG
2	X	**X**	X			X	X	X		**X**					X	X				X			
4	**X**		X																				
5				X																		X	X
6	X			X	X		X	X	X								X	X			X		
7		X		X	X	X			X		X	X	X						X				
8	X																						
12		X	X											X									

Erythrocytes, Deficiency Of- See also Anaemia

	CALC PH	IRID
11	X	
14		X

Eustachian Tubes, Blockage Of

	MERC D	PULS	IOD	SIL	CON	KALI MUR	MERC	ASAR	BELL	CALC	CARB V	FERR PH	GELS	GRAPH	HYDRAST	KALI BIC	LACH	LYC	MERC I R	NIT AC	PETR	SULPH
8		X	X	X	X					X			X	X			X			X		X
14		X	X						X							X						
17	X	X		X	X		X	X			X	X						X	X			
18						X																
21	X	X	X	X		X									X							
24	X						X														X	
27	X																					

Eustachian Tubes, Catarrh- See Catarrh, Eustachian Tubes

Eustachian Tubes, Diseases Of

	MERC D	BAR C	BAR M	CAPS	FERR PH	PETR	PHYTO	SIL	TUB AV
2	X						X		
6	X	X	X					X	
7	X					X			
17					X				
18									X
24	X			X					

Eustachian Tubes, Occlusion Of- See also Catarrh, Eustachian Tube; Inflammation, Eustachian Tube

	MERC D	IOD	NIT AC	PULS	ARS I	GELS	HYDRAST	KALI BIC	KALI MUR	KALI SUL	LACH	MERC	PETR	PHYTO
1		X		X										
2									X					
5				X	X		X			X				
6	**X**	X	X			X							X	
7	X		X					X			X	X		X

Exanthema

	APIS	BELL	BRY	PULS	ARS	ACON	CAMPH	CARB V	MERC	MERC D	NAT SUL	RHUS T
1											X	
7	X		X									X
8	X						X			X		
18		X		X								
19		X	X		X	X						
26				X				X	X			

Excoriation

	AETHUSA	CHAM	LYC	MERC	ARN	CALEND	SANIC	SULPH AC
2	**X**	**X**	**X**	**X**	X		X	
28						E		E

E- External

Exhaustion, Mental- See also Neurasthenia (Includes Brain Fag)

	PH AC	PIC AC	PHOS	ZINC	ANAC	KALI PH	LYC	NUX V	SIL	ARG N	NAT M	ZINC PH	BAR C	CON	GELS	IGN	NAT CAR	AETHUSA	CALC PH	CALC	CIMICI	DIG	KALI BR	PLAT	SEP	STANN	SULPH
1	X	X	X	X	X	X		X	X	X	X	X		X	X	X							X				X
2	**X**	**X**	X	X	**X**	X			**X**		X	X						**X**	**X**								
3																		X									
4	X	**X**				**X**	X					X	X								X						
5					X	X			X															X		X	
6		X	X					X			X					X	X			X							X
7	X	X	X	X			**X**	X						X		X	X		X			X	X		X	X	
8	X	**X**	X	X	X	X	X	X	X	X			X		X	X				X	X		X	X	X		
9								X									X										
10			X			X			X				X		X												
11	X				X		X																				
12	X		X	X				X																			
13				X			X	X			X			X			X					X		X	X	X	X
14	X		X		X		X			X		X		X													
15																					X						
16			X	X			X			X					X			X									
17		X		X		X						X										X					
18				X	X	X					X		X						X								
21	X	X		X	X				X											X							
23		X	X		X					X																	
28	X																										

Exhaustion, Physical- See also Fatigue

	ARS	ARN	CARB V	GELS	AETHUSA	CHINA	MEZ	PH AC	PHOS	SEP	BELL	CALC	KALI CAR	NAT CAR	NAT M	PIC AC	SIL	VER A
1	X			X	X									X		X		
2		X																
3								X							X			
4			**X**		X													
5		X		X		X			X				X		X		X	
6			X	X	X	X	X		X		X	X	X	X		X	X	X
8	X	X																
9	X			X		X		X	X	X	X							
10							X										X	
11	X				X		X											
12		X																
13										X								X
14														X				
16	X																	
17																X		
19				X				X	X									
21			X			X		X		X		X						
22			X										X					
24							X											
25	X	**X**	X							X	X							
26	**X**	X										X						X
27															X			

Exhaustion, Nervous- See Neurasthenia
Exophthalmia- See Exophthalmos
Exophthalmic Goitre- See also Goitre, Hyperthyroidism

	LYCOP	NAT M	IOD	THYROID	BELL	FERR	CACT	SPONG	AMYL N	CALC	VER V	AUR	FUCUS	ADRENAL	ARS	BAR C	FERR IOD	PHOS	PILO	SEC	SPIG	STROPH	SULPH
1	X	X				X								X									
2	X			X		X	X	X									X				X		
3													**X**										
4	**X**	**X**	**X**	**X**	X				X														X
7						X	X																
8	**X**	X	X		**X**	X	X	X	X	X	X	**X**			X	X	X	X		X			X
9		X	X	X																			
10	X							X															
11	X		X		X	X	X			X				X					X				
12			X	X	X	X					X										X		
17	X				X				X											X		X	
19	X	X	X	X				X		X		X	X		X	X		X					
23	X				X						X											X	
24		X		X															X				
25		**X**	X	X																			

Exophthalmos

	BELL	LYCOP	SPONG	AETHUSA	AMYLN	ARS	CAPS	IOD	PHOS	VER A	AUR	OP	BAR C	BROM	CACT	CALC	CANTH	COCCUL	CON	GLON	HYDR AC	HYOSC	KALI MUR	NAT M	THYROID	LAURO		
1		X						X															X					
2		X	X		X				X																			
4	X				X			X																				
6	X	X	X	X	X		X		X				X	X	X	X						X		X				
7	X		X	X		X				X		X					X	X		X								
8	X						X														X							
9	X																											
10	X	X																										
11	X	X																										
12										X																		
13	**X**		X	X		X	X			X	**X**	**X**		X			X	X	X	X	X	X				**X**		
14	X																											
15	X																											
17																							X					
19		X	X			X		X	X		X		X		X	X			X					X	X			
21		X																										
23	X	X																										
24	X		X																						X			
25	X																											

Exostosis (Includes Spurs, Bone)

	CALC FL	HECLA	MEZ	AUR	KALI IOD	PHOS	SIL	DULC	FL AC	LYC	RUTA	AUR M	CALC	MERC	PH AC	ASAF	GUAIAC	RHUS T	SABIN	STAPHYS	SULPH	KALI BIC						
2	**X**	**X**	X			X		X			X							X				**X**						
5	X																											
6			X	X	X	X	X		X	X	X				X	X	X		X	X	X							
7	X		X	**X**	X		**X**	X				**X**	X	**X**														
8	X	X		X	**X**	X	X	X	X	X	X	X	X	X	X	X	X	X	X	X	X	X						
13			**X**	X		**X**	X	X	X	X	X	X	**X**	X	**X**	X	X	X	X	X	X							
14	X									X																		
17	X	X			X																							
18		X																										
19	**X**																											
23	X	X																										
24	X		X						X																			
28		X																										

Exostosis, Jaw

	ANGUST	CALC FL	HECLA
7	X	X	
8	X		
19		X	X
28			X

Exostosis, Thigh

	LAC AC
7	X
8	X

Exostosis, Skull

	PHOS	AUR	ARG M	CALC	CALC FL	KALI IOD	MEZ
6	X	X					
7	**X**	**X**	**X**	**X**	X	X	X
8	X						

Eyes, Diseases Of (Note that only the main remedies from 4 are used here)

	BELL	EUPHR	SULPH	CALC	PULS	ACON	HEP	MERC	CAUST	NAT M	NIT AC	NUX V	ALL C	RHUS T	ARG N	ARN	ARS	AUR	GELS	GRAPH	LACH	PHOS	PHYSO	SEP	SIL
2	**X**	**X**	**X**	**X**		**X**	**X**		**X**	**X**	**X**	**X**			**X**	**X**	**X**	**X**	**X**	**X**	**X**	**X**	**X**	**X**	**X**
3		X											X												
4	X	X	X		X			X						X					X	X					
8	X	X	X	X	X	X	X	X	X	X		X		X		X						X		X	
9	X	X		X		X				X			X		X								X		X
12			X					X																	
13	X	X	X	X	X	X						X													
17													X												
23	X				X		X		X		X							X							
26	X	X	X	X	X		X	X			X			X			X				X				

Eyes, Dryness

	BELL	ACON	ALUM	ARS	OP	SULPH	VER A	PULS	STAPHYS	BERB V	CROC	LYC	NUX M	ZINC	BRY	CAUST	CLEM	EUPHR	MAG CAR	NAT SUL	MANG	RHUS T
4	X		X							X	X									X		
5	X		X							X	X		X									
6		X	X																			
7	X	**X**	**X**	X	X	X								X		X	X	X	X			
8		X		X	X	X	X	X	X			X			X							
9		X																				
10	X																					
11																		X				
13	X			X		X	X	**X**	**X**	X	X	X	X	X	X	X	X		X	X	**X**	**X**
17	X	X	X	X	X	X	X	X	X			X	X	X								
18	X																					
24	X	X			X																	
25	X																					
27	X	X					X															

Eyes, Foreign Bodies In

	SIL	ACON	ARN	CALC	SULPH
7	**X**	**X**		X	
9	X				
19	X	X			
24	X	X			X
25			B		

B- Both Internal and External

Eye, Injury- See Injury, Eye

Eyebrows, Loss/Falling Of- See also Hair, Falling Of, Eyebrows and/or Lashes

	ANANTH	HELL	KALI CAR	SEL	THUJA
1	X		X		
8		X		X	X

Eyelashes, Falling Of- See also Hair, Falling Of, Eyebrows and/or Lashes

	RHUS T	PETR	PH AC	ALOE	ALUM	CALC	EUPHR	MERC	MEZ	SEP	STAPHYS
1	X	X			X						
6										X	
7	X		X				X	X	X		X
8				X							
14		X									
24	X		X								
27						X					

Eyelashes, Ingrowing- See Trichiasis
Eyelid, Cysts- See Cysts, Eyelid
Eyelids, Diseases Of- See also Blepharitis; Chalazion; Entropion; Stye

	GRAPH	HEP	CALC	GUARAN	JATR	MAG PH	MERC	SPIRAE	SULPH																			
2				X	X			X																				
8						X																						
10	X	X					X																					
21	X	X	X						X																			

Eyesight, Weak- See Weakness, Vision
Eye Strain- See Strain, Eyes
Facial Palsy- See Bell's Palsy

Fainting- See also Syncope

	MOSCH	CHINA	ACON	NUX V	OP	VER A	ARS	LACH	NUX M	PULS	BELL	IGN	COCCUL	GLON	CAMPH	SULPH	BRY	CARB V	CHAM	COFF	SEP	HEP	ARN	DIG	HYOSC	IP	PHOS	
1	X	X	X		X	X	X	X	X	X	X	X	X	X	X	X		X			X		X		X		X	
2	**X**		X			X	**X**	X	X			**X**	X			X											X	
3	X	X			X	X			X												X	X						
4	**X**	X					X		X	X			X			X	X											
5	X	X		X		X	X		X	X		X	X		X		X	X			X			X		X	X	
6	X	X	X	X	X	X	X	X		X	X	X	X	X	X	X	X				X			X	X	X	X	
7	**X**	X	**X**	X	**X**	**X**	**X**	**X**	**X**	**X**	X	**X**	**X**	X	X	X			X			**X**	X	X	X	X		
8	X	X	**X**	X	X	**X**		X	**X**	X	X	**X**	X	X	X	X		X	**X**	X		X	X		X	X		
9	X	X		**X**	X		X	X	X	X	X	X			X		X	X		X	X							
10		X	X	X	X	X	X	X		X	X	X	X	X		X	X	X	X	X	X		X		X	X		
11	X		X	X	X						X			X														
12	X	X	X											X	X									X				
13	X	**X**	**X**	**X**	**X**	X	**X**	X	**X**	**X**	**X**	X	X		**X**	**X**	X	X	**X**	X	**X**	**X**	**X**	**X**	**X**	X	X	
14	X	X	X	X	X	X	X	X			X			X	X		X	X			X		X					
15		X	X	X		X	X	X	X		X	X				X			X	X	X		X		X	X	X	
16	X	X		X	X			X											X									
17	X	X	X	X	X	X	X	X	X				X	X	X		X			X		X		X				
18	X	X																X										
19	X			X				X					X	X			X	X						X				
20						X																						
21	X	X	X	X	X	X		X	X	X	X	X	X	X		X	X		X	X		X	X			X	X	
22		X								X									X	X		X						
24		X								X						X				X							X	
25		X	X		X		X				X			X	I									X				
26	X		X	X	X	X			X	X	X	X							X	X		X			X			
27							X																					
28																		X										

I- Inhalation

Fasciitis (Includes Plantar Fasciitis)

	PHYTO	RHUS T	RUTA
19	X		
27	X	X	
29*			X

29* Clark J, et al. A Preliminary Investigation into the Effectiveness of the Homoeopathic Remedy, Ruta graveolens, in the Treatment of pain in Plantar Fasciitis. British J of Podiatry, 2000, 3, 3, 81- 85.

Fatigue, Mental- See Neurasthenia

Fatigue, Physical- See also Exhaustion (Includes Asthenia; Debility; Languor; Lassitude; Lethargy; Malaise; Prostration; Weakness)

	ARS	CHINA	PH AC	PHOS	VER A	GELS	NAT M	CARB V	CALC	SEP	NUX V	KALI CAR	MUR AC	FERR	STANN	BAPT	SULPH	PIC AC	LYC	COCCUL	PSOR	COLCH	ANAC	IOD	NIT AC	PULS	SEC	
1	X	X	X	X	X	X	X	X	X	X	X	X	X	X	X	X	X	X	X	X	X	X		X	X	X	X	
2		**X**	**X**		**X**		**X**	**X**	**X**	X		X		X	X			X	X	X	**X**	X	**X**	**X**				
3	X	X	X	X		X	**X**	X				X	X			X		X			X		X					
4	**X**	**X**	**X**	**X**	X	X	X	**X**		X	X	X	**X**	X	**X**	X	X	**X**	X	**X**	X	X	X	X		X	X	
5	X	X	X	X	X		X	X		X	X	X			X	X		X	X	X	X		X			X		
6	X	X	X	X	X	X	X	X	X	X	X		X	X	X	X	X	X	X	X	X	X	X	X	X		X	
7	**X**	**X**	**X**	**X**	**X**	**X**	**X**	**X**	**X**	**X**	**X**	**X**	**X**	X	X	**X**	**X**	**X**	**X**	X	X	X		X	**X**	X	**X**	
8	**X**	**X**	**X**	X	**X**		X	X	**X**		**X**	X		X		X	**X**	X	X	X	X	X	X			X	X	
9	X	X	X	X		X			X	X	X	X	X		X		X		X	X								
10	X	X	X	X	X	X	X	X			X	X		X	X	X	X	X	X			X		X	X	X	X	
11	X			X	X		X						X					X				X		X				
12	X	X	X	X	X			X	X		X		X	X		X	X						X	X	X			
13	**X**	**X**	**X**	**X**	**X**		**X**	**X**	**X**	**X**	**X**	**X**	**X**	**X**	**X**		**X**		**X**	X	X	X	**X**	**X**	**X**	X	**X**	
14	X	X	X		X	X	X	X	X	X	X			X		X											X	
15	X	X	X		X	X		X	X	X	X		X			X				X					X			
16	X	X	X										X					X										
17	X	X	X		X	X						X	X		X	X	X				X	X	X	X			X	
18	X	X	X	X	X	X	X			X		X		X	X					X	X				X			
19	X	X				X	X	X	X	X	X				X		X		X		X				X			
20	X			X	X	X											X											
21	X	X	X	X		X		X	X	X		X		X				X		X		X				X		
22	X			X	X	X	X	X				X										X						
23	X	X		X	X	X									X	X		X										
24	X	X		X	X	X	X		X	X				X	X	X			X				X			X		
25	**X**	X	X	X		X	X	X	X	X	X	X													X			
26	X	X	X	X	X	X		X	X	X	X		X	X			X									X	X	
27		X				X	X			X			X	X														
29*			X	X		X	X		X																	X		

29* Awdrey R. Homoeopathy and Chronic Fatigue- the Search for Proof. Int J of Alt and Comp Med, Feb 1996, 19- 21.

Favus (AKA Tinea Favosa)

	ARS	CALC	DULC	HEP	RHUS T	SULPH	VINCA	VIOL T	GRAPH	LAPPA	OLEAND	PHOS	PSOR	STAPHYS	MEDO	SULO AC												
2							X								**X**	**X**												
6	X	X	X	X	X	X	X	X		X	X	X																
7	X	X	X	X				X	X				X															
8	X	X	X	X			X	X	X	X	X	X	X	X														
10	X	X	X	X	**X**	X								X														
26	X	X			X	X																						

Felon- See Whitlow

Fever (Includes Hyperpyrexia; Pyrexia)

	BELL	ACON	ARS	BRY	GELS	RHUS T	FERR PH	NUX V	PULS	BAPT	CHAM	HEP	PHOS	MERC	LACH	SULPH	NAT M	CHINA	PYROG	APIS	ARN	DULC	CALC	PH AC	VER A			
1	X	X	X	X	X	X	X	X		X										X				X				
2	X	**X**	**X**		**X**		X				X			X		**X**												
3	X	X	X	X	X	X	X	X	X	X	X	X	X		X	X	X	X	X				X	X	X			
4	**X**	**X**	**X**	X	**X**	**X**	X		X	**X**				X	X	**X**												
5	X	X	X	X	X	X	X		X	X	X	X	X		X			X		X	X		X		X			
6	X	X	X	X	X		X	X	X		X	X		X		X					X							
7	X	X	X	X	X	X		X	X	X	X	X	X	X	X	X	X	X		X	X	X	X		X			
8	X	X	X	X	X	X		X		X	X		X	X			X	X			X			X	X			
9	X	X	X	X	X	X		X				X																
10	X	X	X	X	X		X	X	X			X	X		X	X						X						
11	X	X	X	X								X	X				X	X			X	X		X				
12	X	X	X	X							X		X												X			
13	X		X			X	X		X	X	X						X		X	X								
14	X	X	X	X	X			X		X		X					X				X							
15	X	X		X	X	X								X														
16	X	X	X	X	X					X						X	X	X										
17	X	X	X	X			X		X	X									X			X	X					
18	X	X	X	X	X	X	X			X	X		X						X	X		X						
19	**X**	**X**	**X**	**X**	**X**	**X**	**X**	**X**	**X**	X	**X**	**X**	X	**X**	X	X	**X**	**X**	**X**	X	X		X	X	X			
20	**<u>X</u>**	X					X	X	X																			
21	X	X	X	X	X		X						X	X					X	X								
22	X	X	X	X	X		X		X				X						X			X						
24	X	X	X			X						X			X													
25	X	X	X	X		X		X	X			X		X														
26	X	X		X		X		X	X		X			X	X							X	X	X				
27	X	X		X				X							X					X								

Fever, Hectic

	ARS	PH AC	CHINA	PHOS	SIL	LYC	STANN	BAPT	CALC	HEP	SANG	SULPH	ACET AC	BALS	CALC SUL	CARB V	FERR	IOD	LACH	MERC	PLUM	SEP	STAPHYS	PYROG				
2	**X**	X	**X**				X	X		X				X			X							**X**				
3	X							X	X																			
7	X	X	X	X	**X**	X			**X**	X	X	X	**X**			X	X	X	X	X	X	X						
8	X	X	X	X	X	X	X	X	X		X	X				X			X	X		X	X					
10	X					X															X							
11				X											X													
12		X	X				X			X								X										
15	X	X	X	X																								
17															X													
23					X								X	X														
24	X			X	X	X	X				X	X																
26		X																					X					

Fever, Intermittent– See also Malaria (Includes Fever, Relapsing; Fever, Remittent)

	CHINA	ARS	NAT M	IPEC	CHIN S	BRY	NUX V	RHUS T	PULS	CAPS	CARB V	EUP PERF	GELS	ARN	MENY	ANT C	EUCAL	FERR	IGN	CHAM	SABAD	VER A
4	**X**	**X**	**X**	**X**	**X**		**X**	X	X	X	X	**X**	X		X		X		X			
5	X																					
7	**X**	**X**	**X**	**X**	**X**	X	X	X	**X**	**X**	X	**X**	X	X	**X**	**X**	X	X	X	**X**	X	X
8	X	X	X	X	X	X	X	X	X	X	X	X	X	X	X	X	X	X	X	X	X	X
9	X		X																			
10			**X**											X								
11															X							
12	X	X				X	X	X				X	X									
13	**X**	**X**	**X**	X		X		X	X	X	**X**			**X**	X	**X**		X	X		**X**	**X**
14	X	X	X																			
15	**X**	**X**		**X**		X	**X**		**X**		X		X							X		
16		X			X																	
17																	X					
19		X				X		X														
23	X	X	X	X	X			X		X		X	X				X	X				
26	X	X	X	**X**		X	X		X	X	X			X		X		X	X	X	X	X
28			X																			
29*	**X**	X	X	X	**X**																	

29* Singh K. Evaluation of Ten Homoeopathic Medicines in the Clinical Management of Intermittent Fever. CCRH Quarterly Bull, 1993, 15, 1&2, 9-13.

Fibrillation, Atrial

	DIG	ARS	QUIN	ACON	AGAR M	CACT	CANN S	CRAT	DULC	GELS	HELL	ICTHYOL	KALI N	LAURO	LITH C	SEC	VER A	VER V
5	X																	
9	X		X															
14	X							X										
17	X		X	X	X	X	X		X	X	X	X	X	X	X	X	X	X
19	X	**X**																

Fibrillation, Auricular- See Fibrillation, Atrial

Fibrinosis

	HEP	SIL
6	X	X
8	X	X

Fibrocystic Breast Disease- See Tumor, Breast

Fibroid- See Tumor, Fibroid

Fibroma- See Tumor, Fibroid

Fibrosis

	CALC FL	CAUST	FL AC	SIL	THYROID
17	X	X	X	X	
18	X				
24					X

Fibrositis

	BRY	RHUS T	ARN	CAUST	NUX V	ACON	CHAM	CIMICI	KALM	LAC C	LED	PHOS	RAN B	SIL	THUJA
1															X
9														X	
19	X	X		X	X			X	X	X		X	X		
21	X	X	X	X	X	X	X				X				
29[1]	X	X	X												
29[2]	X	X	X												

29[1] Fisher P. An Experimental Double Blind Clinical Trial method in Homoeopathy. Use of a Limited range of Remedies to Treat Fibrositis. Brit Hom J, 1986, Jul, 75, 3, 142-147.

29[2] Fisher P. An Experimental Double-blind Clinical Trial method in Homoeopathy- Use of a Limited Range of Remedies to Treat Fibrositis. British Hom J, 1986, July, 75, 3, 142-7

Fig Warts- See also Warts

	CINNAB	STAPHYS	LYC	NIT AC	PH AC	SABIN	THUJA	HEP	MERC C	MERC N
1		X				X				
4		X								
6	X		X	X	X		X		X	X
8	X	X	X		X					
14	X			X		X	X	X		

Filariasis

	MERC SU	HYDROC	ARS	CALC FL	CAPS	FERR PH	MEZ	STAPHYS	PSOR	SULPH
1		X								
3	X			X	X	X				
9		X								
10	X									
11			X				X	X	X	X

Fingertips, Cracks- See Cracks, Fingertips

Fissure, Anal

	NIT AC	GRAPH	RAT	PAEONIA	SIL	SULPH	IGN	PLAT	THUJA	ARS	CAUST	NAT M	NUX V	PETR	SEP	AESC	BERB V	LACH	PHOS	CALEND	CHAM	MEZ	RHUS T	CALC PH	LED
1	X	X	X	X	X			X	X								X	X							
2	**X**		**X**	X	X				X					X					X				X		
3	X	X	X	X				X	X											X					
4	**X**	**X**	X	**X**	**X**			X																	
5	X	X	X																						
6	X	X	X		X	X	X	X		X	X	X	X	X	X					X	X		X		
7	X		X	X																					
8	**X**	**X**	X	X	X	X	**X**	X	X	X	X	X	X	X	X	X	X	X	X			X		X	X
9																					X				
10		X																							
11	X	X			X	X			X		X			X	X		X	X	X					**X**	**X**
12																E				E					
13	X				X	X	X		X	X	X	X	X		X	X		X	X			X			
14	X	X	X									X					X								
18	X	X	X	X																					
19	X	X	X	X			**X**			X	X		X		X										
21	X	X	X			X										X									
24	X		X	X		X		X		X		X	X	X							X	X	X		
26					X	**X**	X																		
28	X	X																							
29^	X																								

E- External

29*Bignamini M, et al. Homeopathic Treatment of Anal Fissures using Nitricum acidum. Berlin Journal on Research in Homoeopathy, 1991, 1, 4/5, 286-287.

Fissure, Nipple- See also Cracks, Nipples

	PHYTO	GRAPH	NIT AC	RAT	HEP	LYC	SULPH
1	X			X			
4	X	X		X	X		
6	X	X					
8	X	X				X	
10							X
14		X	X				
18		X	X				
24	X						
25	X						

Fissure, Palms

	ANT C	CALC FL
14		X
18	X	

Fissure, Rectal

	GRAPH	PHYTO	SEP	SULPH
2			X	
8	X	X		
22	X			X
24		X		

Fissure, Tongue

	NIT AC	ANANTH	BELL	CARB V	CHAM	MERC	NUX V	PHOS	RAPH
10	X								
13									X
14		X							
15					X		X		
17	X								
21			X	X		X		X	

Fissures

	PETR	GRAPH	NIT AC	ALUM	ANT C	CALC FL	KALI ARS	KRAM	MERC	NAT M	PAEONIA	RAT	X-RAY
1													X
2		X		X					X			X	
5	X					X							
9	X												
10	X	X											
18	X	X			X								
23	X	X	X				X	X		X	X		
25	X												
28			X										

Fistula

	SIL	NIT AC	CAUST	PHOS	CALC	LYC	FL AC	CALC SUL	SULPH	AUR M	BELL	BERB V	CALC FL	HYDRAST	PETR	CALC PH	CALEND	MYRIST
1	X	X																
2	**X**	X	**X**	X	X		**X**	X		X		X		X	X	**X**	**X**	
3		**X**	X	X					X		X	X	X	X				**X**
4	X																	
5	X	X					X	X					X					
6		X				X												
7	X																	
8	X	X	X	X	X	X	X		X		X							
17										X								
19	X			X				X										
24	X		X	X	X	X									X			
26	X		X		X	X			X									

Fistula, Anal

	SIL	CALC PH	BERB V	CAUST	CALEND	HYDRAST	NIT AC	SULPH	LACH	CALC	AUR M	FL AC	MERC	NUX V	KALI CAR	CALC SUL	GRAPH	HEP	KREO	SEP	STAPHYS	THUJA	IGN	LYC	MYRIST	PAEONIA	PHOS
1	X		X	X	E	X	**X**	X	X			X			X	X											
2	X										X											X				X	
3	X		X							X			X				X										
5	X					X	X											X									
7	**X**	X	**X**	**X**	X	X	X	X	X	**X**	X	X	X	X	**X**		X		X	X	X	X					X
8	X	X	X	X	X	X		X	X	X	X	X	X	X				X	X	X	X		X				
11		X																									
12	X	X		X	E	E		X						X										X			
14	X				E		X																		X		
17		X																									
19			X																								
21	X								X							X											
24	X	X	X	X				X																			

E- External

Fistula, Bone

	SIL	AUR	AUR M	ASAF	ARG	FL AC	HECLA	LACH	MERC	NIT	NIT AC	PH AC	PHOS
6	X												
8	X		X	X	X	X	X	X	X	X	X	X	X
24		X											

Fistula, Breast

	SIL	PHOS	PHYTO
6	X		
24	X	X	X

Fistula, Dental (Includes Fistula, Gums)

	FL AC	SIL	CAUST	SULPH	CALC	STAPHYS	CANTH	LYC	NAT M	PETR	RAT	AUR M	BAR C	CALC PH	MAG CAR	NIT AC
1	X	X														
2			X	X		X										
3	X	X														
4	**X**	X														
5	X															
6		X	X	X	X						X					
7	**X**	**X**	X	X	X	X		X	X			X	X			
8	X	X	X	X	X	X	X			X	X			X		
13	X	X	X	X	X	X	X	X	X	X					X	X
24	X															
26			X	X	X											

Fistula, Gums- See Fistula, Dental

Fistula, Lachrymal

	CALC	FL AC	SIL	PULS	SULPH	BROM	NAT M	NIT AC	PETR	CHEL	LACH	BELL	LYC	STANN	ACON	AGAR M	APIS	AUR M	CALC FL	CAUST	HEP	MERC	MILL	NAT CAR	PHOS	PHYTO	STAPHYS
1		X																									
2			X			X		X		X	X			X		X							X				
3		X	X	X																							
4	X						X																				
6	X	X	X	X	X	X	X		X		X	X								X							
7	**X**	**X**	**X**	X	X	X	X	X	**X**				X				X	X									
8	X	X	X	X	X	X	X	X	X	X	X	X							X		X	X			X	X	X
13	X	X	X	X	X			X		X				X										X			
14	X	X																									
26	X		X	X	**X**								X		X												

Fistula, Rectal

	BERB V	CAUST	SIL	AUR M	CALC PH	CALC SUL	SULPH	THUJA	BACILL	CALEND	FL AC	HYDRAST	KREO	LACH	NIT AC	PAEONIA	PETR	PHOS
1	X	X			X	X	X		X	E	X	X		X	X			
2			X	X				X								X		
3																		X
6	X	X	X			X												
8	X																	
13	X	X	X	X			X	X					X				X	
19	X	X			X													

E- External

Fistula, Vagina

	NIT AC	PULS	CALC	SIL	ANT C	ASAR	LACH	LYC	PETR	THUJA	AGAR M	ASAR C	AUR	BELL	CARB V	CAUST	CON	HEP	KREO	RUTA	SEP	SULPH
3	X	X			X		X		X	X		X										
7	X	X	**X**	**X**		X		X														
8	X	X	X	X	X	X	X	X	X	X	X		X	X	X	X	X	X	X	X	X	X

Flatulence- See also Distension, Abdomen

	LYC	CARB V	CHINA	NUX V	ARG N	PULS	ALOE	CHAM	ASAF	COLOC	SULPH	NUX M	LACH	COCCUL	NAT SUL	PHOS	DIOSC	GRAPH	KALI CAR	POD	RAPH	ALL C	CALC PH	IGN	NAT CAR	SEP	THUJA	VER A
1	X	X	X	X	X	X	X	X		X		X	X	X			X		X		X	X					X	
2	**X**	**X**			**X**			X	X			**X**	**X**			X	X			X	X			X				
3	X	X	X			X			X	X		X															X	
4	**X**	X	X	X	**X**	X	X		X					X	X		X	X					X	X	X	X		X
5	X	X	X	X	X		X	X	X			X			X	X			X	X		X						
6	X	X	X	X		X	X	X	X		X	X	X	X		X		X					X	X		X	X	X
7	X	**X**	**X**	X	**X**	X	**X**	X	X	X	X	**X**	X	X	**X**	**X**	**X**	**X**	X	X	X	X	X	X	X	X	X	
8	X	**X**	**X**	**X**	X	X		X	X	X	X	X	X	X	X	X	**X**	X	X		X			X	X	X		
9	X	X	X	X	X			X	X		X				X										X			X
10	X	X	X	X	X	X					X		X					X				X	X					
11	X	X	X	X		X	X								X								X					
12	X	X		X							X																	
13	X	X	X	X		X	X	X	X	X	X	X	X	X	X	X		X	X				X	X	X	X	X	
14	**X**	**X**	**X**	X	X		**X**	X		X		X		X		X	X				X	X						
15	X	X	X	X		X		X		X			X	X														
16	X	X	X	X	X	X															X							
17	X	X	X	X	X				X	X	X								X			X						
18	X	X	X	X	X		X		X		X	X						X	X		X						X	
19	X	X	X		X		X								X					X								
20	X	X																										
21	X		X		X		X	X			X									X					X	X		
22	X	X				X														X								
23			X		X				X																			
24	X	X	X			X	X	X		X				X						X								
25	X	X	X	X	X			X		X	X																	X
26	X	X	X	X		X					X		X			X												X
27	X		X	X						X																		X
28	X	X																										

Flushing (Of Heat)- See also Menopause

	LACH	BELL	AMYL N	SULPH	SANG	SEP	GLON	PULS	FERR	ACON	SULPH AC	VER V	LYC	CALC	JAB	STRONT C	GRAPH	CHAM	CON	CROT H	GELS	PHOS	IGN					
1	X			X		X									X													
2			X		X						X				X													
4	X	X	X	X	X	X						**X**				X												
5	X	X			X	X	X	X	X					X	X				X		X	X						
6	X	X	X	X	X	X			X		X		X	X					X									
7	**X**	X	**X**	**X**	X	X	**X**	**X**	X	X	**X**	X	X				X	X		X	X		**X**					
8	X	X	X	**X**	X	X	X				X		X		X					X		X						
9	X	X	X		X		X	**X**	X	X		**X**				X												
10		X	X	X				X															X					
11	X			X										X														
12		X								X																		
13													**X**				**X**					X						
14	X	X	X	X	X	X	X		X																			
15				X		X				X								X										
16		X																										
17	X	X	X		X		X				X					X					X							
18	X	X	X	X	X	X	X			X																		
19	X		X	X	X		X	X		X									X	X								
21	X	X	X	X				X	X		X						X											
22		X																										
24		X		X					X									X										
25	X	X	X		X		X	**X**		X		**X**				X												
27	X					X			X																			
28			X																									
29[1]	X		X			X		X						X														
29[2]	X	X		X	X	X																						

29[1] Clover A, et al. Homoepathic Treatment of Hot Flushes. Brit Hom J, 2002, 91, 75-79.
29[2] Bordet MF, et al. Treating hot flushes in menopausal women with homeopathic treatment--results of an observational study. Homeopathy. 2008 Jan; 97 (1):10-5.

Foetus, Malposition Of (Includes Foetus, Breech Presentation)

	PULS	AUR	AUR M																									
2	X																											
6		X	X																									
28	X																											

Foetus, Motion, Excessive

	ARN	OP	HAM	LYC	PULS	CON	CONVAL	CROC	PSOR	SEP	SIL	SULPH	THUJA
8	X	X		X		X	X	X	X	X		X	X
9	X	X	X		X								
13	X	X		X							X		
25	X	X	X		X								

Folliculitis Barbae- See Barber's Itch

Fontanelles, Failure to Close

	CALC	CALC PH	SIL	PULS	ALUM	CALC IOD	MERC	SEP	SULPH
8	X	X	X	X		X	X	X	
10		X	X		X				
14	X								
15	X								
22		X							
26	X		X	X					X

Food Poisoning

	ARS	NUX V	CARB V	BAPT	HYOSC	PULS	PYROG	ALOE	ANTHRAC	ARG N	BRY	CHINA	COLCH	COLOC	CROT T	CUPR	ECHIN	GAMBOG	LYC	MAG PH	NAT M	PH AC	POD	RUMEX	TROMB	VER A
1	X	X	X	X	X	X				X						X					X					
3	X	X	X		X																					
4	**X**																									
5	X	X					X												X				X		X	X
7	**X**								X																	
9	X	X																						X		
10	X																									
11	X			X				X							X			X								
14	X																									
18	X																									
19	**X**												X													
21	X																									
22	X																									
23	X																X									
25	X	X	X			X	X				X	X		X						X		X	X			
28	X																									

Fractures- See also Weakness, Bones (Includes Fractures, Non-Union Of)

	SYMPH	**CALC PH**	**ARN**	**RUTA**	**SIL**	**CALC**	**LACH**	**BRY**	**CALEND**	**EUP PERF**	**HYDRAST**	**SULPH**	**CALC FL**	**LYC**	**NIT AC**	**RHUS T**
1	X	X	X	X		X	X									X
2	**X**	**X**		**X**	**X**					X						
3	X	**X**	X	X		X	X				X					
4	**X**	**X**		X								X				
5	B	X	X	X	X	X							X			
6		X														
7	**X**	**X**		**X**	X	X	X		X							
8	**X**			X	X	X			X			X		X	X	
9	X		X	X												
10	X	X	X													
13	X		X	X	X	X						X		X		
14		X	**X**	X												
15	X															
18	X	X														
19	X	**X**	X	X	X	X	**X**	X		X	X		X		X	
20	X		**X**		X			X		X						
21	X		X													
22	X							X								
24	X	X	X	X	X				X		X					X
26	**X**															
28	X															
29[1]	X		X													
29[2]		X														

B- Both Internal and External

29[1] Oberbaum M, et al. Effect of Arnica montana and Symphytum Officionalis on Bone Healing in Guinea Pigs. International Research Group on Very Low Dose and High Dilution Effects, 1993 Giri Meeting, Brit Hom J, April, 1994, 83, 84-100.

29[2] Werkman C, et al. Comparative therapeutic use of Risedronate and Calcarea phosphoric: allopathy versus homeopathy in bone repair in castrated rats. Brazilian Oral Research, 2006, Jul-Sept, 20, 3, 196-201.

Fracture, Skull

	HYPER	**ARN**	**CALC PH**	**GLON**	**SYMPH**
3				X	
7	X	**X**	**X**		X
14	X				

Frostbite- See also Chilblains

	AGAR M	APIS	NIT AC	PETR	FERR PH	ARS	BELL	CALEND	CARB V	CIST C	HAM	LACH	MAG P AU	NUX M	PSOR	PULS	RAN B	RHUS T	SEC	SIL								
1	**X**							E																				
2			X	X	**X**								X	X														
3	X																											
16	X																											
17	X	X					X											X										
18	X	X	X	X		X			X	X	X				X	X	X		X	X								
21	X	X										X																
28	X																											

E- External

Fungus Haematodes

	PHOS	LACH	SIL	THUJA	CALC	ARS	CARB A	CARB V	LYC	NIT AC	SEP	SULPH	BELL	MERC	NAT M	PULS	STAPHYS											
7	**X**	**X**	X	**X**	X										X	X												
8	X	X	X	X	X	**X**	X	X	X	X	X	X	X				X											
13	**X**	X	**X**		X	X	X	X	X	X	X	X		X														
24	X	X		X																								
26	X																											

Fungus Haematodes, Uterus

	PHOS	CARB A	NIT AC	AUR	BELL	CARB V	CHINA	GRAPH	KREO	LACH	MERC	SEP	SIL	SULPH	THUJA													
2	X									X																		
4	X																											
7	X	X	X																									
8	X	X	X	X	X	X	X	X	X		X	X	X	X	X													

Fungus, Medullary

	CARB A	PHOS	THUJA	NIT AC	SIL																							
8	X	X	X	X	X																							
13	X	X	X																									

Furuncle- See Boils

Galactorrhoea- See also Lactation, Profuse

	PULS	CALC	CON	BELL	BOR	CHINA	PHOS	RHUS T	IOD	LYC	SIL	ACON	BRY	LAC C	LACH	PHYTO
2			X						X							
5	X		X								X					
7	X	**X**	X	**X**		X	X	X	X	X	X				X	
8	X	**X**	X	X	X	X	X	X	X	X	X		X			
9	X				X									X		X
13	X	X	X	**X**	X	X	X	**X**		X		X			X	
14														X		
15		X					X									
21	X		X									X				
22	X															
25	X	X			X											X
26	X	X		X		X							X			

Gall Bladder, Congestion Of- See also Gall Bladder, Obstruction

	BERB V	CARD M	HYDRAST	MANDRA	NUX V	POD	RAPH	RICIN	TARAX
5			X	X	X	X	X	X	X
6		X							
11	X								
14	X								

Gall Bladder, Diseases Of

	CHEL	BAPT	BERB V	CHINA	DIOSC	BELL	BOLET	CALC	CYCL	FERR SUL	HEP	LACH	LYC	MERC	NAT SUL	NUX V	POD	SEP
2		X			X		X			X								
4			X															
5	X			X					X				X					X
9	X																	
11	X														X			
19	X				X													
24	X	X	X	X		X		X			X	X		X		X	X	
25	X																	

Gall Bladder, Obstruction- See also Gall Bladder, Congestion Of

	CHEL	CROT H	LACH
5		X	X
14	X		

Gall Stones- See Calculi, Biliary
Ganglion Cyst- See Cyst, Ganglion
Gangrene

	ARS	LACH	CARB V	SEC	CROT H	SULPH AC	KREO	ANTHRAC	ECHIN	PLUM	SIL	CHINA	BELL	EUPHORB	ACON	APIS	ARN	ASAF	MERC
1	X	X	X	X	X	X	X	X											
2	**X**	**X**	**X**	**X**		X		X	**X**					X		X			
3		X	X	X	X	X													
4	**X**	**X**	**X**	**X**	X												X		
5	X	X	X	X				X											
6	X	X	X	X			X	X		X		X							
7	X	X	X	X	X	X	X	**X**		X	X	X	X			X		X	
8	X	X	X	X	X	X	X			X	X	X	X	X	X		X	X	X
10										X									
11	X	X	X	X		X			X					X					
12	X	X	X																X
13	**X**	X	X	X	X	X	**X**			X	**X**	**X**	X	X	X				
14	X		X	X			X												
16	X	X	X																
17					X				X										
19	X	X		X	X														
21	X	X	X	X					X										
23	X	X		X					X										
24	X	X	X	X	X	X	X	X							X	X	X	X	X
26	X	X									**X**		X						

Gangrene, Genitals

	CANTH	ARS	LAURO	PLUM	SEC
8	X	X		X	X
13	**X**	X	**X**		

Gangrene, Gums

	MERC	MERC C	LACH
7	X	**X**	X
24	X		

Gangrene, Lungs

	ARS	KREO	CARB V	SIL	EUCAL	LACH	CARB A	ARN	CAPS	CARB AC	CHINA	CROT H	DULC	HEP	LYC	OSMIUM	SEC
1	X	X															
6	X	X	X	X						X							
7	X	X					X										
8					X											X	
13						X											
17	X	X	X	X	X	X	X	X	X			X	X	X	X		X
26	X		X	X							X						

Gangrene, Mouth

	SIL	LACH	ARS	CROT H	HYDRAST
7	X	**X**	X	X	X
24	X				

Gangrene, Penis

	LAURO	ARS	CANTH	FL AC	LACH	PLUM
7	X	X		X	X	
8	X		X			X

Gangrene, Throat

	ARS	LACH	ARUM T	AILANTH	CARB V	KALI PH	PHYTO	SULPH	AMM C	ANTHRAC	BELL	CARB AC	CHINA	CHIN ARS	CROT H	KREO	MERC CY	MUR AC	NIT AC	SIL
7	**X**	**X**	X	**X**	X	X	X	X		X			X		X	X		X	X	
8	X	X	X	X	X		X	X	X			X		X			X			
14						X														
17			X																	
26	X	X									X									X

Gangrene, Toes

	SEC	CROT H	LACH
7	X	X	X
13	X		

Gangrene, Tongue

	ARS	LACH	SEC
7	**X**	X	
8	X	X	
10	X		
13	X		X

Gangrene, Uterus

	ARS	SEC	KREO	ACON	APIS	BELL	CALEND	CARB V	CARB A	CHINA	CURARE
7	X	X	X				X				
8	X	X	X						X		X
13	X	X	X	X	X	X		X		X	
26	X	X									

Gastralgia- See also Pain, Abdomen; Pain, Stomach

	ARS	BISM	NUX V	PHOS	BRY	ARG N	GRAPH	PULS	CARB V	LYC	CHINA	CALC	BELL	IRIS V	SEP	SULPH	CHAM	ANT C	FERR	KALI BIC	PETR	SULPH AC	CARB A	COLOC	KALI CAR	VER A
1	X	X	X	X	X	X	X	X	X	X	X	X		X				X	X		X	X				
2		X					X															X			X	
3			X																							
4		**X**		X		X	X														X					
5	X	X			X		X			X										X	X	X				
6	X	X	X	X	X	X	X	X	X		X	X	X		X	X	X		X		X			X	X	X
7	X	X	**X**	X	**X**	X	X	**X**	**X**	**X**		X	**X**	X	X	**X**	X		X	X	X	X	X	**X**	X	**X**
8	X	X	X	X	**X**	X	X	X	X	X	X	**X**	**X**	X	X	**X**	X	X	X				X	X	X	X
9						X																				
10	X	X	X		X		X		X			X	X		X								X			
11	X	X	X	X		X					X			X									X			
12					X																					
13	X	X	**X**	X	X		X	X	X	X	X	X	X		X	**X**	X	X	X	X	X	X	**X**	X	X	X
14	X			X				X			X							X								
15	X		X		X			X			X			X			X	X						X		
18	X			X		X												X		X		X				
19	**X**	X	**X**	**X**	**X**	X	**X**		X	**X**	X	X	X	X	X	**X**		X	X	X			X		**X**	
20	X																									
21				X																						
22	X			X				X						X												
23	X	X	X			X															X	X				X
24	X	X							X						X	X				X						
25	X					X														X						
26	X		X	X	X			X	X	**X**	X	X	X		X		X		X							X

Gastritis (Includes Inflammation, Stomach)

	NUX V	ARS	ANT C	PHOS	BRY	IPEC	ACON	PULS	BISM	BELL	CARB V	CHINA	KALI BIC	LYC	SANG	ANT T	VER A	APIS	ARG N	CHEL	SEP	CANTH
1																			X			
2	**X**	**X**		**X**					X							X						X
3			X											X								
5			X					X														
6	X	X	X		X	X	X	X		X	X	X		X	X			X			X	
7	**X**	**X**		X	**X**				X	**X**					X	**X**	X	X	X			
8	X	X	X	X	X	X	X	X	X	X	X	X	X		X	X	X	X	X	X	X	X
9	X	X	X	X		X		X			X	X	X	X								
10	X	X				X					X	X										
11	X												X									
12	X	X	X	X	X		X	X	X													
13	X	X	X	X	**X**	X	**X**	X	X	X					X		X	**X**		X		**X**
14						X																
18													X									
19	X	X	X	X	X	X		X			X	X	X	X	X	X				X	X	
23	X	X	X						X										X	X		
26	X	X		X	X	X	**X**			X							X				X	

Gastroenteritis

	ARS	POD	ARG N	VER A	PHOS	BRY	CUPR	DULC	IPEC	NUX V	ALOE	BAPT	CROT T	GAMBOG	ANT C	COLOC	CHINA	KALI BIC	PH AC	PULS	SULPH
2						X															
3			X	X																	
5	X	X		X	X		X		X		X				X						
9	X		X	X														X			
11	**X**	X	X		X	X		X	X	X	**X**	**X**	**X**	**X**	X			X	X	X	X
14	**X**	X	X	X																	
17	X		X				X									X					
18	X	X		X			X	X	X	X	X		X	X	X	X	X				
19	X	X	X	X	X	X		X		X		X	X	X			X	X	X	X	X
20					X	X										X					
21	X	X			X			X	X	X		X					X		X	X	X
23		X					X														

Gastromalacia

	KREO	ARS	BISM	CALC	MERC D	ANT C	ANT T	ARG N	BAR C	BELL	BRY	CALC AC	CALC ARS	CAPS	CARB V	FERR	KALI BIC	NUX V	PH AC	PULS	SULPH	VER A
2	X				X																	
7	X	X	X	X	X									X		X						
8	**X**	X	X	X		X	X	X	X	X	X	X	X		X		X	X	X	X	X	X
26	**X**																					

Giardiasis

	CINA	CARB TET	CHELONE	CHEN OIL	GIARDIA	NAT PH	SANTON	TEUCR	THYMOL																			
11	X	X	X	X		X	X	X	X																			
14	X																											
28					X																							

Gingivitis

	MERC	KREO	NAT M	SIL	NUX V	PHOS	BELL	BOR	CHAM	HEP	ACON	AMM C	CAPS	CHINA	IOD	NIT AC	PH AC	PHYTO	STAPHYS	SULPH	CALC							
1							X										X											
5	X	X				X		X						X		X		E										
7		**X**	**X**	**X**	X	X			X		X		X		X			X										
8	**X**		X	X	X	X	**X**	X	X	X		X		X		X	X		X	X	**X**							
9				X																								
10	**X**																			X								
13		X	X	X	**X**					X		X			X													
14	X	X								X	X																	
15	X																											
18	X							X																				
19																			X									
20		X							X																			
21	X	X	X	X		X																						
26	X		X		X		X						X															

E- External

Glanders

	KALI BIC	LACH	ARS	HIPPOZ	MERC	RHUS T																						
2	**X**	**X**		X																								
8	X	X	X		X	X																						

Glands, Diseases Of

	CALC	SIL	SULPH	CARB A	BAR C	BELL	MERC	CON	HEP	IOD	DULC	LYC	SPONG	CIST	CLEM	GRAPH	NIT AC	STAPHYS	BROM	LAPIS	BAD	CARB V	PHOS	RHUS T	SEP			
2			X															X			X							
4	**X**	**X**	**X**	**X**		**X**	**X**	**X**	X	**X**			**X**	X		X			**X**	**X**	X	X						
8	X	X	X	X	X	X	X	X	X		X	X		X	X	X	X	X		X			X	X				
10	X	X	X	X	X	X	X		X		X	X																
13	X	X	**X**	X	X	X	X	**X**	X	**X**	X	X	X	X	X	X	X	X				X	X	X	X			
15		X																										
16	X	X		X	X			X		X					X													
17										X			X															
23	X				X												X		X						X			
24					X																							
26	X	X	X	X		X	X		X		X	X																

Glands, Enlargement- See also Swelling, Glands

	CALC	BAR C	CALC IOD	MERC	ARS IOD	BELL	IOD	CON	KALI IOD	SULPH	ARS	HEP	NIT AC	SIL	ALNUS	BAR M	BROM	CALC PH	CIST	GRAPH	LAPIS	SCROPH	ARUM T	CALEND				
1		X	X				X	X								X												
2	**X**	**X**	**X**	**X**		**X**			**X**		**X**	**X**	**X**	**X**	X	X	X		X	X	X	X	**X**	**X**				
4	X	X				**X**	X	**X**		**X**		X			X													
8	X	X	X		X			X		X	X		X	X				X	X	X								
9							X																					
10																	X											
11							X		X												X	X						
12	X																											
14	X				X																							
15	X			X	X	X				X																		
16					X																							
17									X									X										
24	X		X																									
25				X																								
27				X																								

Glandular Fever- See Infectious Mononucleosis

Glaucoma (Includes Eye, Pressure)

	PHOS	SPIG	GELS	COLOC	BRY	BELL	SULPH	PRUN S	ACON	CEDRON	OSMIUM	AUR	NUX V	PHYSO	EUPHR	ARN	ARS	CHINA	CON	OP	RHOD	LYC
1	X	X	X	X			X	X			X			**X**								
2	X	**X**		X				X		X	X			X								
3	X	X	X	X	X		X	X		X	X											X
4			**X**		X							X					X			X		
5				X								X		X								
6	X	X	X	X	X	X	X	X		X		X	X			X	X		X		X	
7	**X**	X		X	X		X			X												
8	X	X	X	X	X	X	X	X	X	X	X	X	X				X		X		X	
9	X	X	X		X	X			X						X					X		
12	X		X			X							X		X	X		X				
13	**X**	**X**		X	X	X	**X**		X				X		X	**X**	X	X	X		X	**X**
14	X										X			X				X				
21						X																
23	X			X																		
24	X	X	X	X	X	X		X	X	X		X	X		X	X		X	X		X	
25	X	X	**X**		X	X			X											X		
26	**X**																					X
27	X	X	**X**	X	X	X	X	X	X		X									X		

Glossitis

	ACON	APIS	BELL	ARS	MERC	CANTH	LACH	ARN	ARUM T	BAPT	BENZ AC	CROT H	KALI BIC	MERC C	NAT M	NIT AC	PLUM	RHUS T	SULPH
1	X	X	X	X	X	X	X				X	X							
2						X						X							
4				**X**															
5	X	X	X			X			**X**				X			X		X	
6	X	X	X	X			X		X	X			X	X				X	X
7	X	X		X	X		X	X			X			X	X	X	X		X
10	X				X			X							X				
12	X	X	X		X														
13	X	X	X	X	**X**	X	X	X									X		
14		X																	
15		X	X							X									
17	X																		

Glucosuria (Includes Glycosuria)

	PH AC	ARG	CHIO	URAN N	LAC AC	ACET AC	CURARE	SYZYG	THUJA	AMYL N	ARG N	CARB V	CHINA	EUGEN	GLYCERIN	INSULIN	IOD	IRIS V	KALI BR	MOSCH	NAT SUL	PHOS	PLUM	PIC AC	STRY ARS	URAN A		
1	X		X	X					X		X				X													
3							X																					
4	X			X				X																				
5			X	X	X	X								X			X									X		
6		X																	X									
7		X			X					X											X							
10	X	X		X	X											X												
11		X	X																									
12	X																											
13	X								X				X															
14	X	X	X		X	X		X																				
17							X																		X			
23																		X		X				X				
26	X	X										X										X	X					

Gleet

	SEP	NAT M	SULPH	THUJA	AGNUS	TEREB	ALUMEN	FERR	GRAPH	HYDRAST	KALI SUL	MERC	MEZ	NIT AC	PETR	PHOS	NAPHTH											
2	X	X	X	**X**		X	X		X		X		X	X		X	**X**											
3	X																											
4	X	**X**	**X**	X						X		X		X														
6	X	X	X	X	X	X	X	X				X	X	X		X												
7	X	X	X		X	X	X	X	X	X	X		X		X	X												
8	X	X			X	X		X	X						X		X											
11											X																	
12			X	X	X					X		X			X													

Glomerulonephritis- See also Nephritis

	APIS	CANTH	ARS	HELL	MERC	PHOS	SER ANG																					
5	X	X		X	X	X	X																					
21	X	X	X																									

Glossitis- See also Swelling, Tongue

	MERC	APIS	ARS	BELL	LACH	ACON	CANTH	CARB V	CROT H	NIT AC	RAN S	SEP	SULPH AC	ARN	ARUM T	BAPT	CALC	CON	CUPR AC	HEP	MERC C	NAT M	PETR	PLUM	STAPHYS	SULPH		
1	X												X															
2	X	X				X	X				X		X															
3	X	X					X		X																			
6	X	X	X	X	X		X	X		X	X	X		X	X		X	X	X	X		X	X	X	X	X		
8	X	X	X	X	X	X	X	X	X	X	X	X	X	X	X	X	X	X	X	X	X	X	X	X	X	X		
9		X	X		X					X																		
10	X		X					X				X																
17	X	X			X				X							X					X							
21			X	X																								
23		X				X																						
25				X																								
26	**X**	X		X	X	X																						

Glossoplegia

	CAUST	GELS	BAR C	PLUM	DULC	OP	LACH	MUR AC	BELL	HYOSC	ACON	NUX M	ARS	COCCUL	CUPR	ARN	CON	GRAPH	GUACO	HYDR AC	STRAM	ANAC	BOTHR	HEP	LYC	NUX V		
1	**X**	X	X	X	X		X	X																				
2	X			X			X												X				X					
3	**X**	X		X															X									
4	X		X																									
6	X		X	X	X	X	X	X	X	X	X	X	X	X	X	X		X	X	X	X			X		X		
7	**X**	**X**	X	X	X	**X**	X	X		X	X	X		X														
8	X	X	X	X	X	X	X	X	X	X	X	X	X	X	X	X	X	X		X	X	X		X	X	X		
9		X	X																			X						
10	X		X	X	X	X			X		X		X	X	X	X	X											
11	X	X		X	X			X	X								X						X					
13	**X**	X			**X**	**X**		X	X	X	X	**X**								X	X							
14	X		X			X									X													
17	X	X				X																			X			
19				X			X																					
25		X	X																									
26	X				X		X	X	X	X			X					X										

Glue Ear- See also Catarrh, Ear

	KALI MUR	LYC	PULS	CALC	GRAPH	HYDRAST	KALI BIC	KALI SUL	MEDO	MERC	MERC D																	
19	X	X	X					X	X		X																	
21	X	X		X	X	X	X			X																		
28			X																									

Goitre- See also Exophthalmic Goitre (AKA Derbyshire Neck, Struma)

	SPONG	IOD	CALC	BROM	LAPIS	THYROID	NAT M	FUCUS	CALC IOD	LYC	FL AC	NAT CAR	CAUST	KALI IOD	BELL	CALC FL	SULPH	HEP	HYDRAST	LACH	MERC I F	PHOS
1	X	**X**	X	X		X	X	X	X	X									X	X		
2	**X**	**X**	**X**	X	X	X	**X**	X		X	**X**	X	X		**X**							
3	X	X	X	X	X	X		X	X	X									X			
4	**X**	**X**	**X**	X	**X**			X	X		X											
5	X		X	X	X	X																
6	X	X	X	X			X	X	X	X		X	X	X	X	X	X	X		X		
7	**X**	**X**	**X**		X						X									X		
8	X	X	X	X	X		X		X	X			X	X		X	X	X				
9	X	X	X			X	X		X													
11	X	X	X	X	X	X	X	X			X				X				X			
12	X	X	X	X	X	X						X		X			X				X	X
13	**X**	X	**X**	**X**			X			X		X	**X**									
14		X																				
15	X																				X	
16	X	X			X											X						
17	X													X								X
19	X	X	X			X		X						X								X
21	X	X	X								X											
23	X	X		X	X											X						
24	X	X	X	X	X	X	X	**X**	X						X							
25	X	X	X			X	X		X													
26	**X**	X	X	X						X		X	X				X	X			X	
27		X																				
28	X																					

Gonarthrocace

	ARS	CALC	IOD	SIL	ACON	ARN	BELL	BRY	KALI IOD	LACH	LYC	MERC	PULS	SULPH
6	X	X	X	X	X	X	X	X	X	X	X	X	X	X
7	X	X	X	X										

Gonitis- See Inflammation, Knee

Gonorrhoea

	THUJA	CANN S	CANTH	MERC	COP	PULS	ACON	CINNAB	NAT SUL	SEP	CAPS	NIT AC	PETROS	ARG N	MERC C	SULPH	AGNUS	CANN I	HYDRAST	CLEM	CUBEB	KALI SUL	TUSSIL	MEDO	TEREB	GELS	PETR	
1	X	X	X	X	X	X	X	X	X	X	X		X	X		X					X		X	X				
2	**X**	**X**	**X**		X	X	X	X	**X**	X			X	X		X		X	X	X	X	X	X		X	X	X	
3	X			X	X			X							X		X						X				X	
4	**X**	**X**	**X**	**X**	**X**	**X**	**X**		X	**X**	X					X	X				X		X			X		
5								X													X							
6	X	X	X	X	X	X	X		**X**	X	X	X	X	X		X	X	X	X	X	X	X			X	X		
7	**X**	**X**	**X**	**X**	X	**X**	X	X		**X**	**X**	**X**	X	X	X	X	X	X	**X**	X	X	**X**		**X**	**X**	X	X	
8	X	X	X	**X**	X	X	X	X		X	X	X	X	X	X	X	X	X	X	X		X		X	X	X	X	
11	**X**	**X**	X	**X**		**X**	X	X			X	**X**	X		**X**	X		X		X		**X**	X					
12	X		X		X		X							X	X				X								X	
13	X	**X**	**X**	**X**	**X**	X	X	X	X		X	**X**	**X**	X	**X**		**X**								X			
14	X	X				X			X																			
17	X																											
19																								X				
23	X	X	X		X				X			X						X	X	X			X	X				
24				X																								

Gout- See also Tophi; Uricaemia (Includes Lithaemia)

	COLCH	LED	LYC	ARN	BENZ AC	URT U	SULPH	PULS	LITH C	NUX V	SABIN	ACON	BRY	AMM PH	ANT C	GUAIAC	BELL	CAUST	COLOC	GRAPH	KALI IOD	RHOD	CALC	FORMICA
1	X	**X**		X	X	X					X			X	X	X				X	X		X	X
2	**X**	**X**	X		X	**X**	**X**	**X**	X	**X**	**X**			X		X	X				X			X
3	**X**	X			X	X			X					X								X		
4	**X**	**X**	X	X	X	X						X	X	**X**	X			X	X					
5	X	X	X		X	X			X	X			X			X	X							X
6	X		X	X	X		X		X	X	X	X	X	X	X	X		X	X	X	X		X	
7	**X**	**X**	**X**	**X**	X	X	X	X	X	**X**	X		**X**		X	X	X	X	X	X	X	X	**X**	X
8	X	X	X	X	X		X	X	X	X	X	X	X		X	X	X	X	X	X		X	X	
9	**X**	X		X								X					X							
10	X		X							X											X			
11	**X**	**X**	X	**X**	**X**	X	X	X	X		X	**X**	X			X								
12	**X**			X		X	X	X		X		X	X		X						X	X		
13	X	**X**		**X**			**X**				**X**									X				
14	X	X	X					X											X			X		
15	X	X						X		X		X												
16		X	X			X																		
17		X	X				X																	
18		X	X	X	X		X						X										X	
19	**X**	**X**	X	X	X	X	X		X									X		X				
21	X	X	X	X	X	X		X																
22	X																							
23	X	X			X	X			X		X			X								X		X
24	X							X											X					
25	**X**	X		X		X						X		X			X							
26			X												X			X						
28	X																							

Gout, Fingers

	CALC	CALC FL	CLEM	STAPHYS
7	X		X	X
14		X		

Gout, Left Big Toe

	EUP PERF	MANG
6		X
7		X
14	**X**	

Granulatiion

	SIL	CALC	ARS	ALUMEN	BELL	CALEND	GRAPH	HEP	KALI MUR	LACH	SABIN
7	**X**	X	**X**	X					X	X	X
8	X	X			X	X		X			
16							X				

Gravel- See also Calculi, Renal

	LYC	SARS	BERB V	URT U	CANTH	NUX V	OCIMUM	OX AC	PH AC	ACON	CALC	COCCUS	EPIGEA	GALIUM	HYDRANG	LITH C	PHOS	POD	PULS	SEP	SIL	THLASPI	VESICAR	CHIN S	CASC	GRAPH	NM X
1				X																							
2	**X**	**X**	**X**	X			X	**X**	**X**				X	X	X					X			X	**X**	**X**	**X**	**X**
3		X	X	X																							
4	**X**				X		X															X	X				
6	X	X																									
7	X	X										X				X	X				X						
8	X	X				X					X		X	X	X	X	X	X	X		X						
10	X	X																									
11	X	X	X								X									X							
12	X		X		X	X	X	X	X	X								X									
14				X	X																						
15						X				X									X								
16																						X					
24												X															

Grave's Disease- See Exophthalmic Goitre; Hyperthyroidism

Gressus Gallinaceous

	LACH	SIL	AUR	MAG PH
6	X			
7	X	**X**	X	X
10	X			

Gressus Vaccinus

	PHOS	CIC
6	X	
7	**X**	X
10	X	

Growing Pain

	PH AC	CALC PH	GUAIAC	CALC	RHUS T
2			X		
7	X				
8	X	X	X		X
18		X			
21	X		X	X	
25	X	X		X	

Guillan Barre Syndrome

	ACON	CURAR	THUJA
19		X	
21	X		X

Gum Boils- See Boils, Gums; Epulis

Gummata (Includes Gumma)

	KALI IOD	AUR	ARS	AUR FL	BELL	CALC	CARB A	CARB V	CHINA	GRAPH	HEP	KREO	MERC	MEZ	NAT SUL	PH AC	PLUM	RUTA	SIL	THUJA
1	X														X					
2	X																			
6		X	X		X	X		X	X	X			X	X		X	X	X		
8	X	X		X			X				X	X							X	X

Gums, Bleeding- See Haemorrhage, Gums

Gums, Diseases Of- See also Strophulus

	MERC	STAPHYS	CARB V	KREO	MERC C	BRY	DULC	NAT M
2	**X**				**X**			
4	X	X						
6	X							
8	X	**X**	X	X	X	X	X	X
11	X							
12			X					
13	X			X		X	X	
14	X	X	X	X				
18	X							
26	X	X	X					X

Gums, Retracted

	CARB V	ANT C	MERC	CIST	IOD	KALI IOD	PHOS	KALI PH	ARG N	BAPT	BAR C	BOV	CAMPH	CUPR	DULC	LAC C	PH AC	PLUM	SEP	STAPHYS	ZINC
7	**X**	X	X	X	X	X	X	**X**		X			X				X			X	X
8	X	X	X	X	X	X	X		X		X	X		X	X	X		X	X		
9		X																			
14	X		X																		

Gun Shot- See Wounds, Gun Shot

Gynecomastia

	CON	MERC I F	PLUM IOD
3	X		
9		X	X

Haematemesis- See also Haemorrhage, Stomach

	IPEC	PHOS	ARS	ARN	HAM	CARB V	NUX V	ACON	CHINA	FERR	CANTH	MEZ	CROT H	MILL	VER A	LACH	SEC	SULPH	ARG N	BELL	CON	ERIGER	HYOSC	KALI BIC	LYC	PULS	SULPH AC
1	X	X																	X								
2	**X**			**X**	**X**									X													
3	X			X	X										X		X										
4	X	X																	X								
6	X	X	X	X	X	X	X	X	X	X	X	X	X	X	X		X	X		X	X	X	X	X		X	X
7	**X**	**X**	X	**X**	**X**	**X**	X	X	**X**	**X**	X		**X**	X		X	X	X		X		X				X	X
8	X	X	**X**	X	X	X	X	X	X	X	X	X	X	X	X	X	X	X	X	X	X	X	X	X	X	X	X
9	X	X		X			X	X			X																
10	X	X			X							X									X				X		
11		X	X		X							X	X														
12	X		X	X					X	X																	
13	X	**X**	X	**X**	X	X	**X**	**X**	X	X	X	X		**X**	**X**	X		X	X	X			X	X	X	X	
14	X	X	X			X							X														
15			X																								X
19																									X		
21		X																									
22		X	X																								
23		X			X																	X					
24	X	X	X			X	X				X	X				X	X				X			X			
26	**X**	X	**X**	X		X	X	X	X	X					X	X		X					X				

Haematocele

	CON	ARN	CROC	ERIGER	FERR	HAM	IPEC	NUX V	PULS	RHUS T	SABAD	SEC	SULPH	THLASPI	ZINC
2				X											
7						X									
8	X	X	X		X		X	X	X	X	X	X	X	X	X
24	X														

Haematuria- See also Urine, Black

	CANTH	TEREB	HAM	ARN	MILL	LYC	MERC C	PHOS	CALC	PULS	NUX V	NIT AC	SARS	APIS	ARS	CROT H	IPEC	MERC	OCIMUM	CACT	THLASPI	UVA	CHIM U	MEZ	SEC
1	X	**<u>X</u>**	X	X	X			X		X				X		X			X		X		X		
2		**X**	**X**	**X**	X	X						X				X				X	X	X		X	X
3	X	X	X		**X**	X					X	X	X	X							X				
4	X	**X**	**X**			X	X				X			X					X						
5	X						X			X													X		
6	X	X	X	X	X	X		X	X	X	X	X		X	X	X	X	X				X		X	X
7	**X**	**X**	**X**	X		X	**X**	X	**X**	**X**	X	X	X	**X**	X		X	X		**X**	X				X
8	X	X	X	X	X	X		X	X	X	X	X	X		X	X	X	X	X	X	X	X	X	X	X
9	X	X	X									X							X						
10	X	X					X	X			X				X	X		X							
11	X	X	X	**X**	**X**	X	X	X	X			X	X				X					X	X		
13	**X**	X		**X**	**X**	**X**	X	**X**	**X**	**X**	**X**		X		X		X	X	X	X		X		**X**	**X**
14	X	X			X		X	X	X				X			X				X			X		
15	X		X	X																					
16																					X				
18	X	X		X			X	X																	
19	X						X			X			X						X	X					
21	X	X												X								X			
22							X																		
23			X		X																		X		
24	X	X	X	X	X	X		X	X		X		X	X	X	X	X	X						X	
25	X																		X						
26	**X**					X			X	X		X			X		X	X							

Haemaglobin, Deficiency Of

	FERR	FERR PH	VANAD
3			X
8	X		
14		X	

Haemoglobinuria

	PIC AC	PHOS	CHIN S	SANTON
1	X	X	X	X
2	**X**	**X**		
23	X			

Haemolysis- See also Anaemia, Haemolytic (Includes Blood, Tendency to Decompose)

	ARS	ALUM	AMM C	AMM M	CARB V	CHINA	CUPR	KALI PH	LACH	NIT AC	PHOS	SEC
6	X	X			X	X	X	X	X	X	X	X
10	X											
13			X	X								

Haemophilia- See also Haemorrhage

	LACH	PHOS	HAM	SEC	CROT H	MILL	ARN	FERR	CARB V	CROC	ERIG	ARAN D	ARS	CAMPH	CHINA	CINNAM	ERGOT	IPEC	KREO	LAC C	MERC	NAT SIL	NAT SUL	RHUS T	SULPH	SULPH AC	TEREB
1	X	X		X		X		X	X							X			X								
3	X																										
6		**X**	X	X						X	X												X				
7	**X**	**X**	X		X			**X**					X		X												
8	X	X		X	X		X		X	X	X	X		X			X	X		X	X			X	X	X	X
11																						X					
14			X		X																						
16	X					X	X																				
17	X	X			X																						
18						X																					
23	X		X	X																							
24	X	X																									
29*	X		X			X	X																				

29* Kundu T, et al. Homeopathic medicines substantially reduce the need for clotting factor concentrates in haemophilia patients: results of a blinded placebo controlled cross over trial. Homeopathy. 2012 Jan; 101 (1):38-43.

Haemoptysis- See also Haemorrhage, Lungs (Includes Sputum, Bloody; Sputum, Rusty) (Note that only the main remedies from 17 are used here)

	PHOS	ACON	MILL	IPEC	ACALYPH	HAM	BRY	ARN	ARS	BELL	CACT	LED	CHINA	FERR	FERR PH	NIT AC	PULS	HEP	LYC	RHUS T	SABIN	SANG	CALC	DROS	PLUM	STANN		
1				X																								
2	X	X	X		X						X	X			X			X				X			X	X		
3	X		X	X	X	**X**									X													
6	X													X		X												
7	**X**	**X**	X	X	X	X	X	**X**	X	X	X	X	**X**	X		**X**	**X**	X	**X**	X	X		X	X		**X**		
8	X	**X**	X	X	X	X	X	X	X	X	X	**X**	**X**	X		X	X	X	X	X	X	X	X	X	X	X		
9				X																								
10	X						X													X								
11	X	X	X	X	X				X	X	X				X								X					
12	X		X	X		X	X	X										X			X			X				
13	**X**	**X**	**X**	X		X	**X**	**X**	X	X	X	**X**	**X**	**X**		X	X	X	**X**	X	X	X	**X**	**X**	**X**			
14	X	X	X	X											X													
15	X			X						X	X																	
17	X	X	X	X	X	X	X	X	X	X	X	X	X	X	X	X	X		X	X	X	X			X	X		
19	X		X									X			X													
21	X	X							X													X						
23		X	X		X	X																						
24		X	X		**X**	**X**																						
26	X	X		X			X	X	X	X			X	X			X											

Haemorrhage- See also Haemophilia

	PHOS	CHINA	MILL	ARN	IPEC	CROT H	LACH	HAM	CARB V	SEC	ERIGER	NIT AC	ACON	ARS	CROC S	FERR	SABIN	TRILL P	FERR PH	KREO	CINNAM	BELL	CACT	PLAT	RHUS T	BOV	PULS
1	X	X	X	X		X	X		X	X						X				X	X						
2		X	X		**X**	X	X	**X**	X	X		X	X		X	X		X	X	X	X		**X**	X	X	X	
3	X	X	X	X	X	X	X		X	X		X	X		X		X		X	X	X	X		X	X		X
4	X	**X**	X		X	X	X	**X**	X	**X**	**X**	X	**X**	X	X	X	X	**X**			X		X	X		**X**	
5	X	X	X	X	X		X		X	X	X					X											
6	X	X	X	X		X		X	X	X	X	X		X			X			X					X		
7	X	**X**	X		**X**	X	**X**	**X**		X	**X**	X	X	**X**	X	X	X		X	X							
8	**X**	**X**	X	**X**	X		X	X	X	X	X	X	X	X	**X**	X	X	**X**			X	X	X	X	X	X	X
9	X																		X								
10	X					X																					
11	X			X		X	X	X			X								X								
12	X							X					X														
13	**X**	**X**	**X**	X	**X**	X	X	X	X			**X**	X	X	X	**X**	**X**			X	X	**X**	X		X		**X**
14			X	X		X		X	X			X		X	X			X									X
15						X		B																			
16		X																	X			X					
17	X	X	X	X	X	X	X			X									X			X					
18	X	X	X	X							X								X	X							
19			X		X	X	X																X				
21	X			X	X		X		X					X								X					
22	X			X	X				X																		
23		X	X	X	X	X				X	X						X	X		X			X				
24		X	X	X	X		X	X	X	X	**X**	X	X	X	X	X	X	**X**						X		X	
28	X																										

B- Both Internal and External

Haemorrhage, Ante-partum

	CHINA	ACON	ARN	BELL	BRY	IPEC	SABIN	TRILL P
2								X
4	X							
21	X	X	X	X	X	X	X	
24	**X**							

Haemorrhage, Anus, From

	SULPH	CASC	CARB V	HAM	MUR AC	NAT M	NIT AC	PHOS	HIRUDO	ACON	APIS	ARN	CACT	CALEND	CHINA	COLCH	COLLIN	CROC S	CROT H	MILL	SEP	SULPH AC	TEREB
1					X		X																X
2		X							**X**														
5				X		X	X										X				X		
7	**X**	X	X			X		X			X								X				
8	X			X	X			X		X		X	X	X	X	X		X		X		X	
10			X																				

Haemorrhage, Bladder, From- See also Haematuria

	AMYG P	CANTH	CARB V	ERIGER	HAM	MILL	RHUS A
2						X	X
14		X	X				
23	X				X		
24				X			

Haemorrhage, Bowel- See also Haemorrhage, Intestinal/Rectal; Stool, Bloody

	LACH	NIT AC	MILL	ALUMEN	ACET AC	AMM C	AMM M	ANT C	CALC	CANTH	CARB V	FERR	HAM	MERC	PHOS	TEREB
1	X	X			X	X	X						X		X	X
4		**X**	**X**													
6	X	X		X						X			X	X		
8	X	X		X		X	X	X	X	X	X	X		X	X	
10	X			X												
11	X															
12																X
14	X	X	X								X					
24			X		X			X	X			X				

Haemorrhage, Brain

	ARN	LACH	OP	ACON	ANAC	BELL	CAUST	COCCUL	CON	CUPR	GELS	GLON	HAM	HYOSC	IPEC	LAURO	NUX V	PITUIT	PLUM	SEC	SEP	VER V	ZINC	ZINC PH
1		X																						X
6	X	X	X	X	X	X	X	X	X	X	X	X		X		X	X		X		X		X	
14	X																							
17															X			X						
23	X		X										X							X		X		

Haemorrhage, Choroid

	HAM	LACH	ARN	BELL	CHINA	CROT H	PHOS
6	X	X	X	X	X	X	X
7	X	X					

Haemorrhage, Conjunctiva- See Haemorrhage, Eye, From

Haemorrhage, Ear, From

	ARN	CHINA	CROT H	LACH	CALC	CIC	HAM	OP	PHOS	PULS
6		X	X							
7	X	X	X	**X**		X	X	X	X	X
11	X									
14	X		X		X					
24		X								

Haemorrhage, Eye, From

	CROT H	LACH	BELL	CARB V	CHAM	CALC	PHOS	NUX V	ACON	ARN	BOTHR	EUPHR	FERR PH	HAM	IPEC	LED	RHUS T	RUTA	SENEG
1	X																		
5													X						
6	X			X															
7	X	**X**			X	X	**X**	X											
8	**X**	**X**	**X**	X	X	X	**X**		**X**			X		X		X		X	X
12			X							X					X				
13		X	X	**X**	**X**	X		X											
14	X										X								
17																	X		

Haemorrhage, Eye, Into (AKA Haemorrhage, Intraoccular)

	HAM	SULPH AC	CROT H	GELS	LACH	LED
1				X		X
2					X	
4	X					
6	X					
11	X	X	X			
17			X			
19	**X**	**X**				

Haemorrhage, Eyelids

	BELL	ARN	CHAM	SULPH
1				X
10	X		X	
13	**X**	X		

Haemorrhage, Gums

	MERC	CARB V	PHOS	LACH	NIT AC	CALC	STAPHYS	ARS	NAT M	PH AC	KREO	SULPH	CAUST	HAM	ARN	BELL	NUX M	SIL	BAPT	BOV	NUX V	AGAR M	AMM C	ANT C	SULPH AC	TEREB
1	X	X	X	X		X	X			X	X	X	X	X	X				X					X		X
2				X																						
3			X											E												
4					X			X											**X**							
5		X	X	X		X	X				X				X											
6	X	X	X	X	X	X	X	X				X	X			X	X				X		X		X	
7	**X**	**X**	X	**X**	**X**	X	X	X	**X**	X		X		X		X	X	X		X		X				X
8	**X**	**X**	X	X	X	X	X	X	X	X		X	X			X	X	X		X	X	X	X			
9				X							X													X		
10		X		X					X																	
11	X									X	X															
12		X			X									X												
13	X	**X**	**X**		X	X	**X**	X	**X**	X		**X**	X			X	X	X		**X**	**X**	X	X	X	X	X
14	X	X	X			X	X	X			X				X											
15	X	X																	X						X	
16								X																		
17	X	X	X	X	X																					
18	X			X																						
19			X																							
20	X																									
21	X		X						X		X							X								
24	X			X																						
25			X											E	X											
26	X	X	X		X	X			X	X			X													

E- External

Haemorrhage, Intestinal/Rectal- See also Haemorrhage, Bowel; Stool, Bloody

	NIT AC	HAM	ARS	CROT H	IPEC	CARB V	CHINA	ERIGER	PHOS	TEREB	AMM C	MUR AC	PH AC	SEC	COLCH
1	X	X							X	X	X	X			
2				X											
3		X					X			X				X	
4													X		
6	X	X	X		X	X	X	X			X				
7	X	**X**	X	X	**X**		X	X	X	X				X	**X**
8	X		X		X	X			X				X		
11			X	X		X		X							
14				X											
26	X											X			

Haemorrhage, Intracranial- See Haemorrhage, Brain

Haemorrhage, Intraoccular- See Haemorrhage, Eye, Into

Haemorrhage, Kidney- See also Haematuria

	COCCUS	ERIGER	FERR M	LACH	RHUS A	SEC	SENEC
2					X		
7			X			X	X
19		X		X			
24	X						

Haemorrhage, Labor, From- See Labor, Haemorrhage, After; Labor, Haemorrhage, Before

Haemorrhage, Lips

	ARUM T	IGN	LACH	ARS	BROM	BRY	NAT M	ALOE	CARB A	CARB V	CHAM	COBALT	KALI CAR
1	X		X		X		X						
6			X										
7	**X**	X	X		X						X		
13	X	X		X		X	X	X	X			X	X
26		X		X		X				X			

Haemorrhage, Lungs- See also Haemoptyisis

	PHOS	IPEC	ACON	ARN	HAM	CHINA	MILL	ACALYPH	CACT	ARS	CARB V	FERR	FERR PH
2	**X**								**X**				
3								X					
4	X				**X**		X	**X**					
5	X	X		X									
6	X	X	X	X	X	X	X		X	X	X	X	X
14		X									X		
15		X	X	X	X	X							
23	X	X	X				X						X
24	X												
26		X	X	X		X				X		X	

Haemorrhage, Mouth

	DROS	CHINA	KREO	ARN	CARB V	IPEC	PHOS	BELL	LED	CINA	FERR	LYC	ACON	ARS	CROT H	FIC REL	NUX V	PH AC	RHUS T	SULPH AC	TEREB
1															X					X	
6		X			X																
7		**X**	X	X		X	X				X		X								
8	X	X	X	X				X	X		X	X									X
10					X																
11																X					
12	X																				
13	**X**	X	**X**	X		X	X	**X**	**X**	X		X					X				
14	X																				
26	X				X	X	X			X				X				X	X		

Haemorrhage, Mucous Membranes

	ACET AC	ARS H	NAT NIT
3	X		
8		X	
11			X

Haemorrhage, Nipples

	HAM	LYC	MERC	SEP	SIL
6	X				
7		X	X	X	X

Haemorrhage, Nose- See Epistaxis

Haemorrhage, Postpartum

	CHINA	SABIN	SEC	BELL	CANN S	CROC	IPEC	ARN	CINNAM	ERIGER	FERR	KALI CAR	PLAT	TRILL P
2			X		X	X								X
4	X	X												X
6													X	
7	X	X		X	X	X	X	X			X	X	X	
8					X							X		
14									X					
19	X	X	X	X			X			X				
21	X	X	**X**	X		X	X				X			
23									X	X				
24	**X**													
29*								X						

29* Oberbaum M, et al. The effect of the homeopathic remedies arnica montana and bellis perennis on mild postpartum bleeding- a randomised, double-blind, placebo-controlled study- preliminary results. Complementary Therapies in Medicine, 2005, June, 13, 2, 87-90.

Haemorrhage, Rectum- See also Haemorrhage, Bowel; Stool, Bloody

	COLLIN	HAM	NIT AC	ALOE	NAT M	AESC	AMM C	CAPS	MERC	NUX V	HIRUDO	SULPH
1		X		X			X					
3		X	X								X	
5	X		X		X					X		
6	X	X	X			X	X	X	X			X
9	X	X			X							
11	X		X							X		
14		X			X							
24	X	X		X		X		X	X		X	
25	X			X								X

Haemorrhage, Retina

	LACH	CROT H	PHOS	ARN	BOTHR	DUBO M	GELS	BELL	HAM	NAPHTH	NAT SIL
1	**X**	X	X	X	X	X	X			X	X
3	X		X			X	X		X		
4	X	X						X			
5	X		X		X						
6	X	X									
7	X			X							
8			X								
11				X							
14		X			X						

Haemorrhage, Stomach- See also Haematemesis

	HAM	GER MAC	PHOS	CARB V	CHINA	FERR	HYDRAST	SEC	SIL
4		X							
5	X	X			X				
7	**X**		X			X		X	X
9			X						
11							X		
14				X					

Haemorrhage, Tongue

	ARUM T	CROT H	LACH	POD
7	X		X	X
14		X		

Haemorrhage, Umbilicus

	ABROT	CALC PH
1	X	X
3	X	
7	X	X
9		X

Haemorrhage, Ureter- See also Haematuria

	PARIERA
7	X
24	X

Haemorrhage, Urethra- See also Haematuria

	CROT H	MERC	PHOS	SULPH	CALC	CANTH	CHEL	ERIGER	FERR	FERR PH	HAM	KALI IOD	LYC	PULS
3			X								X			
7	X	X	X	X	X	X	X		X	X		X	X	X
24	X	X		X				X						

Haemorrhage, Uterus- See also Menorrhagia

	SABIN	SEC	TRILL P	IPEC	HAM	BELL	CROC S	ERIGER	CHAM	CINNAM	THLASPI	PHOS	CHINA	KREO	LACH	USTIL	CALC	VINCA	ARN	FERR	IOD	MILL	PLAT
1	X		X								X			X			X						
2	**X**										X							**X**					
3												X					X						
4	X	**X**	X	X	**X**			X			X					X		X		X		X	
5	X	X	X		X			X	X			X	X			X			X			X	X
6	X					X	X							X							X		
7										X													
8	X	X	X	X	X	X	X	X	X	X	X	X	X	X	X	X	X	X	X	X	X	X	X
9						X						X											
10				X		X	X		X	X			X	X	X				X	X	X		X
14			X	X	X										X								
16				X			X	X					X										
17				X																			
19	**X**	**X**	X	**X**		**X**	X	X	X	X		**X**	X	X	X	X	**X**			X		X	
21	X	X									X												
22	X																						
23		X	X		X		X	X	X	X	X				X			X					
24	X		X		**X**			X								X					X		
25		X				X				X													
26	X	**X**	X	**X**	X	X			X										X				X
27	X						X																

Haemorrhage, Vagina

	AMBRA	ARG N	IGN	SEP
3	X		X	
7		X		X

Haemorrhage, Venous

	HAM	CARB V	SEC
3		X	
8	X		X
23	X		

Haemorrhagic Shock- See Shock, Haemorrhagic

Haemorrhoids (AKA Piles)

	NUX V	AESC	COLLIN	SULPH	HAM	ALOE	PULS	NIT AC	LYC	ARS	MUR AC	CAPS	LACH	CARB V	GRAPH	IGN	CAUST	POD	KALI CAR	ACON	RAT	BELL	PAEONIA	SEP	AMM C	NAT M
1	**X**	X	X	**X**	X	X	X	X	X	X	X	X	X	X	X	X	X	X	X				X		X	
2	**X**	X	**X**	**X**	**X**	X	**X**		X		**X**	**X**	X	**X**	X	**X**	X	X	X	**X**	X	X	X		X	
3	X	X	X	X	E	X		X	X			X	X				X	X	X		X		X			
4	**X**	**X**	**X**	**X**	**E**	**X**	**X**		**X**	X	X	X	X	X	X	X					X			X		
5	X	X	X		B	X		X	X		X		X					X	X		B		E	X		X
6	X	X	X	X	X	X	X	X	X	X	X	X	X	X	X	X	X	X	X	X	X	X		X	X	X
7	**X**	**X**	**X**	**X**	**X**	X	X	X	X	**X**	**X**	**X**	X	X	**X**	X	**X**	X	X			X		X	X	X
8	**X**	**X**	**X**	**X**	**X**	X	**X**	X	X	**X**	X	**X**	X	X	X	X	X	**X**	X	X		X	X	X	X	X
9	X	B	X	X	B	X	X									X										
10	**X**	X	X	**X**	X	X	X	X	X	X		X		X		X						X				X
11	**X**	**X**	X	**X**	X	**X**		X	X	X	X		X	X		X	X	X		X	X	X	X		X	
12	**X**	**X**	X	**X**	B	**X**	X	X		X		X		X				X		**X**						
13	X	X	X	X	X	X	X	X	X	X	X	X	X		X		X		X	X		X		X	X	X
14	X	X			B	X	X	X	X	X	X	X			X		X				X	X				
15	**X**	X		**X**	**X**		X	X		X								**X**		X						
17	X	X	X																							
18	X	X	X	X	X	X	X	X	X		X		X		X				X		X		X	X		
19	**X**	**X**	X	**X**	X	**X**		X		X	X		X	X	X	**X**	X		X		**X**	X	X	X		X
21	X	X	X	X	X	X	**X**	X		X		X		X	X		X								X	
22	X	**B**	X	X	E			X							X											
23	X	X	X		X	X			X		X												X			
24	X	**X**	**X**	X	X	**X**	**X**	X	X	X	X	X	X	X	X	X	X	X	X	X	X		X	X	X	X
25	X	X	**X**	X		X	X																			
26	**X**	X	X	X	X		**X**	X	X	X	X	X	X	X		X			X	X		X		X		X
27	X		X																							
28		X	X																							

B- Both Internal (oral) and External E- External

Haemorrhoids, Bleeding- See Haemorrhage, Rectum

Hair, Diseases Of

	KALI CAR	ARS	JAB	PH AC	THUJA	WILDBAD
2	**X**		X		X	X
25		X		X		
26	X					

Hair, Dry

	KALI CAR	THUJA	SULPH	PLUM	PSOR	ALUM	CALC	FL AC	PHOS	AMBRA	PHOS AC
1		X						X			
2									X		
5	X	X		X	X		X	X	X	X	
6		X									
7		X	X		X						
8	X		X	X			X				X
10	X		X			X					
13	**X**		X	X	X	X					
14		X									
21	X										
26	X										

Hair, Falling, Of (Includes Alopecia; Hair, Thinning, Of)

	PH AC	FL AC	PHOS	GRAPH	BAR C	LYC	NAT M	SULPH	KALI CAR	ARS	CALC	SIL	SEL	SEP	HEP	NIT AC	THUJA	AUR	CARB V	VINCA	AMBRA	THYROID	PETR	MERC
1	X	X	X	X	X	X	X	X	X				X	X		X								X
2	**X**	**X**			X	X							X	X					X	X		X		
3	X	X	X	X	X	X	X	X	X		X	X		X			X		X	X		X	X	X
4	**X**	X	**X**	X			**X**			X	X				X				X	X				
5	X	X		X	X					X						X	X				X			
6	X	X	X	X	X	X	X	X	X		X	X		X	X	X		X	X		X			
7		X	X	**X**	**X**	X		X		X		**X**			X		**X**				X		X	
8	X	X	**X**	X	X	**X**	X	X	X	X	**X**	X	X	X	X	**X**	X	X	X	X	X		**X**	
9	X	X	X					X	X	X												X		
10	X		X	X	X	X	X		X		X	X			X			X						
11	X	X	X	X		X	X			X			X			X				X				
13	X	X	**X**	**X**	X	X	**X**	**X**	X	X	**X**	X	X	X	**X**	X		X	X		**X**			X
14	X	X	X					X									X							
15	X																							
18													X				X							
19				X																		X		
21	X	X	X		X	X	X		X				X	X				X						
23	X	X																		X				
25	X																					X		
26			X	X	X	X		X	X	X		X			X			X						

Hair, Falling Of, Beard/Whiskers

	GRAPH	NAT M	CALC	ANANTH	PH AC	KALI CAR	PLUM	SEL	SPHING	BROM	CAPS	CARB A	CAUST	NAT CAR	NIT AC
1	X			X					X						
3				X					X						
5	X	X	X		X	X								X	
6		X													
7	X	X		X	X			X		X	X	X	X		X
8	X	X	X				X	X							
10	X	X	X												
13	X	X			X	X	X								
26	X	X	X												

Hair, Falling Of, Body

	SEL	ALUM	ARS	CALC	CARB V	GRAPH	LYC	MERC	NAT M	RHUS T	SABIN	SEC
5	X	X	X	X	X	X	X	X	X	X	X	X
21	X											

Hair, Falling Of, Eyebrows and/or Lashes- See also Eyebrows, Loss/Falling Of; Eyelashes, Loss/Falling Of

	KALI CAR	SEL	GRAPH	PH AC	RHUS T	ALUM	ANANTH	APIS	ARS	CHEL	MERC	STAPHYS	AGAR M	ALOE	BELL	CALC SUL	CAUST	EUPHR	HELL	PHOS	PLUM	SIL	SULPH
1	X	X	X	X	X	X	X																
5	X	X			X		X	X	X	X	X	X				X						X	
6				X																			
7				X	X			X	X	X	X	X						X					X
8	X	X											X	X	X		X		X				
10	X		X																				
13	X	X				X														X	X		
26	X		X																				

Hair, Falling Of, Moustache

	PLUM	NAT M	SEL
5	X		
8	X	X	
13	X		X

Hair, Falling Of, Pregnancy, During Or After- See Pregnancy, Hair, Falling Of, During Or After

Hair, Falling Of, Pubic

	NAT M	SEL	NIT AC	SULPH	NAT CAR	RHUS T	SARS	ZINC	BELL	HELL	IOD	PH AC	SIL	STAPHYS
1		X	X	X							X			
5	X	X	X		X		X					X		X
6	X													
7	**X**	X	X	**X**				X						
8	X					X				X			X	
13	X	X			X	X	X	X	X					

Hair, Greying

	PH AC	LYC	SULPH AC	GRAPH	PHOS	PILO	WEISBAD	ARS H	ASPARA	HYDRAST	JAB	NAT M	NUX V	THUJA	THYROID
1	X	X	X		X	X	X	X				X	X	X	
2			X												
3	X	X			X	X	X		X	X	X				X
7	X	X													
8	X	X	X	X											
9	X														
10	X														
13	X	X	X	X											
14	X														
16	X	X													
21	X	X	X												
26	X														

Hair, Oily/Greasy

	BRY	NAT M	PH AC	KALI SUL	LYC	PULS	THUJA	BENZ NIT	LYSS	MERC	SULPH
2								X	X		
7	X		X								
9		X		X	X	X	X				
13	X		X								
18		X									
19											X
21	**X**	X	X							X	
25				X	X	X	X				

Halitosis (AKA Foetor Oris)

	MERC	**NUX V**	**ARN**	**AUR**	**NIT AC**	**BAPT**	**SULPH**	**ARS**	**CARB V**	**KREO**	**PULS**	**SPIG**	**MUR AC**	**CAPS**	**PETR**	**SIL**	**STANN**	**BELL**	**CARB AC**	**HEP**	**LACH**	**MERC C**	**SEP**
1	X	X		X	X	X				X	X	X	X	X			X			X		X	
2	**X**			**X**	**X**										**X**								
4	**X**				X	X		X					X				X		X				
6	X	X	X	X	X	X	X	X					X	X	X				X				X
7	**X**	X	**X**	X	X	X	X	X	X	X	X	X	X	X	X	X	X	X	X		X		X
8	X	X	X	X	X		X	X	X		X	X			X	X	X	X		X			X
9	X	X							X		X	X	X						X				
10	X			X			X		X														
11			X			X		X		X			X										
12	X	X	X	X	X	X	X	X	X		X		X			X				X	X	X	
13	X	**X**	X	X	X		X	X	X		X	X		X	X	X	X	X			X	X	X
14	X		X	X		X				X						X							
15	X	**X**		X	X	X	X	X	X	X	X		X					X	X	X	X	X	X
16							X																
17	X	X	X	X						X		X		X			X						
18	X	X	X			X																X	
19	X		X		X	X	X	X		X		X		X									
20	X						X																
21	X	X	X	X	X					X	X	X		X						X			
22	X																						
24	X		X			X									X								
25	X	X							X	X	X	X											
26	X	X	X		X		X	X	X							X		X			X		
27	X																						

Hang Nails

	NAT M	**CALC**	**RHUS T**	**SULPH**	**LYC**	**MERC**	**STANN**	**KALI CHL**	**SABAD**	**SIL**	**UPAS**
1	X	X		X							
2								X			X
4	X										
7	X	X	X			X				X	
8	X	X	X	X	X	X	X		X		
10		X	X	X	X						
13	**X**	X	X	X		X	X				
18	X										
26		X	X	X	X						

Hangover- See also Ailments from Alcohol; Alcoholism

	NUX V	CAPS	CHAM	COFF	CUPR	LOB I	PULS	ZINC
2					X	X		
3	X							X
4	**X**	X						
14	**X**							
19	**X**							
20	X							
21	X		X	X			X	
22	X							
27	X							
28	X							
29*	X							

29* Sukul A, et al. Altered solution structure of alcoholic medium of potentized Nux vomica underlies its antialcoholic effect. Brit Hom J, 2000, 89, 2, 73-7.

Hay Fever- See also Rhinitis (AKA Hay Asthma)

	ARS	SABAD	AMBROS	GALPH	KALI IOD	ALL C	EUPHR	ARS IOD	PSOR	STICTA	ARUNDO	GELS	IPEC	KALI BIC	NAPHTHA	NUX V	PULS	LACH	NAT M	SIL	SULPH	ARAL	ARUM T	DULC	NAJA	SANG	SINAP	
1	X	X	X			X	X	X	X	X					**X**						X		X		X	X	X	
2					X	X		X	**X**	X	X	X		X				X				X		X			X	
3		X									X																	
4	**X**	**X**	**X**		X			**X**					X		**X**				X	X		X	X				X	
5	X	X	X		X	X	X	X	X	X	X		X			X		X		X								
6	X	X			X		X			X		X	X	X	X		X	X	X	X		X	X		X	X		
7	X	X					X			X		X	X	X		X		X	X				X	X	X			
8	X	X	X		X		X	X	X	X		X	X	X	X				X	X		X	X	X		X	X	
9	X	X			X	X			X					X		X	X											
11	X		X																									
12	X	O			X	X	X						X	X														
14	X		X																									
15	X				X		X					X	X	X			X											
16		X									X					X					X							
17																					X							
18								X	X																			
19	X	X	X		X	X	X		X	X						X	X		X		X			X	X	X		
21	X	X			X	X	X	X	X	X	X	X				X	X	X		X				X	X	X		
23		X	X			X		X			X				X							X						
25	X	X				X																						
27			X																									
28			X	X																								
29[1]				X																								
29[2]											X						X	X			**X**							
29[3]	X											X				X	X		X	X								

0- By Olfaction

29[1] Ludtke R, Wiesenauer MA. Meta-analysis of Homeopathic Treatment of Pollinosis with Galphimia glauca. Wiener Medizinische Wochenshrift (Klinische Wochenschrift), 1997, 147, 14, 323-327. This study examined 11 clinical trials using Galphimia in the treatment of pollinosis (hay fever), 10 of which confirmed the effectiveness of this remedy for the condition. It's because of these 10 successful trials that the remedy has been placed in this position in the table.

29[2] Goossens M, et al. Evaluation of the quality of life after individualized homeopathic treatment for seasonal allergic rhinitis. A prospective, open, non-comparative study. Homeopathy. 2009, 98, 1, 11-16.

29[3] Van Wassenhoven M. Clinical verification in homeopathy and allergic conditions. Homeopathy. 2013 Jan;102 (1) :54-8.

Hay Fever, Prophylaxis

	ARS	GELS	NUX V	PSOR	ARS IOD	IOD	KALI BIC	NAT M	PULS	SARS	SIL	THUJA																
12	X			X		X	X					X																
16	X			X	X																							
29*	X	X	X					X	X	X	X																	

29*Van Wassenhoven M. Clinical verification in homeopathy and allergic conditions. Homeopathy. 2013 Jan;102 (1):54-8.

Head Lice- See also Pediculosis

	CARB AC	LYC	SABAD	STAPHYS	NAT M	PSOR
1	X	X		X		X
2			X			
3			X		X	
8		X		X		
14	X					

Headache (Note that only the main remedies from 2 and 3 are used here)

	NUX V	BELL	GELS	NAT M	BRY	SIL	GLON	PULS	LACH	ACON	IRIS V	COCCUL	IGN	SEP	ARS	SULPH	CHINA	SANG	ARG N	CIMICI	CALC PH	PH AC	PHOS	LYC	ANAC	CALC
1	X	X	X	X	X	X	X		X	X	X	X	X	X				X	X		X		X	X	X	X
2	**X**	**X**	**X**	**X**	**X**	**X**	**X**		**X**	**X**	**X**	**X**	**X**		**X**	**X**	**X**	**X**				**X**			X	
3	X	X	X	X	X	X	X	X	X		X	X					X	X			X	X				
4	**X**	**X**	**X**	**X**	X	**X**	X	X	X		**X**	X	X				X		**X**	**X**	X					
5	X	X	X	X	X	X	X	X	X	X	X	X	X	X			X	X	X	X	X	X	X	X	X	
6	X	X	X	X	X	X	X	X	X	X	X	X	X	X	X	X	X	X	X	X	X	X	X	X	X	X
7	**X**	**X**	**X**	**X**		**X**	**X**	**X**	X	X	**X**	**X**		**X**	**X**	**X**	X	X	X				X	X	**X**	X
8	X	X	X	X	X	X	X	X	X	X	X	X	X	X	X	X	X	X	X	X	X	X	X	X	X	X
9		X	X	X		X			X										X	X	X	X	X			
10	X	X	X	X	X	X	X	X	X	X		X		X	X	X			X	X		X	X	X		X
11	**X**	**X**	**X**	X	X	**X**	**X**	X	X		**X**	X	X	**X**				**X**	**X**						X	
12	X	X			X		X			X						X				X						
13	X				X	X		X	X			X		X	X	X	X	X	X				X	X	X	X
14	X	X	X	X	X	X	X	X		X	X		X	X			X							X		X
15	**X**	**X**	**X**		X	X	X	X		X	X	X	**X**	X	**X**	X				**X**						
16		X																								
17	X	X		X	X		X	X	X	X		X						X	X							X
18	X	X	X	X	X	X	X	X	X		X		X	X	X	X		X		X	X	X	X	X	X	
19	**X**	X	**X**	**X**		**X**	**X**	X	X		**X**	**X**	X		X	**X**	**X**			**X**	**X**	X	**X**			**X**
20	**X**	**X**	**X**		**X**			X		X	X							X								
21	X	X	X	X	X		X			X			X			X	X							X		
22	X	X	X	X	X		X			X					X											
23	X	X	X	X	X	X	X	X	X	X	X		X	X	X	X	X	X			X	X			X	
24	X	X						X		X									X							
25	X	X	X		X			X							X					X						
26	X	X		X	X	X		X	X	X		X	X	X		X	X						X			X
27			X	X	X	X															X	X				
29*	X			**X**				X	X				X	X	X									X		

29* Muscari-Tomaioli G, et al. Observational Study of Quality of Life in patients with Headache, receiving Homeopathic Treatment. Brit Hom J, 2001, 90, 189-197.

Headache, Frontal (Includes Headache, Forehead)

	BRY	BELL	NUX V	PULS	ACON	KALI BIC	LACH	ARG N	GELS	ALL C	IRIS V	PHOS	STICTA	ARS	ELAPS	HYDRAST	IGN	LYC	SABAD	SEP	SULPH							
1	X						X		X																			
3							X			X																		
4	X	**X**	X					X				X							X									
5		X	X	X							X		X			X				X								
6	X	X	X	X	X	X	X	X				X	X		X	X				X	X							
7	X	X	X	**X**	X		X	X	X	X	X	X	X	X	X		X	X		X	X							
8	X	X		X	X	X		X				X		X				X	X									
9	X	X			X	X	X		X	X						X			X									
10	X	X	X						X												X							
11	X		X								X								X									
12		X			X																							
13		X	X	X	X	X	X			X		X		X	X			X		X	X							
14	X				X	X		X			X		X															
15	X	X		X					X																			
16	X																											
17			X													X		X										
18						X			X				X															
19	**X**																											
20	X	X		X							X			X														
21				X				X									X											
22					X					X																		
24						X	X								X													
25	X																X											
26	X	X	X														X											

Headache, Occipital

	GELS	PETR	PIC AC	NUX V	CIMIC	ONOS	BRY	SANG	SIL	COCCUL	RHUS T	CAMPH	ELAPS	EUP PERF	IGN	SEP	SULPH
1		X															
2		X															
4	X		X		X		X	X		**X**					X		
6		X	X	X	X	X	X	X	X			X	X		X	X	
7	X	**X**	**X**	X							**X**			X			
8	X	X			X	X			X	X	X	X	X	X	X	X	X
9	X	X	X	X	X		X	X	X	X							
10																	X
11			X			X					X						
14	X							X						X			
15	X			X	X												
17	X		X	X								X					
18	X																
19				X	X	X	X										
20	X																
21		X		X													
23	X		X														
24		X				X							X				
25									X								
26																X	X
27			X														

Headache, One-Sided- See Hemicrania

Headache, Parietal

	THUJA	ALL C	ALUM	AMYL N	CANN S	CANTH	CHINA	CHIN A	CINNAB	COCA	COLCH	CYCL	ELAPS	EUP PUR	HEP	HIPPOM	KALM	LAC C	LYC	MEZ	NIT AC	PHOS	PHYSO	PULS	USTIL
7	X	X	X	X																					
8	X				X	X	X	X	X	X	X	X	X	X	X	X	X	X	X	X	X	X	X	X	X

Headache, "Sick" (Includes Headache, Gastric)

	IRIS V	SANG	MUX V	IPEC	BELL	COCCUL	VER A	CHION	PULS	SEP	GELS	GLON	ANT C	ASAR	CALC	CIMICI	KALI BIC	LAC D	NAT SUL	NUX M	SULPH
1	X		X					**X**										X			
2	X	X					X														
3			X	X																	
4	X							X													
6	X	X	X	X			X	X	X												
7	**X**	**X**	X	**X**	X	**X**	X			X	X	X	**X**		X		X	X		X	X
8	X	X	X		X	X			X	X	X	X		X	X	X	X		X	X	
9	X																				
10	X	X			X	X	X			X											
11	X	X			X													X			
12	X	X	X	X	X	X	X		X	X		X	X		X	X	X			X	X
13		X	X			X					X	X		X					X		
14	X			X				X													
15					X						X					X					
17		X																			
18	X																				
19		X			X					X									X		
21	X																				
22	X	X																			
25	X					X															
26			X	X			X		X				X	X							X
28	X																				

Headache, Sun, From- See also Sunstroke

	GLON	BELL	NAT CAR	GELS	KALM	LACH	NAT M	STRAM	ACON	AMYL N	BRY	CALC	COCCUL	IGN	KALI BIC	NUX V	PHELL	SANG	SPIG	SYPH
1	X	X					X													
2	X			X	X			X							X					
3						X											X	X		
4																			X	
7	X	X	X			X		X				X	X	X						X
8		X	X	X	X															
9	X	X		X			X													
10	X	X	X						X											
11	X																			
14	X	X				X														
15		X									X									
17	X				X		X									X				
19	X																			
25	X		X							X										

Headache, Supraobital, Left

	SPIG	ARS	NUX V	ACON	BROM	BRY	CAULO	CHIO	IPEC	KALI BIC	KALI IOD	LACH	LIL T	MERC	JUG R	NUX M	ONOS	PHOS	SEL	SEP	TELL	THER	THUJA
1	X																						
4	**X**																						
6			X																				
8	X	X		X	X		X	X	X		X	X	X	X	X	X	X	X	X	X	X	X	
9		X	X							X													
19						X																	X

Headache, Supraobital, Right

	SANG	CHEL	AGNUS	ARG N	CARB AC	CROT T	IGN	IRIS V	LYC	RAN B
1	X									
4	**X**				X			X		
8	X			X		X	X			
9	X								X	
17		X								
19		X								X

Headache, Temporal

	BELL	CHINA	NUX V	BRY	GELS	CHAM	EPIPHEG	SEP	ACON	AMBRA	AMM C	CARB AC	CINA	DULC	HEP	KALI IOD	LITH C	LYC	MEZ	MOSCH	NUX M	POD	ROBIN	STANN	STROPH
1	X	X									X														
3															X										
4							X																		
7	**X**	X			X	X																			
8	X	X					X	X			X	X	X	X		X	X		X	X	X	X	X	X	
9	X	X		X	X			X	X			X												X	
10		X	X	X		X		X																	X
11					X		X																		
12	X																								
13										X			X	X	X		X	X	X	X	X				
15			X	X					X													X			
16				X																					
17					X					X						X		X							X
18																							X		
19			X																						
25	X		X																						
26	X	X	X			X																			

Headache, Temporal, Left

	ANAC	AMYL N	BROM	CYCL
6	X	X		
19			X	X

Headache, Temporal, Right

	BELL	CACT	CUPR A	GELS	HEP	IRIS V	LYC	PRUN S	PULS	RAN B
5			X							
6	X	X				X			X	
9	X			X						
17					X					
19							X	X		X

Headache, Vertex

	CIMICI	SULPH	CACT	CALC PH	LACH	ALUMEN	BELL	CALC	CHINA	NAT M	PH AC	THUJA
1	X			X		X						
4				X								
6		X									X	X
7	X				X							
8	X		X			X		X				X
9	X	X	X		X					X	X	
10		X					X		X			
14					X							
15	X		X				X					
19	X	X										
25										X		
26		X						X	X			
27				X								

Heartburn (Includes Cardialgia)

	NUX V	PULS	CARB V	ARS	CALC	LYC	SULPH	SULPH AC	CAPS	SEP	NAT M	CHINA	PHOS	KALI CAR	LACH	AMM C	CON	IGN	BERB V	CROC	IRIS V	LOB I	SIL	ARG N	IOD
1	X	X		X	X		X			X															
2		**X**				**X**		X	**X**						X									**X**	
3	X	X	X	X			X																		
4		X					X							X											
5	X					X		X		X								X			X				
6	X		X		X		X	X				X	X	X	X				X				X		
7	**X**	X	**X**	X	**X**	**X**		X	X	X	X		X	X	X	X	**X**		X	**X**	X	X	X	X	X
8	X	X	X	X	X	X	X	X	X	X	X	X	X	X	X	X	X	X	X	X	X	X	X	X	X
9	X			X							X														
10	X	X	X	X	X		X					X													
11	X			X	X														X						
12	X	X	X			X		X	X																
13	X	X	X		**X**	X	X	**X**	**X**	X	**X**	X	X		X	**X**	X			**X**		X	X		**X**
14			X	X																					
15	X	X	X		X	X	X	X				X						X			X				
16	X	X	X		X			X	X																
17																	X					X			
18	X									X				X											
19							X																		
20	X	X																							
21	X			X		X							X												
22	X	X				X																			
25	X										X														
26	**X**	**X**	X	X	X	X	X		X	X		X	X			X		**X**							
28				X																					

Heartburn, Pregnancy, During- See Pregnancy, Heartburn, During

Heart Attack- See Myocardial Infarction

Heart Block

	DIG	CONVAL
3	X	X
17	X	X
19	X	

Heart, Congestion Of

	GLON	ACON	ALOE	ASAF	AUR	NUX M	NUX V	RAUWOLF	RHUS T	SULPH
5			X				X	X		
6	X									
7	X	X		X		X				X
8	X								X	
10					X					

Heart, Dilatation Of- See also Hypertrophy, Heart

	CRAT	PHOS	CACT	ANT T	DIG	STROPH	TAB	ARS	BAR M	LAURO	NAJA	AMM C	ARN	AUR	CONVAL	GRIND	IBER	KALI IOD	KALM	LYC	NUX V
1	X	X				X			X							X					
5					X																
6						X		X											X		
7		X	X	X			X			X	X							X		X	X
8		X	X	X			X			X		X						X		X	X
10		X							X				X								
11	X								X								X				
14	X				X		X														
17	X		X	X	X		X	X			X	X	X	X	X		X		X		
19	X	X		X		X		X		X				X		X					
23	X		X		X	X					X				X						

Heart, Dilatation, Ventricle, Right

	PHOS	ARS	BRY	KALI IOD	LACH	PULS	RHUS T	VER A
6	X	X	X				X	X
7	X			X	X			
8						X		
10	X							
17	X							

Heart, Disease, Ischaemic

	ACON	ARS	CACT	LACH	NUX V	SPIG M
9	X	X	X	X	X	X
17	X	X	X	X	X	X

Heart, Diseases Of (Includes Cardiomyopathy)

	CACT	DIG	CRAT	LACH	ARS	SPIG	NAJA	ACON	ARS I	LYCOP	ARN	KALI CAR	LIL T	AUR	COLLIN	KALM	PULS	LITH C	PHOS	NAT M	SPONG	APOC	GLON	LAURO	AMYL N	AUR M	BRY	
1			**X**			X			**X**	X					X			X										
2	**X**	**X**	**X**	**X**	**X**	**X**	**X**	**X**	**X**	X	**X**	X	**X**		X	X		**X**		**X**		X	X	X	X	X		
3																			X									
4	**X**	**X**	X	**X**	**X**	**X**	X	**X**		X	X		**X**		**X**	**X**	X		X	X		X	X		X			
5		X	X				X		X			X		X					X		X	X						
6	X	X		X	X					X		X			X		X	X	X		X			X				
7	**X**			**X**	X	**X**		**X**		X	X		X	**X**				**X**		X	**X**	X		X	**X**	**X**		
8	X	X		X	X	X	X	X	X	X	X	X	X	X	X	X	X	X	X	X	X	X	X	X	X	X		
9	X	X	X	X	X	X	X	X		X		X	X			X					X		X					
10		X	X	X												X			X									
11			X				X																					
12	X	X			X	X																						
13	X			X		**X**	X	X						X			**X**											
14	X	X	X			X			**X**																	X		
15	X																											
16											X																	
17	X	X		X	X		X		X						X	X								X				
19	X	X	X	X		X	X					X											X					
21	X			X																								
23			X				X			X			X															
24			X		X												X											
25		X	X																									
26	X	X			X			X						X			X			X								
27	X	X	X		X			X				X		X														

Heart, Diseases Of, Left

	ARS
4	X
6	X

Heart, Diseases Of, Right

	PHOS	CARB V	CRAT	LATRO M
4	X			
6	X			
8	**X**	X		
27			X	X

Heart, Diseases Of, Senile

	ARS I	LACH	ARS	ASPAR	STROPH
1					X
8			X	X	
9		X			
10	X				
14	X				
17	X				
24	X				
25		X			

Heart Failure (Includes Cardiac Failure, Congestive Cardiac Failure) (Note that only the main remedies are used from 17)

	CARB V	CRAT	DIG	ARS	STROPH	APIS	CAFF	LACH	NAJA	PHASEOL	ADONIS	ADRENAL	ANT T	APOC	ARN	ARS I	CACT	CAMPH	LAURO	LYCOP	MERC CY	MOSCH
1		X								X		X							X		X	
2		X								X												X
3	X	X	X																			X
4		X			X																	
8	X					**X**															X	
9				X		X																
11			X				X															
14			X		X		X											X				
16	X																					
17	X	X	X	X	X	X	X	X		X	X			X	X	X	X	X				
19	X		X	X	X			X	X		X		X	X	X					X		
21	X		X						X							X	X					
25		X																				
27	X	X		X				X	X			X	X						X	X		

Heart Failure, Left

	ACETAN	ADONIS	ADRENAL	ASPIDO	CACT	CAFF	CALC ARS	CARB V	CHIN A	DIG	IBER	LACH	MERC SU	QUERBR	SARC AC	STROPH	VISC A
11		X	X	X	X	X	X		X	X	X		X	X		X	X
17	X							X				X			X		

Heart Failure, Right

	ADONIS	CRAT	APIS	APOC	ASPIDO	ARS	CACT	CAFF	CARB V	CONVAL	DIG	LATRO M	STROPH
11	X	X	X	X	X	X	X	X	X	X	X		X
17	X												
27		X										X	

Heart, Fatty

	PHOS	AUR	ARN	ARS IOD	ARS	KALI CAR	ADONIS	PHYTO	STRYC PH	VANAD	AUR M	CRAT	CUPR	STROPH	CACT													
1	X	X			X		X		X																			
2								X																				
4	X							X		X		X																
5			X									X																
6	X		X			X					X																	
7	**X**	**X**			**X**	**X**					**X**				**X**													
8	X	X	X										X															
10	X			X																								
14				X																								
16									X																			
17	X	X	X	X	X	X	X	X	X	X			X															
23							X							X														
24	X			X										X														
27										X																		

Heart, Murmurs

	PHOS	CALC	COCCUL	CRAT	LACH	TAR H	ASPAR	CACT	CARB AC	DIG	FERR	GLON	IOD	KALI CAR	KALM	LAURO	NAJA	PSOR	PULS	SPIG	SPONG	STRAM						
2	X																											
7	X	X	X		X	X	X	X	X	X			X	X			X		X			X						
8	X	X	X		X	X					X							X			X							
19	X			X								X			X	X				X								
27				X																								

Heart Valves, Diseases Of (Note that only the main remedies are used from 17)

	SPIG	KALM	SPONG	NAJA	CACT	LITH C	AUR	ARS	DIG	RHUS T	ARS IOD	CRAT GLON	GLON	KALI CAR	KALI IOD	LACH	LYC	ACON	ADONIS	ARN	CALC	LAURO						
1		X		X	X		X			X		X								X								
3							X																					
4	X	**X**		X		**X**																						
6	X		X	X	X	X		X	X	X				X	X	X	X	X		X	X	X						
7	**X**	**X**	**X**	X	X	**X**	X	X	**X**	**X**	X		X	X	X	X	X	X			X	X						
8	X	X	X	X	X	X	X	X		X	X		X	X	X	X	X	X	X			X						
10	X	X	X			X		X																				
11											X																	
17	X		X	X	X	X	X	X	X		X	X	X		X		X		X	X	X							
19	X	X	X	**X**	X		X		X			X	X	X		X			X									
26	X	X	**X**		X																							
27												X																

Heart Valves, Ossification Of

	CALC FL	LAC AC
8		X
25	X	

Heat Rash

	ACON	ARS	AILANTH	APIS	CALC	CHAM	LED	LEPT	OSMIUM	RHUS T	SOL	SULPH
7	X	X	X		X		X	X	X			
10	X	X				X				X		X
21				X							X	

Hectic Fever- See Fever, Hectic

Heels, Cracked- See Cracking, Skin

Hernia

	NUX V	LYC	COCCUL	AESC	CALC	SIL
2	**X**	X	X	**X**	**X**	**X**
3		X	X			
16	X					

Hernia, Bladder

	ALL C	STAPHYS
1		X
7	X	

Hernia, Femoral

	NUX V	CUBEB	PLUM	WEIS
2				X
8		X		
13	**X**			
14			X	

Hernia, Hiatus

	NUX V	LYC	ACON	COCCUL	SULPH	CALC	OP	VER A	PLUM	AUR	BELL	CHAM	LACH	NIT AC	RHUS T	SIL	SULPH AC	ARS	BOR	GELS	MAG CAR	STANN	THUJA
5	X	X																					
6	X	X	X	X	X	X	X	X	X	X	X		X		X	X	X	X	X		X	X	X
7	X					X						X											
8	X	**X**	X	X	X	X	X	X	**X**	X	X	X	X	X	X	X	X	X	X	X	X	X	X
10	X		X		**X**			X				X			X								
11	X			X			X																
12	X		X																				
13	X		X	X	X																		
15	X		X								X									X			
18																	X						
19	X	X																					
21	**X**																						
24	X	X		X		X	X	X	X				X	X		X	X						
25	X					X																	
26	X			X	X					X													
27	X	X																					

Hernia, Incarcerated

	OP	PLUM	VER A
8		X	X
17	X		

Hernia, Inguinal

	NUX V	SULPH AC	SIL	LYC	COCCUL	CALC	AUR	AESC	VER A	ZINC	BELL	GUAIAC	MAG CAR	OP	RHUS T	SPIG	SULPH	CHAM	NIT AC	CARB A	CARB V	LACH	PSOR	ALUM	ASAR
1			X		X	**X**	X	X														X			
2		X														X									
3				X		X					X										X				
6		X					X																		
7	X	X	X	X	X			X		X	X	X	X		X	X				X					
8	X	X	X	X	X	X	X	X	X				X		X		X	X	X	X			X		
13	**X**	**X**	**X**	**X**	**X**		**X**		**X**	**X**		X	X	X	X	X	X	**X**	**X**		X	X	X	**X**	**X**
14	X					**X**																			
21								X																	
24		**X**	X		X					X		X		X											
26	X		X						X								X								
27	**X**			**X**							X			X											

Hernia, Inguinal, Left Side

	ALL C	NUX M	SULPH AC	LIL T
1		X		
6			X	
7	X		X	X
10	X			
14		X		

Hernia, Inguinal, Right Side

	LYC	COCCUL	NUX V	RHUS T
1	X		X	
6	X			
7	X			
8	X	X		
10				X
14	X			

Hernia, Infantile (AKA Hernia, Congenital)

	NUX V	CALC	CHAM	COCCUL	SULPH	VER A
7	X	X	X			
10	X			X	X	X

Hernia, Scrotal

	MAG CAR	MAG M	NUX V
6	X		
8		X	X

Hernia, Strangulated, All Areas

	NUX V	PLUM	ACON	BELL	SULPH	ARS	COCCUL	OP	CALC	LACH	LYC	TAB	VER A	ALUM	COFF	GELS	IPEC	LACH	MILL	PITUIT	RHUS T	SIL	TEREB
1		X																					
2		X																					X
3	X	X	X	X					X									X		X		X	
6	X	X	X	X																			
8	X	X	X	X	X	X	X	X		X	X	X	X		X	X							
9	X																						
13	X		X	X	X	X		X		X			X	X					X		X		
14		X																					
24							X	X				X					X						
26	X		**X**	X	**X**	X	X		X		X												

Hernia, Testicular

	CALC	SIL
1		X
26	X	

Hernia, Umbilical

	CALC	NUX V	AUR	NUX M	COCCUL	LACH	OP	PLUM	SIL	SULPH	VER A	BOR	CINA	GRANAT	NIT AC	STANN	SULPH AC
2								X						X			
3		X	X		X	X				X	X						X
6			X														
7	X	X		X		X	X										
8	X	X	X	X	X			X	X		X	X	X		X	X	
11	X																
14	**X**		X														
21	X	X							X								
24				X			X										
26		X								X							

Hemeralopia

	BELL	VER A	HYOSC	LYC	ANAC	ARG N	CHINA	CHIN A	CYCL	MERC	PULS	RAN B	STRAM	SULPH
8	X	X	X	**X**	X	X	X	X	X	X	X	X	X	X
24			X											
26	**X**	X												

Hemicrania- See also Headache; Migraine

	ARS	SEP	BELL	COFF	NUX V	PULS	ARG N	CHAM	IGN	SANG	ASAR	SIL	ACON	APIS	BRY	CAPS	CHEN A	CHIN A	GRAPH	CIC
2																	X	X		
3		X																		
6	X						X													
7	X						X	**X**			X	**X**		X	X	X	X	X	X	
8	X	X	X	X		X				X	X			X	X	X		X	X	X
9	X		X	X		X			X			X	X		X					
10			X		X	X		X	X	X										
11							X													
12	X		X	X	X				X	X										
13	X	**X**	X	**X**	**X**	**X**		**X**	X	X	**X**	X	X	X		X			X	**X**
14		X					X													
15		X			X															
23	X																X			
25													X							

Hemicrania, Left Side (Includes Migraine, Left side)

	SPIG	SEP	THUJA	ACON	ARG N	BROM	CALC	LACH	NUX V	SULPH
3	X		X							
5	X							X		
6									X	
7					X		X	X		X
8							X			
9	X		X							
10	X									
11	X	X								
13		X		X	X	X				
14	X	X								
17	X									
18						X				
19	X	X	X							
20	X									
21	X		X							
25	X		X							
26	**X**	X		X					X	X

Hemicrania, Right Side (Includes Migraine, Right Side)

	SANG	BELL	IRIS V	SIL	LYC	GELS	AGAR M	BRY	CACT	KALI BIC	PULS	SPIG	NIT AC	PIC AC
3	X											X		
5			X		X			X		X				
6	X	X		X			X		X		X			
7			X										**X**	**X**
9	X			X		X					X			
10	X	**X**		X										
11		X												
13	X	X		X		X	X	X	X	X		X		
14	X		X											
16	X													
17	X													
18	X				X					X				
19	**X**	**X**	X		X		X							
20	X		X			X								
21	X		X		X									
22	X							X						
25	X		X	X	X	X					X			
26	X	**X**												

Hemianopia

	AUR	LYC	NAT M	LITH C	MUR AC	CALC	SEP	STRAM	TITANIUM	BOV	CAUST	CHIN S	CYCL	VER V	ARS	CALC SUL	CIC	COCCUL	LOB I	NAT CAR	NAT SUL	SPIG	STRAM	VIOL O				
1			X				X					X	X															
2	**X**	**X**	X	**X**	**X**				X																			
3	X	X		X	X																							
4	X	X		X	X																							
6		X	X			X	X			X	X	X		X					X					X				
7	X							X																				
8	X	X	X	X	X			X	X				X															
13	X	X	X	X	X	X					X											X						
15														X														
17	X	X	X	X		X	X	X		X					X		X	X		X	X		X					
23	X								X																			
24			X																									
27																X												

Hemianopia, Altitudinal

	AUR	CAMPH	DIG	GELS	LYC	MUR AC	NAT M	ARS	BOV	CALC	CHIN S	LOB I	MORPH	PHOS	PLUM	RHUS T	SEP	STRAM	TITANIUM	VIOL O								
1	X			X																								
3	X																											
4	X																											
6	X		X											X														
7	X	X																										
8	**X**		X	X	X	X	X		X	X	X	X	X		X	X	X	X	X	X								
10	X																											
11	X																											
14	X																											
17	X	X			X	X	X	X																				
24	X																											

Hemianopia Homonymous, Left

	CALC	CIC	NAT CAR	NAT SUL																								
1	X																											
7	X																											
17	X	X	X	X																								

Hemianopia, Homonymous, Right Side

	LITH C	LYC	COCCUL	CYCL	AUR	CALC	NAT M
1	X						
6	X	X		X			
7	**X**	X	X				
8	**X**	**X**		X	X		X
17	X	X	X			X	

Hemiplegia- See also Stroke

	CAUST	ARN	NUX V	RHUS T	LACH	COCCUL	ANAC	BAR C	PLUM	ALUM	BELL	KALI CAR	PH AC	BOTH	ARG N	GRAPH	STANN	STRAM	OLEAND	SULPH AC	CHINA	ELAPS	HYOSC	MERC	PHOS	SEP	STAPHYS	
2					X												X					X						
6	X	X	X	X	X	X	X	X	X	X	X	X	X		X	X	X	X			X		X	X		X	X	
7	**X**	X		X			X											X				X	X					
8	**X**	X	X	X	X	**X**	X		X	X	X	X	X		X	X	X	X		X	X		X	X		X	X	
9		X	X	X				X	X		X			X											X			
10	X	X		X		X	X		X	X	X	X	X		X		X				X			X		X		
11	X	X	X	X	X			X						X					X									
12		X	X																						X			
13	X			X	X	X	X			X		X	X		X					X							X	
14	X													X														
15			X																									
17	**X**	**X**	**X**	**X**	**X**	**X**	X	**X**	**X**	X	X	X	X	**X**		X		X	**X**	**X**		X			X			
23								X											X									
26	X		X		X	X										X												

Hemiplegia, Left Side

	LACH	ARN	RHUS T	BELL	CAUST	NUX V	STANN	ARS	STRAM	ANAC	BAPT	NIT AC	APIS	ACON	BAR M	ELAPS	LYC	OLEAND	OX AC	PETR	SULPH
6	X	X	X	X	X	X	X	X													
7	**X**		X			**X**			X												
8	X	X	X	X	X			X													
10	X	X	X	X	X		X	X													
11	X	X																			
12		X																			
13	X	X		X	X		X		X	X	X	X		X			X		X	X	X
15	X	X																			
17	**X**	X	**X**			**X**	X		X	X	X	X	**X**		X	X		X			

Hemiplegia, Right Side

	CAUST	ARN	BELL	RHUS T	OP	APIS	CALC	PLUM	BOTH	CANTH	CARB SUL	CROT C	CROT H	ELAPS	GRAPH	NAT CAR	PHOS	SIL	STRONT C	SULPH								
1											X																	
6	X	X	X	X																								
7		X	X	X	X	X																						
8	X	X	X	X																								
10	X	X	X	X																								
11	X																											
13	X	X	X		X		X	X									X	X	X	X								
17	**X**	X	X	X	X	X	X	X	X	X		X	X	X	X	X												
19	X																											

Hepatitis

	BRY	MERC	CHINA	PHOS	CHEL	NUX V	LYC	BELL	ACON	LACH	ARS	HEP	KALI C	POD	SULPH	CHAM	MAG M	NAT SUL	NIT AC	CARD M	HYDRAST	NAT M	PULS	SEP	COCCUL	SIL		
1				X						X																		
2									X																			
3	X	X		X				X																				
4	X				X																							
5	X	X	X	X	X		X			X	X			X			X			X	X			X				
6	X	X	X			X	X	X				X	X	X	X								X	X		X		
7	X	X		X	**X**	X	X	**X**	X	X	**X**	X	X	X		X		X	X		X	X			X			
8	X	X	X		X	X	X	X	X	X		X	X	X	X	X			X			X	X			X		
9	X				X	X				X								X										
10				X																								
11	**X**	**X**	X	X	**X**	X	X	X	X	X	X	X	X	X	X	X	X	X	X	**X**		X						
13	**X**	X	X			**X**	**X**	X	**X**	X			X		X	**X**	**X**					X	X	X	X			
14				X																								
15	X	X	X			X		X	X		X	X		X		X												
16			X			X					X																	
17		X																										
18	X	X	X	**X**	X		X				X										X							
19	X		X	X	X	X				X	X		X	X	X		X	X	X	X				X	X			
20		X	X		X	X	**X**	X	X																			
21	X	X	X	X	X					X											X							
23	X			X	X							X							X									
24	X																											
26	X	X	X			X	X	X	**X**	X	X	X	X		X		X						X			X		
27			X	X		X	X	X	X		X							X		X								
28					X																							

Hepatomegaly- Includes Liver, Enlargement of; Swelling, Liver

	CHINA	ARS	MERC	NUX V	CHEL	CHIO	MAG M	LACH	SULPH	DIG	CARD M	POD	LYC	CON	NAT SUL	NIT AC	PTEL	PHOS	AGAR M	BRY	FERR ARS	KALI CAR	LAURO	LEPT	NAT M	NUX M	SIL	VIP
1	X	X				X		X			X	X			X		X			X	X			X	X			X
2						X								X	X						X							X
3			X		X	X						X			X													
4		X	X	X	X		X	X	X	X		X													X			
5	X					X	X			X							X											
6	X	X		X			X		X					X			X					X	X			X	X	
7	**X**		X	X	X	X	**X**		X		X	X	X	X	X	X		X	X			X	X		X	X	X	
8		X	X		X	X	X		X				X				X		X								X	
9				X	X																							
10		X	X	X	X				X																			
11	X	X	X		X	X		X		X	X									X								X
12	X	X	X								X					X		X	X									
13	**X**	X	X	X				X	X				X										X			X		
14	X	X			X	X																						
15	X	X	X	X								X				X								X				
17										X											X							
18	X							X										X										
19	X	X	X	X	X	X	X	X		X	X		**X**			X		X		X		X		X				
20				X																								
21	X																											
24	X													X														
26	X	X		X			X	X	X																			
27										X																		

Herpes (Includes Zona)

	RHUS T	NAT M	SEP	GRAPH	ARS	DULC	RAN B	MEZ	NIT AC	MERC	PETR	HEP	SULPH	BOR	CAUST	CIST	CROT T	TELL	CALC	CANTH	LYC	NAT CAR	STAPHYS	CON	PSOR	SARS	COM	THUJA
1	X	X	X		X	X	X	X	X								X			X					X			X
2	**X**	X	X	X		X			**X**		X		X	X		X		X	X			X		X		**X**	X	
4	**X**	X	X																						**X**			
5	X	X	X	X		X			X		X	X		X						X	X					X		
6	X		X	X	X		X	**X**		X						X	X			X							X	X
7	X	**X**	**X**	**X**	X	X	X			X	X	X	X		X	X	X	**X**	X		X	X	X	X	X			
8	X	X	X	X	X	X	X	X	X	X	X	X	X	X	X	X	X	X	X		X	X	X	X	X	X	X	X
9	X	X					X	X																				
10		X	X																									
12	X	X	X	X	X		X	X					X			X		X					X				X	
13	**X**	X	**X**	**X**	**X**	**X**	X		X	X	X		**X**	X	X	X			X		X	X	X	**X**		X		
14	X						X		X			X																
15	X					X				X																		
17															X													
18	X	X	X					X						X			X			X			X					
19	**X**	**X**	**X**	X	X	X	X	X	X	X	X	X	X	X	X		X	X	X	X	X	X						X
20	**X**	**X**	X	X	X	X					X	**X**																
21				X																								
26	X			X	**X**					X					X													
28		X																										

Herpes, Anus/Perineum

	NAT M	PETR
8	X	X
24	X	X

Herpes, Axilla

	KALI SUL	LYC	SEP
8		X	X
19	X		

Herpes, Back

	CIST	LACH	ZINC
6	X		
8		X	X

Herpes Circinatus (Includes Tinea Corporis)

	SEP	NAT M	NAT CAR	TELL	CALC	BAR C	PHYTO	CLEM	EUP PERF	HYDRAST	LITH C	SULPH	TUB
2	X	**X**	**X**										
4	X	X											
6	X	X	X	X	X					X			
7	**X**	**X**	X	**X**	X	X	X		X		X		X
8	X	X		X	X	X		X					
13	X		X	X									
26	X											X	

Herpes, Cornea

	RHUS T	ARS	CALC	CANN I	EUPHR	NIT AC	PULS	RAN B
19	X	**X**				X		X
27	X		X	X	E		X	

E- External

Herpes, Ears

	SEP	CAUST	CIST	GRAPH	KREO	MAG M	OLEAND	TEUCR
8	X	X	X	X	X	X	X	X
14	X							
24	X							

Herpes, Ears, Behind

	GRAPH	AMM M	LYC	MEZ	NAT M	OLEAND	RHUS T	SEP
8	X	X		X		X		X
19	X		X		X		X	

Herpes, Elbows, Flexures

	CUPR	KREO	NAT M	SEP	THUJA
8	X	X		X	X
19			X		

Herpes, Eyelids

	BRY	CROT T	CLEM	KREO	RHUS T	SEP	SULPH
8	X				X	X	
13	X			X			X
19		**X**	X				

Herpes, Facialis

	DULC	SEP	CALC	GRAPH	NAT M	BAR C	CARB V	CIC	CON	HEP	LYC	MERC	NIT AC	RHUS T	SULPH	ARN	ARS	CAPS	CAUST	KREO	LACH	LED	MAG CAR	NAT CAR	PETR	CROT T
2																					X					
7	X	**X**	X	X	**X**	X	X	X	X	X	X				X			X					X			
8	X	X	X	X	X	X	X	X	X	X	X	X	X	X	X		X	X	X	X	X	X		X	X	
13	X	X	X	X		X	X	X	X	X	X	X	X	X	X		X			X		X				
14																X										
17																X										
19	X		X	X	X							X	X	X					X				X	X	X	**X**
20	X	X																								

Herpes, Fingers (Includes Herpes, Fingers, Between)

	CAUST	GRAPH	NIT AC	NAT CAR	CALC	CANTH	MERC	PETR	RHUS T
8	X	X	X				X		
19	X	X	X	**X**	X	X		X	X

Herpes, Genitalis

	NIT AC	PETR	RHUS T	NAT M	SEP	CROT T	DULC	MERC	SULPH	ARS	CAUST	GRAPH	HEP	PH AC	SARS	SIL	STAPHYS
1		X				X		X			X	X					
3	X			X				X									
5	X	X	X			X											
6		X															
7							X										
8			X		X		X	X	X				X	X		X	
9			X	X													
13	X	X				X	X								X	X	
14	X								X	X				X			
18			X	X	X	X											X
19	**X**	**X**	X	**X**	**X**	X	X	X	X	**X**	X	X	X		X		X
20		X			X		X										
21			X	X													
26	X				X				X								

Herpes, Hands

	CALC	DULC	KALI SUL	KREO	MERC	NAT M	SARS	SEP	STAPHYS	RHUS T	ZINC
8		X		X	X	X	X	X	X		X
19	X		X							X	

Herpes Impetiginiformis

	ARS	BAPT	CHINA	MERC	PSOR	RHUS T
8	X	X	X		X	X
13				X		

Herpes, Iris

	NAT CAR	OSMIUM
2	X	X
8	X	

Herpes, Joints, Flexures

	NAT M	STAPHYS
8		X
19	X	

Herpes Labialis

	NAT M	ARS	RHUS T	DULC	GRAPH	HEP	AGAR M	BELL	CALC	CAUST	CLEM	LYC	MEZ	NIT AC	SIL	SEP	SULPH	TELL	TEREB	THUJA
2																			X	
8	X	X	X																	
9	X																			
17	X			X																
18	X																			
19	X	X	X	X	X	X	X			X	X	X	X	X		X		X		X
26		X	X		X	X		X	X						X		X			
28	X																			

Herpes, Neck

	SEP	KALI SUL	LACH
8	X		X
19		X	
24	X		

Herpes, Neck, Nape

	CAUST	LYC	PETR	SEP	SULPH	CARB A	CLEM	NAT M	NIT
8	X	X	X	X	X				
13	X	X	X	X	X	X	X	X	X

Herpes, Nose

	NAT CAR	NIT AC	SEP	SULPH	AETHUSA	CANTH	LYC	MAG CAR	RHUS T
8	X	X	X						
13				X					X
17			X						
19	X	X			X	X	X	X	
21				X					

Herpes, Phlyctenoides

	ARS	CANTH	RHUS T	SULPH	ACON	BOV	CALC	CLEM	GRAPH	MERC	PHOS	RAN S	SEP	SIL	TELL
8	X	X	X	X	X	X	X	X		X	X	X		X	X
18		X													
26	X		X	X					X				X		

Herpes, Prepuce

	SARS	HEP	NIT AC	PETR	SEP	CAUST	JUG R	KALI NIT	MERC	PH AC	PHYSO	SULPH
1	X											
2	X	X	X	X			X	X			X	
8	X	X		X	X	X			X	X		
26			X		X							X

Herpes, Right Side

	IRIS V	ARS	CANTH	LYC	MERC
6	X		X		X
7	X				
19		X		X	

Herpes Zoster- (Includes Neuralgia, Post Herpetic; Shingles; Zoster)

	MEZ	RHUS T	RAN B	ARS	PRUN S	MERC	APIS	THUJA	CANTH	DOLICH	GRAPH	IRIS V	KALM	ACON	CAUST	NAT M	SULPH	VARIOL	CARB OX	HEP	PULS	ZINC	ANAG	KALI MUR	LACH	RAN S	SEP	
1	X		X	X	X							X				X					X							
2	**X**	X	X	**X**	**X**			X	X	X	X	X	X		X			X	X					X		X		
3	X	X	X	X					E			X																
4	**X**		**X**																									
5	X	X	X	X	X										X							X	X					
7	**X**	X	**X**			X		X		X	X					X				X	X	X		X				
8	X	X	X		X	X		X	X	X	X								X	X	X	X						
9	X	X	X	X			X																					
10		X		X		X								**X**			X			X							X	
11	**X**	**X**	**X**	**X**	**X**	**X**	**X**		X	X			**X**		X												X	
12	**X**	**X**	X	**X**										**X**		X												
13		X						X			X																	
15		X		X										X														
16																		X										
17			X																									
18	X	X	X	X	X		X	X	X				X		X		X						X			X		
19	X	X	X	X	X	X	X	X		X	X	X	X			X	X	**X**										
20	X	X	X	**X**		X	X					X					X								X			
21	X	X	X	X																					X			
23	X		X	X															X									
25		X		X			X																					
27		X																										

E- External

Herpes Zoster, Left Side

	GRAPH	LACH	THUJA
8	X		
18	X	X	X

Herpes Zoster, Right Side

	ARS	IRIS V	KALM	MERC	RHUS T
4					X
8		X			
19	X		X	X	

Hiccough (AKA Hiccups)

	NUX V	IGN	CYCL	CIC	HYOSC	MOSCH	MAG PH	NICCOL	RAN B	TEUCR	VER A	GINSENG	SULPH AC	BELL	BRY	CUPR	RAT	STRAM	TAB	AMM M	IOD
1	X	X			X		X										X			X	
2		X	**X**	**X**	X	**X**		X	X	X		X	**X**		X		X	X	X		X
3	X		X			X	**X**					X	X								
4						X															
5	X	X	X		X	X										X			X		
6	X	X		X	X			X	X	X	X			X			X	X			
7	**X**	**X**	**X**	**X**	**X**	X	**X**	**X**	X	X	X			X	X	X		X		**X**	**X**
8	X	X	X	X	X	X	X	X	X	X	X			X	X	X	X	X	X	X	X
9	X	X	X			X	X					X									
10	**X**											X		X							
11				X																	
12	X												X								
13	**X**	X	X	X	**X**			**X**	X	X	X			X	X	X		X	X	X	X
14																	X				
15	X			X									X		X						
17	X					X				X			X						X		
18		X																			
19																X					
21	X	X	X	X			X														
23									X												
24											X										
25	X	X	X									**X**									
26	X				X						X										

Hip Joint, Diseases Of- See also Coxalgia; Coxarthrocace; Pain, Hip

	SIL	PH AC	CHINA	KALI CAR	HEP	ACON	CALC	COLOC	ARN	BELL	BRY	CAUST	GETTY	KALI IOD	LACH	LYC	MERC	NAT M	NIT AC	PETR	PHOS	PHYTO	RHUS T	STRAM	SULPH	ARG
1	X																									
2	X	**X**	**X**	**X**	X	**X**						X	X												X	**X**
4	X	X																								
7	**X**	**X**	X	X	X		**X**	**X**	X	X	X	X		X	X	X	X	X	X	X	X	X	X	X		
8	X	X	X	X	X	X	X	X	X	X	X		X	X	X	X	X	X	X	X	X	X	X	X	X	

Hirsutism

	THUJA	LYC	NAT M	OL JEC	PHOS	THYROID
1	X			X		
3	X	X	X		X	X
21	X					

Hives- See Urticaria

Hoarseness- See Voice, Hoarseness

Hodgkins's Disease

	ARS	ACON L	CON	ACON	CALC FL	KALI MUR	NAT M	BAR C	ARS IOD	MERC I R	NAT CAR	NAT SUL	NIT AC	PHOS	PSOR
2	**X**	X		**X**	**X**	**X**	**X**								
8	X		<u>**X**</u>					X	X	X	X	X	X	X	X
19	X														
23		X													

Housemaid's Knee- See also Bursitis

	ARN	SIL	STICTA	RUTA	APIS	KALI IOD	RHUS T	BRY	IOD	NAT M	STILL	ACON	AGAR M	BELL	BOV	CALC	CALC PH	GRAPH	LED	SLAG
1	X	X	X																	
2	X	X			**X**	**X**	**X**				**X**						X			X
7	**X**	**X**								**X**										
8	X	X						X	X						X	X				
9			X																	
12	X			X	X	X	B	B	B			B	B	B				X	B	
14			X																	
19			**X**																	
21				<u>**B**</u>																

B- Both Internal and External

Huntington's Chorea- See also Chorea

	AGAR M	GELS	MYGAL	ZIZ
9		X		
16	X		X	X

Hydraemia- See also Anaemia

	NAT SUL	ARS	AUR	CHINA	KALI CAR
1	X				
2	X				
6		X			
8	X		X	X	X

Hydroa- See also Ailments from Sun

	NAT M	CROT T	GRAPH	RHUS T	ARS	CANTH	POP CAN	RHUS V
2	X						X	X
7	X	X	X	X				
8	X	X	X	X	X	X		

Hydrocele

	PULS	RHOD	GRAPH	SIL	ARN	IOD	AUR	SULPH	APIS	CALC	PSOR	BRY	DIG	RHUS T	ABROT	CON	FL AC	NUX V	AMM C	CALC FL	CLEM	LYSS	MERC
1	**X**			X			X								X								
2	**X**	**X**	**X**	**X**			**X**	X			X	**X**	X	X			X	**X**	X				
3	**X**	X	X		X	X	X					X			X					X			
6	X	X	X	X	X	X	X	X	X	X	X		X	X		X							X
7	X	**X**	X	**X**		X		X	X		X						X		X			X	
8	**X**	X	**X**	X	X	X	X	X	X	X	X		X		X	X	X				X		X
9	X	X	X		X	X								X									
13	**X**	X	**X**	**X**	**X**	X		**X**			X							X				X	
14	X			X			X						X							X			
21		X			X							X											
23				X					X														
24	X			X	X			X	X	X						X							
25	X	X	X		X	X				X				X									
26		X	X							X													
27	X	X	X	X		X			X												X		

Hydrocele, Congenital

	PULS	BRY
2	X	X
3	X	

Hydrocephaloid

	PHOS	VER A	ZINC	APIS	CINA	SULPH	CALC	AETHUS	ARG N	ARS	CALC PH	CARB AC	CHINA	FERR PH	HELL	IGN	LYC	MERC	POD	SIL
2		X			X														X	
6	X	X	X	X		X		X	X	X	X		X	X	X	X	X		X	X
7	X	X	X	X	X	X						X						X		
8	X	X	X	X	X	X	X	X	X	X	X	X	X	X	X	X	X	X		X
26	**X**		X				**X**													

Hydrocephalus

	HELL	CALC	APIS	BELL	SIL	SULPH	MERC	ZINC	APOC	CALC PH	BRY	DIG	KALI IOD	HEDERA	IOD	STRAM	TUB	HYOSC	ARN	ART V	BAR C	CARB AC	CUPR	GRAT	LYC
1	X	X	X	**X**		X	X	X	X	X			X	X			X								
2	**X**	**X**	**X**	**X**		**X**		X	X		**X**	X			X					X		X		X	
3		X	X		X	X	X		X					X			X		E						
4	**X**	X	**X**	**X**	X	**X**		**X**	X	**X**		X	**X**		X		X				X				
6		X			X	X				X											X				X
7	**X**	**X**	**X**		X		X	X	X	X	**X**	X	X			X				X		X	X	X	X
8	X	X	X	X					X										X						
9	X																								
10	**X**	X			X	X				X															
12	X	**X**	X	X	**X**	**X**	X					X													
13	**X**	X	X	**X**	X		X	X				X				X		**X**					X		
14	X	X	X				X																		
15	**X**		X	X							X					X		X							
16	X		X								X														
17	X	X	X		X			X							X										
23	X	X												X											
26		X			X	X	X																		

E- External

Hydronephrosis

	PLUM	ARS	EUCAL
1	**X**	X	
23			X

Hydropericardium- See also Pericardial Effusion

	ARS	DIG	APOC	LYC	APIS	BRY	COLCH	LACH
2				X				
4		X						
6	X	X		X				
8	X	X	X		X	X	X	X
10	X							
23			X					

Hydrophobia- See also Rabies

	STRAM	**BELL**	**HYOSC**	**LYSS**	**CANTH**	**LACH**	**GELS**	**XANTH**	**ARG N**	**ATROP**	**CURARE**	**PHOS**	**SCUT**	**TANACET**	**VIP**
6	X														
7	X	X	X	**X**	X	X					X				
8	X	X	X	X		X							X	X	X
9	X	X	X	X	X										
11	X			X				**<u>X</u>**							
13	**X**	**X**	**X**	X	**X**	X						X			
15	X	X	X				X								
17	X														
23		X								X					
25							X		X						

Hydrophobia, Prophylaxis

	BELL	**CANTH**	**STRAM**	**HYOSC**
10	X	X	X	
15	X			
16	X	X	X	X

Hydrosarcocele

	CON	**RHOD**
1		X
24	X	

Hydrothorax (Note that only the main remedies are used from 17)

	APIS	**ARS**	**SULPH**	**APOC**	**COLCH**	**MERC SU**	**HELL**	**LYC**	**BRY**	**DIG**	**KALI CAR**	**LACH**	**MERC**	**SPIG**	**ASPARA**	**CARB V**	**RAN B**	**SENEG**	**SQUILL**	**ADONIS**	**AMM C**	**ANT T**	**FL AC**	**SANG**	**ARS IOD**
2	**X**	**X**	**X**								X							X							X
3		X	X								X		X				X			X			X		
4	X			X						X		X													
6	X	X	X	X	X		X	X	X	X	X	X	X	X	X			X	X			X			
7	**X**	**X**	X	X	X	X	**X**	**X**	X	X		X	X	**X**	X	X	X		X	X		X	X	X	
8	X	X	X	X	X	X	X	X	X	X		X	X	X	X	X	X	X	X		X			X	
9				X		X																			
11						X																			
12							X		X																
16	X																								
17	X	X	X	X	X	X	X	X	X	X	X	X	X	X	X	X	X	X	X		X	X	X	X	X
23					X	X														X	X				
24	X																								
26	X	X			X			X			X					X									

Hyperactivity- See also Restlessness

	COFF	ACON	AGAR M	CALC FL	CINA	FL AC	HYOSC	LYC	MEDO	NUX V	OX AC	PHOS	PSOR	RHUS T	SEP	STRAM
5				X		X		X		X			X		X	
7	X	X	X				X				X					X
14	X															
18												X				
19									X							
27					X											
29*														X		

29* Rocha MPS, et al. Behavior of rats treated with Rhus toxicodendron 200cH. Int J High Dilution Research, 2008, 7, 22, 3-6.

Hyperactivity, Mental

	COFF	PHYSO
5	X	
9		X

Hyperaemia (Includes Blood, Congestion Of)

	BELL	PHOS	GLON	SPONG	STRAM	VER V	AUR	FERR	KALI CAR	LYC	MERC	SULPH	ACON	ARS	CHINA	CHIN A	LACH	OP	PH AC	AMBRA	ARN	CALC	PETR	SENEG	SEP	THUJA
2	**X**																									
4	X																									
6	X				X									X		X	X									
7	X	X	X	X		X	X	X	X	X	X	X	X	X			X		X							
8	X	X	X	X	X	X									X	X		X								
13	X	**X**	X	X	X	X	**X**	**X**	**X**	**X**	**X**	**X**	X		X			X	X	**X**	**X**	**X**	**X**	**X**	**X**	**X**
24	X																									

Hyperaemia, Brain (Includes Congestion, Brain; Determination of Blood to the Head; Hyperaemia, Head; Vasodilation, Brain)

	BELL	VER V	ACON	GELS	GLON	NUX V	PHOS	ARN	CALC	HYOSC	AUR	CHAM	IOD	LACH	OP	IGN	MERC	PULS	FERR	KALI CAR	LYC	SIL	SPONG	STRAM	SULPH	TAB		
1	X	X	X	X	X																							
6	X	X	X	X	X	X	X	X	X	X	X	X	X	X	X	X	X	X	X	X	X	X	X	X	X			
7	**X**			X			**X**		X	X	X																	
10			X		X				X																			
11													X															
12	X			X		X																						
13	**X**		**X**		X	**X**	**X**	**X**	X	X	**X**	**X**	**X**	**X**	**X**	X	X	X	**X**	**X**	**X**	**X**	**X**	**X**	**X**	**X**		
14	X				X																							
15	X	X	X	X		X						X			X	X	X	X										
17	X	X					X	X																				
18	X	X		X										X														
23	X	X	X		X																							
24	X	X																								X		
25	X	X																										
26			X			X		X																				

Hyperaemia, Kidneys

	AUR	JUNI V	VER V
10	X		
23		X	
24			X

Hyperaemia, Liver- See also Liver, Torpidity

	CARD M	POD	PTEL	CHINA	LYC	MAG M	NUX V	SEP
6	X	X	X	X	X	X	X	X
8	X	X	X	X				
11	X							
23	X	X	X		X	X	X	X
24		X						

Hyperaemia, Optic Fundus

	PRUN S	CACT
8	X	X
24	X	

Hyperaemia, Optic Nerve

	BELL	DUB M	GLON
1		X	
8	X		X

Hyperaemia, Retina

	PHOS	BRY	DUB M	PULS	TAR H
1	X	X	X	X	
6					X
8	X				
24	X				

Hyperaemia, Spinal Cord

	ABSINTH	ACON	ARN	ARS	BELL	CUPR	DULC	HYPER	NUX V	RHUS T	SULPH
6		X	X	X	X	X		X	X	X	X
8							X				
23	X										

Hyperaesthesia- See also Erethism; Neuralgia; Pain (Includes Hypersensitivity)

	BELL	**CHAM**	**NUX V**	**HEP**	**COFF**	**CHINA**	**ACON**	**ASAR E**	**COCCUL**	**PHOS**	**ARS**	**HYOSC**	**SIL**	**CON**	**LACH**	**NAT CAR**	**PLUM**	**AUR**	**LYC**	**AMBRA**	**APIS**	**CIMICI**	**IGN**	**OLEAND**	**SPIG**	**TAR H**	**CANTH**	
1	X	X	X	X	X			X	X		X	X	X				X											
2					X												X							X				
4	X								X													X						
6	X		X			X			X	X														X				
7	X	X	X	X	X	**X**	X	**X**	X	X		X		X		X	X	X	X						X		X	
8	**X**	X	X		X		X	X	X			<u>**X**</u>		X	X							X				<u>**X**</u>		
9	X	X	X										X										X					
10	X	X	X										X											X				
11	X																X											
12		X			X						X																	
13	X	**X**	**X**	X	**X**	X	X	**X**	X	**X**	X	X	X	**X**		X		**X**	**X**						X		**X**	
14			X	X																								
15		X					X																					
16				X																								
17		X	X	X	X	X									X	X		X		X	X	X			X			
18	X	X	X	X	X	X	X				X			X	X	X				X			X					
19						X	X								X											X		
20	X			X																								
21	X		X			X																						
22	X	X	X	X						X																		
23								X																				
24																					X							
26		X	X		X	X	X			X	X		X						X				X					
27	X																			X	X							
28		X																										

Hyperaesthesia, Hearing/Auditory Nerve (AKA Hyperacusis)

	BELL	COFF	NUX V	ACON	SANG	ZINC	AUR	BOR	LYC	PHOS	SIL	THERID	OP	NAT CAR	SEP	SPIG	CHINA	ARN	ARS	BRY	CHAM	COLCH	GELS	IGN	SULPH			
6	X	X		X			X		X	X					X	X			X	X			X		X			
7	X	**X**	X	X	X	X			X	X	X	X	**X**	X	X		**X**		X			X	X	X				
8	X	X	X	X	X		X	X	X			X	X	X	X	X		X		X	X	X		X				
9	X		X					X				X																
10	X	X			X						X					X												
11						X				X			X															
12	X																											
13	X	X	X	X	X	X	X		X		X	X		X	X	X	X	X	X	X	X	X		X	X			
14	X				X			X																				
15	X																						X					
17			X			X	X					X																
18	X	X	X					X						X														
20	X							X																				
21		X	X			X	X			X	X		X				X				X							
22	X		X							X																		
24	X	X		X																								
25					X																							
26				X					X									X							X			
27	X					X					X																	

Hyperaesthesia, Olfaction

	PHOS	NUX V	BELL	ACON	HEP	LYC	COFF	AUR	CARB AC	CHAM	CON	SEP	CHINA	GRAPH	SULPH	AGAR M	COCCUL	CALC	COLCH	NUX M	ANAC							
6	X		X		X	X		X				X				X												
7	X	X	X	X	X	X	X	X		X	X	X	X				X		X	X								
8	X	X	X	X	X	X	X	X		X	X	X	X	X	X			X										
10				X											X													
11	X																			X								
13	X	X	**X**	X	X	X	**X**	X		X	X	X	X	X	X	**X**	X	X	X		**X**							
14									X																			
17	X	X		X	X	X	X		X	X	X																	
18		X																										
20			X																									
21									X					X														
22	X	X							X																			

Hyperaesthesia, Retina- See also Photophobia

	BELL	NUX V	PHOS	CON	LACT AC	NAT M	CHINA	EUPHR	GELS	IGN	ACON	ANT T	ARS	CALC	GRAPH	HEP	HYOSC	LAC D	LIL T	MERC	NUX M	PULS	RHUS T	SANG	SULPH
3																			X						
6	X	X	X	X	X	X	X	X	X	X	X	X	X	X	X	X	X			X		X	X		X
7	X	X		X	X	**X**				X															
8			X	X	X				X									X						X	
11			X																		X				
17		X																							
18	X																								
20	X																								
21	X						X																		
22	X	X	X					X																	
24	X																								

Hyperaesthesia, Skin

	SEP	BELL	HEP	LACH	ACON	CIMICI	ARAN D	ARN	CHINA	COFF	GUAIAC	LYC	NUX V	PETR	PULS	SPIG	THUJA
6	X	X	X			X		X		X		X	X		X	X	
8	X			X			X							X			X
15					X				X								
18			X														
19				X													
21		X															
24											X						
26	X																

Hyperaesthesia, Taste

	BELL	CHINA	COFF	CAMPH	LYC	MUR AC
6	X	X	X			X
7	X	X	X	X	X	

Hyperaesthesia, Teeth

	FL AC	ANT C	ARN	COFF	LACH	LYC	MAG PH	MERC	NAT M	PULS	SULPH
7	X					X	X	X	X		X
19	X	X	X		X					X	
28				X							

Hyperaesthesia, Touch- See Hyperaesthesia, Skin

Hyperaesthesia, Uterus

	ATROP S	HELON
7	X	
8		X

Hyperaesthesia, Vision- See Hyperaethesia, Retina; Photophobia

Hypercapnia

	ASPIDO	CARB V
18		X
28	X	

Hyperchlorhydria- See also Dyspepsia

	ROBIN	CALC	CARB V	NUX V	SULPH AC	SULPH	IRIS V	PHOS	ARS	SEP	LITH C	ATROP	BRY	CAPS	CAUST	CHEL	PULS	SAL AC	NAT SUL
1	X			X	X	X	X										X	X	
2	X																		
4	**X**													X					
5	X						X			X						X			
6			X		X			X							X				
7	X		X	X	X		X				**X**			X	X				**X**
8		X		X		X		X											
9		X		X	X														
10		X	X			X			X										
11		X						X				X							
12	X	X		X	X				X							X			
14			**X**			X	X												
15			X	X						X			X						
17					X						X								
18	X																		
23					X							X						X	
24		X																	
26		X	X	X		X		X	X	X			X				X		

Hypercholesterolaemia

	CHEL	CHOLEST	COLCH	IRIS V	NUX V	PHOS	RAPH	SEP	SOLID	TARAX
5	X	X	X	X	X	X	X	X	X	X
29*	X									

29* Baumans V, et al. Chelidonium and cholesterol. Brit Hom J, 1987, 76, 45-46.

Hyperemesis Gravidum- See Morning Sickness

Hyperhidrosis

	MERC	CHINA	HEP	SIL	PH AC	CALC	SEP	VER A	BRY	ARS	JAB	SAMB	BELL	ANT T	CARB V	IPEC	PHOS	SULPH AC	RHUS T	NAT M	TAB
1	X	X	X	X				X			X										
2		**X**			**X**						**X**							X			
3	X				X			X	X												
4	X			X		X			X									X			
5	X	X	X	X	X	X	X	X			X	X	X	X	X	X	X		X		X
6	X		X	X		X	X	X	X	X		X	X	X	X	X	X		X	X	X
7	**X**	**X**	**X**	**X**	X	**X**	**X**	**X**	X	X	**X**		**X**	X	X		X	X	**X**	X	
8	X	**X**	X	X	X	**X**	**X**	X	X	X			X		X		X	X	X	X	
9					X											X				X	X
10	X	X	X				X	X	X	X			X					X	X	X	
11	X	X	X	X	X	X	X				X	X			X					X	
12	X	X	X		X				X			X		X			X				
14	X	X	X			X	X														
15	X	X			X		X		X	X								X			
17	X					X						X		X				X			X
18	X	X		X					X			X	X			X	X		X		
19	X									X		X				X					
21	X					X										X					
22	X		X											X							
23											X										X
24	X	X	X	X				X		X							X				
25	X	X		X	X			X		X			X		X	X					X
26												X			X						
27											X			X							

Hypermetropia- See also Presbyopia

	JAB	ARG N	CALC	CON	CIMICI	DROS	HYOSC	SIL	SULPH	RUTA
2	X									
6		X								
7	X	X	X				X			
8				X	X					
21	X									X
26			X	X		X		X	X	

Hyperpyrexia- See Fever

Hypersensitivity- See Hyperaesthesia

Hypertension (Note that only the major remedies are used from 17)

	GLON	LACH	AUR	BAR C	ACON	CRAT	NAT M	NUX V	BELL	GELS	BAR M	ARS	AUR M	PLUM	VER V	IGN	PHOS	SULPH	ADRENAL	STROPH	LYCOP	NAT IOD	PASS	SEC	RAUWOLF	THUJA	VISC A	
1	X	**X**	X	X	X	X	X		X	X	X	X		X	X	X			X	X				X		X	X	
3	X	**X**	X			X				X	X								X				X				X	
4	X				X									X						X		**X**						
5	X	X	X	X	X			X	X	X				X		X	X						X					
7	X				X			X	X			X	X				X	X										
9	X		X	X		X	**X**	X		X	X				X		X				**X**							
10	X	X	X	X	X	X		X	X		X	X	X	X			X	X		X								
11	**X**		X	X	**X**		X	X			**X**														X			
14	X	X	X	X							X		X	X	X						X							
16						X																						
17	X	X	X	X	X	X	X	X	X	X		X	X	X	X	X			X	X	X	X	X	X	X		X	
18	X	X	X	X	X			X				X	X		X	X	X	X						X		X		
19		X							X																			
21				X																								
24	X		X	X					X				X		X				X			X						
25	X					X	**X**			X								X										
27		X	X			X																						
28		X																										
29[1]		X		X			**X**	X		X		X				X		X								X		
29[2]		X																										
29[3]																									X			

29[1] Campistranous-Lavout JL, et al. Hypertension Trial. Boletin Mexicano, 1999, 32, 42- 47.
29[2] Bernal-Ochoa F, et al. Lachesis muta 200 as a Hypotensive. Brit Hom J, 86, 1991, 35-36.
29[3] Rastogi DP, et al. Rauwolfia Serpentina (Aqua): A New Approach in the Treatment of Hypertension in Homoeopathy. CCRH Quarterly Bulletin, 1996, 18, 1&2, 22-24.

Hypertension, Portal

	AESC	NUX V	SULPH	ALOE	ASAF	APOC	AUR M	CARD M	COLLIN	KALI IOD	KALI MUR	LEPT																
7	X	X	X		X	X		X		X	X																	
18							X																					
27	X	X	X	X					X			X																

Hyperthyroidism- See also Exophthalmic Goitre (AKA Grave's Disease; Thyrotoxicosis)

	IOD	NAT M	LYCOP	BELL	THYROID	CALC	KALI IOD	LAPIS	ADRENAL	ARS IOD	AUR	CACT	CALC IOD	CON	FERR	FUCUS	NUX V	PHOS	SPONG	ARS								
1			X																									
5	X	X			X		X	X		X	X		X	X				X										
9		X			X																							
11	X		X	X		X			X			X			X													
12	X			X											X		X											
17	X	X	X		X				X	X									X									
18	X																											
19	**X**	**X**	X	X	X	X	**X**	**X**			X	X	X	X		X	X	X	X	**X**								
21	X	X	X	X																								
27	X	X				X										X												
28			X																									

Hypertrophy

	CARB A	HYDROC																										
2	X																											
7	X	X																										

Hypertrophy, Heart- See also Heart, Dilatation Of

	CACT	SPONG	ARS	KALM	SPIG	ARN	RHUS T	ACON	DIG	AUR	BROM	CRAT	LYC	NAJA	PULS	KALI CAR	IBER	LITH C	AUR M	IOD	NAT M	VER V						
1	X			X		X	X	X		X		X					X				X							
2	X	X									X	X								X								
3			X							X																		
4	X		X	**X**	X	X	**X**	X			X											X						
5	X	X				X			X																			
6		X	X	X	X																							
7	**X**	**X**	X	**X**	**X**	X	**X**	**X**	**X**	X	**X**		X	X	X	**X**	X	**X**	X	X	X							
8	X	X	X	X	X	X	X	X	X	X	**X**		X		X	X		X		X	X	X						
9		X												X														
10			X	X	X					X			X		X		X		X									
11								X																				
13			X		**X**			X							X													
16	X																											
17	X	X	X	X		X	X	X	X	X	X	X	X	X		X	X	X	X			X						
19	X	X		X	X	X	X		X					X		X												
23						X	X		X			X		X														
24		X																										
26			X		X								X		X													
27												X																

Hypertrophy, Heart, Left

	CACT	IOD	ACON	AUR	GLON	KALM	LACH	PHOS	SPIG	SPONG
6	X	X	X	X	X	X			X	X
7	X	X					X	X		

Hypertrophy, Heart, Right

	PHOS	ARS	IOD	SPONG
6	X			
7	X	X		
8			X	
24	X			X

Hypertrophy, Heart, Ventricle, Left

	AUR M	CALC	CONVAL	GLON	IOD	PHOS
6	X	X			X	X
11			X			
17				X		

Hypertrophy, Heart, Ventricle, Right

	CONVAL	IOD	KALI IOD	PHOS	PULS	SPONG
8		X			X	
11	X					
17			X	X		X

Hypertrophy, Liver- See Hepatomegaly
Hypertrophy, Ovaries- See Swelling, Ovaries
Hypertrophy, Prostate- See Prostate, Hypertrophy
Hypertrophy, Spleen- See Splenomegaly
Hypertrophy, Testes

	BAR M	BUFO	IOD
7			X
8	X	X	

Hypertrophy, Tonsils

	BAR C	**BAR IOD**	**CALC IOD**	**CALC PH**	**HEP**	**IOD**	**MERC**	**MERC I F**	**NIT AC**	**PHYTO**	**PSOR**	**STAPHYS**	**THUJA**
1								X					
14					X								
17											X		
24	X	X	X	X						X			X
25						X							
26							X		X			X	

Hypertrophy, Tongue

	ARS	**CARB AC**	**GRAPH**	**IOD**	**NIT AC**	**PLUM**	**SULPH**
7		X					
8	X		X	X	X	X	X

Hypertrophy, Uterus

	KALI IOD	**APIS**	**AUR M**	**BELL**	**LACH**	**MUREX**	**NAT CAR**	**PLAT**	**SEP**	**USTIL**
7	X		X	X	X	X	X	X	X	X
8	X	X								

Hypervolaemia (AKA Plethora)

	ACON	**BELL**	**NUX V**	**CALC**	**FERR**	**AESC**	**AUR**	**LYC**	**SEP**	**SULPH**	**ARS**	**HYOSC**	**PULS**
2	X			X							**X**		
7	**X**	**X**	X	X			X						
8	X	X	X		X	X		X	X	X			
10		X											
13	X	**X**	X	X	X		X	X	X	X		**X**	**X**
24			X		X	X							
25	X												
26	X	X											

Hypochlorhydria

	CARB V	**HYDR AC**	**MUR AC**	**STRY N**
1	<u>**X**</u>	<u>**X**</u>		X
23			X	

Hypochondria (Includes Hypochondriasis)

	NUX V	CON	ANAC	NAT M	SULPH	LYC	STAPHYS	ARS	SEP	NAT CAR	AUR	CALC	PULS	CACT	PHOS	GRAT	IGN	CHINA	STANN	ARN	BRY	MOSCH	RHUS T	SABAD	VALER	ZINC
1	X	X		X			X		X		X				X											
2	**X**	**X**	X	**X**	**X**	X	X	**X**		X		X				X			**X**			X			**X**	X
4	X		X			X				X																
5																		X						X		
6	X						X		X		X			X												
7		X	X	**X**	X	X	X		X	**X**	X		X	**X**	X	X										
8	**X**	X	**X**	**X**	**X**	X	X	X	X	X	X	**X**	X	X	X	X	X	**X**	X	X	X	X	X	X		X
9	X					X														X						
10		X																								
11			X		X																					
12	X		X					X	X		X		X				X									
13	X		X	X	X	X	X	X	X	X		X	X	X	**X**	X	X	X	X	X	X	X	X	X	**X**	X
21	X	X		X				X				X														
23	X	X			X		X	X									X									
24	X																									
25						X																				
26	X	X											X								X		X			

Hypoglycaemia

	LYC	ZINC
5		X
19	X	

Hypopyon

	HEP	SIL	SULPH	APIS	MERC	PLUM	SENEG	THUJA	ARS	CROT H	GRAPH
2		X				X	X			X	
6	X	X	X					X			
7	X	X	X	X				X			
8	X	X		X	X	X	X				
24	X										X
26	X		X		X				X		

Hypotension (Note here that only the major remedies are used from 17)

	NAJA	CHINA	CARB V	CALC PH	CACT	CRAT	GELS	LYC	NAT M	TUB	VISC A	CAMPH	KALI PH	SEP	ACON	APOC	CAFF	DIG	IPEC	LYCOP	PIC AC	PSOR	SIL	THYROID
1	X	X	X	X			X	X	X	X	X			X		X				X				
3			X	X	X	X		X		X	X		X											
4	**X**											X												
5	X	X				X			X		X	X	X					X			X			
9	X						X																	
10		X	X	X			X	X	X	X			X	X							X	X	X	
11	X																X							X
14		X	X		X	X									X		X							
17	X	X	X	X	X	X	X	X	X	X	X	X		X	X	X		X	X			X	X	X
18		X																	X					
21					X																			
24																				X				

Hypothermia

	CACT	CUPR	DIPHTHER
10			X
17	X		
21		X	

Hypothyroidism (Includes Myxoedema)

	THYROID	BAR C	SPONG	CALC	ARS	GRAPH	CALC PH	AETHUS	ALUM	ARG N	CON	DORYPH	GELS	FUCUS	IOD	KALI CAR	LAPIS A	LYC	NAT M	NUX V	OL JEC O	PRIM O	SEP	SIL	SULPH
1	X																								
2	**X**											X													
3	X		X												X		X				X				X
5	X	X																							
9	X		X																						
11	**X**	**X**		**X**			**X**	X																X	
17	X				X																	X			
18						X																			
19	X			X		X			X	X	X		X			X		X	X	X			X		
21					X																				
23	X																								
24	X																								
27		X	X	X										X											

Hysteria- See Anxiety

Icthyosis

	ARS	ARS I	PLUM	THUJA	PHOS	GRAPH	SEP	SULPH	CALC	CHINA	CLEM	HEP	LYC	PETR	SIL	HYDRAST	NAT CAR	AUR	COLOC	HURA	HYDROC	IOD	LAC C	OENANTH	PIPER M	PLATAN	SYPH	THYROID
2	**X**		**X**	**X**						X						**X**	**X**						X		X	X		X
5		X					X																					
6	X		X	X	X	X	X	X	X		X	X	X	X	X													
7	**X**				**X**					X																		
8	X	**X**	X	X	**X**	X	X	X	X		X	X	X	X	X			X	X	X	X	X						
9		X																									X	
21	X	X	X	X																								
23		X				X		X																X				

Icterus– See Jaundice

Idiopathic Thrombocytic Purpura (AKA Purpura Haemorrhagica)

	PHOS	CROT H	LACH	SULPH AC	ARN	HAM	LED	TEREB	ARS	BRY	PH AC	RHUS T	SEC	KALI IOD
7	X	X	**X**	**X**	X	X	**X**	**X**			X	X	**X**	X
8	X	X	X	X	X	X	X	X	X	X		X	X	X
11	X	X	X	X	X	X	X	X	X	X	X			
12		X	X	X		X			X					
23		X												
26	X				X					X	X	X		

Ileus- See also Obstruction, Intestines; Paralysis, Intestines; Vomiting, Faeces

	OP	RAPH	SAMB	THUJA	NUX V	ACON	ARS	BELL	CHAM	COCCUL	COLCH	CUPR	DIOSC	LYC	NIT AC	PLAT	PLUM	RHUS T	SIL	SULPH	VER A	ZINC	CAST EQ	COLOC	ERIGER	SOL T A	TAB	TANNIN
2	X		X								X												X			X		X
6	X	X	X	X	X	X	X	X	X	X		X	X	X	X	X	X	X	X	X	X	X		X				
8	**X**	X	X	X	**X**	X	X	X	X	X	X	X	X	X	X	X	X	X	X	X	X	X			X		X	
21	X	X																										
24				X																								
26	X																											
29*	X	X																										

29*Barnes J., Resch K-L., Ernst E. Homoeopathy for Post-Operative Ileus: A Meta-Analysis. Journal of Clinical Gastroenterology, 1997, Dec, 25, 4, 628- 633.

Impetigo- See also Ecthyma

	ANT C	**MEZ**	**VIOL T**	**ARS**	**CALC**	**SULPH**	**HEP**	**MERC**	**RHUS T**	**SIL**	**ANT T**	**CIC**	**GRAPH**	**NAT M**	**CROT T**	**IRIS V**	**KALI BIC**	**LYC**	**SEP**	**BAR C**	**CARB S**	**DULC**	**PETR**
2		X	**X**								**X**	**X**				X					X		
3	X																						
4			X								X												
5	X	X	X		X		X						X						X				
6	**X**	X	X	X	X		X	X	X	X	X	X	X	X	X		X	X		X			X
7		X	X		**X**	X	X	**X**	X	X		X	X	**X**	X	X	X	X		X	X	X	X
8	X	X	X	X	X	X	X	X	X	X		X	X	X	X	X	X	X	X	X		X	
9	X	X		X		X				X													
11						X	X																
12	X		X	X							X						X						
14		X	**X**	X			X																
16	X										X												
18	X				X																		
19	**X**	X	X		X	**X**	X	**X**	X	X		X	**X**	X		X			X		X	X	X
20	**X**			X			X	X	X														
21	X	X		X											X								
25	X	X		X		**X**				X													
26		X		X	**X**	**X**		X	X									X	X				

Impetigo, Scrotum

	ANT C	**ANT T**	**CROT T**
4		X	
8	X		
21			X

Impotence- See also Azospermia; Atrophy Spermatic Cord; Debility; Sterility; Weakness, Genital Organs (Includes Erections without Desire; Sexual Desire, Decreased; Sexual Desire, Loss of)

	LYC	AGNUS	SEL	CALAD	PH AC	PHOS	CON	ARG N	SULPH	CALC	NAT M	MOSCH	BAR C	KALI BR	NUX V	STAPHYS	ARN	CAMPH	GRAPH	NUPH	ONOS	PLUM	SIL	YOHIMB	CAPS	MUR AC
1	X			X	X	X	X				X	X		X		X	X		X	X	X			X	X	
2	X	X	X	X	X	X			X	X		X		X	X	X	X			X	X			X		X
3	X	X	X	X		X													X							
4		X						X														X				
6	X	X	X	X		X				X	X	X	X	X				X				X				
7	**X**	**X**	**X**	X	**X**	X	X	X	X	**X**	X	X	**X**	X	**X**	**X**		**X**	X	X		X	X		X	X
8	**X**	X	X	X	**X**	X	X	X	X	X	X	X	X		X			X	X	X					X	X
9	**X**	X	X	X	X		X	X			X				X	X	X						X	X		
10	X				X	X	X															X				
11	X												X													
13	**X**	X	**X**	**X**	X	X	**X**	X	X	**X**	X	**X**	X		X	X		**X**	X			X	X		**X**	**X**
14	X	X	X	X	X	X		X	X												X					
16		X	X																				X	X		
17							X					X									X					
19		X	X																							
21	X		X	X			X	X					X	X			X									
23		X	X		X															X	X			X		
25	X	X					X	X									X									
26	X			X					X	X	X															
27	X	X			X									X												
29[1]	X					X			**X**	X	X												X			
29[2]	X					X		X	X																	

29[1] Gerhard I, et al. Individualised homeopathic therapy for male infertility, Homeopathy, 2002, 91, 133-144.

29[2] de Souza MF, et al. The effect of individualized homeopathic treatment on the semen quality of bulls with reproductive disorders: a case series. Homeopathy. 2012 Oct;101 (4):243-5.

Impotence, Senile

	LYC	AMBRA	SABAL
1	X		
7	**X**		
8		X	
9	**X**		
25			X

Incontinence, Faecal

	ARN	PH AC	BELL	HYOSC	SEC	RHUS T	ALOE	MUR AC	OP	APIS	ARS	CARB V	THUJA	CHINA	OLEAND	COLCH	GELS	PHOS	LAURO	SULPH								
1	X	X		X											X		X											
2					X																							
3							X																					
4	X			X		X		X																				
5							X																					
6	X	X	X	X	X	X		X	X	X	X					X												
7	**X**	X	**X**	**X**	**X**	**X**		X	**X**			X		X	**X**	X		X	X	X								
8	X	X	X	X	X	X	X		X	X	X	X	X	X	X			X	X	X								
9		X																										
10	X		X		X		X	X				X	X			X												
11	X	X								X																		
12						X					X		X															
13	**X**	**X**	**X**	**X**	**X**	X		X	X	X	X	X	X	**X**	X	X		X	**X**	**X**								
14	X		X	X	X		X			X								X										
15			X					X			X																	
16			X					X																				
17	X									X							X											
18							X																					
19		X					X		X								X											
22																	X											
24	X		X									X																
25		X												X														
26	X	X		X		X			X		X	X	X															

Incontinence, Urinary- See also Sphincters, Urinary, Atony (Includes Enuresis; Incontinence, Pregnancy, From; Incontinence, Stress From)

	CAUST	BELL	SEP	PULS	KREO	EQUISET	ARN	GELS	HYOSC	SULPH	CINA	NAT M	NUX V	FERR PH	RHUS T	SIL	APIS	ARG N	ARS	BENZ AC	CALC	ZINC	RUTA					
1	X		X		X	X	X	X	X	X	X	X	X		X	X			X	X	X		X					
2	X		**X**	**X**	**X**	X				X	X			**X**		X				X		X	X					
3	X	X	X	X	X	X	X			X	X	X	X			X		X		X	X	X						
4	**X**					X	X					X	X	X			X											
5	X	X	X	X	X			X	X		X	X	X	X		X	X	X	X			X						
6	X	X					X	X	X								X	X	X			X						
7	**X**	X	**X**	X	X	X	X	X	X	X	X	X			**X**		**X**	**X**	**X**	X								
8	X	X	X	X	X	X	X	X	X	X	X	X			**X**	X		X			X	X	X					
9	X	X	X		X	X		X					X	X		X	X											
10	X	X	X	X			X		X	**X**				X	X	X			X		X		X					
11		X					X												X	X								
12	X	X						X			X		X			X				X	X							
13	X	X	**X**	**X**						**X**		X			**X**							X	X					
14	X	X															X	X	X	X	X							
15		X							X				X															
16		X																										
17	X								X													X						
18	X		X																									
19	X		X	X	X		X	X	X			X			X			X										
20	**X**	X	X	X	X	X																						
21	X	X	X	X	X	X	X	X					X	X														
22	X	X	X	X	X	X																						
23	X		X											X														
24				X																								
25	**X**	X				X		X					X	X			X											
26	X	X	X	X			X		X	**X**	X	X			X						X		X					
27											X																	

Incontinence, Urinary, Coughing/Sneezing, From

	CAUST	PULS	SQUILLA	VER A	NAT M	PHOS	KREO	SEP	ZINC	ANT C	CAPS	PH AC	STAPHYS	THUJA	APIS	ALUMEN	BRY	CHLOR	FERR PH	LACH	NUX V	RUMEX	SCILLA	SULPH				
4	X				X				X														X					
6	X		X			X											X				X							
7	**X**	X	**X**	X	X		X		X			X		X	**X**	X				X								
9	X																											
10	X																											
11			X																									
12				X																								
13	X	X		**X**	X	X	X	X	X	**X**			X	X										X				
17	X	X	X	X	X	X	X	X		X	X	X						X				X						
18	X																											
19	X	X	X					X																				
20	X	X																										
21	X	X																										
22	X																											
25																			X									
26	X	X		X		X					X		X															
27	X				X																							

Incontinence, Urinary, Senile- See also Prostate, Hypertrophy

	CON	BAR C	CAUST	IOD	ALL C	ALOE	BELL	GELS	HEP	SEC																		
6				X																								
7			X		X																							
8				X		X																						
9		X																										
10	X																											
11	X																											
12							X	X																				
14	X								X	X																		
25		X	X																									

Indigestion- See also Ailments From (various foods and drinks); Dyspepsia

	NUX V	**PULS**	**LYC**	**CARB V**	**CHINA**	**ARS**	**BRY**	**IPEC**	**SULPH**	**CALC**	**CHAM**	**ANT C**	**IGN**	**ARG N**	**NAT M**	**ANAC**	**COCCUL**	**GRAPH**	**HEP**	**MERC**	**KALI BIC**	**PHOS**	**LACH**	**NAT CAR**				
1	X					X			X													X						
2						X																						
3	X	X	X											X			X	X										
5	X	X	X		X			X			X	X	X	X	X							X		X				
6	X	X			X	X		X																				
7	X	X	X					X	X	X					X									X				
8	**<u>X</u>**	**<u>X</u>**	X	**<u>X</u>**	**X**	**X**	**X**	**X**	**X**	X	**X**	X	X	X	X	X	**X**	X	**X**	X	X	X	**X**					
9	X	X	X	X		X	X		X	X					X													
10	X	X		X	X		X	**X**								X	X											
12	X	X	X	X			X		X	X	X	X	X						X	X	X							
13			X	X	X				**X**	**X**			X			**X**		**X**	X	**X**			X	**X**				
14	X	X	X	X	X	X		X				X		X														
15	X	X	X	X	X	X	X	X			X	X	X				X		X	X	X		X					
19		X	X		X							X																
20		X																										
21	X	X	X	X	X	X	X			X	X		X	X		X		X			X	X						
22	X	X		X			X				X		X															
23			X								X	X																
24	X				X																							
25	X	X	X	X		X	X		X	X					X													
28	X																											

Indigestion, Senile- See also Dyspepia, Senile

	ABIES N	**CARB V**	**CHINA**
14	X		
15		X	X

Infection

	PYROG	SIL	HEP	ARS	MYRIST	MERC	RHUS T
3	**X**						
5	X	X	X			X	
9		X	X				
11	X						
14					**X**		
16					X		
17		X		X			X
18	**X**	X	**X**	X		X	
19				X			
29[1]		X					
29[2]							X

29[1] Davenas E. Effect on Mouse Peritoneal Macrophages of Orally Administered Very High Dilutions of Silica. Eur J Pharmacology, 1987, 135, 313-319.
29[2] Patil CR, et al. Immunomodulatory activity of Toxicodendron pubescens in experimental models. Homeopathy. 2009, 98, 3, 154-9.

Infection, Ear, Nose and Throat

	LYC	BELL	DULC	HEP	PSOR	SULPH	SULPH IO	ACON	BRY	CALC	CALC PH	CHAM	CIST	FERR PH	IOD	MED	MERC	NAT M	NAT SU	PHOS	PULS	SIL	TUB	TUB AV	VERBASC
5							X								X										
18	X		X	X	X	X	X			X	X					X		X	X			X	X	X	
19	X				X								X												
22		X	X					X				X		X											X
25						X																			
29*	X	**X**		X					X								X			X	X				

29* Haidvogl M, et al. Homeopathic and conventional treatment for acute respiratory and ear complaints: A comparative study on outcome in the primary care setting. BMC Complement Altern Med. 2007 Mar 2;7 (1):7.

Infection, Eye

	CEDRON	PULS
8	X	
20		X

Infection, Fungal (Includes Mycosis)

	SULPH	SIL	SEP	ARS	LACH	LYC	STAPHYS	THUJA	ANT C	CALC	KALI IOD	KREO	NIT AC	PHOS
1				X	X			X						X
5						X								
7							X		X					
8	X	X		X	X	X	X		X			X		
16								X			X		X	
17	X	X	X	X	X	X	X	X		X	X	X	X	X
18	X	X	X											
19	X	X	**X**							X				
21	X													

Infection, Gums- See also Boils, Gums

	AUR	CARB V	HEP	KREO	MERC
5	X			X	
19			X		X
25		X			

Infection, Nails- See Onychomycosis

Infection, Pelvic- See also Ailments from, Labor

	CROT H	PULS	SIL	THUJA
5				X
17	X	X	X	

Infection, Prophylaxis

	ARN	HEP	NOSODE*	PYROG
18		X		X
21	X			
28			X	

* A remedy made from the potentially injective agent

Infection, Respiratory

	PHOS	SIL	ARS	BRY	HEP	KALI IOD	KALI SUL	PSOR	SANG	SENEC	SULPH IO	THUJA	TUB
14				X									
18		X									X	X	
19	X	X	X			X	X	X	X	X			X
21	X												
25					X								

Infection, Respiratory Tract, Upper

	CHAM	CIST	HEP	IP	LYC	NUX V	PSOR	RHUS T
14				X				
17	X		X					X
19		X			X	X	X	

Infection, Salmonella

	BAPT
11	X
21	X

Infection, Sinus

	KALI BIC	KALI IOD	MERC	SAMB
5			X	
14	X			
19		X		X

Infection, Skin (Includes Varicose Ulcers, Infected)

	HEP	PSOR	SULPH	BOR	CALC SUL	CALEND	CAUST	KALI SUL	PYROG	SIL	STAPHYS	TUB
5							X					
9				X								X
18	X				X				X	X		
19			X									
21	X	X										
25		X	X			E		X			X	

E- External

Infection, Throat

	MERC	MERC I F	MERC I R	BELL	HEP	PYROG	SULPH
5					X	X	
9	X						
19				X			X
24	X	X	X				
25	X						
28		X	X				

Infection, Urinary Tract- See also Nephritis

	CANTH	EQUISET	MEDO	BENZ AC	ARS	SEP	TEREB	COP	BELL	SARS	CANN S	LYC	MERC C	PARIERA	RHUS T	SIL	STAPHYS	THUJA	UVA	NUX V	PETROS
1	X																				
5		X	X			X				X				X		X		X			
9		X	X																		
11	X			**X**	X		X	**X**	**X**		X		X		X				X		
14	X								X								X				
18	X	X	X	X	X	X	X					X	X			X	X				
19	**X**		X		X	X	X	X		**X**	X	X		X	X			X	X	**X**	**X**
23				X																	
25		X																			

Infection, Urinary Tract, E coli

	THUJA	COLI	FORMICA	CANTH	ECHIN	EQUISET	METH BL	MERC C	SEP	SIL	SOLID	STAPHYS	TEREB	VANAD
1	X	X	X		X		X							
5	X	X	X	X		X		X	X	X	X	X	X	
17														X

Infectious Mononucleosis

	BAR C	PHYTO	AILANTH	BELL	CALC	CIST	MERC	ARS I	BAR IOD	BAR M	BERB V	CALC IOD	CALC PH	GLAN FE	HYDRAST	LAPPA	SAPO	SIL	SULPH IO	THUJA	TUB
5	X	X	X				X	X	X	X	X	X	X		X	X	X	X	X	X	X
21	X	X	X	X	X	X	X														
22						X															
25	X	X		X	X									X							

Infertility- See Sterility

Inflammation

	ACON	FERR PH	PULS	BRY	ARS	BELL	CANTH	MERC	PHOS	STAPHYS	CUPR	HEP	NUX V	RHUS T	SIL	VER V
2	X	X									X					
3	X					X										
7	**X**	**X**	**X**	**X**	**X**	**X**	**X**	**X**	**X**	**X**	X	X	X	X	X	**X**
9		X										X				
11		X														
13	X		**X**	X	X		X	X	X	X			X		X	
22	X															
29[1]														X		
29[2]														X		

29[1] dos Santos AL, et al. In-vivo study of the anti-inflammatory effect of Rhus toxicodendron. Homeopathy. 2007 Apr;96(2):95-101.

29[2] Patil CR, et al. Dual effect of Toxicodendron pubescens on Carrageenan induced paw edema in rats. Homeopathy. 2009 Apr;98(2):88-91.

Inflammation, Adenoids

	AGRAPH	CALC	HYDRAST	BACILL	CALC PH	SULPH	TUB	PSOR	BAR C	PULS
1	X	X	**X**	X	X		X			
2		X				X		**X**		
3	X		X	X			X			
4	**X**						**X**			
5	X		X							
12		X				X		X	X	X
14	X	X		X	X					
21	X	X			X	X			X	X

Inflammation, Anus

	MEDO	RICIN
3	X	
8		X

Inflammation, Bone- See Osteitis

Inflammation, Bowel- See also Colitis

	APIS	ALOE	APIS	ARG N	CHINA	CROT H	DULC	KALI BIC	LYC	NAT M	NAT SUL	NUX V	PH AC	PHOS	POD	SULPH	THUJA
6	X																
19		X	X	X	X	X	X	X	X	X	X	X	X	X	X	X	X
24	X																

Inflammation, Brain- See also Encephalitis; Meningitis

	ACON	BELL	HYOSC	GLON	OP	SCUT	VER V	STRAM	APIS	ARUM T	BRY	CAPS	CHR OX	CUPR AC	GELS	HELL	KALI BR	MERC	NUX V	ZINC
2						X				X		X	X					X		
3	X	X	X	X																
4	**X**	**X**	**X**	X	X		X	**X**									X			
6									X											
15	X	X	X		X	X	X				X			X	X	X			X	X

Inflammation, Breast- See Mastitis

Inflammation, Caecum- See also Typhlitis

	LACH	VER V	RHUS T
2	**X**	**X**	X
8	X		

Inflammation, Canthi

	ANT C	ARG N	ZINC
14		X	X
26	X		

Inflammation, Cornea

	SULPH	MERC	ARS	CALC	EUPHR	HEP	SYPH	APIS	AUR M	BAR IOD	CALC IOD	CANN I	CANN S	CAUST	ILEX A	KALI BIC	KALI MUR	NUX V	RHUS T	SEP	SIL	SPIG
1															X							
4																	X					
6	X	X	X	X		X		X	X	X	X		X						X	X	X	
8	X						X					X		X		X		X				
13					X																	X
14		X					X															
26	X		X	X	X	X																

Inflammation, Diaphragm (AHA Diaphragmitis)

	BRY	CACT	LYC	ACON	APIS	HEP	NUX V	STRAM	BELL	CHAM	COCCUL	DIG	DULC	NUX M	SULPH	BISM	COLCH	COLOC	CUPR	HAM	HYOSC	MORPH S	PARRAF	PULS	RHUS T	TAB	VER A	VER V
2						X		X								X							X					X
5		X																										
6	X	X	X	X	X	X	X	X	X	X		X	X		X		X								X	X		
7	X	X	X	X	X	X	X	X	X			X		X	X			X		X		X					X	
8	X		X		X								X	X					X									
13	X			X			X			X	X										X			X				
23		X																										
26			X								X																	

Inflammation, Duodenum (AKA Duodenitis)

	CHAM	CHINA	HYDRAST	KALI BIC	LYC	MERC	POD	PULS	ACON	ARG N	ARS	BELL	IOD	IRIS V	KALI SUL	NUX V	PHOS	URAN N
6	X	X	X			X		X	X							X		
7					X		X			X	X	X	X	X	X		X	X
8		X	X	X	X	X	X	X										
14	X			X														

Inflammation, Elbow

	ANT C	ARG N	ARN	LAC AC	PHOS	PULS
7	X					
8				X		
14		X	X		X	X

Inflammation, Eye- See also Conjunctivitis (Includes Episcleritis; Scleritis; Uveitis)

	ACON	BELL	EUPHR	MERC	ARG N	ARS	PULS	SULPH	APIS	CANTH	CINNAB	HEP	NUX V	ANT T	PLUM	RHUS T
1			X													
2				X						X	X		X	**X**	**X**	**X**
4	**X**	**X**									X					
6	X	X		X			X	X					X			
8		X				X			X	X		X		X		
12	X	X						X								
13	X	X	X	X	X	X	X	X	X	X	X	X	X		X	X
14	X	X	X	X	**X**		X		X			X				
15			X	X		X	X									
19			X													
21					X											
24	X		X													
26	**X**					X		X								

Inflammation, Genitals, Female

	ACON	ASAF	MERC	RHUS T	ARS	BELL	FERR PH	KALI CAR	KREO	LYC	MERC C	PETR
7	X	X	X	X	X	X	X	X	X	X	X	X
8	X	X	X	X								

Inflammation, Glands- See Adenitis

Inflammation, Glands, Inguinal

	SIL	DULC	MERC	BAD	CLEM	LITH C	MERC I R
1	X						
7		X		X	X	X	X
10	X						
13	X	X	**X**				

Inflammation, Glands, Lymphatic- See also Lymphadenitis

	ARS	BAR C	BELL	HEP	MERC	MERC C	MERC I R	SIL
6	X	X			X			
7				X				X
8			X				X	
13						X		

Inflammation, Glands, Sublingual

	MERC	CANTH	IOD	KALM
7	**X**	X	X	X

Inflammation, Glans Penis- See Balanitis
Inflammation, Gums- See Gingivitis
Inflammation, Heart- See also Endocarditis; Myocarditis; Pericarditis; Rheumatic Carditis

	CACT	DIG	BRY	ARS I	CANN S	NAJA	SPIG
2			**X**				
7	X					X	X
8		X					
14	X	X		X	X		

Inflammation, Intestine, Small

	ACON	ARS	CHAM	CHINA	LYC	LYSS	MERC	NUX V	TEREB
6	X		X	X	X	X	X	X	X
19		X							

Inflammation, Kidneys- See Nephritis
Inflammation, Knee (AKA Gonitis)

	BRY	COCCUL	SULPH	IOD	SIL	CALC	LED	NUX V	PULS	ACON	ARN	ARS	BAR M	BELL	CALC FL	CHINA	FERR	LACH	LYC	MERC	PHOS	RHUS T	STICTA
7	**X**			X									X	X									
8	X	X	**X**	X	X	X		X			X	X				X	X	X	X				
13	X	**X**	X				X	X	**X**													X	
14	X	X			X		X								X								X
26	X		X	X	X	X				X										X	X		

Inflammation, Labia

	AMBRA	APIS	COCCUS	SEP	THUJA	ACON	CALC	CARB V	CON	FERR	KALI CAR	KREO	MERC	NIT AC	NUX V	STAPHYS	SULPH
2		**X**	**X**														
13	**X**			**X**	**X**	X	X	X	X	X	X	X	X	X	X	X	X

Inflammation, Lachrymal Duct- See Dacryocanaliculitis

Inflammation, Lips

	ACON	BELL	MERC	MERC D	MUR AC	SULPH
7	X	X	X	X		
8					X	
10						X

Inflammation, Lungs

	ACON	AGAR M	BRY	CORNUS	FERR	KALI IOD	MILL	PHOS	TEREB	SANG
7	X	X	X	X	X	X	X		X	X
15								X		

Inflammation, Lymph Nodes- See Lymphadenitis
Inflammation, Lymph Nodes, Cervical- See Lymphadenitis, Cervical
Inflammation, Mastoid- See Mastoiditis
Inflammation, Meibomian Glands

	DIG	EUPHR	HEP	CHAM	PULS	STAPHYS	ACON	ARS	CALC	MERC	NUX V	SEP	STICTA	STRAM	SULPH
4	X														
6			X												
7	X	X	X			X									
8		X	X	X	X		X	X	X	X	X	X	X		X
13	X	X		X	X	X								X	

Inflammation, Mouth- See Stomatitis
Inflammation, Mucous Membranes

	ACON	ARS	MERC	NUX V	APIS	BELL	BRY	NIT AC	SULPH
7	X	X	X	X	X	X	X	X	
8								X	
13	**X**	**X**	**X**	**X**	X	X	X		**X**

Inflammation, Muscle- See Myositis
Inflammation, Nail Pulp

	BELL	CALEND	CON	HELL	KALI CAR	LYC	NAT M	PH AC	TEUCR
2		X							
13			X	X	X	X	X	X	X
21	X								

Inflammation, Nerves- See Neuritis

Inflammation, Nipples

	CHAM	GRAPH	SIL
6		X	
7	X		X
8	X		
14	X		
21	X		

Inflammation, Nose- See also Rhinitis

	SEP	SULPH	AUR	EUPHR	FL AC
1				X	
2	**X**	**X**			**X**
8	X	X			
13	X	X	X		
14			X	X	

Inflammation, Ovaries- See Ovaritis

Inflammation, Palate

	NUX V	RAN B	ACON	APIS	BAPT	BELL	CALC	CHAM	COLCH	GELS	KALI BIC	LACH	MERC
7			X	X		X			X	X		X	
13	**X**	**X**					X	X					X
15					X						X		

Inflammation, Pancreas- See Pancreatitis

Inflammation, Penis- See Balanitis

Inflammation, Prepuce (Foreskin)- See Posthitis

Inflammation, Prostate- See Prostatitis

Inflammation, Rectum-See Proctitis

Inflammation, Retina- See Retinitis

Inflammation, Scars

	HEP	SIL	SULPH AC
5	X		X
21		X	

Inflammation, Scrotum

	PH AC	ARS	MUR AC	NAT SUL	NAT M	PLUM	RHUS T
1				X			
7							X
8	X						
13	X	X	X		X	X	

Inflammation, Serous Membranes

	BRY	APIS	DIG
7	X	X	
8			X
18	X		

Inflammation, Soft Palate

	NIT AC
6	X
21	X

Inflammation, Spermatic Cord- See Chorditis
Inflammation, Spinal Cord- See Myelitis
Inflammation, Spleen- See Splentitis
Inflammation, Tendons- See Tendonitis
Inflammation, Testes- See Orchitis
Inflammation, Throat- See also Pharyngitis Pain, Throat; Tracheitis;

	BELL	MERC	CANTH	CAPS	LACH	NIT AC	ACON	BAR C	HEP	PHYTO	PULS	ARG N	LYC	DULC	FERR PH	SENEGA
4										X						
7	**X**	X	X	**X**	**X**	X	**X**	X	X	X	X	**X**	X	X	**X**	
8	X		X								X					
12	X	X														
13	**X**	**X**	X	X	X	**X**	**X**	X	X	X	X	X	**X**	**X**	X	**X**
17						X										
19																X
24	X		X	X												
26		X			X			X	X							

Inflammation, Thyroid- See Thyroiditis
Inflammation, Tongue- See Glossitis

Inflammation, Tongue, Tip Of

	RHUS T	SULPH	ARS	PHYTO	ARG N	LACH	SQUILLA	ALOE	BELL	CARB A	CARB V	CAUST	KALI BIC	LATH	MERC I F	MORPH	NUX V	POTHOS	RHUS V	VER A
4	**X**																			
5	X		X	X	X														X	
6	X	X	X		X	X	X									X	X			X
10	X	X		X						X	X	X								
11	X																			
13	X	X		X		X							X		X			X		
15									X											
17	X	X	X											X						
18	X																			
19	X																			
21								X												
24	X						X													

Inflammation, Umbilicus

	CALC	PHYSO	SAC LAC
2		X	X
6	X		

Inflammation, Urethra- See Urethritis
Inflammation, Uterus- See Metritis
Inflammation, Uvula- See Uvulitis
Inflammation, Vagina- See Vaginitis
Inflammation, Veins- See Phlebitis
Inflammation, Vulva- See Vulvitis
Inflammatory Bowel Disease- See Inflammation, Bowel

Influenza

	ARS	GELS	BRY	EUP PERF	RHUS T	ACON	NUX V	BELL	BAPT	CAUST	SABAD	CAMPH	MERC	SULPH	CHINA	INFLUENZ	PHOS	ALL C	DULC	PYROG	STICTA	ARN	CARB V	IPEC	PULS	ARS IOD	SANG	
1	**X**	X	X	X	X			X	X	X				X		X			X				X			X		
2		X	**X**	**X**	X	**X**		**X**	**X**	X	X	X		**X**	X			X	X	X	X		X				**X**	
3	**X**	X	X	X	X	X				X	X			X						X								
4	**X**	**X**	X	**X**	**X**	X			X	X		X					X	**X**	**X**		**X**					X		
5		X		X	X	X						X				X					X	X						
6	X	X	X	X	X	X	X	X			X		X				X								X		X	
7	X	X	X	X						X	X	X	X				X	X	X		X		X	X	X			
8	X	X	X	X	X	X	X	X		X	X	X	X	X	X		X	X			X	X	X	X	X	X	X	
9	**X**	X	X	X	X	X	**X**	X			X					X												
10	X	X	X	X	X	X	X			X	X		X	X	X													
11	**X**	**X**	**X**	**X**	**X**	**X**	X	**X**	X	X	X			X	X		X	X	X			X		X	X	**X**		
12	X	X	X	X		X	X	X	**X**			X		X													X	
13	X		X		**X**	X	**X**	X		X	X	**X**	X		X								X		X			
14	X	X	X	X	X	X										X												
15	X	X				X	**X**	X	X			**X**	X		X								X	X				
16	X	X	X	X	X	X	X		X											X								
17	X	X	X		X	X	X	X			X	X	X	X	X	X		X	X			X		X	X	X	X	
18		**X**	X	**X**	**X**	X		X	X											X								
19	**X**	**X**	**X**	**X**	**X**	X	**X**	**X**	X	X			**X**	X	X					**X**	X	X						
20	X	**X**	X		X	X	X	X																				
21	X	X	X	X	X	X	X	X	X											X								
22	X	X	X	X			X										X											
23	X	X		X							X																	
25	X	X	X			X	**X**									X												
26	X		X		**X**	X		X		**X**			X		X		X					X		X				
29[1]		X		X				X								X												
29[2]	X																											

29[1] Vincent S, et al. Management of influenza-like illness by homeopathic and allopathic general practitioners in france during the 2009-2010 influenza season. J Altern Complement Med, 2013 Feb; 19 (2):146-52.

29[2] Mathie RT, et al. Homeopathic treatment of patients with influenza-like illness during the 2009 A/H1N1 influenza pandemic in India. Homeopathy, 2013 Jul; 102 (3):187-92.

Influenza, Prophylaxis

	INFLUENZ	OSCILLO	ACON	ARS	BAPT	GELS	NAT M	PYROG
9	X							
11	X							
16	X	X	X	X	X	X	X	X
17	X							
18	X	X						

Ingrowing Toenails- See Toenails, Ingrowing

Injuries- See also Wounds; Bruising

	ARN	RUTA	RHUS T	CALEND	HYPER	APIS	LED	SYMPH	HEP	CALC PH	BELLIS	LACH	MILL	STAPHYS	SULPH AC	ACON	ALL C	BRY	CALC	CIC	CON	HAM	PHOS	PULS
1	X	X	X	X	X		X	X		X							X							
2						X						X												
3	X																							
4	**X**										X													
5	X			E							X													
6	X																							
7	**X**	X	X	X	X				X			X	X	X	X	X				X	X			
8	**X**	X	X	X	X	X	X	X	X	X		X	X	X	X	X	X	X	X	X	X	X	X	X
9	X	X		X	X			X																
10	X	X	X	X	X	X	X	X		X	X			X					X					
12	X															X								
13	**X**	X	**X**	X	X				**X**			X		X	**X**					X	X		X	**X**
14	X	**X**	X	E	X		X			X			X				X	X	X			X		
16	X																							
17	X												X											
21	X	X	X			X					X											X		
22	X	X	X		X	X	X	X	X									X					X	
24	**X**																							
28	X																							
29[1]	X																							
29[2]	X																							
29[3]	X																							

E- External

29[1] Schmidt CA. Double Blind, Placebo- Controled Trial: Arnica montana Applied Topically to Subcutaneous Mechanical Injuries. Journal of the American Institute of Homeopathy, Winter 1996, 89, 4, 186-193.

29[2] Alecu A, et al. Effect of the homeopathic remedy Arnica montana 7CH on mechanical trauma in mice. Cultura Homeopática, 2007, 20, Jul-Sept, 16-18.

29[3] Chakrabarti J, et al. Cytogenetical Effects of Sonication in Mice and their Modulations by Actinomycin D and a Homeopathic drug, Arnica 30. Ind J of Exp Biol, 2001, December, 39, 12, 1235-42.

Injury, Abdomen

	ACON	APIS	ARN	BELLIS	BRY	CALEND	HAM	RHUS T
5				X			X	
7	X	X	X		X	X		X

Injury, Back

	HYPER	RUTA	ACON	ARG N	ARN	CALC	CIC	CIMICI	CON	KALI CAR	NAT M	NIT AC	NUX V	PRUN S	RHUS T	ZINC
7	X	X	X	X	X	X	X		X				X	X		X
19	X							X		X	X	X			X	
27	X	X														

Injury, Bladder

	ARN	STAPHYS	OP
18		X	
19	X		
21	X	X	X

Injury, Blood Vessels- See also Bruising

	ARN	BELLIS	HAM	LYSS	RHUS T
1		X			
7	X		X	X	X

Injury, Bones/ Periosteum- See also Fracture; Pain, Bones; Pain, Periosteum

	RUTA	SYMPH	CALC PH	ARN	CALC	CALEND	PH AC	PULS	SIL	HECLA	MAG SUL	PHOS	PHYTO	RHUS T	STAPHYS
1	X		X												
4		**X**		X											
5			X		X					X	X				
6									X						
7	X	X	X												
8	X	X			X	X	X	X	X			X	X		X
9	X	X													
10		X													
12	X														
13	**X**	X		X	X	X	X	X							
14	**X**		X												
17	X			X											
19	**X**														
20	X														
21	X														
22	X													X	
24		X													
25	X	X													
26	B														
27	X														
28	X														

B- Both Internal and External

Injury, Brain- See also Injury, Head

	ARN	NAT SUL	CIC	HELL	HYPER	OP	CALC	LACH	NAT M	NUX V	SULPH
4	X										
8		X	X	X		X					
9					X						
11	**X**										
13	X		X								
14	X										
16			X								
18		X									
21	**X**	X		X	X						
24		X									
27	**X**	X									
28		X									
29*	X	X	X	X		X	X	X	X	X	X

29* Chapman EH, et al. Homeopathic Treatment of Mild Traumatic Brain Injury. J Head Trauma Rehab, 1999, Dec, 14, 6, 521-42.

Injury, Breast

	CON	ARN	BELLIS
4	X		
5	X		X
9	X		
19	X		
21		X	
24	**X**		

Injury, Cartilage

	RUTA	ARN	ACON	APIS	BRY	CAUST
1	X					
14	**X**	**X**	X	X	X	X

Injury, Chest

	ARN	ACON	APIS	BRY	CHAM
7	X		X		X
21	X	X		X	

Injury, Coccyx

	HYPER	BELLIS	ARN	CARB A	KALI BIC	NAT SUL	RUTA	SIL
1	X							
4	X							
5	X		X			X	X	
7	X							
10		X						
14	X							
17	X							
19	X	X		X	X			X
22	X							
24	X							

Injury, Cornea

	SIL	ACON	CAD	CON	EUPHR	HAM	STAPHYS
7	X	X		X		X	X
8			X				
19	X				X		

Injury, Crush, Finger- See also Injury, Finger

	HYPER	ARN	ARIST CL	SEC
4	X	E		
14	X			
16	X			
19	X		X	X
21	X			
22	X			
24	X	E		

E- External

Injury, Crush, Toes- See also Injury, Toes

	HYPER	SEC
4	X	
19		X
21	X	
24	X	

Injury, Ear

	ARN	RUTA	BELL	CHIN S	HEP	HYPER	LED	SEC	SYMPH
14	X	X	X		X		X		
17	X	X		X		X			X
19								X	

Injury, Eye

	SYMPH	LED	ARN	HYPER	ACON	HAM	CALEND	RUTA	CON	EUPHR	NIT AC	STAPHYS	PHYSO	PULS	SIL	TAMUS	BERB V	CIC	GUARAEA	LACH
1			X	X		X														
2	X												X							
3	X		X	X																
4	X	**X**							X											
5	X	**X**				X		X												
7	X	X	X		X	X	X			X		X		X	X		X		X	X
8											X									
9								X			X									
10	X																			
14			X															X		
15																X				
17				X																
18	X	X	X			X		X												
19	X			X	X					X		X								
21	X	X	X	X	X		X													
22		X		X	X		E													
24	X								X											
28	X																			

E- External

Injury, Finger- See also Injury, Crush, Finger (Includes Injury, Fingertip)

	HYPER	ARIST CL	ASAF	RUTA
8			X	X
14	X			
16	X			
19	X	X		

Injury, Gland

	CON	IOD	KALM	PETR	PHOS
4	X				
8	X	X	X	X	X
12	X				
19	X				
24	X				

Injury, Gunshot

	AMM C	ARN	CALEND
8	X		
19		X	
24			X

Injury, Head

	ARN	NAT SUL	CIC	HELL	HYPER	ACON	BELL	OP	PHOS	AMMC	BAR M	CALC	CON	CUPR	HYOSC	LED	MERC	NAT M	RHUS T	RUTA	SIL	SULPH	SYMPH	VER A
3		X						X																
6	X									X	X						X							
7	**X**	X			X																			
8		X																						
9	**B**	X			X	X	X		X									X		X			X	X
14			X																					
16				X																				
17	X	X	X										X	X										
18		X																						
19	X	X	X																					
20	X	X																						
21	**X**	X	X	X																				
24	X	X	X	X	X	X	X	X							X	X								
26	X		X						X			X							X		X	X		

B- Both Internal and External

Injury, Joints

	RUTA	ARN	RHUS T	AGNUS	BELLIS	BRY	SULPH AC	SYMPH
4	**X**							
5			X					
7			X					
8				X				
9	X	X						X
14	**X**							
16							X	
20	X	X			X	X		
24	X							

Injury, Ligaments- See also Injury, Tendons/ Ligaments

	RHUS T	RUTA	ARN	BELLIS
8	X			
9		X		X
17		X		
18		X		
20	**X**		**X**	
24	**X**			
25		X		

Injury, Muscle

	ARN	BELLIS	RHUS T	CALC	CIMICI	CON	DULC	EUPHR	HEP	LACH	NUX V	PULS	SULPH	SULPH AC
8	X			X		X	X	X	X	X	X	X	X	X
19	X	X												
20	**X**	X	X											
21	X		X											
24					X									

Injury, Nails

	LED	RHUS T
7	**X**	X

Injury, Nerves

	HYPER	ALL C	BELLIS	LED	BRY	CALEND	CIMICI	HELON	MAG PH	NAT SUL	SPIG	SYMPH	XANTH
1	X												
2								X					X
3	X												
4	**X**												
5	X		X										
7	**X**					X			X				
8	**X**												
10	X				X								
14	X	X		X									
15	X												
16	X												
17	X	X											
18	X									X			
19	**X**		X										
22	X			X									
24	X						X				X	X	
28	X												
29*	X												

29* Mohammadi R, et al. Homeopathic treatment for peripheral nerve regeneration: an experimental study in a rat sciatic nerve transection model. Homeopathy. 2012 Jul;101 (3):141-6.

Injury, Spinal Cord (Includes Concussion, Spinal)

	HYPER	ARN
4		X
7	X	
14	X	
19	**X**	
21	X	X
27	X	

Injury, Spine

	HYPER	ARN	CALC	CARB A	CIC	CON	NIT AC	RHUS T	RUTA	TELL	BRY	KALI BIC	MAG PH	NAT SUL	NUX V	SIL	ZINC
1	X																
2	X						X										
3	X		X	X				X									
4	X																
5	X									X							
7	X	X				X											
8																	X
14	X	X			X	X											
16	X																
17	X									X							
19	X	X	X	X			X	X	X		X	X	X		X	X	
21		X															
24	X				X												
27	B	X							X					X			

B- Both Internal and External

Injury, Teeth

	ARN	ACON	BRY	HYPER
19	**X**	X	X	X

Injury, Tendons/Ligaments- See also Injury, Ligaments

	RUTA	RHUS T	ARN	ANAC	CALC	SYMPH	AGNUS	AMM C	ANT C	BRY	CARB A	CARB V	HYPER	LYC	MAG P AU	NAT M	NUX V	PETR	PHOS	SEP
1	X	X	X	X																
2									X											
4	**X**	**X**																		
8	X	X	X		X		X	X		X	X	X	X	X	X	X	X	X	X	X
14	**X**				X															
18	X	X																		
19	**X**		X	X																
20		**X**																		
21	X																			
22	X					X														
24	X					X														
25	X																			
28	X																			

Injury, Testes

	ARN	CON	HAM	PULS
7	X		X	X
19		X		

Injury, Toes- See also Injury, Crush, Toes

	ASAF	HYPER	RUTA
8	X		X
14		X	

Injury, Tongue

	HYPER	CALEND	CAUST
1		X	
7	X		X
19	X		

Innutrition- See also Digestion, Diseases Of; Digestion, Weakness (Includes Imperfect Nutrition; Malnutrition)

	CALC	CALC PH	SIL	ARS	NAT M	SABAL	SULPH	ALFALFA	CHINA	FERR IOD	FERR	FERR PH	MERC I R	LYC	NAT PH	PLUM	SANIC	VANAD	XANTH
1																			X
2						X												X	
4			X																
9					X						X	X							
10	X		X	X	X		X										X		
11	X		X												X				
12	X	X					X			X									
14						X		X											
15									X										
17	X												X						
22		X																	
23		X																	
24		X		X															
27														X		X			

Insomnia- See also Sleeplessness

	COFF	NUX V	GELS	PULS	ACON	IGN	CHAM	ARS	COCCUL	KALI PH	PASS	CHINA	OP	SULPH	HYOSC	CYPRIP	LYC	BELL	AMBRA	CALC	KALI BR	NAT M	AUR	CIMIC	CINA	PHOS	RHUS T	
1	X		X	X		X				X				X		X												
2	X				**X**					X	X					X				X	X							
3	X		X							X	X					X												
4	**X**	X	**X**	X	X	X	**X**			X	X	X	X		**X**			**X**						X		X		
5	X	X	X	X		X		X		X					X	X			X		X	X					X	
6	X	X	X	X	X	X			X			X	X	X	X			X										
7	X	X	X	X	X	X	X	X	X			X		X		X	X	X		X		X			X	X	X	
8	X	X	X	X	X	X	X	X	X			X	X	X	X	X	X	X	X	X	X	X			X	X	X	
9	X	X	X	X	X		X		X		X		X	X	X		X				X			X				
10		X			X		X																X					
14	**X**	X			X		X	X				X							X				X					
16	X		X	X					X		X							X										
17	X	X				X	X	X			X																	
18	X	X	X		X	X		X		X			X		X				X			X			X	X		
19	X																											
21	X	X	X	X	X	X	X	X	X			X	X				X			X	X		X		X		X	
22	X	X	X	X				X	X																			
23	X									X	X	X	X						X					X				
24	X																											
25	X	X		X			X		X		X						X							X				
27	X			X		X				X				X						X			X					
28	X																											
29[1]		X																										
29[2]		X																										
29[3]	X																											
29[4]		X												X			X					X						
29[5]	X	X																										

29[1] Sukul A, et al. Reduction of Alcohol induced Sleep time in Albino Mice by Potentised Nux Vomica prepared with 90% Ethanol. Brit Hom J, 1999, 88, 58-61.

29[2] Ruiz G, et al. Homoeopathic Effect on the Sleep Pattern of rats. Brit Hom J, October 1997, 86, 201-206.

29[3] Ruiz- Vega G, et al. An Evaluation of Coffea cruda effect on Rats. Brit Hom J, 2000, 89, 122-126.

29[4] Naudé DF, et al. Chronic primary insomnia: efficacy of homeopathic simillimum. Homeopathy, 2010, Jan, 99, 1, 63-8.

29[5] Bell IR, et al. Effects of homeopathic medicines on polysomnographic sleep of young adults with histories of coffee-related insomnia. Sleep Med. 2011 May;12 (5):505-11.

Insomnia, Pregnancy, During- See Pregnancy, Insomnia From

Insomnia, Senile

	ACON	BAR C	PHOS
7	X	X	
9	X		
12			X
14	X		

Intermenstrual Flow- See Menses, Irregular

Intertrigo

	LYC	SULPH	GRAPH	CAUST	CHAM	MERC	CALC	CARB V	HEP	PETR	ACON	BELL	CHINA	HYDRAST	PULS	RHUS T	SEP	SIL
2	X			X				X										
6	X	X			X	X										X		
7	**X**	**X**	X	X	X	X	X	X	X	X	**X**	X		X	X			X
8	X	X	X	X	X	X	X	X	X	X	X	X	X		X	X	X	X
12	X	X			X	X	X							X				
13		X	X						X	X			X				X	
14			X	X														
18			X															

Interstitial Cystitis- See Cystitis, Interstitial
Interstitial Keratitis- See Keratitis, Interstitial
Interstitial Nephritis- See Nephritis, Interstitial

Intestines, Dryness

	ALUM	BRY	OP	PLUM
1	X		X	
7			X	X
11		X		
14	X	X		
17	X			
22		X		

Intussusception, Intestines/ Bowel

	PLUM	VER A	ACON	BELL	NUX V	OP	THUJA	COLOC	ARS	CUPR	ALUM	BRY	KALI BIC	PHOS	RHUS T	VERIN	ARN	CARB V	LACH	LOB I	LYC	MERC	MERC C	SULPH
1	X	X	X			X																	X	
2	X	X					X							X		X								
3	X	X	X			X			X															
6	X		X	X	X	X	X	X	X	X	X		X	X		X		X						
7	X	X	X	X	X	X		X	X			X	X		X		X		X	X	X	X		
8	X	X					X			X														
21				X	X			X							X									
24	X	X		X	X	X	X	X		X	X													
26			X	X	X		X		X			X												X

Iritis

	MERC C	ARN	HEP	RHUS T	ACON	ASAF	AUR	BELL	CLEM	EUPHR	KALI IOD	NIT AC	BRY	COLOC	SPIG	TEREB	THUJA	CEDRON	CINNAB	GELS	MERC	SULPH
1	**X**	X	X	X			X					X					X	X				
2	X					X				X					X	X						
4	**X**	X		X	X			X	X	X			**X**			X	X			X		
6	**X**	X	X	X	X	X	X	X	X	X	X	X	X	X	X	X	X	X	X	X	X	X
7	X	X				X		X	X	X		X		X				X			X	
8	X	X	X	X	X	X	X	X	X	X	X	X	X	X	X	X	X		X	X		X
11											X											
12		B			X		X	X	X						X				X		X	X
14	X		X				X															
17			X			X					X											
21	X			X	**X**																	
23				X							X	X	X	X								
24			X																			

B- Both Internal and External

Irritable Bladder

	NUX V	ARN	BELL	BENZ AC	BRY	CAUST	CHAM	COLCH	COP	EQUISET	FERR PH	IGN	OX AC	PARIERA	PULS	RHUS T	SAB	STAPHYS	SULPH
4														X					
6	X	X			X			X			X		X			X	X		X
8				X						X									
14																		X	
15			X				X					X							
21	X					X			X						X				

Irritable Bowel Syndrome (AKA IBS)

	SULPH	COLOC	ARG N	LYC	NUX V	ANT C	ARS I	CANTH	GRAT	HELON	IGN	IRIS T	LIL T	MAG PH	NAT CAR	NAT M	THUJA
8										X							
18	X	X		X	X						X	X		X			X
19	X	X	X	X	X	X	X		X				X		X	X	
21		X	X					X									
27	**X**																

Ischias- See Coxalgia

Ischuria- See Urine, Retention

Itch- See Pruritis

Jaundice (Includes Icterus)

	CHEL	MERC	CHINA	NUX V	PHOS	DIG	POD	CHAM	CARD M	HYDRAST	ACON	ARS	CHIO	LACH	BRY	MYRICA	SULPH	BERB V	CROT H	LYC	SEP	LEPT	NIT AC	CON	BELL	IOD	CALC	
1	<u>**X**</u>	X		X	X	X			X			X	X	X		X												
2	X	**X**	**X**		**X**	X	X	**X**	X	X	X	X	X	X	X		X	X	**X**		X	X		X		**X**		
3			X	X			X	X	X	X			X				X				X							
4	<u>**X**</u>	X	X	X	X	**X**	X	X	X				X	X	X	**X**												
5	X		X	X	X	X	X	X	X	X		X	X		X			X	X	X	X	X	X	X		X		
6	X	X	X	X	X	X	X	X	X	X	X	X		X	X	X	X	X	X	X	X	X	X	X	X	X	X	
7	**X**	**X**	**X**	**X**	**X**	X	**X**	X	X	X	X	X	X	**X**	X	X	X	X	X	X	X	X	**X**	X	**X**	X	**X**	
8	X	X	X	X	X	X	X	X	X	X	**X**	X	X	X	X	X	X	X	X	X	X	X	X	X	X	X	X	
9	X			X																X								
10	X	<u>**X**</u>	X	X	X	X		X						X			X		X								X	
11	**X**	X	X	X	X		X	X	**X**	X	**X**		**X**		X	**X**		**X**		X		**X**						
12	X	X	X	X	X	X	X	X		X	X	X											X		X			
13		X	X	X		X	X				X	X		X	X		X			X	X		X	X	X	X	X	
14	X		X		X	X							X			X												
15		<u>**X**</u>	**X**	X	X		**X**	<u>**X**</u>	X	**X**	X	X			X								X					
16	X	X	X	X											X													
17					X	X			X					X														
18		X			X					X		X		X														
19	X		X			X	X	X	X			X	X			X	X			**X**	X	X						
20	X	X																										
21	X	X			X						X							X										
23	X			X		X				X	X		X			X		X					X					
24			X				X			X														X				
26		**X**	**X**	X		X	X	X			**X**	X					X				X				X			

Jaundice, Conjunctiva

	CHINA	CROT H	CANTH	CHAM	CHEL	CHIN S	CHIO	DIG	DOLICH	ELAT	GELS	HYDRAST	LACH	MERC	MYRICA	NAT SUL	PHOS	PLUM	POD	SEP	VER A							
7	**X**	**X**	X	X	X	X		X	X	X	X	X	X		X	X	X	X	X	X	X							
8														X														
11							X																					

Jaundice, Neonatal

	CHAM	MERC	CHINA	ACON	NUX V	CHEL	NAT SUL	POD	BRY	CROT H	KALM	LUPUL	MYRICA	SEP	THYROID
3	X	X	X												X
5			X	X			X							X	
7		**X**	X	**X**	X										
10	**X**	X	X		X										
11						X			X		X	X			
15	**X**														
16	X	X	X		X			X							
19						**X**	X						X		
21	**X**									X					
26		X		X				X							

Jaw, Diseases Of

	ABSINTH	CALC	CHLOR	CUPR	HYDR AC	OP	PHOS	RHUS T
2		X					X	
8			X					
14	X			X	X	X		X

Jaw, Dislocation, Easy- See also Dislocation, Easy

	PETR	PULS	STAPHYS
2	**X**		X
8		X	

Jejunum, Diseases Of

	POD
7	X
8	X

Joints, Deformed, from Arthritis

	CAUST	BENZ AC	CALC	CALC FL	HEP	KALI MUR
14	X		X			X
19	X	X		X	X	

Joints, Diseases Of

	CALC	ACON	ARG	BENZ AC	BERB V	CALC PH	HEP	IOD	KALI IOD	LED	MERC	PHOS	BACILL	BOV	BRY	CAUST	DROS	PH AC	RHUS T	SABIN	STAPHYS	SULPH
2	**X**	**X**	**X**	**X**	**X**	**X**	**X**	**X**	**X**	**X**	**X**	**X**	X	X								
7																			X	X		
8	X																	X			X	X
10																	X					
14																X						
27															X							

Keloid

	SIL	GRAPH	FL AC	CUPRE L	THIO	NIT AC	CALEND	CAUST	CIC	HYDROC	LYSS	MALAND	SULPH	THUJA	TUB	VACCIN
1	X		X	X											X	
2	**X**			X		**X**						X	X			X
5	X	X	X					X								
9	X		X				B									
18		X												X		
19		X			X				X		X					
21	X	X	X													
28					X					X						

B- Both Internal and External

Keratitis

	GRAPH	EUPHR	SULPH	APIS	HEP	KALI BIC	THUJA	ACON	ARN	CALC	CHIN A	CINNAB	CON	CROT H	CROT T	HAM	KALI IOD	RHUS T
2						**X**					X			X	X			
4			X		**X**								X					
5																		X
6		X	X					X	X							X		
7	**X**	X		**X**			**X**			X	X	X						
8	X	X	X	X	X	X	X	X	X	X		X	X	X	X	X	X	X
11																	X	
24	X																	

Keratitis, Interstitial

	AUR	HEP	LOB E	MERC	NAT M	NIT AC
1		X		X	X	X
2			X			
8	X					
11	X					

Keratoconjunctivitis

	GRAPH	MERC C	MERC D	ZINC
7		X	X	X
8	X			

Kidney, Congestion

	TEREB	HELL	HELON	ALOE	APIS	ARG N	AUR M	BERB V	CANTH	COLCH	EUCAL	HYDRAST	JUNI C	LESP C	NUX V	PHOS	PULS	SOLID	URT U
1	X																		
5	X		X	X				X			X	X	X	X				X	X
7	X		X		X		X		X	X					X		X		
8	X	X				X										X			
10	X	X																	

Kidney, Diseases Of

	TEREB	BERB V	APIS	CANTH	LYC	PLUM	ARS	MERC C	NUX V	BELL	DIG	AUR M	CHEL	CHINA	COLCH	KALI CAR	OCIMUM	PARIERA	PULS	SARS	SEC	SENEC	FERR
2	**X**			**X**		**X**	**X**	**X**		**X**						X	X					X	**X**
3	**X**		X			X						X				X							
4	**X**	X	X	X		**X**	X	X		X	**X**												
5					X																		
6																			X				
7	X	X	X	X	X		X	X				X	X	X	X				X		X	X	
8	**X**																				X		
9	X	X	X						X				X	X									
10	X			X	X												X						
11		X			X																		
12							X				X												
13		X			X	X			X						X					X			
14			X																				
17			X																				
27		**X**																X					
28				X					X									X		X			

Kidney, Failure (AKA Renal Failure)

	OP	ACON	AMM C	APIS	ARN	BELL	CAMPH	CARB AC	CUPR AR	GLON	HELL	MORPH	TEREB
11	X		X					X	X	X	X	X	
21	X	X		X		X	X						X
25					X								

Kidney, Fatty

	PHOS	ARS	MERC C	KALI IOD	PLUM	TEREB
1	X		X			
4	X					
7	X	**X**		X	X	X
10	X	X	X			
12	X					
17	X					
24	X					

Kidney, Floating

	CALC IOD	SEP
1	**X**	X

Kidney Stones- See Calculi, Renal

Kleptomania

	ARS	BRY	KALI CAR	LYC	NUX V	PULS	SEP	SULPH	TAR H
2									X
13	X	X	X	X	X	X	X	X	

Knee, Diseases Of

	AGNUS	KALI CAR	PULS
2	X	X	
8			X

Labour, Breech Presentation

	PULS	ACON	CAULO
1	X		X
3	**X**		
7	**X**	X	
8	**X**		
16	X		
21	X		
26	X		
28	X		

Labour, Delayed

	CAULO	GELS	PULS	ACON	ARN	BELL	CHAM	CIMIC	PITUIT	SEC	VISC A
1									X		
2											X
4	**X**	**X**	X	X	X			X		X	
22	X										
25		X	X			X	X				

Labour, False

	CAULO	BOR	CIMICI	CINNAM	COFF	GELS	KALI PH	MITCHEL	NUX V	PULS	SEC	VIB P
8		X	X	X		X	X					
21	X				X				X	X	X	
22	X											
23								X				X

Labour, Haemorrhage, After- See also Haemorrhage, Uterus

	CANN S	CHINA	BELL	CHAM	FERR	IPEC	NIT AC	PLAT	SABIN	ALUMEN	ARN	CANN I	CROC	HAM	HYDRAST	HYOSC	KALI CAR	SEC	THLASPI	TRIL P	USTIL
1		X															X				
2	X																	X		X	
7	X	X	**X**	**X**	**X**	**X**	**X**	**X**	**X**	X	X	X	X	X	X	X			X		X

Labour, Haemorrhage Before

	SEP	TRILL P
2		X
3	X	

Labour, Pain, after Delivery

	CHAM	ARN	NUX V	PULS	CUPR	SABIN	SEC	CAULO	COFF	XANTHO	BELL	BRY	CIMICI	GELS	OP	RHUS T	IGN	SEP	VIB OP	DIOSC	LACH
1																			X		
2	X	X			X	X	X	X		X					X	X			X		**X**
4	X	X	X	X	X	X		X		X			**X**	X				X			
7	**X**	**X**			X	X	X	X	X	X	**X**	X		X		X	X			**X**	
8	X	X	X	X	X	X	X	X	X	X	X	X	X	X			X	X			
10	X	X	X	X			X														
13	X	**X**	X	**X**	X	X	X				X	X			X	X					
15	X		X																		
21	X		X	X					X												
26	X		X	X					X						X						

Labour, Painful (Includes Labour, Too Strong)

	CHAM	COFF	BELL	NUX V	PULS	CIMICI	CUALO	GELS	ACON	SEC	ARN	KALI CAR	LYC	SEP	CON	AUR	CALC	CAUST	COFF T	KALI CAR	OP	PHOS	PLAT	POD	RHUS T	SEP	VER A	
1							X																					
2		X											X															
3	X	X	X		X	X																						
4	**X**	X	**X**	**X**		X	**X**		X	X	X	X																
5				X		X		X		X	X	X																
7	X	X	X	X		X	X	X											X			X					X	
8	X	X	X	X	X	X	X	X	X	X	X			X	X	X		X		X			X			X		
9					X	X	X	X	X		X																	
10	X	X	X	X	X				X	X																		
13	**X**	**X**	X	X	**X**			**X**	X	X		X	X	**X**	X		X							X	X			
14	**X**																											
16											X																	
18						X	X																					
21		X	X	X																								
25	X							X																				
26	X	X	X	X	X				X	X			X								X							

Labour, Pains, Ceasing- See also Labour, Slow; Labour, Stopped

	BELL	OP	PULS	NUX V	SEP	THUJA	KALI CAR	SEC	CAMPH	CARB V	CAULO	CHAM	GELS	NAT M	PLAT	RUTA	SULPH											
7	X	X	X	X	X	X		X	X	X	X		X															
8	X	X	X	X	X	X	X				X	X	X	X	X	X	X											
13	**X**	**X**	**X**	X	X	X	**X**	**X**	X	X		X		X	X	X	X											

Labour, Pains, False

	CAULO	PULS	CIMICI	BELL	GELS	NUX M	NUX V	VIB OP	OP	COFF	DIOSC	ACON	BOR	BRY	CHAM	CINNAB	CINNAM	DULC	HYOSC	KALI CAR	KALI PH	SEC	SEP					
1	X	X						X																				
2	X	**X**						X																				
3	X		X																									
4	**X**	X	X																									
7		**X**	X	X	X	X			X	X	**X**					X												
8			X		X								X				X				X							
10		X					X					X		X				X										
13		**X**		**X**		X	X		**X**											X								
14	X				X			X																				
16	X																											
18																						X						
26		X		X		X	X			X					X				X				X					
27	X																											

Labour Pains, Irregular/Spasmodic

	BELL	CHAM	IPEC	PULS	CAUST	HYOSC	IGN	NUX V	SEC	CAULO	COCCUL	COFF	CUPR	GELS	KALI CAR	NUX M	OP	SEP
7	X	X	X	X	X				X	X		X				X	X	
8	X	X	X	X	X	X	X	X	X	X		X	X	X	X			X
10	X	X	X	X		X	X	X			X							
13	X	X	X		X	X	X	X	X		X		X	X	X	X	X	X
25				X														

Labour, Premature

	CIMICI	BAR C	CALC	CALC PH	SIL	TRILL
15				X		
16	X	X	X		X	X

Labour, Slow (Includes Labour, Difficult; Dystocia; Labour. Prolonged)

	CAULO	PULS	SEC	BELL	GELS	CAUST	COFF	NAT M	NUX V	ANAC	ARN	AUR	BERB V	CARB V	CHAM	CIMICI	CINNAB	COCCUL	COFF T	HYOSC	IGN	JAB	KALI CAR	LYC	OP	SEP	USTIL	VISC A
1																											X	
2																												X
3		X	X	X	X			X	X													X						
4		X																										
6					X																							
7	**X**		X	X	X	**X**	X	X			X	X			X	X	X		X	X	X		X	X	X	X		
8				X						X			X					X										
10			X						X																			
14						X																						
21		X					X																					
22	X													X														
25		X	X																									
28	X																											
29*	X																											

29* Eid P, et al. Applicability of Homoeopathic Caulophyllum thalictroides during labour. Brit Hom J, October, 1993, 82, 245-248.

Labour, Stopped- See also Labour, Pains, Ceasing

	OP	SEC	CARB V	GELS	PULS	BELL	CAMPH	CAULO	CAUST	GUAREA	SEP	THUJA
5	X			X								
6	X											
7	X	**X**	X	X	X	X	X	X		X	X	X
8		X										
14									X			
21	X	X			X							
22			X									

Labour, To Facilitate

	CAULO	CIMICI	ACON	ARN	GELS	SEC	CALC FL	CAUST	CALEND	CHINA	COLLIN	PYROG
2			**X**	**X**	X		**X**		**X**	**X**	**X**	**X**
3	**X**											
8	X	X	X	X	X	X		X				
9	X				X							
10	X					X						
14								X				
16	X	X		X			X					
18	X	X										
22	X											
23	X	X	X			X						
25	X											
27	X											
28	X											

Labour, Weakness Of

	PULS	CARB V	CAULO	NAT M	SEC	GELS	KALI CAR	NUX M	THUJA	CIMICI	ARN	BELL	CAMPH	CHAM	CHINA	GRAPH	NUX V	OP	RUTA	SEP	CANN S
7	X	X	X	**X**	**X**	X	X	X	X	X			X			X					
8	X	X		X	X	X	X	X	X		X	X	X	X	X	X	X	X	X	X	
13	**X**	X	**X**	X	X	X	X	X	X	**X**		X		X	X	X	X	X	X	X	**X**
14			X																		
22		X																			
25	X										X										

Lachrymal Duct Blockage- See also Epiphora

	SIL	CALC	NAT M	PULS	RHUS T	AMBROS	EUPHR	FLAC	MERC I F	PETR	THIO
1	X	X						X		X	
3					X						X
7	X	X	X		X						
8			X						X		
14				X		X	X				
19	**X**			X							
20	X										

Lachrymation, Deficient- See Eyes, Dryness

Lachrymation, Profuse/Frequent- See also Epiphora

	EUPHR	ALL C	PULS	NAT M	ARS	SABAD	CALC	KALI IOD	BELL	GRAPH	SPIG	ACON	NUX V	MERC	RHUS T	ARG N	BRY	HEP	SULPH	LYC	PHOS
1	X	X	X							X					X						
2	X																				
3	X	X		X			X														
4	X	X	X			X	X	X	X	X			X				X				
5	X	X	X	X		X		X		X			X							X	X
6	X	X		X	X	X	X	X	X	X		X			X	X		X		X	
7	X	X	X							X	X		X	X		X		X	X		X
8	X		X	X	X		X		X	X	X	X	X	X	X		X	X	X	X	X
9	X	X	X	X	X	X						X					X				
10	X	X	X		X						X	X		X							
11	X					X															
12	**X**				X				X												
13	**X**	X	X	X	X	X	X	X	X	**X**	**X**	X	X	**X**	**X**	X		X	X	**X**	**X**
14	X	X			X		X				X					X					
15	X		X								X								X		
16	X			X		X															
17	X	X		X	X	X	X	X					X				X				
18	X	X		X				X													
19	X	X	X	X		X		X													
20	X								X												
21	X	X				X									X						
22	X	X	X																		
23								X													
24	X	X	X	X				X	X			X		X	X	X					
25	X			X	X		X										X				
26	X		X		X		X		X		X	X		X				X	X		
27					X								X								
28		X																			

Lachrymation, Profuse, Right

	TEUCR	ELAPS	HYOSC	IRID
7	X	X	X	
8				X
17	X			

Lactation, Absent- See Agalactia

Lactation, Deficient- See also Agalactia (AKA Hypogalactia)

	CALC	PULS	ASAF	AGNUS	CHAM	URT U	ACON	BRY	CHINA	RHUS T	RICIN	CALC PH	CAUST	LAC C	PH AC	SABAL	SEC	ZINC	BELL	DULC	IOD	LAC D	MERC	SEP	STICTA	SULPH	PHELL
1	X		X	X	X	X					X					X	X									X	
2	X														X	X		X								X	
3	X	X	X	X	X								X														
4		**X**																									
5	X		X			X			X		X				X							X					
6		X																									
7	X	X						X	X	X		X	X		X		X				X						
8	X	X	X	X	X	X	X	X	X	X				X				X	X	X	X		X		X		
9	X		X	X		X						X		X			X					X					
10	X	**X**					X	X											X								
13	**X**	**X**	X		X	X		X	X	X			X	X				X		X			X		X		**X**
15							X			X																	
18				X							X																
22												X															
23			X	X							X																
25			X	X	X		X									X											

Lactation, Disorders Of

	ACON	ASAF	BRY	CHINA	PHOS	PULS	SIL	CALC	CHIM	GALEG	IOD	LAC V D	LACT V	MEDUSA	PH AC	PHYTO	RHEUM	RICIN	SABAL	URT U
2	**X**	**X**	**X**	**X**	**X**	**X**	**X**	X	X	X	X	X	X	X	X	X	X	X	X	X

Lactation Disorders- Milk Coagulates

	BOR	LACH
8	X	X
26	X	X

Lactation Disorders- Milk Quality Poor (Includes Milk Distasteful; Milk Sours Easily; Milk Thin)

	CINA	MERC	PULS	BOR	CALC	CARB A	CHAM	NUX V	SIL	CALC PH	CHINA	IOD	KALI BIC	LACH	RHEUM	RICIN	STANN	SULPH
8	X	X	X	X	X	X	X	X	X	X		X	X	X		X		
13	X	X	X	X		X	X	X									X	
21					X													
26	X	X	X						X		X				X			X

Lactation, Profuse- See also Galactorrhoea (Includes Weaning)

	PULS	CALC	LAC C	BELL	BRY	PHYTO	ARN	CHINA	CHION	CON	CYCL	IOD	LAC V D	MERC	PHELL	PIPER N	RHUS T	SOL O	SPIRA	URAN N	URT U	USTIL						
1	X		X						X				X	X														
2										X		X				X		X	X	X		X						
3	**X**	**X**		**X**	**X**																X							
4						X																						
5	X	X	X		X		X				X				X													
6						X																						
7	X		X	X																								
8	**X**	X		X	X																							
9	X		X																									
10	X	X						X									X											
14			X																									
15	X			X	X																							
22	X																											
24						X																						
26	X	X																										

Larynx, Tuberculosis- See Tuberculosis, Larynx
Larynx, Spasm- See Spasm, Larynx
Laryngismus- See Spasm, Larynx
Laryngismus Stridulus- See Spasm, Larynx

Laryngitis

	ACON	HEP	PHOS	SANG	LACH	BELL	CAUST	CARB V	DROS	ARG N	KALI BIC	ALL C	ARG	IOD	KALI IOD	RUMEX	SAMB	SULPH	BROM	MERC	ANT T	NUX V	SEL	APIS	MANG	CALC	DULC	GELS
1	X		X	X	X		X	**X**		X	X	X				X	X						X		X			
2	**X**	**X**	**X**	**X**	**X**		**X**	X	X			X	X	**X**	**X**			**X**			**X**		X	**X**	**X**			
4	**X**	**X**		X		X							X	X			X	X										
5	X	X		X		X	X	X				X			X	X	X		X							X	X	X
6	X	X	X	X	X	X	X	X	X	X	X	X		X	X	X		X	X	X	X	X			X	X	X	
7	**X**	X	X	X	X	X	X	X	**X**	X	X		X	X	X			X	X	X	**X**			X	X	X		**X**
8	X	X	X	X	X	X	X	X	X	X	X	X	X	X	X	X	X	X	X	X	X	X	X	X	X	X	X	
9			X		X							X	X			X				X			X					
11	**X**	**X**	X	X	X	X	**X**	X	X	X	X	X	X		X	**X**	X			X		X	X				X	
12	X	X	X	X							X			X					X		X							
13	X	X	X	X		X			X					X						X								
14	X	X	X	X		X		X	X	X	X																	
15		X		X	X																							X
16	X	X		X							X			X					X									
17	X	X	X	X	X	X	X	X	X	X	X	X	X	X	X	X	X	X	X	X	X	X	X	X	X	X	X	X
18	X					X																						
19										X									X									
20			X						X																			
21	X	X	X	X	X		X	X																X				X
22			X								X	X																
23	X		X		X					X			X										X	X				
24	**X**	X	X	X	X	X	X	X	X	X	X	X	X		X	X	X	X		X		X					X	
25	X	X	X			X	X	X		X																		
26	**X**			X	X	X	X		X				X				**X**	X				X				X		
27																						X						

Larynx, Diseases Of

	PHOS	ALL C	SEL	MANG	ACON	CIMICI	ALUM	AMBRA	AMM BR	ANT T	ARG	ARUM M	ARUM T	ASCL T	CUPR	EPILOB	FERR PIC	IOD	KALI BIC	KALI CAR	LACH	MERC CY	PARIS	SAMB C	STANN	STILL		
2									X							X				X				X		X		
3	X	X				X		X																				
6															X													
7				**X**															X				X					
8	X				X		X						X				X				X							
9	X	X	X								X	X										X			X			
12																		X										
17			X							X				X														

Lead Poisoning- See also Ailments from Lead

	OP	PLAT	PLUM	NUX V	ARS	BELL	SULPH AC	ALUMEN	ALUM	CAUST	ZINC	AETHUSA	ANT C	CHAM	COCCUL	COLOC	HYOSC	KALI IOD	KAOLIN	NAT SUL	POD	STRAM
1		X		X			X															
2		X								X									X			
6	X	X		X	X	X			X		X		X		X						X	
7	X	X	X	X	X	X	X				X					X				X		
8	X	X	X		**X**			X														
9			X																			
10	X																					
13	**X**	**X**		X		X			X					X			X					X
16	X						X	X										X				
17			X							X												
19			X																			
23												X										

Lens, Opacity- See Cataract

Leprosy

	HYDROC	ARS	COM	GRAPH	LACH	SULPH	ANT T	ARS I	BACILL	HOANG	HURA	PHOS	PIP M	SEP	SIL	THYROID	ANAC	CALC	CALO	CARB A	CARB V	CARB AC	CAUST	HYDRAST	KALI IOD	NAT CAR	BUFO
1	**X**			X			X	X	X	X	X					X						X					
2			X		X					X	X		X			**X**								X			
4	X																										
7		X		X	X	X	X					X		X	X			X		X	X	X	X		X	X	
8	X	X	X	X	X	X						X	X	X	X		X	X	X	X	X		X		X	X	
9	X																										
11	**X**	X						X																			**X**
12	X	X	X	X	X	X						X		X	X		X										
14	X							X	X																		
17						X																					
23	X		X						X	X	X		X						X					X			
24							X																				

Leucocythemia

	PIC AC	CALC	NAT M	NAT SUL	NUX V	ARS I	CEANOTH	ARAN D	ARS	CALC PH	CHINA	DIADEM	IPEC	KALI PH	NAT PH	THUJA
2	**X**	**X**	**X**			**X**	**X**									
7	X	X	X	X	X					X	X	X				
8	X		X	X	X			X	X				X	X	X	X
23	X	X														

Leucoderma- See Vitiligo

Leucorrhoea (AKA "Whites")

	PULS	KREO	SEP	CALC	ALUM	CHINA	GRAPH	HYDRAST	NIT AC	SULPH	NAT M	BOR	ARS	MUREX	PHOS	MAG M	MERC	THUJA	CARB A	PLAT	HELON	LACH	SIL	AMM C	NAT CAR	AGNUS	CAUST	FERR
1	X	X	X	X	X	X	X	X	X			X		X	X	X	X		X			X		X	X			X
2	X	**X**	**X**	**X**	X	X	X	**X**		**X**	**X**		X	X		**X**	X		X		X					X	X	
3		X									X	X			X									X		X		
4	**X**	**<u>X</u>**	**X**	**X**	**X**		X	X	**X**	X		X	**X**				X			X	X						X	
5	X	X	X	X	X			B	X		X	X			X			X			X							X
6	X	X	X	X	X	X	X	X	X	X	X	X	X	X	X	X	X			X	X	X	X	X	X		X	X
7	**X**	**X**	X	X	**X**	X	**X**	**X**	**X**	**X**	**X**	X	X	**X**	X	X	**X**	X	X	**X**	X	X	X	X	X		**X**	X
8	X	X	X	X	X	X	X	X	X	X	X	X	X	X	X	X		X	X	X	X	X	X	X	X	X	X	X
9	X	X	X	X	X	X	X	X	X	X		X								X						X		
10	X	X	X	X	X	X			X	X	X		X	X		X	X		X	X		X	X		X			
11	X	X																X										
12			X	X																								
13	**X**	**X**	X	**X**	**X**	**X**	**X**	X	X	**X**	**X**	X	X	X	**X**	**X**	**X**	X	**X**	X		X	X	**X**	**X**	X	**X**	X
14	X		X	X	X	X				X				X				X					X					
15	X		X	X		**X**		X		X			X										X					
17	X																											
18		X	X				X	X			X		X					X			X							
19			X			X					X																	
20		X	X	X			X		X			X																
21	X	X	X	X	X	X	X	X	X	X		X			X		X		X									
23	X	X	X		X		X	X			X			X				X			X							
24	X			X			X												X			X						
25	X	X	X	X	X	X			X			X								X								
26	**X**		**X**	X		X	X		X	**X**	X				X	X							X	X	X			X
27	X	X			X							X										X						
28		X																										

B- Both Internal and External

Leukemia

	ARS	NAT M	NAT SUL	CALC	THUJA	CEANOTH	CHINA	NUX V	PHOS	PIC AC	ARAN D	ARS I	CALC PH	CARB V	CROT H	IPEC	KALI NIT	NAT ACET	NAT CAR	NAT NIT								
1	X	X	X	X		X	X		X			X																
3			X																									
6	X	X	X	X	X			X						X		X	X	X	X	X								
7		X	X	X	X		X	X		X	X		X															
8	X	X	X	X	X		X	X		X	X		X	X	X	X												
11	X	X			X	X			X	X		X					X	X	X	X								
17						X			X						X													
28	X																											

Leukemia, Myeliod, Acute- See Leucocythemia

Leukoplakia (AKA Leucoplakia)

	THUJA	CAUST	HYOSC	KALI CHL	LAC C	NUX M	PHYTO	SULPH AC
21		X	X			X	X	
27	X			X	X			X
28	X							

Libido- See Sexual Desire

Lichen- See also Scleroderma (AKA Lichen Simplex; Neurodermatitis)

	SULPH	ARS	APIS	PHYTO	ARS I	RUMEX	AGAR M	ANANTH	ANT C	BELL	BRY	DULC	JUG C	LED	JUG R	TILEA
2	X	**X**	**X**	X	**X**	**X**	X					X	X			X
4			X													
6	X	X		X		X		X	X	X	X			X	X	X
7	X			X			X	X				X				
12	X	X	X						X				X	X	X	
18					X											
26	X	X								X	X					

Lichen Planus

	SULPH IO	ARS	ANT C	JUG C	LED	RUMEX	AGAR M	BELL	CALAD	CHIN A	IGN	IOD	KALI BIC	KALI IOD	KREO	LYC	JUG R	PLANTAG	PHYTO	SARS	STAPHYS	SULPH
2	X																					
6	X	X	X		X		X			X		X	X	X			X			X	X	
11	X	X	X	X	X	X		X	X						X	X		X	X			X
21	**X**	X		X		X																
29*											X											

29* Mousavi F, et al. Ignatia in the treatment of oral lichen planus. Homeopathy. 2009, Jan, 98, 1, 40-4.

Lice, Eyelids- See Phthiriasis

Lice, Hair- See Head Lice; Pediculosis

Lice, Skin- See Pediculosis

Lienitis- See Splenitis

Lientaria

	CHINA	FERR	OLEAND	CALC	GAMBOG	PH AC	PHOS	AMBROS	ALSTON	ARN	ARS	ASAR	CAHINC	CALC PH	CHAM	FERR PER	MAG CAR	MERC	PEPSIN	PSOR	RAPH	RAT	RHOD	SIL	SULPH
2	**X**	X	X		X	X	X	X	X						X	X				X	X		X		
8	**X**	X	X	X	X	X				X	X	X	X	X			X		X			X		X	
23	X																								
26	**X**	X		X			X											X							X

Limbs, Inco-ordination- See Locomotor Ataxia

Lipoma

	BAR C	PHYTO	CALC	CROC	LAPIS	URIC AC	BELL	AGAR M	GRAPH	PHOS	THUJA
2						X					
3	X	X			X	X					X
7	**X**	X	X	X			**X**				
8	X	X	X	X	X			X	X	X	

Lips, Cracked- See Cracking, Lips

Lips, Diseases Of

	ZINC	ARS	EUPHR	LACH	NAT M	PH AC	SULPH IO
2	X		X		X		X
8	X	X		X		X	

Lithaemia- See Gout

Lithiasis- See also Calculi (Various organ specific)

	LYC	CALC	BERB V	SARS	SEP	UVA U
8	**X**	X	**X**	**X**	**X**	**X**
18	X	X				

Liver, Congestion- See Liver, Torpidity

Liver, Diseases Of

	CHEL	NUX V	LYC	BRY	CHINA	PHOS	POD	LACH	MAG M	SULPH	CARD M	BELL	MERC	BERB V	CHIO	NAT SUL	SEP	TARAX	ACON	ARS	LEPT	MYRICA	PULS	CALC	HYDRAST	KALI CAR	NIT AC	
1	X	X	X	X	X	X	X	X		X	X				X	X		X		X	X	X						
2	**X**	**X**		**X**	**X**	X	**X**	X	**X**		X			**X**	X			X			**X**	X			**X**	**X**		
3			X		X		X		X		X				X	X												
4	**X**	X			X					X					X	X		**X**				X	X					
5	X	X	X	X	X									X			X								X			
6		X	X		X	X	X	X	X	X		X		X						X			X			X	X	
7	**X**	**X**	X	**X**	X	**X**	**X**	**X**	X	X	**X**	**X**	**X**	**X**	X	X	**X**	X	X	X	**X**	X	X	**X**	X	X	**X**	
8	X	X	X	X	X	X	X	X	X	X	X	X	X	X	X	X	X	X	X	X	X	X	X	X	X	X	X	
9	X	X			X	X			X									X										
10	**X**	X	X	X	X	X	X	X		X		X	X				X		X									
11	**X**																											
12	X	X		X																								
13		**X**						X	X	**X**		X	X										X	X				
14	X		X																									
16				X		X	X						X						X	X					X		X	
17	X			X																								
18			X								X						X											
19	**X**	**X**	**X**	X	X	**X**	X	X	**X**	**X**	X	X	X	X	X	**X**	X		X	X	X	X	X	X		X	X	
20																			X									
21	X																											
24			X	X																								
26		X	X	X				X		X		X	X											X				
27			X								X																	
28	X																											

Liver, Enlargement Of- See Hepatomegaly

Liver, Failure

	APIS	BELL	OP	ZINC	CAMPH	CARB AC	HELL	MUR AC	PH AC	STRAM
11	**X**	**X**	**X**	**X**	X	X	X	X	X	X

Liver, Fatty

	PHOS	CHEL	CALC	MAG M	SULPH	VANAD
1	X					
4	**X**					
5	X	X		X		
6	X					
7	**X**	X	X			
8	X	X	X	X	X	
10	X					
14	X					
17	X					X
19	X				X	
23	X					X
24	X					

Liver Spots- See also See Skin, Discoloration

	LYC	SEP	PLUM	MEZ	APIS	CARD M	CURARE	NUX V	SULPH	ANT C	ARS	CAUST	CON	DULC	GUAREA	LACH	MERC	NAT CAR	NAT HYPO	NIT AC	PHOS	THUJA
1	**X**	X	X		X	X	X															
2	**X**	**X**					X								X							
3	X		X	X	X														X			
4		**X**				X																
5	X	X						X					X	X		X	X			X	X	X
6	X		X																			
7	X		X					X	X		X											
8	**X**		X						X	X		X						X				
10		X																				
19				X																		

Liver, Torpidity- See also Hyperaemia, Liver; Obstruction, Liver (Includes Bile Flow, Reduced; Liver, Stagnation Of)

	MERC	NUX V	LYC	POD	CHIO	CHEL	PHOS	SULPH	SEP	BRY	VER A	AESC	ALOE	ARS	CARD M	HYDRAST	IRIS V	LACH	LED	MAG M	NAT M	NAT SUL	PTEL					
1				X	X			X		X																		
2									X														X					
3	X			X	X																							
4	**X**		**X**	**X**	X	X				X			X				X											
5	**X**	X	X	X	X	X			X	X		X	X	X	X	X	X			X		X						
6			X			**X**			X										X		X							
7		X		X	X		X	X			X				X	X		X	X			X	X					
8		X	X				X	X			X			X				X			X							
10	**X**	X	X	X				X																				
11	X					X																						
14	X	X	X		X	X	X																					
17											X																	
18		**X**					X																					
19												X								X								

Lochia, Offensive

	SEC	BAPT	BELL	CARB V	KREO	SEP	CHR AC	ARS	BRY	CARB A	CHINA	RHUS T	SIL	STRAM														
2	X													X														
7	**X**	X	X	**X**	**X**	X	**X**		X	X	X	X	X															
8	X	X	X	X	X	X																						
10			X																									
15		X						X																				

Lochia, Profuse

	COFF	MILL	SEC	BRY	CROC	CALC	CHINA	PLAT	PULS	TRILL P	USTIL	ACON	ARN	ART V	BELL	CARB A	CHAM	ERIGER	HEP	IPEC	LIL T	NUX V	RHUS T	XANTH				
2		X																										
3					X																							
7	X	X	**X**	X						X	**X**			X				X						X				
8	X	X		X						X							X				X							
10												X																
13	X	X		X	**X**	X		X	X							X			X				X					
15							X								X					X								
21	X		X			X			X				X									X						
26			X				X	X																				

Lochia, Protracted

	CHINA	CALC	CAULO	SEC	CROC	LIL T	RHUS T	CARB A	KREO	BELL	BENZ AC	HELON	SEP	TRILL P
2												X		
3					X									
7	X	X	X	**X**		X	X	**X**	**X**		X		X	X
8	X		X			X								
10					X					X				
13	X	X	X	X			X							
21	X	X												

Lochia, Scanty

	ACON	BELL	COLOC	BRY	CHAM	DULC	GUAREA	PLAT	PULS	SEC	STRAM
7		X	X	X		X	X		X	X	X
21	X	X	X		X			X			
26	X										

Lochia, Suppressed

	ACON	BRY	CHAM	PULS	HYOSC	MILL	BELL	CAULO	CIMICI	COLOC	DULC	NUX V	OP	PLAT	SEC	ZINC	CARB AC	IGN	VER A	VER V
2					X	X										X				
3				X																
7	X	X	X		X	X	X	X	X						X	X	X			X
8	X	X	X					X	X	X		X	X					X		
10		X	X	**X**							X			X						
13	X	X	X	X	X	X	X			X	X	X	X	X	X				X	
26	X																			

Lockjaw- See Tetanus

Locomotor Ataxia- See also Titubation (Includes Clumsiness; Inco-ordination; Staggering Gait)

	ARG N	GELS	NUX V	ALUM	BELL	PHOS	PLUM	PIC AC	CAUST	CON	SEC	STRAM	SIL	PHYSO	ARS	AGAR M	COCCUL	LACH	RHUS T	SULPH	TAR H	ZINC	ZINC PH	ALUMEN	IGN			
1				X										X		X							X					
2	**X**	X	**X**	X		**X**	X	**X**	X			X	X	X	**X**			X			X			**X**	**X**			
3	X			X			X																					
4	**X**		X	**X**	**X**		**X**	**X**			**X**		**X**									X						
6	X	X		X	X	X		X			X	X		X	X			X		X	X							
7	X	X	**X**	X	X	**X**	X	X	X	X		X	X	X			X	X	X	X		X			X			
8	X	X	X		X	X				X		X			X				X	X	X	X		X				
9	X	X	X				X		X			X	X				X		X					X	X			
10		X			X			X		X								X										
11	X		X	X	X	X	X	X		X	X		X	X	X								X					
13		X	X	X	X				X		X	X				X			X	X	X							
14	X		X						X	X						X	X						X					
16										X																		
17		X	X		X	X		X		X	X					X						X						
19	**X**	X				X			**X**								X											
21		X							X																			
23	X			X	X		X				X												X					
27	X					X	X																					

Lumbago (Includes Pain, Back, Lower; Pain, Back, Lumbar)

	RHUS T	NUX V	BRY	SULPH	ACON	AESC	ANT T	BELL	BERB V	DULC	ARN	CIMICI	PULS	SEP	CALC	COLOC	KALI CAR	NAT M	RUTA	CHAM	LYC	SABIN	CALC FL	GNAPH	AGAR M	ARS	KREO
1	X	X		X		X			X	X					X	X		X				X	X				X
2	**X**	**X**	**X**	**X**	**X**	**X**	**X**		**X**	**X**	**X**						X						**X**	X	**X**		
3	**X**	X			X	X	X	X			X		X											X			
4	**X**	**X**	X	X	X	X						**X**		**X**								X	X	X			
5	X	X	X			X			X	X	X	X		X		X	X		X	X		X					
6	X	X	X	X	X	X	X	X	X			X			X		X	X		X	X	X			X	X	X
7	**X**	**X**	**X**	X	X				X	X	X		X	**X**	X	X	X	X		X	X	X			X	X	X
8	X	X	X	X	X		X	X	X	X	X	X	X		X	X	X	X	X		X		X				
9	**X**	X	X	X	X	X			X		X		X	X		X	X	X	**X**			X	X	X		X	X
10	**X**	X	X	X	X			X	X	X	X		X		X					X	X	X			X		X
11	X	X	X	X		X		X								X			X	X	X			X		X	
12	X				X		X				X	X															
13										**X**			**X**		X			X									
14	X		X				X					X		X		X			X	X			X		X		
15		X	X	X	X			X				X	X	X													
16	X	X	X				X	X	X									X									
17										X									X					X			
18	X		X	X									X	X		X				X				X		X	
19	X			X		X		**X**	X	X				X	**X**		X	X	X		X				X		
20												X															
21	X	X	X	X	X	X	X	X		X	X	X	X		X		X				X	X					X
22						X																					
23	X	X					X																				
24	X	X		X		X		X																			
25	X	X	X	**X**	X		X				X	X		X				X	**X**				X				
26	**X**	X		X	B			X	X				X		X	X				X	X					X	
28	X																										

B- Both Internal and External

Lumbricoides- See Worms, Tape

Lungs, Congestion Of- See also Catarrh, Lungs

	PHOS	ACON	CARB V	FERR PH	ANT T	BRY	VER V	DIG	TEREB
5	X			X					
6	X		X		X				
7	X	**X**							**X**
8			X					**X**	
10			X	X		X			
11	X	X		X			X		
12		X				X	X		
21					X				

Lungs, Diseases Of

	ANT T	ARS	HEP	SULPH	PHOS	BRY	ACON	LYC	CALC	CARB V	ARS IOD	BELL	IOD	KALI BIC	KALI IOD	LAURO	NIT AC	PULS	SIL	CAPS	CROT H
2	**X**	**X**	**X**	**X**			**X**	**X**		X	**X**	**X**			X					**X**	**X**
5	X																				
7								X	X							X					
8	X	X	X	X	X	X	X	X	X	X		X	X	X	X		X	X	X		
10	X	X	X		X																
12	X	X	X	X	X	X	X			X			X	X		X					
14		X																			
17											X										
19	X																				
21						X															
26		X	X	X	X	X			X								X		X		
27				X	X													X			

Lungs, Hepatisation

	CACT	BROM	CAMPH	CHEL	KALI CAR	KALI IOD	KALI MUR	LYC	PHOS	SULPH	TEREB
6		X									
7	X		X	X	X	X	X	X	X		
8	X										X

Lupus

	ARS	HYDROC	THUJA	HYDRAST	HEP	KALI BIC	SIL	SULPH	RAD BR	CAUST	KREO	NIT AC	PHYTO	CALC
1	X								**X**					
2	**X**	**X**		**X**	**X**	**X**		**X**			X		X	**X**
3	X	X	X						**X**					
4	**X**			X										
6	X	X	X			X	X	X		X				
7	**X**	X	**X**	X	X	X	X				X	X	X	
8	X	X	**X**		X	X	X	X		X	X	X	X	X
9		X												
12	**X**													
19	X													
23		X		X										
24	**X**			X	X		X			X				
27	X		X									X		

Lyme Disease

	LED
19	**X**

Lymphadenitis (Note that only the main remedies are used from 17)

	BELL	GRAPH	PHYTO	HEP	IOD	SULPH AC	ARUM T	AUR	BAR C	BAR M	CALC	CALC IOD	CARB A	CIST	CON	DULC	HELL	KALI CAR	LAPIS	MERC	NIT AC	RHUS T	SPONG	SIL	CALC FL	CHAM
1	X	X		X	X						X	X	X											X		
4	X	X			X														X				X		**X**	
5		X	X	X							X	X	X	X										X		
6								X							X		X					X				
8				X																						
13	X					**X**												X		X	X					**X**
17	X	X	X		X	X	X	X	X	X				X	X	X	X	X	X	X	X	X	X			
18			X				X		X							X										
21										X																
25			X																							

Lymphadenitis, Cervical (Note that only the main remedies are used from 17)

	SULPH AC	ARUM T	AUR	BAR C	BAR M	BELL	CIST	CON	DULC	GRAPH	HELL	IOD	KALI CAR	LAPIS	MERC	NIT AC	RHUS T	SPONG	CALC FL
4										X		X		X				X	**X**
5							X												
6			X					X			X						X		
13	X					X							X		X				
17	X	X	X	X	X	X	X	X	X	X	X	X	X	X	X	X	X	X	
18		X		X					X							X			
21					X														

Lymphangitis

	APIS	BELL	HEP	BUFO	ARS	GRAPH	HYPER	RHUS T	SULPH	AUR M N
8	**X**	X	X		X	X		X	X	**X**
9	X	X	X			X		X		
10							X			
16							X			
18				X						
19	X			X					X	
21		X	X							
24					X					

Lymphatic System, Diseases Of

	BELL	CALC	SIL	BAR C	CARB V	CHINA	DULC	FERR	GRAPH	LYC	MERC	NAT M	PETR	PULS	RHUS T	SEP	SULPH
7	X	X	X	X	X	X	X	X	X	X	X	X	X	X	X	X	X
8	X	X	X	X	X	X	X	X	X	X	X	X	X	X	X	X	X
9	X	X	X														

Lymph Nodes, Swelling Of- See Swelling, Lymph Nodes

Lymph Nodes, Neck, Swelling Of- See Swelling, Lymph Nodes Cervical

Lyssophobia

	LYSS	ARG N	GELS
2	X		
23	X		
25		X	X

Malaria

	CHINA	ARS	NAT M	EUP PERF	IPEC	SULPH	CHIN S	GELS	NUX V	RHUS T	CEDRON	MENY	NAT SIL	VER A	PULS	ARN	BRY	CAPS	CARB V	MALARIA	AMM PIC	APIS	CHIN A	BELL	CALC	CIMEX	FERR ARS	LYC
1	<u>X</u>	X	X	X			X	X	X	X	X	X		X	X		X			X		X				X	X	
2						X							X															
3	X	X	X	X	X		X	X	X	X		X		X				X		X			X	X		X	X	
6	X	X	X	X	X	X	X	X	X	X	X	X		X	X	X	X	X	X			**X**		X	X	X		X
7	**X**	**X**	**X**		**X**			X		X			X			X	X											X
8	<u>**X**</u>	**X**	**X**	X		X		X			X		X			X					X		X					
9	X																											
10	<u>X</u>	X	**X**	X	<u>**X**</u>	X		X	X	X				X	X	X	X	X	X			X		X	X			
11	X	X	**X**	X	X		**X**	X	X		**X**	**X**	**X**	X					X	X	**X**		**X**					
12	<u>X</u>	X	X	X	X				X		X								X									
14	X	X	X	X																								
16		X	X	X	X	X																						
17	X	X	X			X	X						X												X			X
21	X	X				X	X																					
23		X	X				X					X						X			X						X	
29[1]																				X								
29[2]		X		X																								
29[3]	X	**X**	**X**	X		X			X	X					**X**													

29[1] Rastogi DP, et al. Research Studies in Malaria and role of Malaria officionalis. CCRH Quarterly Bulletin, 1993, 15, 3&4, 7-11.
29[2] Lira Salazar G, et al. Effects of Homeopathic Medications Eupatorium perfoliatum and Arsenicum album on parasitemia of Plasmodium berghei-infected mice. Homeopathy, 2006, Oct, 85, 4, 223-8.
29[3] Van Erp VM, et al. Homoeopathic Treatment of Malaria in Ghana. Brit Hom J, 1996, 85, 2, 66-70.

Malaria, Prophylaxis

	ARS	CARB V	CHIN S	MALARIA	NAT M
12		X			
16				X	X
21	X		X		

Malum Pottii- See Pott's Disease

Mania

	STRAM	HYOSC	VER A	LACH	BELL	CANTH	NUX V	SULPH	ARS	ACON	OP	PLAT	ANAC	CANN I	MERC	CALC	CAMPH	CUPR	PHOS	PULS	AGAR M	KALI BR	TAR H	BAR M	CIMICI	CROC S	NUX M	
1	X	X	**X**	X	X		X	X			X	X			X	X	X	X		X			X	X				
2	**X**	**X**	X		**X**	X		X		**X**				**X**	X			X						X		X		
3	X	**X**	X	X												X								X				
4	**X**	**X**	X	X	**X**	X	X	X	X	X		**X**	**X**			X	X			X	**X**	X			X		X	
6	X	X	X	X	X	X	X			X	X	X	X				X				X				X			
7	**X**	**X**	**X**	**X**	**X**	**X**	**X**	**X**	**X**		**X**		**X**		**X**							**X**	**X**		**X**		**X**	
8	X	X	X	X	X	X	X	X	X	X	X	X	X	X	X	X	X	X	X	X	X	X	X			X	X	
9	X	X		X	X								X															
11		X																										
12	X		X																									
13	**X**	X	X	X	X	X	**X**	X	**X**	X	**X**	X		X		X	X	X	X	X	X					X	X	
14	X	X	X	X		X		X						X					X			X						
15	X																											
17			X																					X				
18				X																			X					
21		X			X									X					X									
23	X		X	X		X			X																X			
26	X	X	X	X	X		X		X	X	X	X			X			X	X	X						X		

Manic Depression

	IGN	GELS	MOSCH	NUX M	PLAT	CAMPH	CANN I	CIMICI	CROC	HYOSC	LACH	NAT M	THLASPI															
1			X	X					X			X	X															
4		X																										
10		X																										
11	X			X	X			X		X																		
14	X					X	X																					
15	X																											
18	X		X								X																	
27					X																							

Marasmus- See also Emaciation (Includes Atrophy of Children; Marasmus Infantum)

	CALC PH	ABROT	IOD	CALC	NAT M	BAR C	MAG CAR	SARS	HEP	SULPH	ARG N	ARS	LYC	OL JEC A	VER A	OP	PHOS	PSOR	SANIC	TUB
1	X	X	X	X	X	X	X													
2								X	X							X				
3	X	X	X	X	X	X														
4	**X**		**X**	**X**	**X**	**X**	**X**		**X**	**X**		X					X			
6											X				X		X			
7	X	X	X	**X**	**X**			X		X		X	X	X		X				
8	X	X	X	X	X	X	X	X	X	X	X	X	X	X	X	X	X	X		
9	X	X									X									
10	X	X	X	X	X	X	X		X	X	X	X	X					X		X
11			X					X						X						
16	X	X																		X
19															X					
23		X				X	X	X						X						
25															X					

Mastalgia- See also Neuralgia, Breast (Includes Pain, Breast, of Cancer)

	CON	BRY	PHYTO	BELL	PULS	CARB A	CALC	APIS	CIMICI	LAC C	HYDRAST	IOD	PHELL	ARS	AST R	LACH	MUREX	RAN B	SULPH
1	X		X								X								
2	X						**X**			X							X	**X**	
3	X	X		X					X									**X**	
4	**X**	X	**X**			X			X				X				X		
5		X	X		X														
6	X	X	X					X				X							
7	X	X	X	X	X		X	X		X	X	X	X						
8	X	X	X		X	X							X						
9	X	X	X	X	X				X	X									X
10	X	X	X	X	X	X	X	X			X	X		X	X	X			
13				X													X		X
14	X	X	X			X				X				X	X				
17	X								X										
18	X		X		X		X			X		X			X				
21	X	X		X	X	X	X									X			
22			X																
23													X						
24	X	X	X	X		X		X						X		X			
25	X	X		X	X				X		X								X
26		X		X															
29*		X						X											

29* Berrebi A, et al. Treatment of Pain due to Unwanted Lactation with a Homeopathic Preparation given in the Immediate Post-Partum Period. J Gynecol Obstet Biol Reprod (Paris), 2001, June, 30, 4, 353-357.

Mastalgia, Left

	CIMICI	RAN B
4		X
9	X	
17	X	
25	X	

Mastitis

	BELL	BRY	PHYTO	SIL	HEP	MERC	SULPH	CON	ACON	APIS	LACH	PHOS	PULS	GRAPH	CARB A	ARN	CALC	CHAM	CIMICI	RHUS T	CARB V	BELLIS	CIST	CROT T	LAC C	LYC		
1	X		X		X	X		X														X						
2																		X										
3	X																											
4	X	X		X		X	X	X	**X**																			
5	X	X	X		X			X		X	X		X		X		X		X						X			
6	X	X	X	X	X	X	X			X	X	X		X		X				X								
7	X	**X**	**X**	X	X	X		X		X	X	X	X					X		X			X	X		X		
8	X	X	X	X	X	X	X		X	X	X	X	X		X		X	X			X			X		X		
9	X	X	**E**	X	X		X		X										X						X			
10	X	**X**		X	X		X							X		X	X											
13	X	X	X	X	X	X	X	X				X			**X**						**X**		X					
14			X								X																	
15	X			X	X				X													E						
18	X	X	X																									
21	X	X	X	X	X																							
23	X	X												X														
24	X	X	X	X	X	X	X			X		X	X	X						X								
25	X	X	X	X	X	X	X		X										X									
26	X	X				X																						
29*	X	X	X	X				X								X												

E- External

29* Vershney JP et al. Comparative Efficacy of homeopathic and allopathic systems of medicine in the management of clinical mastitis in Indian dairy cows. Homeopathy, 2005, 94, 81-85.

Mastoiditis

	CAPS	AUR	BELL	FL AC	HEP	SIL	AMM PIC	ASAF	BAPT	BRY	KALI MUR	MERC	MERC IOD	NIT AC	ONOS	PHOS
1			X										X			
5	X	X		X		X										
6	X															
7	X															
9	X			X												
16	B									X	X					X
17	X	X	X				X	X						X	X	
19		X			X				X							
24	X	X			X	X						X				

B- Both Internal and External

Mastodynia- See Mastalgia; Neuralgia, Breast

Measles

	PULS	ACON	EUPHR	GELS	BELL	BRY	ARS	KALI BIC	SULPH	FERR PH	IPEC	DROS	PHOS	MORBIL	VER V	CAMPH	RHUS T	APIS	CARB V	COFF	CUPR	DULC	LACH	STRAM	ANT C	MERC	SIL
1	X		X			X	X	X				X						X									X
2	**X**	**X**	**X**	X	**X**	X	**X**	**X**	**X**	X		X			X	**X**	**X**		X		X	X	X				
3	X	X	X		X	X	X	X	X	X				X			X										X
4	**X**	**X**	**X**	**X**	X	**X**	**X**	X	X	X												X	X	**X**			
5	X		X	X	X					X				X													X
6	X	**X**	X	X	X	X	X	X	X		X	X	X		X	X		X	X	X			X	X	X	X	
7	**X**	X	X	X	X	**X**	**X**	**X**	X	X	X	**X**	X		X	X	X	X	X	X	X		X	X		X	
8	**X**	**X**	X	**X**	**X**	**X**	X	X	**X**	**X**	X	X	**X**		**X**	X		X	X	X	X	X	X	X	X	X	
9	X	X	X	X		X				X				X													
10	X	X	X		X	X	X		X		X			X							X						
11		X	X	X	X	X	X	X	X	X	X	X	X										X				
12	X	**X**		X	X	X	X	X	X		X		X		X	X	X				X						
13	**X**	X		X	X	X	X	X	X		X	X	X				X			X		X			X		
14	X	X	X	X	X	X	X	X																			X
15	X	X	**X**	X	**X**	X	X	X			X		X		**X**												
16	X	X		X	X	X								X				X		X				X			
17	X			X					X										X							X	X
18	X		X	X	X																						
19																									X		
20	X	**X**					X	X		X							X	X									
21	X	X	X		X																						
22	X	X	X	X	X	X		X		X												X					
23		X	X	X			X							X		X											
25	X	X	X	X		X				X				X													
26	**X**	X	X		X	X	X		X		X	X	X		X	X			X	X	X	X			X	X	
28	X													X													

Measles, German (Includes Rubella)

	PULS	ACON	BELL	FERR PH	ATROP	COFF	GELS	MORBIL	PHYTO	RHUS T	SULPH IO
2					X						
5	X	X	X				X			X	X
14	X	X	X	X							
16	X	X				X		X			
18	X										
20	X	X	X	X							
21									X		
22	X	X	X	X							

Measles, Prophylaxis

	MORBIL	ACON	ARS	PULS	BRY
9	X				
10	X	X	X	X	
16	X	X	X	X	X
25	X				
28	X				

Megrim- See Migraine

Meibomian Glands, Diseases Of

	GRAPH	MERC
6	X	
8		X
24	X	

Melaena- See Stool, Bloody

Melanosis

	AUR	PHOS	SANIC
2	X		
8		X	X

Memory, Deficient

	ANAC	BAR C	LYC	SULPH	CALC	PH AC	ZINC	LACH	MEDO	NUX V	SEP	KALI BR	NAT M	MERC	NUX M	PHOS	AUR	CON	OLEAND	HYOSC	KALI PH	LAC C	PLUM	RHUS T	BOV	HELL	STRAM	
1	X		X	X	X	X		X	X		X	X			X		X	X	X			X		X	X	X	X	
2	**X**	**X**		**X**			**X**												X									
3	X		X																									
4	X	X	X	X	X	X				X	X		X			X												
5	X	X	X		X	X			X	X		X			X	X	X				X							
6	X	X	X	X	X	X		X		X	X		X	X		X			X	X			X		X		X	
7	**X**	X	X	X	X		X	**X**	X	**X**	**X**	**X**	X	**X**	**X**	X	X	X	X	X	X	X		X	X	X	X	
8	**X**	X	**X**	**<u>X</u>**	**X**	X	X	**<u>X</u>**	X	**X**	X	X	**<u>X</u>**	**X**	X	X	X	**X**	**X**	**X**		X	X	**X**	X	**X**	**X**	
9	X	X	**X**			X				X	X	X	X		X					X		X	X	X				
10	X	X	X	X	X	X			X	X						X	X	X			X							
11	X	X	X	X	X				X												X							
12						X	X																					
13	**X**	X	X	**X**	X		**X**	**X**			**X**		**X**	X	**X**	X	**X**	X	X	**X**		X	X	X	**X**	X	X	
14	X	X	X	X	X	X												X			X	X						
17	X	X					X	X																				
18	X	X				X	X		X			X									X							
19	X																											
21	X			X	X		X		X					X									X			X		
22	X																											
24	X	X		X	X																		X					
25			**X**									X																
27	X				X									X														

Memory, Deficient, Ageing Related/Senile

	LYC	BAR C	ANAC																									
1		X																										
6	X																											
7	X																											
8			X																									
9	X																											
14	X	X																										
27		X																										

Meniere's Disease

	SAL AC	CHIN S	NAT SAL	CARB SUL	CHENO	SIL	THERID	CHINA	LACH	BRY	CON	PHOS	ARN	CROT H	ACON	BELL	CAUST	CIC	COCCUL	COLCH	GLON	KALI BR	LED	NAJA	NAT SUL	TAB		
2		**X**	**X**	X			X	**X**	**X**								X						X		X	X		
4	X									X			X															
5	X	X	X	X	X	X	X		X		X	X		X										X				
6		X	**X**			X					X							X				X				X		
7	X													X						X								
8	X	X	X	X			X		X	X	X		X	X	X	X	X	X		X		X	X	X				
9	X		X	X	X	X	X	**X**		X									X									
11	X	X			X		X																		X			
14				X	X	X																						
17	X	X	X	X		X	X		X				X															
18	X				X																							
19	X	**X**	**X**			X						**X**			X	X												
21	X	X							X																			
23	X		X	X																	X							
24		**X**	X		X			X			X								X									
25	X							X		X																		
27		X	X									X									X							
28	X																											

Meningitis (Includes Cerebrospinal Meningitis; Leptomeningitis Spinalis; Meningococcal Meningitis)

	BELL	APIS	HELL	BRY	CIC	ACON	CUPR	ZINC	OP	VER V	SULPH	GELS	HYOSC	STRAM	CALC	GLON	ARN	PHOS	CROT H	MERC	ANAC	LACH	COCCUL	DIG	HYPER	IODOFOR	PLUM	PULS
1	X	X	X	X	X	X	X	X	X	X	X	X	X		X	X			X									
2	**X**	**X**	**X**	**X**	**X**	**X**	X	**X**	X	X	X	**X**	X	X		X	**X**		**X**	X			X	X	X	X		
3	X	X				X		X													X					X		
4	**X**	**X**	**X**	X	**X**	X	X	**X**		**X**	X	X			X											X		
5		X										X																
6	X	X	X	X	X	X	X	X	X		X	X		X	X	X	X	X		X		X	X	X	X		X	
7	**X**	**X**	**X**	X	X	**X**	X		X	X	X	X	**X**	**X**	X	**X**	X		X	X	**X**	**X**	X	X			X	X
8	**X**	X	X	X	X	X	X	X	X	X	X	X	X	X	X	**X**	X	X	X	X	X	X	X	X	X		X	X
9		X	X	X	**X**		X			X							X											
10	**X**	X	**X**	X			**X**	X			X		X	X	X	X		X										X
11	**X**	**X**	**X**	**X**	**X**		**X**	X	**X**																			
12	X	X	X	X		X			X	X			X		X		X					X						
14	X	X			X		X												X									
15	X		X	X		X		X	X	X		X	X	X													X	
16	X	X		X																								
17	X	X	X	X	X		X	X	X		X			X				X								X		
18		X																										
19	X				X				X																			
21	X			X		X											X											
23	X		X		X					X			X								X				X			
26	**X**	X	X	X		X	X				X				X	X		X		X								
27								X						X				X										

Meningitis, Tubercular

	CALC	PHOS	BACILL	BELL	BRY	IODOFOR
10	X	X				
16			X			X
26	X	X		X	X	

Menopause

	LACH	SEP	CIMICI	SANG	SULPH	PULS	AMYL N	BELLIS	CALC	SULPH AC	IGN	ACON	COCCUL	CYCL	GLON	USTIL	KALI CAR	BRY	CAULO	CON	GELS	GRAPH	VER V	MUREX
1	**X**	X	X	X	X	X		X	X						X									
2	**X**	**X**	**X**	X	X		X	X		X	**X**			X		X	**X**							X
3	**X**	X	X	X	X			X											X		X			
4	**X**	X	**X**	X			X	**X**				X			X	X			X				X	
5	X	X	X						X	X					X		X			X		X		
6	X	X							X	X				X		X				X				
7	**X**	**X**	X		X		**X**			X	X		X	X				X		X	X			**X**
8	X	X		X	X	X					X	X	X	X		X		X		X	X			X
9	X		X	X		X	X	X				X		X	X				X				X	
10	**X**				X	**X**					X		X					X						
11	X		X																					
13	X	X		X	X	X				X	X		X											
14	X	X		X			X								X									
15		X	X			X						X	X								X		X	
16	X																							
17	X	X	X	X								X												
18	**X**	X			X																	X		
19	X	X					X		X							X								
21	X	X				X	X		X	X							X	X				X		
23	X			X	X																			
25	**X**		X			X	X	X											X				X	
27	X	**X**				X																X		
28	X	X																						
29[1]	X	X															X							
29[2]	X	X			X				X															

29[1] Jacobs J, et al. Homeopathy for menopausal symptoms in breast cancer survivors: a preliminary randomized controlled trial. J Alt Compl Med, 2005, Feb, 11, 1, 21-7.

29[2] Nayak C, et al. Management of distress during climacteric years by homeopathic therapy. J Altern Complement Med. 2011 Nov;17(11):1037-42.

Menorrhagia

	CALC	SABIN	BELL	CHINA	CROC S	PHOS	PLAT	NUX V	LACH	SEC	CARB V	IPEC	KREO	SIL	SEP	TRILL P	FERR	USTIL	CHAM	LYC	ALET	AMM C	ARS	COCCUL	IGN	BOV	BRY	VER A
1	X	X	X	**X**	X	X	X	X	X	X	X	X	X	X	X	X	X	X	X	X	X	X		X	X			
2		X			**X**	X	X			**X**						X		**X**			X			X				
3	X																											
4	**X**		X				X	X		X			**X**								X	X						
5				X		X	X		X											X								
6	X	X	X		X	X	X	X		X	X	X	X	X	X	X	X		X	X		X		X	X		X	X
7	**X**	**X**	X	**X**	X	X	X	X	X	X	X	X	X	X	X	X	**X**	X	X	X	X	X	**X**	X	X	X	X	X
8	**X**	X	**X**	X	X	**X**	**X**	X	X	X	X	**X**	X	X	X	X	X	X	X	X	X	X	X	X	X		**X**	X
9		X	X	X	X	X	X	X	**X**		X		X		X			X					X			X		
10	X	X	X	X	**X**	X	X	X		X		X		X					X					X	X			
12	X																											
13	**X**	**X**	**X**	**X**	**X**	**X**	**X**	**X**		**X**	**X**	X	X	**X**	X		X			**X**		X	**X**		X	X	X	**X**
14	X	X	X	X	X			X	X	X	X	X		X	X	X			X		X	X	X				X	
15	X		X	X			X					X																
16	X																											
18	X	X		X	X	X		X		X	X			X		X			X							X		X
19	X		X	X					**X**				X			X	X	X			X			X				
21	X	X	X	X	X				X			X		X	X		X											
23		X						X							X		X									X		
24	X					X																						
25		X	X	X	X	X	X		**X**		X		X		X			X					X			**X**		
26	X	X	X			X	X	X			X	X					X		X	X					X		X	X
28		X																										

Menses, Absent- See Amenorrhoea

Menses, Arrested- See also Amenorrhoea (Includes Menses, Suppressed)

	PULS	ACON	SEP	SULPH	BELL	DULC	FERR	GRAPH	LYC	OP	SIL	APIS	CALC	CHAM	NAT M	NUX V	PHOS	SENEC	VER A
1				X					X								X	X	
3	X	X																	
6	X	X	X	X	X	X	X	X	X		X	X	X	X	X	X	X	X	X
7	X	X	X	X		X		X	X	X	X	X		X	X	X			
8		X	X	X	X	X			X	X									X
10	**X**	X	X	X	X		X	X		X			X		X				X
12	X						X												
14	X						X												
15	X	X	X					X			X		X			X			
17	X																	X	
25																	X		
26	X	X	X		X	X					X			X					
27												X							

Menses, Delayed

	PULS	SEP	SULPH	GRAPH	PHOS	LACH	NAT M	MAG CAR	LYC	CAUST	CON	IOD	KALI CAR	ACON	CALC	DULC	BELL	BRY	CIMICI	HEP	IGN	SIL	VIB OP	XANTH	KALM	NAT SUL	SENEC	
1	X	X	X	X		X		X	X				X		X									X				
2																											**X**	
3	X							**X**																				
4	X	X	X	X	X					X	X	X				X												
5	X					X			X																			
6	X			X	X	X																						
7	X	X	X	X	X	X	X	X	X	X	X	X	X		X	X	X			X	X	X		X		X		
8	**X**	**X**	**X**	**X**	**X**	X	X	X	**X**	X	**X**	X				X			X	X		X		X	**X**		X	
9		X	X		X		X							X														
10	**X**	X	X	X	X	X	X			X					X		X	X										
13	**X**	X	X	**X**	X	X	**X**	**X**	X	**X**	X	**X**	**X**	X		X	X			X	X	X			X	**X**		
14	X	X	X																				X					
15	X	X			X									X	X				X		X							
16			X																				X					
17	X																											
18		X		X		X		X																				
21	X	X	X	X			X						X					X					X					
22	X																											
24	X			X	X																							
25	X	X	X		X		X							X				X	X									
27						X																						

Menses, Before, Diseases Related To- See PMS
Menses, Early- See also Menses, Premature

	CALC	NUX V	PHOS	AMBRA	BELL	COCCUL	SABIN	SIL	KREO	CARB V	FERR	PLAT	AMM C	BRY	SEP	AMM M	CANTH	CHAM	KALI CAR	ARS	CARB A	CHINA	RHUS T	BOV	CROC	MAG SUL	PULS	
1	X	X	X	X	X	X			X		X	X	X		X	X			X		X							
3				X																								
4	**X**	X	X		X	X		X				X	X															
6	X	X	X				X	X	X				X	X	X	X												
7	**X**	X	X	X	X	X	**X**	X	X	X	**X**	X	X	**X**	X	X	X	X	X	**X**	**X**	X	**X**	X	X	X	**X**	
8	X		X	X	X	X	X	X		X	X						X	X	X			X	X		X		X	
9		X							X	X							X											
10	X	X	X		X		X								X													
13	**X**	**X**	**X**	**X**	X	**X**	X	**X**	X	**X**	X	**X**	X	**X**	X	**X**	**X**	**X**	**X**	**X**	**X**	X	**X**	**X**	**X**	**X**	X	
14	X	X		X	X									X						X		X				X		
15		X						X																				
18			X				X											X						X				
19	X		X	X		X					X																	
21		X																										
24	X																											
25			X						X	X		X																

Menses, Irregular/ Intermittent (Includes Menses, Between)

	PULS	SEP	COCCUL	CALC	IOD	LACH	NUX M	SEC	CAULO	CHAM	CHINA	CON	CYCL	FERR	HAM	NAT M	NUX V	SABIN	STAPHYS	SULPH	AMBRA	PHOS
1			X										X									
2															X			X			**X**	
3		X																				
4			X	X																		
6	X			X					X						X							
7	X	X	X	X	X	X	X	X		X		X		X			X		X			
8	X	X	X		X	X	X	X	X	X			X	X	X		X	X	X	X		**X**
9	X										X	X				X				X		
10		X	X																			
12	X	X																				
13			X		X		X															
14	X	X			X		X									X	X					
15	X	X																				
18		X						X					X						X			
19	X			X		X		X						X				X			X	X
21	X	X									X											
25	X										X	X				X				X		
27						X			X													

Menses, Intermenstrual Flow- See Menses, Irregular

Menses, Painful- See Dysmenorrhoea

Menses, Pregnancy, Continue Through

	COCCUL	CROC S	PHOS	PLAT	SULPH
10	**X**	**X**	X	X	X

Menses, Premature- See also Menses, Early

	CALC	CARB V	PHOS	CALC PH	SABIN	BRY	NUX V	PLAT
1	X	X		X	X			
3	X			X				
8	**X**	**X**	**X**		X	**X**	**X**	**X**
9			X					

Menses, Profuse- See Menorrhagia

Menses, Prolonged- See also Menorrhagia

	NUX V	PHOS	SEC	CALC	KREO	LYC	PLAT	SABIN	FERR	IGN	PULS	ACON	CHINA	CROC	MILL	SEP	SULPH AC	ARS	CARB A	IPEC	NAT M	RHUS T
1	X																					
6		X	X	X	X	X	X		X	X				X		X						
7	X	X	X	**X**	X	X	X	**X**	**X**		**X**	X		X	X		X	**X**	**X**		**X**	**X**
8	**X**	**X**	X		X	X	X	**X**		**X**	X		X				X			**X**		
9												X	X									
14				X																		
15	X															X						
18		X	X											X								
19															X							

Menses, Scanty (Includes Oligomenorrhoea)

	PULS	SEP	GRAPH	NAT M	LACH	SULPH	CON	PHOS	KALI CAR	ALUM	SIL	CALC	COCCUL	CAUST	DULC	FERR	MAG CAR	CARB V	CYCL	VIB OP	AMM C	LYC
1	X		X	X	X	X	X		X	X		X	X				X		X			
2	X																					
3	X			X	X																	
4	X	X	X	X		X	X	X			X		X		X							
5	X	X	X	X					X		X	X							X			
6	X	X	X	X	X	X	X		X			X		X			X		X			X
7	**X**	**X**	X	**X**	**X**	X	X	X	X	X	X		X	X	X	X	X	X	X	X	X	
8	**X**	X	**X**	X	X	X	**X**	X		X	X		X	X	X	X	X	**X**				X
9	X	X		X		X	X	X				X				X						
10	**X̲**	X			X								X									
12	X															X						
13	X	X	**X**	**X**	X	**X**		**X**	**X**	**X**	**X**		X	X	X	X		X			**X**	**X**
14	X	X				X				X					X					X		
15		X	X																			
16																				X		
18			X		X												X					
21	X	X	X		X															X		
24	X	X	X		X																	
25	X	X		X			X	X				X										
26	X	X	X	X		**X**		X	X	X	X			X				X			X	
29*	X	X		X								X										

29* Cardigno P. Homeopathy for the treatment of menstrual irregularities: a case series. Homeopathy. 2009 Apr; 98 (2):97-106.

Menses, Short

	PULS	SULPH	GRAPH	NAT M	BAR C	PHOS	LACH	ALUM	AMM C	DULC	BERB V	CON	MERC	PLAT	SEP	THUJA	VIB OP
1			X				X										
7	**X**	X	X	X	X		**X**		X	X	X	X	X	X	X	X	
8	**X**	X	**X**	**X**	X	X	X			X							
9	X	X		X		X									X		
13	X	X	X		X	X		X	X	X	X	X	X	X			
14		X						X									X
18																X	X
25					X												
26	X	X	X	X		X		X	X								

Menstruation, Diseases Of

	PULS	NAT M	ACON	CIMICI	ARS	BELL	CALC	CAULO	CAUST	CHAM	CHINA	CON	FERR	GRAPH	HAM	IPEC	KREO	LITH C	LYC	NIT AC	PLAT	SEP	SULPH	AMM M	APIS	BOV	CYCL	KALI IOD
2		**X**	**X**	**X**	**X**	**X**	**X**	**X**	**X**	**X**	**X**	**X**	**X**	**X**	**X**	**X**	**X**	**X**	**X**	**X**		**X**	**X**	X	X	X	X	X
6	X																				**X**							
8	X	X	X	X	X	X	X	X	X	X	X	X	X	X	X	X	X	X	X	X	X	X	X	X	X	X	X	X
14	X	X																										
24	X																											

Mercury, Ailments From- See Ailments From, Mercury
Mesenteric Artery, Aneurism- See Aneurism, Mesenteric Artery
Mesenteric Glands, Diseases Of

	IOD	BAC TEST	CALC	CALC IOD	CON	GRAT	KISSING
2		X				X	X
8	X		X		X		
12	X						
24	X			X			

Meteorism- See Distension, Abdomen

Metritis

	BELL	PULS	ACON	CANTH	NUX V	SABIN	SEP	ARS	COLOC	BRY	CON	LACH	RHUS T	SEC	LYC	CHAM	KALI CAR	MERC	SULPH	VER V	LAC C							
1	X	X	X		X	X	X	X	X	X	X	X	X			X												
2		X																										
4	X					X																						
6	X	X	X	X	X	X	X	X	X	X	X	X	X	X		X	X	X	X	X	X							
7	**X**	X	X	X	X	X	X	**X**	X	X	X	X		X	**X**		X	X	X	X	X							
8	X	X	X	X	X	X	X	X	X	X	X	X	X	X	X	X	X	X	X	X	X							
9				X																								
13	**X**	**X**	**X**	**X**	**X**		X	X	**X**	X	X	X	X	X	X	X	X	X	X		X							
16						X																						
23			X	X																X								
26	**X**				X		X						X	X	X													

Metralgia- See also Cramp, Uterus; Hyperaesthesia, Uterus; Pain, Genitalia, Female

	SEP	BELL	LACH	PLAT	CON	MUREX	PULS	SABIN	MAG PH	IGN	KREO	NUX V	CIMICI	AUR M	BRY	CHAM	COCCUL	FERR	IPEC	LYC	NAT M	VIB OP						
1	X	X	X	X	X	X	X	X			X																	
2	**X**								X													X						
4							X		**X**				**X**				X											
6	X	X	X	X	X	X	X	X		X		X	X	X	X	X		X	X	X	X							
7	X	X	X	X	X	X	X	X		X	X	X			X	X	X	X			X	X						
8	**X**	X		X	X	X	X	X	X	X		X	X		X	X	X		X	X	X							
10	X	X	X	X	X	X					X			X				X	X	X								
14								X			X																	
15		X		X						X		X																
16																						X						
17		X																										
20			X						X																			
21														X														
25	X																											
27			X																									

Metrorrhagia

	SABIN	HAM	SEC	TRILLP	NIT AC	BELL	CALC	CROC S	IPEC	PLAT	CHINA	ERIGER	BOV	FERR	LYC	PULS	PHOS	APOC	CAULO	RHUS T	SEP	SULPH	CHAM	COFF	HYOSC	NUX V	STRAM	
1	X															X												
2			X	X	X			X					X		X			X		X				X				
3				X	X								X															
4		X																										
6	X	X	X	X	X	X	X	X	X	X	X	X		X	X	X	X	X	X	X	X	X			X	X		
7	**X**	**X**	**X**	**X**	**X**	**X**	**X**	**X**	**X**	**X**	**X**	**X**		**X**	X	**X**	**X**		**X**		X	X	X	X		X	X	
8	X	X	X	X	X	X	X	X	X	X	X	X	X	X	X	X	X	X	X	X	X	X	X	X	X	X	X	
10	X						X										X											
11		X																										
13	**X**	X	**X**	X	X	**X**	**X**	**X**	**X**	**X**	**X**	**X**		**X**	X	**X**	X	X	**X**	X	X	X	**X**	**X**	**X**	**X**	**X**	
14	X	X	X																									
17																											X	
18													X															
19						X							X															
23				X	X								X					X				X						
24							X																					
25										X																		
26	X	X	**X**	X		X		X	**X**	X	**X**	X		X	X					X	X		X		X			

Migraine- See also Headache; Hemicrania (Includes Megrim)

	IRIS V	IGN	NAT M	BELL	SIL	SANG	CYCL	GELS	NUX V	PULS	SEP	CALC	LAC D	LYC	SPIG	TONGO	ARS	AUR	BRY	KALI BIC	PHOS	SCUT	THUJA					
1	X	X		X			X									X						X						
2	X															X												
3	X	X	X	X	X		X									X						X						
4									X		X																	
5			X	X	X	X	X	X	X	X	X		X	X				X			X							
6			X																									
7		X			**X**			X				X	X				X		X	X	X							
8	X	X	X	X	X	X	X	X	X	X	X	X	X		X		X			X	X		X					
9	X	X	X	X	X	X		X	X	X	X			X	X				X	X								
12																		X										
14	X	X		X							X												X					
16																						X						
18	X	X				X	X	X					X	X			X		X	X								
19	X	X	**X**	**X**	X	X	X		X			X	X		X			X	X		X							
20	X					X																						
21	X		X		X	X				X				X	X								X					
22	X																											
23	X											X				X	X					X						
25			X		X	X				X				X	X								X					
26		X		X	X				X			X																
28																X												
29[1]		X	X							X	X							X										
29[2]		X	X	X	X		X	X																				
29[3]	X	X		X				X																				

29[1] Straumshein P, et al. Homeopathic Treatment of Migraine. Brit Hom J, 1998, 87, 3-5.
29[2] Brigo B, Serpelloni G, Homoeopathic Treatment of Migraine. Berlin Journal on Research in Homoeopathy, 1991, 1, 2, 98-106.
29[3] Danno K, et al. Homeopathic treatment of migraine in children: results of a prospective, multicenter, observational study. J Altern Complement Med. 2013 Feb; 19 (2):119-23.

Migraine, Left Sided- See Hemicrania, Left

Migraine, Right Sided- See Hemicrania, Right

Miliary Eruptions- See also Sudamena (Includes Milaria)

	ACON	ARS	BRY	CHAM	IPEC	BELL	SULPH	AMM C	CALC	NAT	RHUS T	JAB	MERC	PH AC	ANT C	CARB V	CAUST	HELL	HEP	LACH	MEZ	PULS	VER A	CACT	CALAD			
2	**X**	X	X	X				X				**X**												**X**				
6		X	X						X		X			X				X										
7	X	X	X	X	X	X			X	X	X																	
8	X	X	X	X	X	X	X	X		X	X	X	X		X		X		X	X	X	X						
13	**X**	X	X	**X**	**X**	**X**	**X**	X	X	X			**X**	**X**	X	X	X	X	X	X	X	X	X		**X**			
26	X				X		X									X							X					

Milk- See Ailments from Milk; Lactation

Milk Crust- See Cradle Cap

Milk Fever- See also Fever; Pain, Breasts, Swelling, Breasts

	BRY	ACON	BELL	ARN	RHUS T	CHAM	COFF	CALC	IGN	MERC	OP	PULS
2	X					X		X				
3	X	X	X									
4	X											
7	X	X	X			X						
8	X	**X**	X	X	X		**X**					
10	X	X	X	B	X	X						X
13	**X**	X	**X**	X	**X**	X	X		X	X	X	
15					X							
24	X											
25		X		X								

B- Both Internal and External

Milk Leg- See Phlegmasia Alba Dolens

Miosis

	OP	MERC C	ACON	ARN	BELL	COCCUL	PHYSO	PULS	SEP	VER A	ANAC	ARS	CAMPH	CHAM	CHEL	CIC	IGN	MEZ	NAT M	NUX V	SIL	SULPH	ZINC
1		X						X	X														
8				X	X	X		X	X	X	X	X	X	X	X	X	X	X	X		X	X	X
9	X					X																	
11	X						X																
12	X	X		X																			
13		X			X	X		X	X	**X**	X	X	X	X	X	X	X	X		X	X	X	X
14							X																
15																				X			
17	X				X																		
19	X		X																				
20			X																				
21	X																						
24		X	X	X			X												X				

Miscarriage- See Abortion, Threatened

Mitral Valve Insufficiency

	CACT	KALI CAR	SPONG	CONVAL	SPIG	ADONIS	APIS	AMYL N	ARS IOD	CRAT	DIG	KALI BIC	LAURO	LITH C	NAJA	QUEBR	RHUS T	STROPH	VISC A	ZINC
1					X				X						X					
4				X																
5	X			X		X				X	X		X			X		X		
6	X																			X
7	X	X	X		X		X	X				X		X			X			
8			X																	
10		X																		
11	X																		X	
17		X	X																	

Mitral Valve, Diseases Of

	CONVAL	DIG	ARS	ARS IOD	CAFF	KALI CAR
1				X		
4	X					
5						X
11		X			X	
17	X	X	X			

Mitral Valve Regurgitation

	ADONIS	LAURO	STROPH	APOC	LYCOP
8					X
11	X		X		
17		X			
19	X	X	X	X	

Mitral Valve Stenosis- See Stenosis, Mitral Valve

Moles (Includes Melanocytic Naevi)

	CALC	SIL	SULPH	NAT CAR	SABIN	THUJA	CARB A	CARB V	CAUST	FL AC	GRAPH	HEP	LYC	MERC	NIT AC	PHOS	PLAT	PULS	RHUS T	SEC	STAPHYS
2				X	X													X			
8		X	X	X										X						X	
9					X																
11	X	X				X	X		X	X	X	X	X		X						X
12						X															
13	X		X																		
26	X	X	X					X								X	X		X		

Moles, Uterus

	CALC	CANTH	SABIN	SEC	SIL	ACON	ARS	BELL	CAULO	CHINA	FERR	GRAPH	HYOSC	KALI CAR	LYC	MERC	NAT CAR	NIT AC	PH AC	PULS	SEP	SULPH
1	X	X	X	X	X													X	X			
8	X	X	X	X	X	X	X	X	X	X	X	X	X	X	X	X	X			X	X	X

Mollities Ossium- See Osteomalacia

Molluscum (Includes Molluscum Contagiosum; Molluscum Fibrosum)

	CALC	SULPH	SIL	CINNAB	DULC	MEDO	THUJA
2	X	X	X				
7		X					
18				X	X		X
19						X	
28	X						
29*	X						

29* Manchandra RK, et al. Double Blind Placebo Controlled Trials of Homeopathic Medicines in Warts and Molluscum Contagiosum. CCRH Quarterly Bull, 1997, 19, 3&4, 25-29.

Mononucleosis- See Infectious Mononucleosis

Morning Sickness (Includes Nausea of Pregnancy)

	NUX V	IPEC	SEP	SYMPHOR	KREO	ANAC	PULS	TAB	CARB AC	COLCH	PHOS	ALET	ARS	NAT M	LAC AC	NUX M	CER OX	IRIS V	LOB I	NAT PH	PETR	SULPH	ASAR E	CHEL
1	X	X	X	**X**	X					X	X	X			X	X							X	
2			X		X	X	X	X			X	X					X	X	X		X			
3	X		X	**X**		X				X				X										
4	X			**X**		X			X								X			X				
5	X	X	X		X			X							X	X							X	X
6	X																							
7	**X**	X	**X**		**X**		X	**X**	X	X	X		X	X	**X**	**X**		X	X		X	X	**X**	**X**
8	X	X	X	X	X	X	X		X		X	X	X	X	X	X					X	X		
9	X	**X**	X	X	X	X			X			X					X		X	X				
10	X	X	X				X						X	X										
14		X		X																				
15	**X**	X			X		X						X											
17								X																
18	X	X	X		X			X		X								X	X					
19		X	X	**X**	X		X	X	X	X	X							X						X
21	X	X	X				X							X							X	X		
22	X					X				X	X	X								X				
23				X																				
25	X	X	X	**X**	X	X			X			X					X			X				
26		X	X																			X		
28	X			X																				

Moreton's Neuroma- See Neuroma

Morvan's Disease

	LACH	SIL	THUJA	AUR M	SEC
2	**X**	**X**	**X**	X	X

Motion, Involuntary- See also Tremor, generally and specifically

	HELL	STRAM	BELL	COCCUL	ART V	CAMPH	CAUST	CIC	COLCH	CUPR	GELS	HYOSC	LACH	LYC	MERC	MYGALE	PLUM	RHUS T	SIL	VER V	ZINC
3																	X				
6		X	X	X		X			X		X	X						X		X	
7	X	X		X									X								
10	X	X					X			X				X					X		
11	X	X	X					X													
14	X																				
17					X											X					
18																					X
19															X						

Motion, Involuntary, Fingers

	KALI BR	CUPR AC	CUPR	IGN	MOSCH
7	X	X			X
10			X	X	
19	X				

Motion, Involuntary, Hands

	CUPR	MERC	STRAM	BOR	CHAM	HYOSC	IGN
7		X	X	X		X	
10	X						X
26	X	X	X		X		

Motion, Involuntary, Head

	BELL	CIC	CAMPH	CAUST	CHAM	CUPR	LYC	ZINC
7	X	X	X	X		X	X	X
10					X			
11	X	X						
16					X			
21								X
26	X	X	X	X		X	X	

Motion, Involuntary, Leg

	HELL	CUPR	HYOSC	IGN	CAUST	IPEC	SEC
7	X				X		
10	X	X	X	X			
14	X						
26		X	X	X		X	X

Motion, Involuntary, Limbs

	BELL	CUPR	MYGALE	OP	STRAM	ZINC
7	X	X		X		X
10	X					
17			X			
21					X	

Motion Sickness- See also Airsickness, On Descent; Seasickness (Includes Nausea, Air Travel, From; Nausea, Car Travel, From)

	COCCUL	PETR	TAB	NUX V	BOR	VER A	BELL	ARS	BRY	IGN	SEP	COLCH	CARB AC	ACON	APOC	ARN	FERR	HEP	IPEC	IRIS V	KREO	LYC	NUX M	OP	RHUS T	SIL
2				X								X				X										
3	X	X	X	X	**X**		X																			
5	X	X	X							X																
7	**X**	**X**	X	X		X		X	X		X	X	**X**			X	X	X	X	X		X	X	X		X
8	**X**	X	X	X		**X**	X	**X**	X	X	X	X			X		X	X					X			X
9	X	X	X	X	X																X				X	
10	X	X		X		X	X																	X		
14	X																									
15	X			X		X	X																			
16	X	X			X									X												
17			X																							
18	X	X	**X**	X	X				X	X									X			X				
19	X	X	X								X		X		X					X						
20	X	X	X	X																						
21	X	X	X	X	X									X											X	
22	X																									
25	X	X	X	X	X																X					
26	X	X						X																		
28	X	X	X																							

Motion Sickness, Air Sickness, Prophylaxis

	BELL	BOR
10	X	
16	X	X

Motor Neurone Disease

	PLUM	STRYCH	ZINC	ABROT	ARG N	CAUST	GELS	IOD	LYC	NAT M	NUX V	PHOS
9				X		X	X	X	X	X		
11	X	**X**	**X**		X						X	X
17	X											

Mountain Sickness- See Altitude Sickness
Mouth, Cracked, Corners Of- See Angular Stomatitis; Crack, Mouth, Corner Of
Mouth, Diseases Of

	BELL	MERC C	BOR	KALI BIC
2	X	X		
4			X	
8				X

Mouth, Dryness- See Xerostomia
Mucous Membranes, Diseases Of

	ARS	BELL	KALI BIC	NAT M	PULS	ALUM	CALC	CAPS	CARB V	CAUST	DULC	IPEC	MERC	NUX V	PHOS	SENEG	STANN	SULPH
6	X			X														
7	X			X	X													
9			X															
11		X																
12			X															
13	X	X			X	X	X	X	X	X	X	X	X	X	X	X	X	X

Mucous Membranes, Dryness Of

	BRY	NAT M	STICTA	NUX M	BELL	ACON	ALUM	TEREB	ALUM OX	AESC	COR R	GRAPH	MERC C	PHYTO	OP	SENEG	SINAP	SULPH
3	X																	
5	X	X					X											
7		X	X	X		X		X										
8	X	X	X					X	X		X	X		X	X	X		
9	X			X														
14	X	X																
17	X			X	X		X						X				X	
18	X	X	X	X	X	X				X								
19			X															
20																		X
24		X			X													
27		X																

Multiple Sclerosis

	PHOS	PLUM	TAR H	ARG N	LATH	NUX V	CAUST	GELS	AUR	NAT M	PHYSO	AGAR M	ARS	CROT H	IGN	OX AC	PIC AC	RHUS T	SIL
1		X	X																
6	X		X	X		X					X								
7	**X**	X	X			X	X										X	X	X
8	X	X	X	X	X	X	X	X			X			X	X	X	X	X	X
9		X		X	X			X	X							X			
11	X	**X**		**X**	**X**	X			X		X			X					
12	X				X														
14			X																
17													X						
19	X	X		X	X	X	X	X	X	**X**		X	X		X				
21	X		X									X							
27	X						X	X		X									

Mumps

	BELL	PULS	MERC	PHYTO	ACON	RHUS T	CARB V	PAROTID	PILO	ARS	BRY	SULPH	JAB	LACH	TRIFOL P	ABROT	APIS	BAR C	CALC	COCCUL	KALI BIC	LYC	MERC I F	MERC C	PILO M
1	X	X	X					X	X							X							X		
2	**X**	**X**	X	X	**X**		X		X				X	X	X						X			**X**	
3	X	X		X			X	X	X							X							X		
4	**X**	X	**X**			**X**								X											**X**
5	X	X						**X**					X		**X**		X	X	X						
6	X	X	X			X	X			X		X		X						X		X			
7		X	X	X		X	X			X				X				X	X		X				
9	X	X			X	X		X				X													
10	X	X	**X**				X			X	X	X	**X**							X		X			
11	X		X	X		X									X										
12	X	X		X	X																		X	X	
14	X	X			X						X					X	X								
15		X	X		X																				
16	X			X				X	X																
18		X	**X**									X													
20	**X**	X	X	X	X	X	X		**X**	X	X										X				
21	X		X	X	X																				X
22	X	X									X						X								
25	X	X			X	X						X													
26	**X**		**X**			X	X				X							X	X	X		X			
28		X																							

Mumps, Prophylaxis

	PAROTID	PILO	MERC	PILO M	RHUS T	TRIFOL P
9	X					
10		X				
15			X			
16	X	X				X
22					X	
25	X			X		
28		X				

Muscae Volitantes- See also Vision, Diseases Of

	PHOS	AGAR M	RUTA	NIT AC	CHLF	COCCUL	CROT H	LACT V	MERC C	PHYSO	TAB	TEREB	THUJA	CHINA	NUX V	BELL	CON	CURARE	HYOSC	ITU	PARAF	ZINC
2	**X**			**X**	X			X					X	**X**	**X**			X		X	X	
6	X																					
7	X	X		X	X	X	X	X	X	X	X	X	X									
8		X	X				X			X	X	X										
12						X			X							X	X		X			X
24			X																			
26		X	X																			

Muscles, Atrophy- See Atrophy, Muscle
Muscles, Weak- See Amyotonia; Myasthenia
Muscular Dystrophy

	IOD	PLUM	ABROT	ALUM	ANT T	AST R	ARS	CALC	CAUST	CHINA	CUPR	CUPR AR	EUPION	GELS	JAB	LYC	MAG PH	NAT M	ZINC
9	X	X	X	X		X			X					X		X	X	X	
16	X	X					X				X	X							X
19								X											
27					X					X			X		X				

Myalgia

	RHUS T	BRY	GELS	ARN	CIMICI	CAUST	SANG	EUP PERF	DULC	BAPT	CALC	SIL	ACON	ANT T	COLCH	MACROT	VER V
1			X							X							
2		**X**	**X**		**X**	**X**			**X**				**X**	**X**	**X**	**X**	**X**
4	X	X	X		X	X	**X**	X	X								
5				X						X							
7	X	X		X	X												
8	X		X	X	X		X										
9	X	X															
10		X	X		X	X	X					X					
11			X					X									
12		X	X		X												
13	X					X					X	X					
14	X	X	X		X						X						
15		X															
16	X	X				X	X		X								
17					X												
18	X	X	X	X				X									
19	X							**X**									
20	X	X															
21	X		X														
22	X			X													
23				X													
24	X						X										
25				X													
27		X				X											
28	X	X															
29[1]				X													
29[2]				X													

29[1] Tveitin D, et al. Arnica and Muscle Soreness. FACT, 1998, 3, 4, 155-156.
29[2] Tuten C, et al. Reducing Muscle Soreness with Arnica Montana. Alt and Comp Ther, 1999, 5, 6, 369- 372.

Myasthenia

	CALC	ANAC	CURARE	FERR	PLUM	STRAM
1	X	X		X	X	X
10	X					
19			X			

Myasthenia Gravis

	CAUST	FERR	GELS	PLUM	SYPH
1	X				
9			X	X	X
14	X	X			

Mycosis- See Infection, Fungal

Mycosis, Nails- See Onychomycosis

Mydriasis

	BELL	GELS	CALC	HYOSC	OP	STRAM	VER V	CINA	HELL	NUX V	LACHNAN	AETHUSA	ARG N	ARN	BUFO	CANN I	CEDRON	CHINA	CIC	CON	CROT H	HEP	HYDR AC	IOD	KALI IOD	SEC	SULPH	
5	X																											
6	X					X	X	X	X							X			X									
7	X	X	X	X	X	X		X	X	X				X			X	X		X	X			X	X			
8	X	X	X	X	X	X	X	X		X	X			X								X				X	X	
9	X	X																						X				
10	X					X																						
11									X			X				X												
12	X																											
14	X		X		X														X									
15	X			X	X	X	X																					
16	X																						X					
17	X	X	X	X		X							X		X			X			X					X		
18	X						X																					
19	X	X					X						X		X													
20	X																											
21	X											X																
22	X																											
24	X	X	X	X	X			X		X	X						X			X		X	X		X		X	
25	X				X																							
27	X	X	X																									

Myelitis

	OX AC	PIC AC	RHUS T	ARS	BELL	DULC	HYPER	PHOS	ARN	LATH	MERC	NUX V	PHYSO	SEC	SULPH	ACON	CIC	PLUM	SIL	CALC	VER A	BRY						
1	X				X		X		X								X	X				X						
2	**X**	X		**X**		X						**X**		X		**X**	**X**	**X**										
3	X			X	X	X	X		X	X				X				X	X									
6		X	X	X	X		X	X			**X**		X	X	X				X		X							
7			X		X	X	X	X	X		X	X			X	X				X	X							
8	X	X	**X**	X	**X**	X	X	**X**	X		**X**	**X**	X	X	**X**	X	X		**X**	**X**	X	**X**						
10	X									X			X															
11		X											X															
14			X																									
17		X		X						X																		
23	X	X								X																		
25			X			X																						
27								X																				

Myelitis, Transverse

	ACON	ARN	ARS	BELL	CIC	CROT H	DULC	LACH	MERC	NUX V	OX AC	PHOS	PLUM	SEC	STRYCH	ZINC P
1	X	X	X	X	X	X	X	X	X	X	X	X	X	X	X	X
17	**X**	**X**	**X**	**X**	**X**	**X**	**X**	**X**	**X**	**X**	**X**	**X**	**X**	**X**	**X**	**X**

Myocardial Infarction

	CACT	LACH	ACON	DIG	ARS	ARN	CRAT	LATRO M	SPIG	CROT H	NUX V	MORPH	NAJA
9	X	X	X	X	X				X		X		
11	**X**	X	X	**X**	X	**X**	**X**	**X**				**X**	**X**
14	X	X				X			X				
17	X	X		X	X	X	X			X			
19	X	X	X					X		X			
21	X		X					X					
25	X	X	X	**X**	X		X		X		X		

Myocardial Ischaemia

	LACH	ACON	ARS	CACT	DIG	NUX V	SPIG M
9	X	X	X	X	X	X	X
17	X						

Myocarditis- See also Inflammation, Heart (Note that only the main remedies are used from 17)

	ARS I	DIG	SPIG	CACT	BRY	ARS	LACH	NAJA	VER V	ACON	ADONIS	APIS	AUR	CARB V	PHOS	VIP
1			X													
4	X	X	**X**	X	**X**				X							
7		X	**X**	X	X	X	X	X	X	X		X		X		
8	X	X	X	X			X	X	X			X		X	X	
9	X	X														
10	X															
14	X	X														
16				X												
17	X	X	X			X					X		X		X	X
19													X			
21		X					X									X
23						X		X			X					
24	X															
26					X					**X**						

Myopia

	PHYSO	PHOS	NIT AC	CARB V	CALC	CHINA	PETR	PH AC	AGAR M	ANGUST	CON	ANAC	CYCL	GELS	HYOSC	RUTA	SULPH AC
1	**X**	X			X	X		X	X								
2	**X**		X				X		X	X							X
3	X												X				
5	X																
7		X	**X**	X						X	X	X		X	X		
8		X	X	X	X	X	X	X			X	X	X		X	X	X
9	X																
13		X	X	**X**	X	X	X	X	**X**	X	**X**	X	X		X	X	X
14	X													X			
21	X	X															
23	X																
24		X			X									X		X	
25	X																
26		X		X		X	X	X									

Myositis

	BRY	RHUS T	CALC FL	ARN	CALC PH	CAUST	PH AC	PHYTO	SANG	SYMPH	THUJA
1	X	X		X							X
3			**X**		X		X			X	
9		X									
10	X								X		
24	X										
27						X		X			

Myositis, Ossifying

	CALC FL	CALC PH	FL AC	SYMPH	THUJA
1	**X**	X	X	X	X

Myotonia

	RHUS T
1	**X**

Myringitis- See Tympanic Membrane, Inflammation
Myxoedema- See Hypothyroidism

Naevi

	THUJA	CALC	FL AC	LYC	PHOS	SIL	SULPH	VAC	ACET AC	CARB V	FERR PH	HEP	RAD BR	ARS	BOR	CALC FL	CARB A	CAUST	GRAPH	IOD	LACH	MERC	NIT AC	SEP	STAPHYS			
1	B				X			X					X															
2	X	**X**	X	**X**	**X**			X	X		X																	
3	X		X	X				X					X															
5	X																											
8	X	X	**X**	X	X	X	X		X	X	X	X		X	X	X				X	X	X						
9	X																											
10		X					X																					
11	X	X	X	X		X						X					X	X	X				X		X			
12	B																											
21	X				X																							
26		X				X	X			X														X				

B- Both Internal and External

Naevi, Vascular (AKA Telangiectasia)

	LYC	CALC	CARB V	PHOS	BELL	CONDUR	FERR PH	FL AC	PLAT	PULS	SEP	SIL	STRONT	SULPH	THUJA													
6	X	X	X	X	X	X	X	X	X	X	X	X	X	X	X													
7	X	X	X	X																								
8	X																											

Nails, Diseases Of- See also Hang Nails; Inflammation, Nail Pulp; Injury, Nails; Onychogryphosis; Onychomycosis; Paronychia; Toenails, Ingrowing; Ulceration, Nails and Surrounds (Includes Onychia)

	SIL	GRAPH	ANT C	THUJA	NIT AC	SEP	ALUM	FL AC	SULPH	CAUST	HEP	ARS	LACH	AMBRA	CALC	DIG	MAG P A	NAT M	NAT SUL	OX AC	SEC							
1	X	X	X	X	X		X	X		X			X	X	X		X											
2	**X**	**X**	**X**		**X**		**X**			X		**X**								X	**X**							
3	X	X	X	X	X	X		X									X			X								
4	X																											
5	X	X	X	X	X	X	X	X		X		X	X	X	X	X		X	X	X	X							
6		X		X		X																						
7	X	X	X	X	X	X						X		X		X		X										
8	X	X	X	X		X	X	X	X	X	X		X						X									
9		X				X																						
10	X				X		X		X																			
11	X	X	X								X																	
13	**X**	**X**	X	X	X	X	X	X	**X**	X	X	X	X		X	X		X										
14	X	X	X	X							X								X									
18	X			X																								
21	X	X	X	X							X						X											
23								X																				
24								X	X																			
26	X	X			X	X	X		X																			

Nails, Falling Of

	HELL	MERC	THUJA	ANT C	ARS	BOR	GRAPH	HEP	SIL	SEC	SEP	SQUILL	USTIL
1	X												
7													X
8	X	X	X	X	X						X	X	
13		X	X				X		X	X			
14						X		X					

Nail, Fungal Infection Of- See Onychomycosis

Nappy Rash

	CALEND	MEDO	SULPH	CALC	MERC	RHUS T
14	E					
18		X				
21		X	X	X	X	X
22	E					
27			X			

E- External

Narcolepsy- See also Stupor

	BAPT	AETHUSA	ARN	CIMEX	HYDR AC	HYOSC	INDOL	LACH	MAG CAR	NAT SUL	OP	PULS	SULPH
1	X	X	X	X		X	X		X	X		X	X
9								X					
17					X								
19	X										X		

Narcotics, Ailments From– See Ailments from Narcotics

Nasal Septum, Perforation Of

	KALI IOD	AUR	AUR M	KALI BIC	MERC C	MERC I R
1	X					
8		X	X			
11	X					
12						X
14	X			X	X	
17	X	X	X		X	
24				X		

Nausea (Includes Biliousness)

	IPEC	NUX V	ARS	BRY	PULS	ANT C	COCCUL	PHOS	SEP	VER A	TAB	IRIS V	PETR	ANT T	LYC	BELL	CUPR	IGN	ACON	CHAM	SANG	FERR	THER	COLCH	KALI BIC	NAT M	RHUS T
1	**X**	X	X	X	X	X	X		X				X					X		X	X		X	X		X	
2		**X**		**X**								**X**		X	**X**							**X**	X				
3	X		X	X	X																						
4	X	X	X	X	X	X	X		X			**X**	X					X					X	X			
5	X	X	X			X	X		X		X		X	X	X			X					X	X	X		X
6	X	X	X	X	X	X	X	X	X	X	X			X		X	X	X	X		X		X	X		X	X
7	**X**	**X**	**X**	X	**X**	**X**	**X**	X	X	**X**	X	**X**	**X**	**X**	X		X		X	**X**		X			X	**X**	**X**
8	X	X	X	X	X	X	X	X	X	X	X	X	X	X	X	X	X		X	X	X	X	X	X	X	X	X
9	X	X	X	X	X	X	X	X	X	X	X	X	X		X	X		X			X				X		X
10	X	X	X	X	X	X	X	X	X	X						X		X	X	X	X	X		X		X	
11	X	X	X	X	X			X	X	X		X				X	X										
12	X		X	X		X						X		X					X	X		X					
13	**X**	**X**	**X**	**X**	**X**	**X**	**X**	**X**	**X**	**X**	**X**	X	**X**	X	**X**	**X**	**X**	**X**	X	**X**	X	X	**X**		X	**X**	**X**
14	**X**		X	X		X	X	X	X	X		X		X			X				X				X	X	
15	X	X	X	X	X	X	X					X		X	X	X		X		X	X				X		
16	X	X														X											
17	X	X		X	X		X	X	X		X		X	X	X	X			X		X	X	X			X	X
18	X	X		X		X	X	X	X		X						X	X						X	X		
19	**X**	**X**	**X**	X	X	X	**X**	**X**	**X**	**X**	**X**	X	X	X	X		X		X	X	X	X	X	X	X		
20	X	X	X	X	X		X			X	X	X	X			X											
21	X	X	X	X	X						X			X								X		X	X		
22	X	X	X					X		X		X					X				X						
23	X		X			X					X		X				X										
24	X	X			X			X		X	X								X					X			
25	X	X	X	X	X	X		X		X	X		X		X			X					X				X
26	**X**	**X**	X	X	X	X	X	X	X	X			X		X	X	X	X	X	X		X					X
27	X																			X						X	

Necrosis

	MERC CY	SIL	BACILL	CAD IOD	COCCUL	FL AC	KALI IO	LACH	SAL AC	THER
1		X			X	X	X			
2		X	X						X	X
11	X									
16				X						
17	X									
19								X		

Necrosis, Bone

	SIL	PHOS	CALC	SULPH	FL AC	ASAF	CALC FL	AUR	ARS	MERC	MEZ	SABIN	ANGUS	AUR M	BOTHR	CALC IOD	CALC PH	CARB AC	EUPHORB	HEP	KALI IOD	LYC	NIT AC	PLUM	SEC	THER	THUJA
1	X						X										X		X								
2	X														X												
4	X				X		X																				
6	X	X	X	X	X	X		X		X	X					X				X	X	X	X				
7	X	X	X	X	X	X	X							X				X									
8	X	X	X	X	X	X	X		X			X														X	
9								X																			
10	X	X	X	X																							
13	X	X				X			X	X		X	X											X	X		X
14								X																			
24		X									X																
26	X		X	X																							

Necrosis, Bone, Jaw

	ANGUST	EUPHORB	PHOS	SIL
1	X	X		X
14			X	

Necrosis, Bone, Jaw, Lower

	PHOS	ANGUST	SIL	SYMPH
7	X		X	
8	X	X		
10				X
14	X			

Necrosis, Bone, Jaw, Lower, Left

	PHOS	SYMPH
1	X	
7	X	
10		X

Necrosis, Bone, Jaw, Upper

	MERC C	CALC FL	FL AC	SIL
3		X	X	X
7	X			
8	X			

Necrosis, Bone, Mastoid

	CAPS	SIL
6	X	X
24	**X**	

Necrosis, Ossicles

	AUR	FL AC	NIT AC	SIL
1		X		
6	X		X	X

Necrosis, Tibia

	HECLA	PHOS
7	X	
14		X

Nephralgia- See also Colic, Renal

	BERB V	CANTH	TEREB	APIS	BELL	CANN S	COLCH	ACON	ARN	BENZ AC	HEP	NUX V	SULPH	ARG N	ARS	COCCUS	HELON	LYC	OCIM	RHUS T	KALI CAR
1	X	X	X	X	X					X											
2			X														X				
4	X	X	X	X	X			X													
5		X	X																		
6			X						X		X				X					X	
7	X	**X**	X			X	**X**			X	X	X					X	X		X	X
8	X	X		X		X	X		X			X		X	X	X			X		
9	X																				
10	X	X	X	X	X	X	X	X	X	X	X		X	X	X			X	X	X	
11	X									X								X			
13	X	X	X		X	**X**	X	X			X	X	X								**X**
14	X		X	X													X		X		
16	X																				
19		X	X										X			X					
20	X																				
21	X	X						X													
23	X													X							
24	X	X	X						X							X					
25	X																				
26		X			X							X	X								

Nephralgia, Left

	BENZ AC	ALL C	APIS	BERB V	HYDRANG	KALI ARS	KALI CAR	LACH	LACHNAN	MILL	PARIERA	THUJA
10	X	X	X			X						X
13	X								X			
19	X			X	X		X	X			X	
24										X		

Nephralgia, Right

	SARS	NUX V	LYC	BELL	CANN I	OCIM	PHYTO	TEREB
6		X						
10	X				X			
11	X							
13							X	
14	X							
19	X	X	X	X		X		X
21		X	X					

Nephritis

	CANTH	ACON	ARS	PHOS	TEREB	APIS	MERC C	PLUM	MERC	KALI CHL	CANN S	HELL	NUX V	BELL	COLCH	BERB V	APOC	HEP	LYC	ARN	BENZ AC	SULPH	BRY	CHEL	HELON	CHIM
1	X			X			X	X		X		X					X		X		X					
2		X						X	**X**	X	X												X	X		X
3	X	X	X		X	X		X	X			X			X										X	
4	X	X	**X**	**X**	X		**X**	X		X							X									
5	X		X	X	X	X	X	X				X					X								X	
6	X	X	X	X	X	X	X	X	X			X	X	X	X			X	X		X	X	X	X	X	
7	X	X		X	**X**				X		X		X	X		X			X	**X**	**X**		X	X		X
8	X	X	X	X	X	X	X	X	X		X	X	X	X	X	X	X	X	X	X	X	X	X		X	X
9	X						X			X						X										
10	X	X	X	X	X	X	X	X	X	X	X	X	X	X	X	X		X	X	X	X	X	X	X	X	
11	**X**	X	**X**	X	**X**	**X**	**X**	**X**	X	**X**	X	X				**X**		X	X							**X**
12	X	X	**X**	X	X	X	**X**	X	X			X	**X**		X		X					**X**		X		
13	**X**	X							X		**X**			X	X			X				X				
14	X		X	X	X	X				X																
15	X	X											X	X	X					X						
16			X																							
17								X																		
19	X	X	X			X							X	X		X		X								
21	X	X	X			X																				
23	X		X	X		X	X										X									
24									X																	
26		**X**									**X**															
27					X					X																
28	X																									

Nephritis, Interstitial

	AUR M N	GLON	LYC	METH BL	PHOS	PLUM	RHUS AR	SENEG
10					X			
17								X
23	X	X	X	X		X	X	

Nephritis, Right Side

	OCIM	TEREB
14		X
27	X	

Nephrotic Syndrome

	ARS	AM BENZ	APIS	APOC	CALC	DIG	EUP PUR	FERR	FERR PH	NAT M	SIL	TEREB
11	X	X	X	X		X	X					X
21	X							X	X			
29*					X					X	X	

29* Pai PN. Nephrotic syndrome. Brit Hom J, 1969, 58, 94.

Nerve Conduction Delayed

	ALUM	COCCUL	PLUM
19	**X**	X	X

Nerves, Diseases Of

	MAG PH	HYPER	ARG	AUR	KALI PH	PHOS
7	X	**X**			X	
10			X	X		X
22	X					

Nettle Rash- See also Urticaria

	DULC	ANT C	APIS	RHUS T	ACON	ARS	ASTAC F	NAT M	SULPH	ARUM DR	BELL	ELAT	FERR SUL	KALI SUL	IGN	LATRO K	MEDUSA
2	**X**	**X**	**X**			**X**	**X**	**X**	**X**	X		X	X	X		X	X
6			X	X											X		
14	X																
15	X	X		X	**X**						X						

Neuralgia- See also Hyperaesthesia; Pain

	ACON	ARS	CHAM	MAG PH	SPIG	BELL	CHINA	COFF	COLOC	KALM	NAT M	PHOS	PULS	SULPH	CAUST	GELS	MEZ	RHUS T	CIMIC	IGN	MERC	RAN B	STAPHYS	BRY	HYPER	SANG	VER A
1		X	X	X	X	X	X	X			X						X	X	X	X			X			X	
2	**X**	**X**	**X**	**X**	**X**	**X**	**X**	X	**X**	**X**		**X**	**X**	**X**	X	X	**X**					**X**	**X**		X	X	
3			X	X	X											X										X	
4	**X**	**X**	**X**	**X**			X		**X**		X			X				X			X						
5					X			X							X										X		X
6											X																
7	X	X	**X**	**X**	**X**	**X**	X	**X**	**X**	X	X	**X**	X	X	**X**	**X**	X	X		X	X		X				X
8	**X**	**X**	X	X	**X**	**X**	**X**	X	X	X	**X**	**X**	**X**	**X**	X	X	X	**X**	X	**X**	**X**	X	X	**X**		X	X
9	X			X		X			X													X			X	X	
10	X	X	X			X		X											X					X			
11											X																
12	X	**X**		X		X	X	X	X	**X**	X	X	X	X	X	X		X	X	X	X	X		X			X
13	**X**	X	X			X	X	**X**				X	X	X	X			X		**X**	**X**		X				X
14	X	X	X	X	X		X					X													X		
15	X	X	X		X	X	X									X			X					X			
17		X	X	X	X					X			X														
18	X								X																		
19					X		X	X																			
21	X	X		X	X				X								X					X					
22				X																							
23			X			X	X	X		X							X		X								
27										X															X		

Neuralgia, Abdominal- See also Gastralgia

	COLOC	CUPR	DIOSC	NUX V	SIL
1	X				
4	X			X	
8			X		X
9		X			

Neuralgia, Arms- See Pain, Arms

Neuralgia, Aural- See Otalgia

Neuralgia, Brachial

	TEREB	VER A	HYPER	ACON	BRY	CALC FL	KALM	MERC	NUX V	RHUS T	SULPH	ALL C	BELL	BELLIS	CAFF	CALC	CCAL PH	CHAM	COCCUC	CORN F	INDIG	LYC	PARIS	THUJA
2	X		X														X				X		X	
8	X																							
17	X	**X**	X	**X**	**X**	**X**	**X**	**X**	**X**	**X**	**X**	X		X	X			X	X	X				
26		X											X			X						X		X

Neuralgia, Breast- See also Mastalgia

	MUREX	CALAD	CON	ARG	BELL	CALC	CANTH	CHAM	CIMICI	CROT T	KALI CAR	NIT AC	PHOS	PHYTO	RHUS T	TAB	FERR	HYDROC	PHELL	SIL
6	X	X	X	X		X	X		X	X	X	X	X		X	X	X		X	X
7	X	X	X		X			X						X						
8	**X**	X	X	X	X	X	X	X	X	X	X	X	X	X	X	X		X		

Neuralgia, Cervico-Brachial

	ACON	RHUS T	ARN	ARS	FERR	GRAPH	IGN	LYC	PHOS	SEP	STAPHYS	SULPH	VER A	BRY	CHINA	KALM	NUX V	SANG	SPIG
6	X	X	X	X	X	X	X	X	X	X	X	X	X		X				
8	X	X	X	X	X	X	X	X	X	X	X	X	X						
11	X	X												X		X	X	X	X

Neuralgia, Cervico-Occipital

	ACON	BELL	CALC	CAUST	IGN	KALM	LACH	NUX V	PULS	SPIG	SULPH	BRY	CHINA	RHUS T
6	X	X	X	X	X	X	X	X	X	X	X			X
7												X		
8	X	X	X	X	X	X	X	X	X	X	X		X	

Neuralgia, Ciliary- See also Pain, Eye

	MEZ	PRUN S	SPIG	CEDRON	CINNAB	CROT H	NAT M
1	X						
2		X	X	X		X	
4	**X**	**X**	X				X
8				X			
11		X					
13	X						
14	X		X		X	X	
17		X					
19	X		X				
23		X	X	X	X		X
24				X			

Neuralgia, Crural

	STAPHYS	XANTH	COFF	CHAM	COLOC	GNAPH	LIMUL	MAG PH	PHYTO	POD	SULPH
2		X									
5	X	X		X	X	X	X	X			
6	X		X						X		
8	X	X	X							X	X

Neuralgia, Ear- See Otalgia

Neuralgia, Eye- See also Pain, Eye

	SPIG	BELL	CHINA	CINNAB	ASAR	CAUST	CHEL	COLOC	CROT H	GUIAIAC	HAM	HEP	HYOSC	IGN	KALI IOD	KALM	MAG PH	NATM	PH AC	PLUM	PRUN S	RAN B	RUTA	SIL	THUJA			
1								X																				
3															X													
5																					X							
7	X	X	X	X			X		X		X			X		X	X	X						X				
8	X	X	X		X	X				X		X	X						X	X					X			
11	X			X																								
14																							X					
17																						X						
19	X																											

Neuralgia, Facial (Includes Prosopalgia)

	ACON	SPIG	BELL	MAG PH	COLOC	CHAM	ARS	MEZ	PULS	PHOS	PLAT	CHINA	KALM	NUX V	STAPHYS	CAUST	VERBASC	CAPS	CALC	MERC C	VER A	BRY	CEDR	LACH	GELS	MAG CAR	AUR	
1	X	X	X	X	X	X		X		X	X			X	X		X									X		
2												X							X	X								
3	X			X	X																							
4	**X̲**	**X**	X						**X**														X					
5	X	X	X	X	X	X		X					X			X										X		
6	X		X	X		X	X	X	X	X	X	X		X	X	X	X						X	X	X	X		
7	X	X	**X**	X	X	X	X	X	X	X	X	X		X	**X**	**X**		X	**X**	X	**X**			X	X		X	
8	X	X	X	X	X	X	X	X	X	X	X	X	X	X	X	X	X	X	X		X	X						
9		X	X	**X**		X							X														X	
10	X	X	X		X	X	X		X							X				X		X		X				
11	X	X	X	X	X	X	X	X			X	X	X				X	X					X		X			
12	X	X	X	X	X		X			X			X															
13	X	X	X		X	X	**X**	X		X	X	X		X	**X**	X		**X**	**X**		**X**	X					**X**	
14	X	X	X	X			X	X		X	X									X				X	X			
15									X											X								
18	X	X	X	X	X	X	X	X					X	X									X			X		
19		X		X													X											
21		X			X		X						X				X											
23	X	X			X																							
24	X																											
26	X	X	X		X	X		X	X	X	X	X		X	X			X			X	X						
29*				X					X																			

29* Mojaver YN, et al. Individualized homeopathic treatment of trigeminal neuralgia: an observational study. Homeopathy. 2007 Apr; 96(2):82-6.

Neuralgia, Facial, Left Sided (Includes Prosopalgia, Left Sided)

	SPIG	COLOC	LACH	NAT CAR	CHEL	CHINA	COLCH	DULC	GLON	HELL	IGN	KALI BIC	KALI CY	KALI MUR	MAG CAR	MAG PH	MEZ	PLANTAG	PULS	SULPH	THUJA	VALER
1	X	X													X						X	
6				X						X												
7	X	X			X	X		X	X	X						X	X					
8	X	X	X				X				X	X	X	X				X	X	X		X
9	X																					
10		X	X																			
14	X																					
21	X																					
24				X																		
26			X																			

Neuralgia, Facial, Right Sided (Includes Prosopalgia, Right Sided)

	BELL	CACT	KALM	MAG PH	ARAN D	CANTH	CARB AC	CAUST	CHIN S	COCCIN	KALI PH	KALM	MEZ	PHOS	PULS	VERBASC
1	X															
5					X											
6			X													
8		X	X	X		X	X	X	X	X	X		X	X		X
11		X														
12	X															
19				X												
21												X			X	
26	X															

Neuralgia, Head- See also Headache

	ABROT	AESC	BELL	COLOC	KALI CY	NIT AC	SCUT	SPIG	STANN	VER A	ZINC PH
1				X	X		X				
8	X	X				X		X	X	X	
12			X								
14											X

Neuralgia, Heart- See Pain, Heart
Neuralgia, Herpetic- See Shingles
Neuralgia, Hip- See Coxalgia

Neuralgia, Infraorbital- See also Pain, Eye

	ARG N	CHINA	BELL	GELS	IRIS V	MAG PH	NUX V	ARS	COLOC	HYDROC	MAG CAR	OSMIUM	PLAT	VERBASC	ZINC
1	X	X				X									
4			**X**					**X**							
6		X		X		X	X								
7	X			X	X				X	X					
8	X	X	X		X		X				X		X	X	X
14												X			

Neuralgia, Infraorbital, Left

	ARG N	ARS	GLON	LACH
6				X
7		X	X	
8	X			

Neuralgia, Intercostal

	RAN B	MEZ	ARN	CIMICI	RHUS T	MAG PH	ARS	BRY	ASC T	CALC	CARB V	CAUST	CHEL	CHINA	MERC	PHOS	SEP	SPIG	SULPH	ZINC
2						**X**			X											X
4	X	**X**	X	X	X															
5	X		X		X			X					X							
6		X	X	X	X		X	X		X	X	X		X	X		X	X	X	
7	X	X				X							X			X				X
8	X		X	X	X	X	X	X		X	X	X		X	X	X	X	X	X	
9	X	X																		
12	X						X													
17	X								X											
18		X																		
19		X																		
21	X																			
24				X																

Neuralgia, Jaw

	PHOS	AMPHIS	CALC	CAUST	CIMICI	COFF	EUPHORB	KALI CY	MEZ	RHOD	VERBASC	STAPHYS
6	X				X							
7	X								X			
11		X	X	X			X	X		X	X	
12						X						X

Neuralgia, Left Sided

	COLOC	SPIG	LACH	ACON	ARS	ASAF	COLCH	LOB I	MAG CAR	MEZ	NAT M	VERBASC	ZIZ
1		X											
6	X		X			X				X			
8		X					X	X					X
11	X	X	X	X								X	
12	X				X						X		
18	X	X							X				

Neuralgia, Malar, Right

	CAPS	CIMICI	PARIS
4	X		
5		X	X

Neuralgia, Maxillary

	CIMICI	HEP	NAT M	SANG	SULPH
6	X	X	X	X	
12					X

Neuralgia, Neck- See also Pain, Neck

	TAB
6	X
7	X

Neuralgia, Orbital- See also Pain, Eye

	ASAF	BELL	GELS	SPIG	ATROP S	CARB AC	CEDRON	CHEL	CHINA	CINNAB	HEP	HYDROC	KALI BIC	MAG PH	NAT M	PLAT
2	X											X				
4				X												
7		X			X											X
8						X	X	X	X				X		X	
10				X												
12			X													
14		X	X							X	X					
17	X															
18														X		

Neuralgia, Ovaries- See also Ovaralgia

	HAM	LIL T	COLOC	CIMICI	BELL	XANTH	LYC
1		X				X	
4	X	X	X				
7		X	X				**X**
8	X	X	X	**X**	X		
12	X			X	X		
23	X					X	

Neuralgia, Periodic

	CHINA	BOLET	CHEL	CHIO	COLOC	GELS	KALI BIC	NAJA	NICC SUL	PARTHEN	TOXICOP	SULPH
2									X	X	X	
8	<u>**X**</u>						X					X
23		X	X	X	X	X		X				

Neuralgia, Post-herpetic– See Herpes Zoster
Neuralgia, Rectum- See Pain, Rectum
Neuralgia, Right Sided

	MAG PH	BELL	SANG	IRIS V	CACT	CAUST	COLOC	EUP PUR	HEP	KALM	MERC	PULS	RHOD	SULPH	ZINC
1	X		X												
6		X				X	X						X		X
8	X	X						X	X	X					
11	X		X		X						X	X			
12	X	X												X	
18	X														
19				**X**											

Neuralgia, Shoulder

	STAPHYS	ANAC	PHYTO
5		X	
7	X		
8	**X**		
12			X

Neuralgia, Spermatic Cord- See also Pain, Spermatic Cord

	OL AN	OX AC
1	X	X
7	X	
23		X

Neuralgia, Stump- See also Pain, Stump (Post-Amputation) (AKA Phantom Limb Pain)

	ALL S	HYPER	SYMPH	AMM C	AMM M	ASAF	CALC	SABAL	STAPHYS
1	X								
3	X								
4	X	X							
7	X								
8	X		X		X	X	X		
14	X								
17	X								
19	X	X							X
21		X							
24			X						
28	X	X		X				X	

Neuralgia, Subcostal

	ARG N	ZINC
2		X
14	X	

Neuralgia, Supraorbital (Includes Pain, Eye, Over)

	KALI BIC	CEDRON	STANN	ARS	MAG PH	TEREB	ARG N	CARB V	IRIS V	LACH	SANG	SEP	SULPH	URAN N
1		X	X		X		X							
2						X								
4		X	X											
6		X	X		X			X						
7	X		X	X	X	X	X	X	X	X	X			X
8	X			X		X				X				X
9	X			X					X					
10													X	
13												X	X	
14	X													
15												X		
17		X									X			
18	X													

Neuralgia, Supraorbital, Left (Includes Pain, Eye, Left, Above)

	SPIG	SULPH	ACON	ARS	EUGEN	KALI IOD	LAC FEL	NUX V	SIL	THUJA
1				X		X				
7					X			X		
8										X
10		X	X						X	
19							X			
21	X									
24	X									
26		X								

Neuralgia, Supraorbital, Right

	CARB AC	CHEL	CHINA	GELS	KALI BIC	LYC	RAN B	SANG	SIL
7	X	X	X						X
18					X	X			
21							X		
22								X	
25				X					

Neuralgia, Teeth- See Toothache

Neuralgia, Temporal

	IRIS V
6	X
7	X

Neuralgia, Testes– See also Pain, Testes

	HAM	COLOC	AUR	BERB V	BELL	CALC	CLEM	IGN	MAG PH	OL AN	OX AC	SABAD
1	X	X	X					X	X	X		
7	X	X		X	X							
8	X	X	X	X		X	X				X	X
12	X											

Neuralgia, Tongue- See also Pain, Tongue

	AGAR M	ARS	MANG AC	MANG
1	X	X		X
8			X	

Neuralgia, Uterus

	BELL	CHAM	KALI CAR	PLAT	PULS	CIMICI	COCCUL	CON	GELS	ASAF	SABAD	SEP
1								X				
7	**X**	X	X				X		X	**X**		
8				X	X	X	X					
12						X						
13	**X**	**X**	**X**	**X**	**X**			X	X		**X**	**X**

Neurasthenia (Includes Nervous Exhaustion)

	PH AC	KALI PH	PIC AC	PHOS	GELS	NAT M	SIL	ZINC	ARS	NUX V	CHINA	IGN	ANAC	SEP	CALC	ARG N	ARN	AVENA	COCCUL	OX AC	SEL	LACH
1		X	X			X	X	X				X	X	X	X	X			X			
2	X	X	X					X										X		X		**X**
3	X	X				X						X	X					X				
4	**X**	X	**X**	**X**	**X**	**X**	X	**X**	X	X		X	X	X		X	X	X		X	X	X
5					X																	
6	X	X	X	X	X	X	X	X	X	X	X	X		X	X		X		X		X	X
8	X	X	X	X	X	X	X	X	X	X	X	X	X	X	X	X	X		X		X	
9	X		X	X					X	X	X						X			X		
10	X	X	X	X	X	X	X		X				X									
12	X			X					X	X	X											
13	**X**			**X**			**X**		X	X	**X**	X			**X**				X			
14	X					X																
15	X			X	X					X	X			X								
16	X																					
17		X	X																	X		
18	X	X			X			X													X	
21					X																	
23		X	X					X								X		X				
24							X															
27		X																				

Neuritis

	HYPER	ACON	ARS	BELL	RHUS T	PHOS	LED	PLUM	ARN	CIMICI	ALL C	CACT	CALC	CAUST	COLOC	HEP	KALM	LACH	MAG PH	MERC	NUX V	PHYSO	PULS	SIL	SULPH	ANANTH		
1		X		X				X											X			X						
2			X																									
4	**X**	**X**		X	X		X	X	**X**	**X**												X				**X**		
6											X																	
7	X	X	X	**X**	X	**X**						X				X	X			X	X		X	X	X			
8		X	X	X	X	X	X		X			X	X	X	X	X	X	X		X	X		X		X			
10			X		X	X	X	X		X			X	X										X				
14	X										X																	
17	X																											
21		X	X												X			X	X									
23	X																											
24	X																											

Neuritis, Multiple- See Polyneuritis

Neuritis, Optic

	ARS	APIS	BELL	PHOS	NUX V	PLUM	PULS	NAT M	AUR	CARB SUL	GELS	HAM	LACH	MERC	TAB	THYROID	VER V											
1			X				X					X	X				X											
2	**X**														X	X												
3	X	X		X	X					X																		
6						X																						
7			X	X			X																					
8			X																									
11		X												X														
19	X			X	X	X		**X**	X		X																	
21		X																										

Neuritis, Peripheral

	BEN D	NUX V	PLUM																									
2	X																											
17		X	X																									

Neuritis, Rheumatic

	RHUS T	CACT	FERR PH	KALI MUR																								
4	**X**		X	X																								
8		X																										

Neuroma (Includes Moreton's Neuroma)

	ARN	CALC	HYPER	STAPHYS	BENZ AC	CALEND	RUTA	SIL
1	X		X	X				
7		X						
28	E	X	X	X	E	X	E	E

E- External

Night Terrors

	CALC	BELL	KALI BR	KALI PH	STRAM	ACON	CINA	SIL	ARS	AUR	BAPT	BRY	CAUST	CHAM	HYOSC	IGN	LYC	NIT AC	NUX V	PHOS	PULS	SOL NIG	SULPH	SYPH
2	X			X						X												X		
3																								**X**
5	X		X	X	X		X	X	X				X	X		X						X		
6																	X							
7	X							X			X	X		X				X					X	
8	X	X			X	X		X	X	X		X	X			X	X	X	X	X	X		X	
9			X				X								X									
10		X													X				X					
11				X							X													
12	X	X					X																	
14		X		X		X																		
18			X		X															X				
19					X																			
21			X																					
27																					X			
28						X																		

Night Sweats- See Perspiration, Night

Nipples, Cracked- See Cracks, Nipples

Nipples, Retracted

	SARS	ARS I	HYDRAST	LAPIS	NUX M
7		X			X
8	X				
9	X				
13	X				
24			X	X	

Nocturia- See Enuresis, Nocturnal

Nodes

	STILLING	SIL	AMM PH	BENZ AC	KALI BIC	KALI IOD
2	X	**X**			**X**	**X**
5				X		
8	X	X	X	X		
23	X		X			

Nodes, Arthritic (Includes Nodules)

	LED	BENZ AC	LYC	CAUST	CALC	GRAPH	AMM PH	ANT C	AUR	DIG	RHOD	SABIN	STAPHYS	BRY	CALC FL	CARB A	CARB V	GUAIAC	LITH C	SIL
6	X	X				X	X													X
8	X	X	X	X	**X**	X	X	X	X	X	X	X	X	X		X	X	X		X
9	X	X																		
12								X												
13	**X**	X	**X**	X	X	**X**		X	**X**	**X**	**X**	**X**	**X**	X		X	X			
14	X																			
17																			X	
19		X	**X**	X											X			X	X	
24															X					
25	X						X													
26		X	X	X	X															

Nodes, Bone

	STILLING	KLAI BIC	CALC FL	NUX V	AUR	CAUST	FL AC	GUAIAC	HEP	KALI IOD	LED	PHOS	PHYTO	RHUS T	SIL
1	X														
2	X	**X**		**X**											
3		X	X									X		X	
4								X			X				
7			X			X			X	X			X		
8	X				X										X
14							X								

Nodes, Eyelids

	STAPHYS	CON	SIL	THUJA
1	X	X		
3	X	X		
4	X			
7	X		X	X

Nodes, Fingers

	CALC	DIG	GRAPH	LED	STAPHYS	AGNUST	ANT C	LYC	RHOD
5							X		
13	**X**	**X**	**X**	**X**	**X**	X		X	X

Nodes, Gums

	PH AC	BERB V	NAT SUL	PLUM	STAPHYS
1	X				
13	X	X	X	X	X

Nodes, Joints

	BENZ AC	LED	LYC	RHOD	SABIN	STAPHYS	LITH C	AMM PH	BRY	CALC	CARB A	CAUST	FORMICA	GUAIAC	SIL
7	**X**	X	X	X	X	X	**X**		X	X			X		X
8	X		X	X	X	X		X			X	X		X	
14		X													

Nodes, Leg

	ANGUST	AUR	PHYTO	STILL
7	X		X	
8		X		X

Nodes, Wrist

	CALC	LED	RHOD
13	**X**	**X**	X

Noma

	ARS	ALUMEN	CARB V	KALI PH	GUAREA	CALC	CHINA	CON	ELAT	HELL	SEC	SIL	SOL T A	SULPH
2	X	X		X									X	
6	X		X	X			X			X	X			
8	X	X	X		**X**	X		X	X			X		X

Nose, Bones, Diseases Of

	MERC I R	ASAF	AUR	RHEUM	SIL
3	X			X	X
8	X	X	X		

Nosebleed- See Epistaxis

Nose, Congestion (Includes Nose, Blocked; Nose, Obstructed; Nose, Stopped)

	NUX V	ARUM T	DULC	LYC	SAMB	SIL	ARS	AMM C	CARB V	KALI BIC	NAT M	CALC	CASUT	PULS	SULPH	ALL C	HYDRAST	KALI IOD	NAT CAR	AMBRA	AUR	GRAPH	MANG					
5	X			X	X					X		X		X		X	X	X			X							
6	X												X															
7	**X**	**X**	X	X	**X**	X		X	X		X	X			X	X	X	X			**X**	X	X					
8		X		X				**X**					X		X				X	X								
10	**X**		X	X			X		X																			
13	X	X	X	**X**	X	X	**X**	**X**	X	X	X	**X**	**X**	X	**X**			X	X	**X**	X	**X**	**X**					
14	X	X	X					X		X				**X**														
15	X						X										X											
17		X	X		X	X	X	X	X										X	X			X					
18			X		X					X							X											
19				X		X				X			X		X	X		X										
21	X	X				X					X																	
22											X			X														
24		X				X	X				X	X				X			X			X						
25	X		X		X		X		X																			

Nose, Diseases Of

	NUX V	KALI BIC	SIL	ARN	BELL	BOR	CAPS	CARB A	GRAPH	OX AC																		
2	**X**	X	X	**X**	**X**	**X**	**X**	**X**	X	**X**																		
9	X	X	X																									

Nose, Dryness Of

	BELL	STICTA	BRY	CALC	NAT M	PHOS	SIL	SULPH	ARS	KALI BIC	NUX M	SAMB	AGAR M	AMBRA	BAR C	CAMPH	CIMEX	COCCUS	DROS	KALI CAR	LYC	MEZ	NIT AC	NUX V	RHUS T	SANG	SPONG	ZINC
7		**X**				X	X	X	X	X	**X**	**X**					X			X			X	X	X		X	
8																			X									
9	X																											
10	X		X													X												
11	X																											
12		X																										X
13	**X**	X	X	**X**	**X**	**X**	**X**	**X**	X	X	X		X	X	X		X	X	X	X	X	X	X		X			X
17	X	X	X	X	X	X	X	X	X	X		X	X	X	X	X		X			X	X		X		X	X	
21				X	X																					X		
22			X																									

Numbness

	ACON	OX AC	PLAT	CON	COCCUL	PHOS	RHUS T	AMBRA	NAT M	SEC	IGN	ARS	NUX V	CARB V	CIC	GRAPH	LYC	PLUM	CALC PH	CARB A	CHAM	CHINA	KALI CAR	OP	PETR	PULS	SIL	TAR H
1	X	X	X	X		X	X	X		X	X	X			X													X
2	**X**	**X**	**X**	**X**		**X**				**X**	**X**	**X**			**X**			**X**										
3	X	X		X				X	X	X					X						X							
4	X																											
5			X																									
6		X											X	X														X
7	**X**		X		X	X	X	X	X		X		X	X		**X**	**X**			**X**	X	X	**X**	X	X	X	**X**	
8	**X**	X	**X**	X	X	**X**	X	X		X	X	X	**X**	X	X	X	X	X	X	X	X	X	X	X	X	X	X	X
9	X		X	X	X		X									X	X									X		
10								X																				
11																			X									
13	X			X	**X**	X	X	X	X	**X**	**X**		**X**	**X**		X	X			**X**		X	**X**	X	X	X	**X**	
14	X			X					X			X							X									X
15	X						X																					
17	X	X			X		X		X										X			X			X			
18																					X							
19		X	**X**	X	X	X			X									X										
21	X																	X						X				
22		X																										
24												X																
27		X																										

Numbness, Arm, Left

	RHUS T	ACON	CACT	LACH	CIMICI	GLON	KALM	SUMBUL	AMBRA	ARG N	ARN	AUR	BAR C	BUFO	CINNAB	DIG	LAC C	LATRO M	MILL	NAJA	NUX V	PALLAD	PULS					
1	X	X	X								X	X																
4	X	X					**X**									X							X					
5	X				X																							
6	X			X																								
7	X	X	X	X	X	X		X	X				X	X			X				X							
11							X																					
13		X				X									X				X			X						
14			X	X																								
17		X	X		X			X		X																		
19	X		X	X		X												X		X								

Numbness, Arm, Right

	ACT S	CHINA	HEP	KALI BIC	LYC	MERC I F	NAT M	NIT AC	PHYTO																			
1	X																											
4									X																			
7		X	X		X		X	X																				
13				X		X																						

Numbness, Arms

	COCCUL	LYC	NUX V	PHOS	KALI CAR	AMBRA	ARG N	GRAPH	SEP	ACON	CROC	RHUS T	SIL
1	X												
7	**X**	**X**	X	X	X	X		X	X	**X**		**X**	
13		**X**	X	X	**X**	X		X	X		**X**		**X**
14	X			X			X						
17			X										
19							X						

Numbness, Extremities

	SEC	ACON	PHOS	PLUM	APIS	BELL	CAUST	CROT H	GELS	GRAPH	HOANG	IGN	LATRO M	LED	LYSS	NAT M	NUX V	OENANTH	OP	PETR	RHUS T	SEP	SULPH	TEREB	VER V
1	X										X			X										X	
4	X								X																
5																		X							
6	X		X	X	X																				
8				X				X		X			X		X					X		X			
9							X																		
12		X																							
14		X														X									
15																									X
19												X													
21			X																						
26	X					X											X		X		X		X		
27		X																							

Numbness, Face

	ACON	ARS	COCCUL	GELS	PLAT
14	X				X
17	X				
19		X	X	X	

Numbness, Feet

	PHOS	ALUM	COCCUL	HELON	NAT M	ARS	PHYSO	ACON	CAUST	COCA	COLOC	NUX V
1							X			X		
3		X										
6	X	X		X								
7	X		X	X		**X**		X	X	X	X	
8	**X**			X			**X**					
9											X	
10		X										
13			X		X							X
14					X			X				
15												X
19	X		X		X				X			
24						X						

Numbness, Fingers

	SIL	PHOS	ACON	CAUST	NAT M	LACH	PARIS	LYC	AMYL N	APIS	BAR C	BELL	CARB A	CIMEX	CON	DIG	FERR	IOD	LATH	MUR AC	SEC	ANAC	RHUS T
1			X		X	X															X		
4	X																						
5	X	X		X		X	X			X											X		
6	X	X										X											
7	X	X	X	X			X	**X**	X		X		X	X	X	X	X	X		X			**X**
8	X								X			X										**X**	
9					X																		
10	X																						
13		X	X	X	X		X	X			X		X	X		X	X	X		X			
14			X		X	X				X													
19		X		X											X				X				
21																			X				

Numbness, Forearms

	ARG N	FL AC	NUX V
1		X	
13			X
19	X		

Numbness, Genitals, Male

	AMBRA	GRAPH	BAR C	BERB V	MERC	PLAT
5	X	X			X	X
7		X				
8			X			
13	X			X		

Numbness, Hand, Left

	CUPR AC	GRAPH	LYC	MERC SU	RHUS T
6	X				
7		X	X		X
13				X	

Numbness, Hand, Right

	CYCL	DULC	FERR PH	GELS	HEP	SEC
6						X
7		X	X	X	X	
13	X					

Numbness, Hands

	PHOS	COCCUL	COCA	COLCH	HYOSC	LACH	NUX V	ACON	APIS	CAUST	LYC	MEZ	RAPH	CROC
1		X	X			X							X	
6	X				X									
7	X	X	X	X		X	X	X		X	X	X		
8			X	X	X									
10									X					
13	X				X		X				X	X		**X**
14	X	X		X		X		X	X				X	
15							X							
19	X	X								X				

Numbness, Head

	ARS	ASAF	GRAPH	STAPHYS
3		X		
8			X	
19	X			X

Numbness, Heels

	ALUM	IGN
1	X	X
4	X	
6	X	
8	X	
17	X	

Numbness, Legs

	COLOC	NAT M	ACON	NUX V	PIC AC	PLUM	LYC	RHUS T	ARG N	CALC	CALC PH	CON	CROT H	DIADEM	GNAPH	HYPER	KALI CAR	LAC C	MERC C	MORPH	ONOS	OP	OX AC	PHOS	PULS	SULPH	TAR H
1																				X							X
4					X																			X			
6				X		X																					
7	X	X	X	X			**X**	**X**	X	X	X		X	X		X	X		X			X			X		
8			X		X																						
9	X	X																									
14		X																X									
17																					X		X			X	
19						X						X			X												
25	X																										

Numbness, Left Sided

	LACH	SUMBUL
9		X
19	X	

Numbness, Limbs

	ACON	HYOSC	PHOS	AMBRA	ARS	GLON	NAT M	NUX M	NUX V	OX AC	PLUM	PULS	RHUS T	SEC	SEP	VER V
1		X								X						
3				X												
4			X													
6		X				X	X			X				X		X
7	X		X	X	X	X	X	X			X	X	X	X	X	
8			X		X			X	X						X	
10	X											X				
11	X															
12											X					
14													X			
15									X							X
16		X														

Numbness, Lip

	NAT M	PLAT
19		X
21	X	

Numbness, Mouth

	ACON	AMBRA	BOV	INDIGO	JATR	MAG SUL	NAT SUL	PLAT
13		X	X	X	X	X	X	
19								X
21	X							

Numbness, Nose

	NAT M	MEDO
17	X	X
21	X	

Numbness, Shoulder, Left

	RHUS T	ARN
1	X	X
4	X	

Numbness, Single Parts

	ALUM SIL	AMBRA
1	X	
10		X

Numbness, Soles

	RAPH	ALUM	BRY	LIMUL	OLEAND	SEP
1	X	X				
5				X		
13			X		X	X
14	X					

Numbness, Sole, Left

	CUPR AC
6	X
7	X

Numbness, Spine

	NUX V
4	X
7	X

Numbness, Toes

	CON	ACON	CAUST	CHAM	PHOS	CALC	CHEL	GRAPH	PIC AC	SEC	SIL
4											X
5	X	X	X		X	X	X	X		X	
7	X		X	X							
10		X									
13				X	X						
14									X		
19	X										

Numbness, Tongue (Includes Numbness, Tongue, One-Sided)

	NAT M	GELS	HELL	HYOSC	ZINC	ACON	BENZ AC	CALC PH	COLCH	CROT H	FL AC	IGN	LITH M	NUX M	RHEUM
1			X	X											
3													X		
6	X				X										
7		**X**	X	X		**X**		X	X	X	X			X	X
8					X		X								
14	X														
19	X	**X**										X			
21	X														

Nyctalopia- See also Blindness, Night

	SIL	PHOS	SULPH	HELL	NUX V	BELL	ACON	BOTHR	CON	CYCL	GELS	FERR	HYOSC	MERC	NIT	PETROS	RAN B	STRAM	STRYCH	VER A
1								X												
2				X	X	**X**							X			X	X		X	X
7	X	X		X								X								
8	X	X	X		X		X		X	X	X			X	X			X		
24	X	X	X																	
26	**X**	X	X																	

Nymphomania- See Sexual Desire, Increased

Nystagmus

	AGAR M	BELL	HYOSC	MAG PH	PHYSO	GELS	RAT	IOD	NUX V	AMM M	ARG N	BENZ N	CALC	CIC	COCCUL	IGN	JAB	KALI BR	KALI IOD	PETR	PULS	RHUS T	SANTON	STANN	STRAM			
1				X																								
2	X					X						X							X									
6		X	X		X																							
8	X	X	X	X	X		X		X					X		X	X	X			X		X					
9								X			X																	
13			X				**X**			**X**										X		X		X				
17	X	X		X				X	X				X		X										X			
19	**X**					**X**																						
24	X				X																							

Obesity (AKA Adiposis; Adiposity; Polysarcia)

	CALC	GRAPH	CAPS	FERR	FUCUS	THYROID	PHYTO	AMM BR	ANT C	AUR	SULPH	CALC ARS	AMM M	AMM C	ARS	ASAF	BLATTA	CUPR	KALI BIC	KALI CAR	LYC	PULS	THUJA					
1	X	X			X	X			X	X			X															
2	**X**	X	X		X	X	**X**	X		X		**X**				X												
3	X	X	X		X	X	X	X	X								X											
4	X	X																										
5	X	X																										
6	X			X							X																	
7	**X**	**X**	**X**	**X**			**X**	X		X	X	X	X		X	X		X	X	X	X	X	X					
8	X	X	X	X	X			X	X	X	X	X	X	X	X	X		X			X	X	X					
9	X	X	X			X	X																					
10	X	X												X					X									
11	X																											
13	**X**		**X**	**X**					X		X							X			X	X						
14		X				X																						
17		X	X										X	X														
18	X	X							X		X									X			X					
19		X			X	X											X											
21	X	X	X	X				X												X								
22		X																										
23		X			X					X		X					X											
24					X														X									
25	X					X	X																					
28	X	X																										

Obstruction, Intestines- See also Peristalsis, Reduced

	PLUM	OP	NUX V	ACON	COLOC	CUPR	LACH	ARS	BELL	BRY	CAUST	RHUS T	CHAM
1	X	X	X	X			X		X		X	X	
2	**X**	X											
6	X				X	X							
7	X	**X**					X				X		
8	X	X	X	X	X	X	X	X	X	X		X	
15	X	X	**X**	**X**				**X**		X			**X**
24	**X**	**X**	**X**		X	X							

Obstruction, Liver

	CHEL	CHIO	BRY	CHINA	NUX M
1		X	X		
9	X				
13				X	X
14	X				
19		X			

Obstruction, Portal Circulation- See also Circulation, Portal, Poor

	NUX V	SEP	AESC	CARB V	SULPH
6		X			
8	X	X		X	X
10	X				
18		X			
19	X		X		

Odontalgia- See Toothache

Oedema- See also Swelling (AKA Dropsy)

	APIS	ARS	APOC	DIG	HELL	CHINA	TEREB	LYC	COLCH	PHOS	RHUS T	BRY	DULC	KALI CAR	NAT M	SULPH	CALC	LACH	STROPH	CANTH	FERR	ACON	CARD M	LED	MERC
1	X	X	X	X	X	X	X	X	X	X	X		X					X	X		X				
2	**X**	**X**	**X**	**X**		X	**X**	X	X	X	X	X	X	X	X		**X**	X	**X**			**X**	X		
3	X	X	X		X	X	X	X		X	X					**X**									
4	**X**	**X**	**X**	**X**	**X**	X	X	X	X		X			X				**X**	X	X					
5															X		X								
6	X	X				X	X	X	X	X	X	X	X				X			X			X	X	X
7	**X**	**X**	X	**X**	**X**	X	**X**	**X**	**X**	X	X	X	X	X	X	X	X	X		X			X	X	X
8	**X**	**X**	**X**	X	X	X	X	**X**	**X**	X	X	X	**X**	X		X		X		X				X	X
9	X	X	X	X	X				X			X			X						X				
10	X	X			X		X		X	X	X			X					X						
11	X		X	X			X	X															X		
12	X	X	X	**X**	X							X				X				X					
13	X	**X**	X	**X**	**X**	**X**	X	**X**	X	X		X	**X**	X	X	**X**	X	X		X	X	X		X	X
14	**X**	X		X		X	X				X										X	X			
15	X	X			X	X				X												X			X
16	X	X	X	X		X																			
17	X		X	X															X						
18	X											X		X											
19			X																					X	
21	X	X													X						X				
22	X																								
23	X		X	X	X																				
24	**X**													X											
25															X										
26	X	X	X		X	X		X	X				X			X					X	X			X
27	X																X						X		
28	X		X																						

Oedema, Abdomen- See also Ascites

	ANT C	APIS	ARS
4	**X**		
11		X	
21			X

Oedema, Ankles- See also Swelling, Ankles

	ARS	FERR	STRONT C	ACETAN	ANT T	APIS	CRAT	CHINA	HAM	LACH	MEDO	MUR AC	VIP	URT U
1	X	X									X		X	X
4												X		
12	X	X						X						
14			X											
17			X	X										
19					X									
21	X					X			X					
25							X			X				

Oedema, Cardiac

	DIG	ADONIS	CACT	COLLIN	LAC D	LACH	ACON	ARN	CAFF	CRAT	IBER	KALI MUR	LYC	NAT M	PRUN S	STROPH
7	X		X	**X**	**X**	**X**						X		X	X	
10													X			
11	X	X					X		X	X						X
14	X															
16			X													
17		X									X					
27								X								

Oedema, Cardiac, Origin Of

	ARS	DIG	LACH	LYC	APOC	LAC D	CONVAL	AUR M	ADONIS	APIS	ARS I	BRY	CACT	CARB V	CHIN ARS	COLCH	CRAT	FL AC	HELL	KALI MUR	NAT M	PHASEOL	PRUN S	RHUS T	SQUILL	STROPH	VIP
1	X	X	X		X	X	X				X											X					
3	X			X																				X			
4	X	X																									
5		X			X				X								X									X	
6	X		X												X												
7	**X**	X	**X**	**X**	X	**X**	X	**X**		X		X	X			X		X	X	X	X		X		X		
17																											X
26	X			X										X													

Oedema, Cerebral

	APIS	ARS	BELL	CUPR AR	DIG	HELL	LYC	MERC	NAT M	ZINC
4	X				X		X			
6		X								
8		X								
12	X		X			X		X		
14				X					X	
18	X									
26										X

Oedema, Chest

	ARS	DIG	APIS	HELL	BRY	MERC SU	CARB V	COLCH	KALI CAR	SENEG	SPIG	AMM C	AUR	CHINA	DULC	FL AC	LYC	OP	RAN B	SANG	SQUILLA	STANN
1			X																X			
4						X																
12	X	X		X	X																	
13	X	X	X	**X**	X	X	**X**	**X**	**X**	**X**	X		X	X	X	X	X	X		X	X	X
15	X	X	X									X										

Oedema, Conjunctiva

	APIS	ARG N
4	X	
8		X

Oedema, Extremities- See also Swelling, Extremities

	APIS	CACT	ARS	CHINA	COCCUL	FERR	SENEC	STROPH
1	X	X		X				
4	X							
8			X		X		X	
9	X							
10								X
11						X		
12	X							
14	X							
16		X						
25	X							

Oedema, Eyes- See also Swelling, Eyes, Around

	APIS	ARS	KALI CAR	ARG N	ARS I	EUPHR	GRAPH	KALI IOD	MERC C	PHOS	PRUN S	RHEUM
1		X			X							
6	X	X								X		X
9		X						X				
10	X		X									
11	X											
14	X	X	X	X		X	X		X			
18											X	
28	X											

Oedema, Eyelids- See also Swelling, Eyelids

	KALI CAR	APIS	ARS	CROT H	MERC C	RHUS T	CALC	GRAPH	KALI BIC	PHOS	PHYTO	TELL
4	X											
6	X	X		X		X	X					
7	X	X	X	X	X	X		X	X	X	X	X
14					X							
18		X	X									
19	X											

Oedema, Eyelids, Lower

	BRY	PHOS	ARS	ASPARA	CACT	DIG
5		X				X
6	X	X				
8				X	X	
18			X			
24	X					

Oedema, Eyelids, Upper

	APIS	KALI CAR	CON	NAT CAR	PHOS
4					X
5	X	X	X	X	
6		X			
17	X				

Oedema, Eyes, Under

	APIS	ARS	PHOS	BRY	KALI CAR	OLEAND	PULS
1	X						
4		X					
6			X				
13	X	X	X	X	X	X	X

Oedema, Face

	APIS	ARS	PHOS	OP	LYC	CALC	FERR	MERC	AMM C	BELL	BRY	KALI CAR	APOC	AUR	CHAM	COCCUL	COLCH	CROT H	HELL	IPEC	SEP	VER V	CHINA	HYOSC	NAT CAR	SAMB	SPIG	
1	X	X																										
3	X		X									X	X															
4	X		X																									
6	X	X	X	X	X	X	X	X	X					X		X				X								
7		X	X		X			X									X	X	X									
8	X				X		X											X										
9	X	X				X																						
10				X																	X							
11	X						X																					
12		X																										
13	X	**X**	**X**	**X**	X	X		X	**X**	**X**	**X**	**X**		X	X	X	X		X	X	X		**X**	**X**	**X**	**X**	**X**	
14		X																				X						
15	X	X		X						X	X																	
17																						X						
24													X															
26															X													

Oedema, Feet

	ARS	MERC	APIS	LYC	CHINA	FERR	ARG	NIT AC	PHOS	PLUM	RHUS T	STROPH	SULPH
1	X		X									X	
3		X											
4	X												
6		X		X			X	X					
7	X		X	X	X	X		X	X	X			
8	**X**	X		X	**X**	**X**			X		X		X
10							X				X		
12	X												
14		X											
17												X	
21	X		X										
26										X			X

Oedema, Foot, Left

	KALI ARS	KALI CAR
6		X
10	X	

Oedema, Glottis

	APIS	CHINA	STRAM	ARS	ARUM T	CHLOR	CROT H	BELL	IGN	KALI IOD	MERC	SANG	STAPHYS	CHIN ARS	HIPPOZ	HYOSC	IOD	KALI BR	PILO	VIP
4						**X**														
7	**X**	X	X	X	X		X	X		X										
8	**X**	**X**	**X**	X	X		X	X	X		X	X	X			X		X		
17	X	X	X	X	X	X	X	X	X	X	X	X	X	X	X		X		X	X

Oedema, Hand, Left

	CACT
6	X
8	X
19	X

Oedema, Hands

	ARS	BOV	CACT	CALC ARS	GRAPH	LYC	NAT CHL
1					X		X
6						X	
8			X	X			
12	X						
18		X					

Oedema, Hepatic Origin

	LYC	ARS	CHINA	MUR AC	APIS	APOC	AUR M	CARD M	CHIM	FERR	FL AC	LAC D	MERC
1	X			X		X						X	
3	X	X			X								
4	X			X									
7	X		X				X	X	X		X		
26	X	X	X							X			X

Oedema, Joints (AKA Hydrarthrus)

	IOD	PULS	ACON	ANT C	ARS	BRY	CALC	CON	DIG	KALM	LYC	MERC	RHUS T	SIL	SULPH
8	X	X		X	X	X	X	X	X	X	X	X	X	X	X
12	X	X	X												

Oedema, Knee

	APIS	SULPH
4	X	
26		X

Oedema, Labia

	APIS
14	X
24	X

Oedema, Larynx

	APIS	KALI IOD	SANG	KALI HYD	LACH	ACON	ARS	ARUM T	BELL	CANTH	CHINA	PHOS
1		X										
5	X											
6	X		X		X	X	X	X	X	X	X	X
7	X	X	X									
8		X										
9	X											
14				X								
17	X		X	X	X							

Oedema, Legs

	LYC	ARS	SULPH	APIS	BRY	CHINA	COLCH	DIG	FERR	HELL	SENEC	ACET AC
3			**X**		**X**							
4	X							X				**X**
6	X	X					X			X		
7	X	X		X		X	X	X	X	X	X	
8	X	X	X			X						
10		X		X								
12									X			
17	X											
24				X							X	
26			X		X							

Oedema, Limbs

	APIS	ARS	AUR M	COLCH	DIG	EUP PUR	GRAPH	HAM	MEDO	SENEC	STANN	THYROID
1									X			X
7	X				X	X	X	X		X	X	
8		X		X								
17			X									

Oedema, Lungs (Note that only the main remedies are used from 17)

	AMM C	ANT T	KALI IOD	ARS	PHOS	LACH	CARB V	IPEC	APIS	KALI CAR	KALI PH	NAT M	SANG	STROPH	VER A	BELL	DIG	PULMO V	SULPH	TUB
1			X											X				X		
2	X		X		X	X					X	X			X			X		X
3			X																	
5							X													
6	X	X	X	X	X	X	X	X					X			X	X		X	
7	X	**X**	X	**X**	X	**X**		X	X			X			X					
8	X	X	X	X	X	X	X	X		X	X				X	X			X	
10	X	X												X						
11	X	X		X	X				X	X			X							
14	X	X	X																	
16		X																		
17	X	X	X	X	X	X	X	X	X	X	X	X	X	X			X			X
19	X						X													
21	X			X																

Oedema, Neck

	APIS	MERC I F
6	X	
8		X

Oedema, Ovaries

	APIS	LACH	ARS	CALC	BELL	BRY	CHINA	COLOC	GRAPH	IOD	KALI BR	LIL T	LYC
1	X												
7	**X**	X	**X**	**X**			X			X		X	X
8	X	X	X		X		X	X	X	X	X		X
13	X	X		X	X	X		X	X		X	X	
26	X					X							

Oedema, Ovary, Right

	APIS	IOD
1		X
6	X	

Oedema, Penis

	RHUS T
1	X
6	X

Oedema, Pericardium- See Hydropericardium

Oedema, Pharynx

	APIS	RHUS T
17		X
18	X	

Oedema, Pregnancy During- See Pregnancy, Oedema During

Oedema, Renal Origin

	APIS	ARS	COLCH	TEREB	APOC	ASC T	CANTH	COCHIN	LYC	PHASEOL	UREA	VESICAR
1	X	X		X						X	X	X
2	X	**X**		X	X							
7	X		**X**			X						
22	X											
26		X	X				X	X	X			

Oedema, Scrotum

	RHUS T	ARG	ARS	APIS	FERR SUL	NAT SUL
1	X					
6	X	X				
7	X		X		X	X
8	**X**		X			
10		X				
24				X		

Oedema, Throat

	APIS	LAC C	MUR AC	NAT ARS	RHUS T
1	X				
8	X	X	X		X
17				X	
18	X				

Oedema, Tongue

	APIS	KALI IOD
1		X
3	X	

Oedema, Uterus

	APIS	ARS	SULPH	LYC	CALC	CAMPH	CHINA	CON	DIG	MERC	SEP	HELON	AESC T	BELL	BROM	BRY	CANTH	COLCH	DULC	FERR	HAM	HELL	KALI CAR	KREO	LED	PHOS	PULS	RHUS T
1		X			X			X																X			X	
7	X	X	X	**X**		X	X		X	X	X	**X**		X														
13	X	X	X	X	X	X	X	X	X	X	X		X		X	X	X	X	X	X	X	X	X		X	X		X
26	X		X																									

Oedema, Uvula

	APIS	PHYTO	BAR M	INDIUM	KALI BIC	KALI IOD	KALI MAN	MERC CY	NAT ARS	NUX V	PHOS	RHUS T
6	X											
8	X		X	X	X	X	X		X	X	X	X
10	X											
17		X						X				
18	X	X										

Oesophagitis

	ARS	ACON	RHUS T	CARB V	BELL	NIT AC	PHOS	AMM C	ARS	ASAF	CANTH	COCCUL	LACH	MEZ	SEC	SULPH AC	CARB AC	MERC C
2		X		X				X							X	X		
6	X	X	X		X	X	X		X		X		X	X				
7	**X**	X	**X**	X		X	X											
8	X			X				X		X	X	X	X					
11	**X**	X			**X**	X	X									X	**X**	**X**
13	X		X	X	X				X	X		X		X	X			
26	X	X	X															

Oesophagus, Diseases Of

	IGN	ARN	ARS	ASAF	BELL	CANTH	CARB V	COCCUL	EUPHORB	LAURO	MERC	MEZ	NAJA	NAT ARS	NAT M	RAPH	RHEUM	RHUS T	SABAD	SEC	SENEG	SCHIN	SINAP A	SULPH	VER A
2	X													X		X	X				X	X	X	X	
8		X	X	X	X	X	X	X	X	X	X	X	X		X			X	X	X					X

Oligomenorrhoea- See Menses, Scanty

Omodynia- See also Rheumatism

	CALC	BRY	FERR	SANG
6		X		X
8	X		X	

Onychia- See Nails, Diseases Of

Onychogryphosis

	GRAPH	SIL	SULPH	SABAD	ALUMEN	ANT C	CALC	MERC	SEP
8	X	X	X	X	X	X	X	X	X
10	X	X	X						
13	X	X	X	X					
14	X								
19		X							
21	X								
26	X	X	X						

Onychomycosis

	GRAPH	SIL	THUJA	ANT C	CALC	CALEND	HEP	MYRIST	NAT SUL	SEP	SULPH
3						X					
8	X	X					X		X		
18		X	X								
19	X				X			X		X	X
21	X	X	X	X							

Ophthalmia- See also Conjunctivitis

	RHUS T	ARG N	SULPH	ACON	ARS	BELL	EUPHR	PULS	HEP	CALC	ARN	KALI BIC	MERC	SPIG	CON	CROT T	GELS	LYC	MERC C	SIL	APIS	NIT AC
2			X									X				X						
4	**X**	X			X	X	X	X		X		X			X							
6	X	X	X	X	X	X		X	X	X		X			X	X		X	X	X	X	X
7	**X**	**X**			**X**		X	**X**	X	X	X	X	**X**		X	X			X		**X**	
8	X	X	**X**	X	X	**X**	X	**X**	**X**	X	X	X	**X**	X	X	X	X	X	X	X	X	**X**
10	X		X	X	X	X			X	X	X						X					
12	X	X	X	X	X	X	X		X		E		X	X			X	X	X	X		X
14		X	X				X															
15			X	X		X					X			X			X					
17		X																				
23	X	X		X			X							X								
24								X														
26	X		X	**X**	X	X	X	X	X	X			X	X				X		X		

E- External

Ophthalmia Gonorrhoica

	NIT AC	ACON	PULS	ANT T	ARS	BELL	HEP	MERC	MERC C	SULPH	THUJA	TUSSIL
6	X	X	X		X	X	X		X			X
7	**X**	X		X				X		X	X	
8	**X**		X									

Ophthalmia Neonatorum

	ARG N	MERC	ACON	NIT AC	PULS	APIS	CALC	CHAM	EUPHR	RHUS T	SULPH	SYPH	THUJA	DULC	HEP	LYC	MERC C	ARS	BELL	BRY	CALC HP	IGN	KALI SUL	NUX V	PHOS
2	**X**																								
4		**X**		**X**																			X		
6		X			X			X								X									
7	**X**	X	X	**X**	X	**X**	**X**	X	X	X	X	X	**X**		X				X	X		X		X	
8	X	X	X	X	X	X	X	X	X	X	X	X	X	X	X		X	X			X				X
9	X											X													
14	X		X			X											X								
26		X	**X**	X			X		X	X	X			X		X									
27	X				X																				

Ophthalmia, Purulent

	ARG N	MERC	HEP	SULPH	APIS	EUPHR	NIT AC	PULS	RHUS T	ALUMEN	ARG	ANT T	ARS	CALC	CALC SUL	CANN I	CARB V	CHAM	CHLOR	CINNAB	GRIND	KALI BIC	LYC	NAT M	PHYTO	PSOR	THUJA	
1	X		X						X																			
6	X	X	X	X	X	X	X	X	X		X	X	X	X		X	X	X		X		X	X	X	X		X	
7	**X**	**X**	X	**X**	X		X												X		X					X		
8	**X**	X								X																		
12	X																											
14	X	X				X		X							X													

Ophthalmia, Phlyctenular- See Keratoconjunctivitis

Ophthalmia, Rheumatic

	ACON	ANT T	BRY	LED	MERC	PULS	SPIG	VER A	CALC	PHYTO	APIS	ARUNDO	BOR	CHAM	CHINA	COCCUL	COCHL	COLCH	COLOC	EUPHR	MEZ	PSOR	RHUS T					
7	**X**	**X**	**X**	X	X	X	X	X	**X**	**X**	X	X	X	X	X	X	X	X	X		X	X						
8		X		X																								
26	**X**		X		X	X	X	X												X			X					

Ophthalmia Senilis

	ALUM	APIS
4	X	
7		X

Opisthotonos

	CIC	NUX V	STRAM	BELL	IGN	OP	CUPR	IPEC	VER V	STANN	RHUS T	ANGUST	KALI BR	PASS	PLAT	STRYCH	LED
1	X	X	X	X			X										
2										X							
4	X	X			X		X										
6	X		X					X	X			X			X		
7	X				X			X	X				X				
8	**X**	**X**	X	X	X	X	X		**X**	X	X		X	X	X	X	**X**
13	**X**	X	**X**	X	**X**	**X**	X	**X**		X	**X**	X		X			
16	X																
17	X	X	X	X		X										X	
19	X	X	X			X											
24		X		X													
27	X																

Optic Disc, Diseases Of

	DUBO M	DUB	PLUM
1	X		
8		X	X

Optic Nerve Atrophy

	PHOS	NUX V	AGAR M	ARG N	ARS	CARB SUL	PLUM	SANTIN
1	X		X		X	X		
3	X							X
4	X							
7	X	X						
8		**X**		X			X	

Optic Nerve, Congestion

	SULPH
8	X
24	X

Orchitis

	PULS	CLEM	SPONG	AUR	HAM	RHOD	CON	RHUS T	BELL	MERC	ACON	ARN	PHYTO	NUX V	STAPHYS	NIT AC	BROM	GRAPH	IOD	LYC	THUJA	ARG N	GELS	KALI IOD
1	X	X	X	X		X	X			X		X					X	X	X		X			
2		**X**	**X**		**X**								X											
3	X	X	X	X			X	X	X		X	X	X			X								
4	**X**	**X**	X	X	X	**X**															X		X	
5	X	X	X	X	X		X		X								X							
6	X	X	X	X	X	X	X	X	X	X	X	X	X	X	X	X	X	X	X	X	X	X	X	X
7	**X**	**X**	X	X		X	**X**	X	X	X	**X**		X	X	X							X		X
8	**X**	**X**	X	X	X	X	X	**X**	X	X	X	**X**	X	X	X	X	X	X	X	X	X	X	X	X
9	X		X			X		X				X						X	X					
11	X	X	X	X	X			X					X											
13	**X**	**X**	X	X			X		X	X				**X**	X	**X**				X				
14	X				X	X																		
18	X																							
19			X																					
23	X	X	X		X	X					X													
24	**X**																							
26	X	X	X	X				X	X	**X**	X	X		X	X					X				

Orchitis, Right Side

	AUR	MERC
1		X
4	X	

Orthopnoea

	CONVAL	APIS	ACON FE	ANT T	ARS	AUR	CHAM	CUPR	LOB I	STRY ARS	VER V
4					X						
8		X		X			X	X	X		X
11	X										
17	X	X	X			X				X	
23	X										

Ossification, Arteries- See also Arteriosclerosis; Calcification

	CALC FL	LAC AC	LITH C	SANIC
2			X	X
8		X		
25	X			

Osteitis

	MERC	SIL	PH AC	AUR	CALC	MEZ	STAPHYS	PHOS	ASAF	NIT AC	SULPH	LYC	SYMPH	MANG	CHINA	HECLA	PHYTO	PULS	RHUS T	RUTA	STILLING	STRONT C	HEP
1		X	X	X			X						X	X						X	X	X	
3													X			X			X	X			
4	**X**									X												X	
5		X		X				X									X						
6	X		X		X				X														
7	X	**X**	X	X	**X**	X	X		X	X	X	X	X				X						
8	X	X	X	X	X	X	X	X	X	X	X	X			X			X					
10	X		X			X		X															
13	**X**	**X**	X	**X**	X	**X**	**X**	X	**X**	**X**	X	**X**		**X**	X			X	X				**X**
23																X					X		
26	X	X	X		X	X	X	X			X												

Osteitis Deformans

	CALC PH	HECLA	KALI IOD	MERC C	RHUS T	SIL	SULPH
2		X					
3	X		X	X	X		
13							X
16						X	

Osteoarthritis

	BRY	ARN	CALC	CALC FL	LED	RHUS T	PULS	CALC PH	SIL	BENZ AC	COLCH	NAT SUL	ACON	CAUST	CHEL	DULC	MEDO	SULPH	FORM AC	HECLA	KALI CAR
5			X	X				X	X			X		X		X	X				
9	X	X	X			X					X										
11	**X**	X			**X**	X				X					X				**X**	**X**	
12	X						X		X				X					X			
19	X	X	**X**	**X**	**X**	X	X	**X**	X	**X**	**X**	**X**		X	X	X	X	X			**X**
21	X	X			X	X	X	X					X								
29[1]		E																			
29[2]		E																			
29[3]	X			**X**		X	X														

E- External

29[1] Knuesel O, et al. Arnica montana gel in osteoarthritis of the knee Adv Ther, 2002, Sep- Oct, 19, 5, 209-218.

29[2] Widrig R, et al. Choosing between NSAID and arnica for topical treatment of hand osteoarthritis in a randomised, double-blind study. Rheumatol Int. 2007, Apr, 27 (6) :585-91.

29[3] Pinto S, et al. Lipid peroxidation, erythrocyte antioxidants and plasma antioxidants in osteoarthritis before and after homeopathic treatment. Homeopathy. 2008 Oct;97 (4):185-9.

Osteochondritis, Knee

	BERB V	AUR	CALC PH	KALI BIC
3	**X**			
5		X	X	X

Osteogenesis Imperfecta (Includes Bones, Brittle)

	CALC PH	CALC	BUFO	CALC FL	CALC IOD	LAC AC	SIL	RUTA
1	X	X		X	X		X	
3		X						
7						X		
8	X		X					X
10	X							

Osteoma (Includes Osteomata)

	CALC FL	HECLA	MEZ	CALC	CALC IOD	CALC PH	LYC	MERC	MERC I F	PHOS	PHYTO	SEP	SIL	SULPH
1									X					
2			X								X			
4	X	X												
7			X											
8	X	X		X	X	X	X	X		X		X	X	X
10	X													
16		X												
23	X													
24		X												
27		X												

Osteomalacia- See also Weakness, Bones (Includes Bone, Softening of; Mollities Ossium)

	CALC	SIL	MERC	PHOS	CALC PH	ASAF	BELL	GUAIAC	LYC	SEP	STAPHYS	SULPH	ARN	FL AC	HEP	MEZ	NIT AC	PULS	RHUS T	RUTA	SYMPH
2			X					X													
6	X	X		X	X								X	X					X		X
7	X	X	X	X	X	X	X	X	X	X	X	X									
8	X	X	X	X	X	X	X		X	X	X	X	X	X	X	X	X	X		X	X
12	X																				
13	X	X	X	X		X	X	X	X	X	X	X			X	X	X	X	X	X	
14	X																				
27	X	X	X	X	X																

Osteomyelitis

	SIL	MERC C	ACON	AUR	BELL	BRY	ECHIN	GUNPOW	MEDO	MERC	NAT M	PH AC	PULS
1	X						X		X				
2												X	
8		X											
9	X			X									
14	X		X		X	X					X		
17	X												X
21								X					
24										X			

Osteophytes

	CALC FL	CALC	FL AC	SIL
10	X			X
18	X			
19		X		
24	X		X	

Osteoporosis- See also Weakness, Bones

	CALC	CALC FL	CALC PH	SIL	SYMPH	VERMIC
18	X			X		
28						X
29[1]					X	
29[2]	X	X	X			

29[1] Sakakura CE, et al. Influence of homeopathic treatment with comfrey on bone density around titanium implants: a digital subtraction radiography study in rats. Clin Oral Implants Res. 2008, Jun, 19 (6) :624-8.

29[2] Harkin C. Effect of Homeopathic Calcium on Bone Density. Homeopathic Links, Spring, 2008, 21, 44-49.

Osteosarcoma- See also Cancer, Bone; Enchondroma

	HECLA	CALC FL	SIL
1	X		
2	X		
8	X	X	
16			X

Otalgia- See also Otitis

	CHAM	PULS	BELL	MERC	ACON	HEP	PLANTAG	NUX V	DULC	SIL	SULPH	ARN	CAPS	SPIG	ARS	CALC	GELS	GUAIAC	MANG	PHOS	RHUS T	FERR PH	VERBASC
1	X	X	X	X	X	X							X	X			X						X
2	**X**	**X**					**X**							X				X					
3	X	X	X			X	X						X					X					
4	X	X					X					X											
5													X										
6	X	X	X	X	X	X	X	X		X	X	X	X		X	X	X			X	X		
7	**X**	**X**	**X**	**X**			X	X	**X**			X		X			X	X	X				**X**
8	X	**X**	**X**	X	X	X		X	X	**X**	**X**	X	X	**X**		X		X		X	X		X
9						X																	
10	X	X	X	X	X	X		X			X										X		
12		X	X												X								
13	X	X	X	X				X	X	X				X	X			X	X	X	X		
14	X	X	X	X	X		E								X	X							
15	X	X	X	X	X																		
17	X	X	X														X		X				
18					X																	X	
19	X		X		X														X			X	
20	X	X	X	X		X				X												X	
21	X	X	X			X			X								X						X
22	X	X		X	X	X			X													**X**	
23	X				X		X																
24	X	X	X	X	X		X	X			X	X	X		X	X				X	X		
25	X	X		X	X	X	E				X												
26	X	**X**	X	X				X	X	X	X	X				X				X			
27	X																						
28		X																					

E- External

Otalgia, Left Side

	KALI BIC	VERBASC
6	X	
22		X
27	X	

Otalgia, Right Side

	BELL	MAG PH
22	X	X
25	X	

Otitis

	PULS	BELL	MERC	CHAM	KALI BIC	FERR PH	ACON	DULC	SULPH	CALC	KALI MUR	HEP	PSOR	CACT	CAPS	MERC D	PLANTAG	SIL	TELL	ARS	HYDRAST	KALI CAR	KREO	LACH	PIC AC	SANG
2														X			**X**					X			X	
3	X	X	X		X						**X**		X		X				**X**							
4	**X**	**X**	X	**X**		**X**	X	X	**X**	X	X		X				X									X
5	X	X	X	X	X	X				X	X					X		X		X	X					
7	**X**	X	**X**	X	X	X	X	X	**X**	**X**		X	X	X	X	X		**X**	X		X	X	X	X	X	X
8	X	X	X	X	X	X	X	X	X	X		X	X	X	X	X	X	X	X	X			X	X	X	X
10	**X**	X	X	X			X	X	X	X		X														
12		X																								
13	X	X	X		X																	X	X			
15	X								X			X														
18		X	X	X	X	X	X	X			X	X	X	X	X	X				X	X			X		
19	X																									
20	X				X																					
22		X		X		X	X	X																		
23											X															
28	X																									

Otitis Externa

	BELL	PULS	MERC	ACON	HEP	SIL	ARS	CHAM	GRAPH	PIC AC	RHUS T	TELL	ANT C	ARN	BAR C	BOR	CACT	CALC	CALC PH	FERR PH	LACH	LYC	MANG	MYRIST	SULPH
4		**X**																							
5														X					X					X	
7		X																							
8	X	**X**	**X**		X	X	X			X	X				X	X	X	X					X		X
9										X															
11	X			X	X	X					X		X												
14	X																								
19									X			X									X				
20	**X**	X	X		X	X		X												X		X			
21	X		X	**X**					X																
24	X			X			X	X				X													
26	X	X	X																						

Otitis Interna- See also Tympanitis

	BELL	GELS	HEP	LACH	MERC
8		X			
26	X		X	X	X

Otitis Media

	PULS	BELL	CHAM	MERC	ACON	HEP	SIL	SULPH	CAPS	CALC	LYC	KALI BIC	MERC D	TELL	GRAPH	KALI MUR	ARS	FERR PH	CHINA	PSOR	CAUST	LACH						
1									X																			
4	X			**X**		**X**	**X**	X	**X**				X	**X**	X	X				X	**X**							
5	**X**	X	**X**		X	X			**X**								**X**											
6	X	X	X	X	X	X	X		X	X	X	X	X	X	X		X	X	X	X	X	X						
7	**X**		X								X		**X**															
8	X	X	X	X	X	X	X	X	X	X		X		X	X		X		X	X	X							
9	X	X	X		X	X																						
12	X	X	X	X	X			X																				
13	X	X		X	X	X	X			X																		
14		X														X												
17	X	X	X	X	X	X	X		X					X		X		X										
19	**X**	**X**	**X**	**X**	X	**X**	**X**	**X**		**X**	**X**	**X**	X	X	X	X		**X**		X		**X**						
21	X	X			X																							
24		X													X	X			X									
25	X	**X**	X	X	X																							
27	X	X	X	X		X	X	X		X		X	X															
28	X																											
29[1]	**X**	X	X	X		X	X	X	X	X	X						X	X	X									
29[2]	X	X	X		X		X				X	X										X						
29[3]	X		X					X		X																		
29[4]	X		X	X			X	X			X																	

29[1] Frei H, et al. Homoeopathy in acute otitis media in children. Brit Hom J, 2001, Oct, 90, (4); 180-2.
29[2] Friese K.H. et al. The Homoeopathic Treatment of Otitis Media in Children. Int J. Clin. Pharmacol. Ther. 35, 7, July 1997, 296-301.
29[3] Jacobs J, et al. Homeopathic treatment of acute otitis media in children. Paediatric Infectious Diseases Journal, 20, 2, Feb 2001, 177-183.
29[4] Sinha MN, et al.. Randomized controlled pilot study to compare Homeopathy and Conventional therapy in Acute Otitis Media. Homeopathy. 2012 Jan;101(1):5-12.

Otorrhoea

	PULS	MERC	CALC	HEP	SIL	SULPH	LYC	GRAPH	CAUST	AUR	PSOR	CARB V	NIT AC	TELL	ASAF	BELL	KALI BIC	BOR	ARS	CALC SUL	ELAPS	HYDRAST	PETR	PHOS	BAR M	CHAM	NAT M
1	X	X	X	X	X			X		X	X		X	X			X			X	X	X					
2							X		X		X	X						**X**					X				
3	X	X		X		X									X											**X**	
4			X	X	X							X						X									
6	X	X	X		X	X	X	X	X	X	X	X		X	X		X	X	X		X				X		
7	X	**X**	X	X	**X**	**X**	**X**	X	**X**	X	**X**		X	X	X	X			X			X		X	**X**		X
8	X	X	X	X	X	X	X	X	X	X	X	X	X	X	X	X	X				X	X	X	X		X	X
9	X																										
10	X	X	X	X		X	X									X											
12	X	X	X	X	X	X	X	X	X	X				X					X					X			
13	X	X	X	X	X	X	X	X	X				X		X	X		X					X	X		X	**X**
14	X		X	X	X														X								
15	X	X	X	X	X	X				X		X	X			X											
17										X															X		
18																			X			X					
19								X			X			X						X			X				
21		X						X																			
22																	X										
23													X							X							
24	X	X	X			X	X	X	X	X	X	X		X	X		X	X			X						
25	X	X				X																					
26	X	X	X	X	X	X	X	X	X			X	X			X											
27	X	X		X	X		X										X			X							

Otorrhoea, Left Ear

	FERR	ARS	GELS	SULPH
6	X			
7	X	X	X	X

Otosclerosis

	CALC FL	GRAPH	FERR PIC	THIO
17	X	X	X	X
21	X	X		
27	X			

Ovaralgia- See also Pain, Genitalia, Female

	COLOC	APIS	LIL T	BELL	PLAT	POD	ARS	BRY	CANTH	CON	LACH	CIMICI	IOD	NAJA	STAPHYS	THUJA	BUFO	CHAM	GOSS	HAM	HELON	PLUM	SENEC	TEREB	ZINC	ZINC VAL	PULS	
1			X		X	X	X			X	X						X	X										
2		**X**				X													X					X			**X**	
4	X		X				X					X		X		X										X		
5	X				X					X						X					X							
6				X			X	X	X	X			X									X	X		X			
7	X	X	X	X		X	X	X	X				X	X		X	X			X	X			X	X			
8	X		X	X	X	X					X	X		X	X			X	X	X		X				X		
9									X																			
10		X																										
13	X	X	X			X		X			X				X													
14	X		X						X			X	X															
18			X																									
20	X			X																								
21					X										X													
22	X	X																										
24		X																					X					
26	X	X		X	X			X		X	X																	
27	X	X																										

Ovaralgia, Left

	LACH	ARG	LIL T	THUJA	USTIL	BROM	COLOC	NAJA	VESPA	LYC	PHOS	PLAT	POD	ZINC	ABROT	AMM BR	APIS	ATROP S	CARB AC	FERR	GRAPH	HAM	KALI BR	LAC C	LAC D	STRAM	THLASP	
1	X	X							X		X																X	
2				X					X																			
3	X																											
4	**X**	X	**X**		X			X						X														
5	X	X	X	X								X																
6	X	X					X			X																		
7	X		X			X	X	X			X	X	X			X		X				X	X	X	X			
8	X	X	X			X	X		X	X			X	X	X		X			X	X					X		
9					X														X									
13	X			X																								
13						X																						
19	X				X																							
20	X																											
21				X				X																				
25					X																							
27	X																											

Ovaralgia, Right

	PALLAD	POD	APIS	BRY	LYC	ARS	BELL	CENCHR	COLOC	IOD	LACH	MERC	ARG N	FERR	GLON	GRAPH	LAC C	LACT AC	LOL	MUREX	NAJA
1	X			X				X		X	X	X					X		X		
3		X							X			X									X
4		X				**X**			X							X					
5	X	X	X	X	X			X													
6	X	X																			
7	X	X	X	X			X			X			X					X			
8	X	X	X	X	X	X	X				X			X	X						
13			X																		
18																				X	
21	X				X																
27	X																				

Ovaritis

	APIS	PLAT	BELL	CANTH	ACON	IOD	LACH	SABIN	ANT C	ARS	COLOC	HAM	PULS	AMBRA	BRY	CHINA	MERC	PALLAD	STAPHYS	THUJA	LYC
1	X	X	X	X	X	X	X	X		X	X							X			
2	**X**												**X**								
4	X	X	**X**							X		E									
5		X					X														
6		X	X	X	X	X	X	X	X	X	X	X	X		X	X	X		X	X	
7	X	X	X	X	X	X	X	**X**	X					X				X			**X**
8	X	X	X	X	X		X	X	X	X	X	X		X	X	X	X	X	X		X
11																				X	
13				**X**	X	X			X					X		X	X		X		
14	X					X															
18													X								
23	X											X								X	
26	X										X				X						

E- External

Ovaritis, Left

	LACH	THUJA	APIS	ARG	CAPS	COLOC	GRAPH	HAM	LAC C	LIL T	POD	ZINC	ZIZIA
4		X				X							
5		X											
6	X												
7	X		X					X					
11		X											
13	X	X		X	X		X		X	X	X	X	X
14	X												

Ovaritis, Right

	BELL	APIS	LYC	PALLAD	AESC	ARG	HAM	IOD	LAC C	POD
1	X	X								
4	**X**			X						
6		X								
7			X			X				
8								X		
13	X	X	X	X	X		X		X	
17										X

Ovarian Atrophy- See Atrophy, Ovaries
Ovarian Cysts- See Cysts, Ovaries

Ovaries, Congestion

	APIS	ACON	BELL	HEP	KALI IOD	LAC AC	SEP
7	X		X	X	X		X
8	**X**					X	
9		X					

Ovary, Congestion, Right

	APIS	LYC	PALLAD	BELL	IOD
1	X				X
4	X				
7	X	**X**	**X**	X	

Ovaries, Diseases Of

	LYC	NAJA	APIS	CIMICI	CANTH	COLOC	CON	HAM	HEP	IOD	KALI BR	LACH	LIL T	PALLAD	PLAT
1	X														
2		**X**			**X**	**X**	**X**	**X**	**X**	**X**	**X**	**X**	**X**	**X**	**X**
4			**X**	X											
7	**X**														
8	X	X	X	X	X	X	X	X	X	X	X	X	X	X	X
17		X		X											

Ovary, Diseases Of, Left

	USTIL	LACH	ARG	ALUMEN	APIS	BROM	COLOC	LIL T	MERC	NAJA	THUJA																	
2	X																											
4					X																							
7		**X**	X	X																								
8	X	X	X			X	X	X	X	X	X																	
19	X																											

Oxaluria

	OX AC	NM X	SENNA	BERB V	CAUST	NIT AC	TEREB	ALOE	BENZ AC	KALI HP	KALI SUL	LYC	LYSID	MEDO	NAT PH	NAT SUL	SOLID	SULPH										
1	**X**				X		X											X										
2	**X**	**X**		**X**									X															
3	**X**	**X**	X																									
5	X		X	X	X	X	X	X			X	X		X	X	X	X											
16	X																											
23	X		X			X			X	X																		

Oxyuriasis- See Worms, Pin

Ozaena

	AUR	KALI BIC	CALC	PULS	ELAPS	ASAF	MERC C	NIT AC	KALI IOD	PETR	IOD	ALUM	AUR M	GRAPH	HEP	SEP	CAD SUL	HYDRAST	CALC FL	LACH	NAT CAR	SANG	STICTA	THUJA	PSOR			
1	**X**	X	X	X	X		X		X	X								X		X				X				
2	**X**	**X**			X	X		**X**			**X**	X	X			X	**X**	**X**	X		X		X	X	**X**			
3	X		X			X	X			X			X				X											
6	X	X	X	X	X	X					X			X							X				X			
7	X	X	X	X	X	X	X		X	X		X	X	X					X		X	X	X					
8	X	**X**	X	X	X	X	X	X	X	X	X	X	X	X	X	X		X	X	X		X	X	X				
11									X																			
12	X	X						X			X											X	X					
13	**X**	X	X	X		**X**				X		X		X		X				X								
14	X	X	X	X	X		X		X						X		X			X								
17	X	X	X	X	X	X	X	X	X	X	X	X	X		X	X	X	X	X		X	X		X	X			
19	X														X													
20		X																										
21			X																									
23					X			X																				
24	X	X		X										X	X													
26			X	X				X								X												
28							X																					

Paget's Disease

	HECLA	CALC PH	SIL
27	**X**	X	X

Pain- See also Hyperaesthesia; Neuralgia

	CHAM	HEP	BRY	GELS	RHUS T	NUX V	MAG PH	ACON	BAPT	EUP PERF	PHYTO	VER A	ARN
9	**X**	**X**	X	X	**X**	X	**X**		X	X	X	X	**X**
10			X	X	X								
12									X				
14			X	X	X			X		X			
15						X							
17	X						X						
19	X	X											
21	X	X											
22	X	X						X					
24											X	X	
25			X	X		X							
28	X												

Pain, Abdomen- See also Gastralgia; Tormina (Includes Enteralgia)

	ARS	BELL	COLOC	NUX V	BRY	SULPH	CHAM	PHOS	PLUM	PULS	VER A	ACON	DIOSC	LACH	MAG PH	MERC	SEP	LYC	ALOE	APIS	IOD	CANTH	COCCUL					
1	X	X		X	X				X		X								X									
2													X															
3	X	X				X							X		X													
4	X				X				X		X						X						X					
5								X																				
6		X	X	X			X	X						X		X			X	X	X	X	X					
7	X	X	X	X	X	X	X	X		X		X	X	X		X	X	X	X	X		**X**	X					
8	X	X		X			X	X			X	X		X			X					X						
9		X		X		X				X					X													
10	X	X		X	X	X	X	X	X	X			X	X			X				X							
11	X					X			X							X					X							
12	X		X	X						X	X	X									X							
13	X	X	X	X	X	X	X	X	X	X	X	X		X		X	X	X	X	X	X	X	X					
14	X	X	X	X			X	X	X		X				X			X		X								
15		X	X		X					X				X		X				X								
16		X										X																
18	X					X	X			X	X																	
19	**X**	**X**	**X**	**X**	**X**	X	**X**	X	X			X	X		X	X	X	**X**	X				**X**					
20	X	X	X												X													
21	X	X	X	X	X		X					X		X	X	X		X			X							
22			X																									
23			X										X		X													
24	X	X	X	X	X				X		X		X					X	X	X		X						
25					X	X				X							X											
26	X	X	X			X		X																				

Pain, Achilles Tendon (Includes Arthralgia, Tendo Achilles)

	CAUST	CIMICI	MUR AC	RHUS T	RUTA	ANAC	ANT C	ARIST M	BENZ AC	CALC	CANN S	COLCH	KALI BIC	MYRICA	NAT	NAT M	PULS	SEP	STAPHYS	SULPH	TET	UPAS	ZINC					
2								X						X							X	X						
5	X	X			X				X																			
7	X	X								X	X	X						X										
8	X		X	X		X	X								X	X	X		X	X			X					
14		X		X	X								X															
21			X																									

Pain, Ankle

	PHYTO	PULS	PROP	CALC	CANN I	CAULO	POD	RUTA	ABROT	ACON	AGAR M	ALL C	AMM C	ANT T	ARG	CALC PH	CARB A	CAUST	COLCH	COLOC	HELL	LAC D	LITH C	MANG M	VISC A
1		X	X																					X	
2			X																						
3			X																						
4		X																							
7	X			X		X	X			X	X	X		X		X	X		X		X		X		
13		X						X					X		X					X					
14	X				X				X													X			
15							X																		
17	X				X																				
21				X		X		X										X							X

Pain, Anus (Includes Anus, Constriction Of)

	ALOE	SULPH	NIT AC	ARS	NAT M	RAT	GRAPH	LACH	PLUM	CAPS	HAM	IGN	IRIS V	KALI CAR	LYC	MERC	NUX V	PAEONIA	SIL
1	X	X	X			X	X			X			X					X	X
4	X	X	X			X	X											X	X
5			X		X									X	X				
6		X	X	X	X	X		X	X			X	X	X		X	X		
7	X	X	X	X	X	X	X	X		X	X	X	X	X	X	X	X	X	X
8			X		X				X			X							
9	X										X		X						
10	X			X															
11	X	X	X	X			X												X
12									X										
13	X	X	X	X	X	X	X	X	X					X	X	X	X		
14		X	X	X	X	X			X	X		X							
15		X									X								
17								X											
20															X				
21	X										X								
22		X																	
24	X				X	X	X			X							X	X	
25	X																		
26		X		X												X			

Pain, Appendix- See also Appendicitis

	APIS	ARS	BRY	CROT H	IRIS T	LACH	RHUS T
8				X			
18					X		
25	X	X	X			X	X

Pain, Arm

	EUP PUR	GELS	PULS	SPIG	ACON	ARN	CALC	CANTH	CAUST	COCCUL	LED	SEP	STAPHYS
1				X							X		
7	X		X			X	X	X	X			X	X
8			X										
9		X											
11	X												
13			X		X	X	X	X	X	X	X	X	X
14	X			X						X			
15		X											
17				X	X								
25		X											

Pain, Arm, Forearm (Includes Arthralgia, Forearms)

	CALC	CARB V	NIT AC	PH AC	RHOD	STAPHYS	CAUST	RHUS T	SEP	SULPH
8	**X**	X	X	X	X	X	**X**	**X**	**X**	**X**
13	X	X	X	X	X	X				

Pain, Arm, Left

	CACT	RHUS T	CRAT	KALM	LATRO M
1	X		X		
4	X				
6		X			
7	X	X			
10				X	X
14	X		X		
17	X			X	
19	X	X			X
21	X				

Pain, Arm, Right

	PHYTO	SANG	ACON	APIS	FERR	LEPT	LIL T	NIT AC
3	X							
6	X							
7			X	X		X		X
8	X	X			X			
10		X						
14	X							
17	X							
21							X	

Pain, Arms, Upper (Includes Arthralgia, Arm, Upper)

	BRY	COCCUL	HEP	LACHNAN	FERR	PHYTO	ARS	ASAF	BELL	CHINA	IGN	KALM	MAG P A	MERC	MEZ	MUR AC	NIT	PH AC	PULS	SARS	SEP	STANN	STAPHYS	SULPH	VAL
4												X													
8	**X**	X			**X**	**X**	X	X	X	X	X		X		X		X		X		X	X		X	X
9				X																					
12																X									
13	X	X	X											X				X		X			X		
24			X																						
25				X																					

Pain, Axilla

	JUG C	CARB V
2	**X**	
3	X	
7		X

Pain, Back

	KALI CAR	RHUS T	NUX V	LYC	SEP	AESC	ARN	CIMICI	PULS	BERB V	CALC	BELL	BRY	GELS	PHOS	SULPH	ANT T	NAT M	ACON	PHYTO								
1						X				X	X																	
2	**X**					X	**X**																					
3	X	X	X			X	X	X	X	X	X				X		X											
4	X	**X**		X	**X**			X		X	X	X	X		X	X	X	X	X	X								
5	X				X	X												X										
6	X	X		X	X	X		X		X	X	X	X	X	X	X			X	X								
7	X	X	**X**	X	**X**		X		**X**		X		**X**	X	X			**X**										
8	X	X							X					X			X		X									
9			X						X			X		X				X										
10		X	X	X	X			X	X	**X**		X	X		X	X												
11	X	X		X		X								X														
12		X	X	X		X		X									X		X	X								
13	X		X	X	**X**		X		**X**		X		X		X	X	**X**											
14				X		X	X	X		X	X		X					X										
15		X	X					X						X					X									
16		X																										
17	X	X															X			X								
18			X				X	X																				
19	**X**	**X**	**X**	X	X	X	X	X		X	**X**	**X**	X		X	X		X		X								
21	X	X			X		X																					
22	X									X																		
24							X		X							X			X	X								
25			X		X	X						X		X														
26	X	X	X	X					X			X				X												
27	X			X																								

Pain, Back, Pregnancy, During- See Pregnancy, Back Pain, During
Pain, Back, Lower- See Lumbago
Pain, Back, Lumbar- See Lumbago
Pain, Bladder- See Cystalgia

Pain, Bone

	EUP PER	RUTA	MERC	ASAF	AUR	RHUS T	NIT AC	PH AC	KALI IOD	MEZ	STAPHYS	MANG	BAR C	CALC	FL AC	KALI BIC	NAT M	ARG	CUPR	STILLING
1		X		X					X			X			X					X
2	**X**	**X**				X						X								
3	X	X		X																
4	X	**X**	**X**		X	X	X		X								X			**X**
5		X														X				
6	X	X	X	X	X	X	X	X	X	X	X				X					X
7	X	X	X		X	X	X	X		X	X		X	X	X		X	**X**	X	
8		X	X	**X**	X		X	**X**		X	X	X	X	X			X	X	X	
9	X			X	X	X					X					X				
10	X	X				X							X							
11	X								X											
12	X		X		X		X													
13		X	**X**	**X**	X	X	**X**	X		X	X	**X**	X	X					**X**	
14	**<u>X</u>**			X				X	X							X	X	X		
15			X																	
18	X																			
19	**X**																			
21	X	X			X			X	X	X					X					
22	X															X				
24		X	X				X			X				X						
28	X																			

Pain, Bone, Arms

	ARS	AUR	LYC	MEZ
6	X			
7			X	X
24		X		

Pain, Bone, Cranial

	BELL	GUAIAC	HEP	NIT AC	PULS
4				X	
6	X	X	X		
15					X

Pain, Bone, Facial

	AUR	AETHUS	CAPS	CINNAB	COLOC	HELL	HEP	KALI CAR	KALI IOD	KALM	MERC	MERC C	MERC I F	MERC I R	MEZ	NAT M	NIT AC	NIT	NUX V	PHOS	PHYTO	SIL	ZINC
1					X																		
4	X																						
5	X			X						X													
7								X									X				X		
8														X									
12											X												
13		X	X			X	X						X			X		X	X				X
14									X			X								X			
18															X								
21																						X	

Pain, Bone, Frontal

	KALI IOD	KALI BIC
4	X	
14	X	X

Pain, Bone, Legs

	ARS	AUR	GUAIAC	LED
6	X			
7			X	X
24		X		

Pain, Bone, Malar

	ACT R	AGAR M	CALC CA	CAUST	CIMICI	CUPR AC	HYOSC	IRIS V	KALI IOD	PLAT	POLYPOR	STRYCH	ZINC
2	X		X								X	X	X
6										X			
7		X		X		X	X	X	X				
8					X								

Pain, Bone, Mastoid

	AUR	CANTH	CAPS	ARN	CINA	GELS	PHOS	PLAT
1	X	X	X					
4			X					
6	X							X
7		X			X	X		
17							X	
24				X				

Pain, Bone, Nasal

	KALI IOD	MERC	AUR	CARB A	COLCH	INDIG	KALI BIC	MEZ	NAT M	NIT	SIL	VER A
4	X											
13		X	**X**	X	X	X						
14	X	X					X		X	X	X	X
18								X				

Pain, Bone, Skull

	IPEC	AUR	EUP PERF	KALI BIC	ARG N	NIT AC	ACON	ANT C	CANTH	CINNAB	MEZ	PH AC	PHOS	RHOD	RUTA	STAPHYS
6													X			
8		X														
9			X	X												
10	X															
13	X	**X**		X	**X**	**X**	X	X	X	X	X	X		X	X	X
14	X		X													

Pain, Bowel- See also Pain, Abdomen

	ACON	ARS	BRY	COLOC	IGN	IRIS V	CAPS	CHAM	HYDRAST	LACH	MERC	NUX V	RHUS T	SULPH
6	X	X	X	X	X		X					X	X	X
10		X					X		X				X	X
11			X			X				X	X			
12	X		X					X						
14										X				
15	X	X			X	X		X	X		X	X		
18				X	X									
21						X								
24				X										

Pain, Breast- See Mastalgia

Pain, Calf (Includes Arthralgia, Calves)

	BRY	CANN I	EUPHR	GNAPH	LYC	NUX V	ARS	CHAM	SEP
1				X					
8	X		X		X	X	**X**	**X**	**X**
12	X								
13			X		X				
14		X		X					
17		X				X			

Pain, Cancer

	CONDUR	ACON	ARS	CARC	CALC OX	CEDRON	EUPHORB	MORPH	SIL	ACOHOL	APIS	ARS BR	CALC AC	CALC ARS	CAMPH	CARB AC	CAUST	CHIM	CHOLEST	ECHIN	HYDRAST	NIT AC	NUX V	ORNITHO	PHOS	TAR C
1			X								X						X					X			X	
2													X													
3		X										X		X		X			X					X		
4						X		X	X																	
8	**X**									X																
9		X		X			X								X								X			
10					**X**																					X
12		X	X																							
14				X														X								
15	X																				X					
16	X		X	X			X	X												X						
24	X					X			X																	

Pain, Caecum

	HYDRAST	NAT SUL
10	X	
16		X

Pain, Cartilage

	ARG	LOB SYPH	RUTA
1	X		
2	X	X	X
19	X		

Pain, Cervix

	CARB A	ARG	CAULO	CON	MUREX
1		X		X	
4	X				
5			X		
6					X
19	X				

Pain, Cheek

	ACON	SANG	SPIG
4	X		
5		X	
14			X

Pain, Chest- See also Pain, Heart; Pleurisy (Note that only the main entries are used for 13)

	BRY	ACON	ARS	PHOS	ARN	RAN B	SULPH	CACT	KALI CAR	SENEG	PULS	BELL	CALC	CARB V	LACH	NUX V	SPIG	CAUST	EUP PERF	KALM	NIT AC	CHINA	COLCH	GELS	OX AC	RHUS T	STANN	
1		X		X	X	X		X	X	X					X											X		
2	**X**	**X**	**X**		**X**	**X**	**X**				**X**															X		
3						**X**																						
4	**X**	X			**X**	**X**		X	X							X				X	X							
5				X						X																		
6	X	X	X	X	X		X	X	X	X	X	X	X	X		X	X		X	X		X			X			
7	X	X	X	X	X	X	X	X	X	X	X		X	X	X	X	X	X	X		X	X	X	X		X	X	
8										X			X															
9	X		X																									
10	X	X											X							X								
11	X		X						X										X									
12	X	X	X	X																				X				
13	X	X	X	**X**	X	X	X			X	X	X	X	X	X	X	X	X			X	X	X		X	X	X	
14	X	X	X	X	X	X						X		X					X	X			X		X			
15	X	X	X	X				X				X	X	X		X		X						X				
16	X						X																					
17	X		X	X	X		X	X	X	X	X				X		X	X		X				X			X	
18		X																										
19	X	X			X		X	X	X						X										X			
20			X																									
21	X	X		X				X				X					X						X					
22	X																											
24																			X		X							
25	X		X	X													X											
26	X	X		X	X		X		X		X	X		X	X	X		X			X	X						
27			X																									

Pain, Coccyx- See Coccydynia

Pain, Coition, During, Female

	SEP	NAT M	KREO	ARG N	PLAT	BERB V	FERR	LYC	LYSSIN	MERC C	AGNUS	APIS	BELL	CAULO	FERR PH	HYDRAST	STAPHYS											
1	X	X	X	X	X	X	X	X	X	X						X	X											
4	X		X		X							X	X															
6	X	X	X		X			X							X													
7	X	**X**	X	**X**		X			X	X																		
8	X	X		X			X				X			X														

Pain, Deltoid

	AUR	CAULO	FERR	LAC C	PHYTO	SANG	ZINC OX	ZINC VAL																				
2							X	X																				
8	X	X	X	X	X																							
10						X																						

Pain, Diaphragm- See also Inflammation, Diaphragm

	STANN	NUX V	ACON	AGAR M	APIS	ASAF	ATROP	BRY	DIG	HOMAR	IGN	IPEC	LYC	MEZ	NAT M	NUX M	RHUS T	SIL	SPIG	STRAM	VIOL T							
2	X									X																		
6		X							X		X			X			X	X										
7	X	X	X	X	X		X	X				X				X				X								
13						X							X		X				X		X							

Pain, Ear- See Otalgia

Pain, Elbow

	ARG	LACHNAN	ARN	BRY	CARB V	CAUST	CORNUS	GRAT	IOD	LED	OL JEC A	PHOS	PULS	RAPH	SPIG	SULPH	VISC A	ZINC OX										
1								X																				
2														X				X										
7	X			X	X	X	X		X		X																	
9		X																										
13										X					X	X												
14	X		X									X	X				X											
25		X																										

Pain, Epigastrium

	CARB V	NUX V	ARS	BRY	CHAM	CHINA	KALI CAR	LYC	PHOS	PULS	ANAC	ARG N	CALC	CAMPH	CAUST	CINA	COCCUL	COLCH	CUPR	DIOSC	HYDRAST	HYOSC	IOD	KALI BIC	LACH	SANG		
1		X				X		X											X							X		
4																							X					
6			X	X			X								X		X	X		X	X							
7	X	X	X	X	X	X	X	X	X	X		X	X	X	X	X		X	X	X	X	X	X	X	X	X		
9											X													X				
10	X																											
11	X								X	X			X			X												
13					X									X														
18		X																							X			
19			X				X					X																
25	X										X																	
26	X	X		X	X	X		X	X	X							X					X						

Pain, Epiglottis

	MERC C	CHAM	MERC	WYETHIA																								
4				X																								
7	X	X																										
8	X		X																									

Pain, Eustacian Tube- See Otalgia

Pain, Extremities

	RHUS T	ACON	AGAR M	ALUM OX	BRY	CAUST	CEDRON	LAC C	NAT SUL	PHYTO	VER A																	
1									X																			
6	X				X	X	X																					
8			X	X							X																	
10										X																		
14	X	X						X																				

Pain, Extremities, Lower

	ABROT	AGAR M	GELS	NIT AC																								
3	X																											
4				X																								
8		X																										
11			X																									

Pain, Eyes- See also Neuralgia, Eye; Neuralgia, Infraorbital; Pain, Orbit (Note that only the main remedies from 13 are used here)

	SPIG	BELL	RUTA	BRY	GELS	EUPHR	MERC	MERC C	PHOS	SULPH	ALL C	ARS	CALC	EUP PERF	NUX V	SANG	AUR	COLOC	HEP	PRUN S	ACON	ASAF	CHEL	CIMICI	CON	KALI IOD	PULS	
1	X	X	**X**	X		X	X	X			X				X	X									X			
2	**X**		X																									
3			X			X	X	X													X				X			
4	X		X	**X**	X	X		X		X	X								X			X						
5						X												X										
6	X	X		X		X	X		X	X	X	X	X		X	X	X	X	X	X		X	X		X	X		
7		X						X						X				X	X				X			X		
8	X	X	X		X		X		X	X					X		X							X				
9	X	X	X	X	X	X			X		X		X														X	
10	X				X		X			X			X	X		X					X						X	
11						X		X									X											
12	X	X										X												X				
13				X			X		X	X		X	X		X			X				X					X	
14	X	X	X		X		X	X		X	X	X		X			X	X	X				X	X				
15	X				X																			X			X	
17				X				X				X				X			X	X					X			
18			X			X					X			X						X								
19												X				X										X		
20	X																											
21		X		X	X									X	X						X							
22														X		X												
24	X	X	X	X	X				X	X			X		X		X			X		X	X			X		
25	X	X	X	X	X	X			X				X															
27		X		X	X		X		X											X	X							
28			X																									

Pain, Eye, Left

	SPIG	CROC S
1	X	
6		X
11	X	

Pain, Eye, Above- See Neuralgia, Supraorbital
Pain, Eye, Above, Left- See Neuralgia, Supraorbital, Left
Pain, Eye, Right

	BELL	SANG	CARB V	COM	CROT H	HEP	HYOSC	LAC C	MEDO	PRUN S	RAN B	SEP	ZINC
1		X											
6	X					X	X						X
7				X	X				X		X		
10												X	
13	X	X						X					
15			X										
19										X			

Pain, Eyelids

	ARS	APIS	CAUST	COBALT	COLOC	EUPHORB	HEP	LYC	MEDO	SIL	TONGO
4								X			
6		X			X						
7			X			X			X		
8				X							
12	X										
13	X									X	X
14							X				

Pain, Face- See Neuralgia, Face; Prosopalgia

Pain, Feet (Includes Arthralgia, Feet; Arthralgia, Tarsal Joints; Feet, Burning, Feeling of; Neuralgia, Feet; Podalgia)

	SULPH	RHUS T	PULS	LED	ARN	ARS	BRY	CHAM	KALI CAR	COLCH
1			X							
2		**X**		**X**	X					**X**
3	X			X				X		
7	X		X		X	X			X	
8	X	X	X	X	X	X	X		X	X
10	X									
13	X	X		X	X		X		X	
14							X			
18	X									
21	X	X	X					X		
24	X									
25		X	X			X		X		

Pain, Fingers

	SULPH	AMBRA	AMM M	ANT C	BENZ AC	CARB V	CAULO	CAUST	HEP	HYPER	KALM	LYC	MANG	PETR	PH AC	SEP	SIL
3				X								X					
7	X				X	X	X	X	X		X			X			
8	X	X	X			X		X	X			X	X	X	X	X	X
13	X	X	X		X					X	X		X		X	X	X
14				X						X							
22							X										

Pain, Fracture Of- See also Pain, Bone

	RUTA	SYMPH	BRY	CALC	CHAM	COLCH	HYPER	MERC	RHUS T	STICTA
3	X		X	X	X	X	X	X	X	X
18		X								
19	X	X								

Pain, Gall Bladder- See also Cholecystitis

	BERB V	BAPT	BELL	CHEL	BRY	CHINA	COLOC	FERR SUL	HYDRAST	LEPT	LYC	MAG PH	MANDRA	MORG P	NAT SUL	NEPENTH
1															X	
2								X								
5	X		X	X	X	X	X					X	X			X
6		X								X						
11	X	X												X		
14	X															
18				X					X							
19											X					
24	X	X	X													

Pain, Genitalia, Female- See also Pain, Vagina; Pain, Uterus; Pain, Ovaries

	CALC	CARB V	AMBRA	ARS	CAUST	KALI CAR	KREO	LAC C	NAT M	NIT AC	NUX V	PLAT	SULPH	THUJA
6	X	X							X				X	
7	X	X	X	X	X	X	X	X	X	X	X	X		X
13	X	X	X	X	X	X	X	X	X	X	X	X	X	X

Pain, Genitalia, Male- See also Pain, Testes; Pain, Penis

	ARN	ANAC	BOV	CALC	CANN S	CANTH	COLOCIN	KREO	JAC CAR	MAG	MERC D	NIT AC	PULS
2							X						
7	X			X							X		
13	X	X	X		X	X		X	X	X			

Pain, Glands, Axillary

	ANTHRAC	ASAR	BAR C	BELL	CARB A	KALI CAR	MERC	SIL
7	X				X	X		
15				X			X	
26		X	X					X

Pain, Glands, Cervical

	MERC	CALC	PHYTO	PULS	SEP	ALUM	AMM M	ARN	ARUM T	BELL	CAPS	CAUST	CON	HELL	KALI CAR	LYC	MERC C	NAT M	NIT AC	PH AC	SEL	SPIG
5																	X					
8											X											
10				X																		
12	X																					
13	X	X		X	X	X	X	X		X		X		X	X	X		X	X	X	X	X
15	X																					
17			X		X																	
18									X													
19		X	X																			
21	X																					
24	X												X									
25	X																					

Pain, Glands, Inguinal

	CALC	MERC	ARS	BELL	BERB V	DULC	GRAPH	MEZ	TAB	THUJA
13	**X**	**X**	X		X	X	X	X	X	X
15				X						

Pain, Glands, Parotid

	BELL	SABAD
13		X
21	X	

Pain, Glands, Salivary

	ACON	IGN	MERC I F	MERC I R
12			X	
13	X			
14				X
19		X		

Pain, Glans Penis

	ARS	COP	LYC	RHUS T	SARS
1	X	X		X	X
7		X	X	X	X
13	X		X		

Pain, Groin

	BERB V	CAULO	CIMICI	EUPIO	IRIS F	LAURO	MERC	SIL	TEREB
2				X					
3					X			X	
8			X						
9	X								
10		X							
11							X		
13						X			
24									X

Pain, Growing

	GUAIAC	SIL
2	X	
8		X

Pain, Gums- See also Teething

	MERC	CHAM	STAPHYS	BELL	HEP	CALC	NIT AC	ARN	ARS	NAT M	NUX V	CARB V	CAUST	DOLICH	KREO	LACH	NUX M	PHOS	PULS	SULPH	TEREB	SIL
1		X						X							X							
2							**X**							X								
4															X						X	
5							X															
6	X	X	X	X	X	X		X	X	X	X	X	X			X	X	X	X	X	X	X
7	X		X		X		X					X		X		X						**X**
8	X		**X**	X		**X**		X	X	X	X		X			X	X	X	X	X		
9				X																		
10		X								X	X									X		
12	X																					
13	X	X	X	X	X	X			X	X	X		X	X			X	X				
14				X	X		X	X							X							
15		X																				
21	X																					
24																					X	
26	X	X	X		X	X			X			X							X			

Pain, Hands (Includes Arthralgia, Hands)

	SULPH	LED	PULS	RHUS T	CALC	RUTA	ACON	ACT SP	AMBRA	APIS	ARS	CARB V	CAUST	CHAM	CINA	GRAPH	HEP	KALM	LACH	NAT M	NUX V	PETR	PHOS	RHOD	SPONG	BRY	SEP
1	X	X	X					X																			
2		**X**	**X**	**X**		**X**																					
3										X																	
4								X																			
7	X				X		X			X	X	X			X	X	X	X	X	X		X	X		X		
8	**X**			X	**X**				X			X	X	X		X	X		X	X	X	X	X	X	X	**X**	**X**
13	X					X			X				X		X			X						X			
14	X	X					X																				
23			X	X							X			X							X						

Pain, Hands, Palm Of

	FL AC	PHOS	RHUS T	SULPH
6		X		
8	X			
12			X	
13				X

Pain, Heart

	CACT	SPIG	LACH	LIL T	ACON	NAJA	SPONG	KALM	LITH C	AUR	GLON	LAURO	CIMICI	OX AC	VER V	KALI CAR	APIS	ARN	ARS	BRY	LATRO M	AMBRA	COLCH	TAR H
1	X	X	X	X	X	X		X		X			X											
3	X	X													X									
4		**X**	**X**	**X**		X		**X**	X		X			X										
5	X	X					X			X			X					X				X		
6	X	X	X	X	X		X		X	X		X	X	X		X				X				X
7	X	X	X	X	X	X	X	X			X	X				X	X	X		X			X	
8	**X**	X	X	X	X	X	X		**X**	X	**X**	X		X	X	**X**	X		X	X		X	**X**	**X**
10	X		X	X	X		X	X		X							X	X	X		X		X	
11	X				X	X															X			
12	X	X													X									
13	X		X					X	X													**X**		
14	X	X	X	X		X	X	X	X		X			X	X			X	X					
15	X	X	X		X								X		X									
17	X	X	X	X	X	X	X	X	X	X	X	X	X	X		X	X		X	X	X			X
19	**X**	X	X	X		X	X					X									X			

Pain, Heels (Includes Arthralgia, Heels)

	GRAPH	CYCL	PETR	VALER	PHYTO	PULS	SEP	SIL	TART AC	AMM M	ANT C	CAUST	CHEL	FERR	LED	LYC	MEDO	NAT CAR	SABIN	CALC CA
1			X			X			X								X			
2		X		**X**					X										X	**X**
3	X	X			X	X		X	X											
5			X	X	X		X						X			X	X			
7			X											X				X		
8	**X**		X			X	X	X		X	X	X			X	X		X	X	
9		X		X	X							X			X					
10		X																		
13	X						X			X										
14	X										X		X	X						
21								X												

Pain, Hip- See Coxalgia

Pain, Hypochondria- See also Pain, Abdomen

	ARS	BRY	CALC	CARB V	CHEL	GRAPH	KALI BIC	KALI CAR	LYC	MERC	POD	SULPH	ZINC	ACON	BOR	CROT T
7	X	X	X	X	X	X	X		X		X	X				
8								X		X						
13	X	X	X	X	X	X	X	X	X	X	X	X	X	**X**	**X**	**X**
24													X			

Pain, Ileo-Caecal- See also Pain, Abdomen; Typhlitis

	BELL	RHUS T	MERC	BRY	PLUM	FERR PH	GINSENG	IRIS T	LACH	BAPT	COLOC	KALI MUR	KALI PH	MAG PH
1	X	X	X		X	X		X					X	X
3	X							X	X					
4	X	**X**		X		X						X		
6	X	X	X		X		X							
9				X					X		X			
10	X	X	X	X	X		X							
11										X				
16	X													
24	X		X											

Pain, Increased Sensitivity To- See Hyperaesthesia

Pain, Intercostal

	RAN B
1	**X**

Pain, Interscapular

	NAT ARS
2	X
17	X

Pain, Intestinal- See also Pain, Abdomen

	APIS	BRY	CHEL	IRIS V	PHOS	VERIN
2						X
8			X			
11				X		
13	X					
22					X	
24		X				

Pain, Jaw

	ACON	AMPHIS	ARUM T	CAUST	DOLICH	PHOS	PSOR	SPIG
1			X					
2		X			X			
6						X		
13							X	
14	X							X
21				X				

Pain, Jaw, Lower

	NUX V	AUR	ARUM T	CARB A	CAUST	COLCH	GELS	GUAIAC	KALM	LACH	MERC C	PHOS	RHUS T	SPIG
7	X	X		X	X	X	X	X	X	X	X	X	X	
8	X		X											
15														X

Pain, Jaw, Lower Left

	ARUM T	MAG P AR
1		X
8	X	

Pain, Jaw Upper

	KALM	ACT SP	AGAR M
1		X	X
4	**X**		

Pain, Joint, Sacroiliac- See Lumbago

Pain, Joint, Temperomandibular

	ARUM T	RHUS T	ACON	CAUST	MEZ	SPHING	SPIG	SPONG	XANTHO
2	**X**					X	X	X	X
3	X								
4			X	X					
6		X							
7		X			X				

Pain, Joints- See also Rheumatism; Rheumatoid Arthritis; Synovitis (Includes Arthralgia)

	BRY	RHUS T	PULS	LED	MERC	BELL	ARN	RUTA	COLCH	LYC	ACON	APIS	CAUST	CHAM	NUX V	ARS	SULPH	ARG	CAUL	IGN	NAT M	MANG
1											X			X				X				
2	**X**																					
4	X		X	X								X										
5							X	X				X										
6										X												
7	X	X	X	X	X	X	X		X	X		X		X		X	X	X				
8	X	X	X	X	**X**	X	X	X	**X**	**X**			X		X	**X**	**X**			X	X	**X**
9	X	X						X					X		X							
10	X	X	X		X	X		X						X								
11	X								X		X								X			
12	X					X																
13			**X**	X	**X**				X	X	X				X		X			X	X	X
14		X											X	X						X		
15		X		X	X		X								X							
18	X											X										
19	X	X	X	X			X	X					X			X		X	X		X	
20	X																					
21		X	X								X											
22	X	X																				
24		X																				
25						X																
27																			X			

Pain, Joints, Elbow

	BRY	ANT C	ARG	CALC	CAUL	CAUST	GRAPH	KALM	LED	LYC	MERC	MEZ	PETR	PHOS	PULS	RHUS T	RUTA	SEP	STAPHYS	SULPH	VER A
8	**X**	X	X	X	X	X	X	X	X	X	X	X	X	X	X	X	X	X	X	X	X

Pain, Joints, Fingers

	CAUST
8	X
19	X

Pain, Joints, Small

	CAULO	ACT SP	COLCH	CIMICI	LED	RHOD
1		X				
3		X				
4				X		
10			X			
11			X			
12					X	X
22	X					
23	X					
27	X					

Pain, Joints, Wrist

	ARS	BRY	CAULO
8	**X**	**X**	**X**

Pain, Knee- See also Gonarthritis

	PULS	BRY	SULPH	CALC	RHUS T	BENZ AC	BERB V	CAUST	DIOSC	APIS	HELL	KALI IOD	STAPHYS	CHINA
1	X													
2						**X**	**X**		**X**					
3	X		X	X			X		X			X		
4	X									X		X		
7	X		X	X	X			X		X	X	X	X	
8	X	**X**	**X**	**X**	**X**			**X**			X		X	**X**
9	<u>**X**</u>													
11		X												
13	X		X								X		X	X
14		X				X		X		X				
17			X						X					
21				X		X	X							
22		X												
24					X									
25	**X**	X			X									

Pain, Kidneys- See Nephralgia

Pain, Labia

	KREO	APIS	ARS	CALC	SAC LAC	SIL	SULPH
1	X						
2					X		
11	X						
14		X	X				
26				X		X	X

Pain, Labour- See Labour, Painful

Pain, Labour, After- See Labour, Pain, After Delivery

Pain, Larynx- See also Laryngitis

	PHOS	BELL	HEP	SPONG	CARB V	ALL C	BRY	LACH	ACON	ANT T	ARG	CHAM	EUP PERF	HYDR AC	IGN	KALI BIC	NUX V	BROM
1				X		X												
4	X	X	X	X			X						X					
5																X		
6	X	X																
7	X	X	X	X	X			X	X	X	X	X		X	X	X	X	
8	X	X	X							X				X				**X**
9		X											X					
10	X																	
11		X																
13	X			X	X			X				X		X	X			X
14	X	X	X	X	X				X								X	
15	X				X			X								X		
17	X		X	X	X		X			X		X			X			
18	X					X												
19		X				X												
21	X					X												
22																	X	
24	X	X	X	X		X	X				X		X					
25	X	X	X		X		X	X	X		X							

Pain, Leg, Left

	NAT CAR	CIMICI	APIS	CARB AC
6	X			
7	X	X	X	X

Pain, Leg, Right

	KALI CAR	ASC S	CIC	COCCUS	KALI IOD	POD	RHOD	RHUS T
1	X							
7	X	X	X	X	X	X		X
21							X	

Pain, Legs (Includes Arthralgia, Legs)

	KALI CAR	RHUS T	DIOSC	BRY	CHAM	CON	GELS	RHOD	SEP	CARB A	ARS	ASAF	BELL	CALC	CARB AC	CAUST	FERR	LYC	MERC	MEZ	NUX V	PH AC	PHYTO	PULS	SULPH			
1			X																									
2			**X**							**X**																		
3			X												X													
7	X	X		X	X		X		X	X	X	X		X	X	X			X	X	X	X	X	X	X			
8	X	X		X		X		X	X			X	X	X		X	X	X	X	X	X	X		X	X			
9					X		X																					
13	X	X		X				X									X	X										
14	X																						X					
16						X																						
17						X					X																	
18									X																			
21		X						X					X															
25					X		X																					

Pain, Ligaments

	RHUS T	CUPR	RHOD																									
7		X																										
11	X																											
14	X																											
17	X																											
21			X																									

Pain, Limbs

	BRY	RHUS T	DULC	ACON	ARS	GELS	EUP PERF	ARN	CARB V	CHINA	PH AC	PHYTO	SEP	CALC	CAUST	CIMIC	GUAIAC	LACH	LYC	MERC	PULS
4	X		**X**			X					X	X									
6	X	X		X	X	X	X	X	X	X		X	X	X	X	X	X	X	X	X	X
7	X	X	X		X	X	**X**	X	X	X		X	X	X	X		X	X	X	X	X
8		X																			
10	X				X				X												
11	X										X										
12	X										X					X					
13				X														X			
14				X				X													
15	X		X	X	X	X			X				X			X					
16		X																			
17			X			X															
20	X																				
21							X														
22							X														
24	X	X										X					X				
26	X	X	X	X	X			X		X	X		X	X	X				X	X	X
27										X											

Pain, Lip

	ARS	APIS	CARB A	CIC	MUR AC	SULPH	RHUS V
2							**X**
7	X	X	X	X	X	X	
10	X						
13	X		X	X	X	X	
14		X					

Pain, Liver (AKA Hepatalgia)

	BRY	CHEL	MERC	NUX V	CHINA	LACH	LYC	ACON	ARS	PHOS	SULPH	BELL	BERB V	CALC	CHIO	POD	CARB V	DIG	LEPT	MYRICA	PTEL	SEP	KALI CAR	MAG M	CARD M	NAT SUL		
1	X	X			X	X	X		X	X	X			X	X		X			X	X				X	X		
3		X													X													
4	**X**	**X**	**X**			X	X			X	X				X			X	X	X	X	X	X					
5	X	X		X						X			X			X			X		X	X		X				
6	X	X	X	X	X	X	X	X	X	X	X	X		X		X	X		X	X	X	X	X		X			
7	X	X	X	X	X	X	X	X		X	X	X	X	X	X	X	X	X	X		X		X	X	X	X		
8	X		X	X	X				X				X					X										
9						X							X													X		
10	X	X	X	X	X		X		X		X	X																
11	X	X	X				X	X	X						X				X	X					X			
12	X	X	X	X				X																				
13	X		X	**X**	X	X	**X**	X	X	X	X		X	X		X	X	X				X	**X**	**X**		X		
14		X					X			X					X		X			X								
15	X		X	X	X			X				X				X												
17																		X										
18	X	X				X			X	X																		
19	X	X	X	X	X	X	X	X	X	X	X	X	X	X	X	X			X	X	X	X	X	X	X	X		
20		X		X	X			X				X																
21	X	X	X			X																X						
24		X		X	X	X							X	X		X												
26	X		X	X	X	X	X	X	X		X	X		X			X							X				
27																		X										

Pain, Loins- See also Pain, Kidneys

	NUX V	ACON	BRY	SULPH	ANT T	BELL	BERB V	POD	PULS	RHUS T	AESC	ALOE	BAPT	BUFO	CANTH	CARB AC	CAULO	CAUST	CHAM	DULC	IOD	KALI TAR	LYC	PH AC	PLUM	RUTA	SEC	SEP
4					X																							
6																					X							
8																				X					X			
9				X			X									X	X											
10	X		X	X		X			X									X	X								X	
11							X																					
12		X	X		X						X	X												X				
14										X					X								X					
15	X	X	X			X		X	X	X			X															X
17								X						X								X				X		
18	X																											
24	X	X																										
25				X																								

Pain, Lung, Right

	ANISE	PHOS
8	X	
10		X

Pain, Lungs, Apices

	BRY	MYRTUS	PHOS
4	X		
8		X	X

Pain, Mouth

	MERC	LACH	NAT M	ARS	ARUM T	HEP	HYDRAST	NIT AC	APIS	IGN	IPEC	MERC C	MEZ	PHOS	SULPH AC	VER A
2		X			**X**	**X**	X	**X**								
3		X														
4	X			X												
6			X		X											
7	X	X	X	X		X	X	X	X	X	X	X	X	X		X
8		X				X									X	
9									X							
11				X								X				
12	X		X													
13	X		X	X	X					X	X		X	X		X
15							X								X	
26	X															

Pain, Muscles- See Myalgia

Pain, Nails, Under

	BELL	GRAPH	HEP	SEP	ANT C	BERB V	CAUST	HYPER	MERC	MYRIST	NIT AC	SQUILLA	SULPH	TEUCR
1										X				
2				**X**										
3						X								
13		X	X		X		X		X		X	X	X	
14	X		X					X						X
21	X	X												

Pain, Neck- See Neuralgia, Neck

	CIMICI	GELS	CAUST	BRY	LACHNAN	BELL	CALC PH	DULC	APIS	ARS	CALC	CHEL	FERR	GLON	GRAPH	GUAIAC	HELL	KALM	LACH	PULS	SIL	SULPH	VER V
1	X	X					X																
3	X				X								X										
4																		X			X		
5			X				X				X				X	X							
6		X							X				X						X				
7		**X**	**X**						X			X		X	X		X		X		X	X	X
8					X									X									
10																		X					
11	X	X	X	X	X	X		X								X				X			
12	X					X																	
13				X		X											X			X			
14	X	X		X	X							X											
15		X				X																	X
17										X	X												
18	X																						
19	**X**		X				X															X	
20								X															
21	X	X	X	X	X			X															
22		X																					
27				X						X													

Pain, Neck, Nape Of

	GRAPH	AMM C	ANT C	BRY	CARB V	CAUST	CHINA	DAPHNE	DULC	GELS	HEP	IGN	MERC	POD	PULS	RHOD	RHUS T	SARS	SPIG	STAPHYS	VER V
10											X		X								
13	**X**	X	X	X	X		X	X				X		X	X	X		X		X	
15										X									X		
17																	X				X
21						X			X												

Pain, Nerve- See also Neuralgia

	HYPER	CEDRON	RHOD
5	X		
8		X	X
21	X		
22	X		

Pain Nerve, Ulnar

	KALM
1	X
11	X

Pain, Nipples

	SULPH	ARN	PHYTO	CHAM	CROT T	GRAPH	SIL	HAM	PHELL	LYC	CAST EQ	MERC	PULS	CALEND	SEP	AGAR M	BOR	CALC	CON	HELON	HYDRAST	IGN	NUX V	PHOS
1			X		X		X		X		X						X							
2	X	**X**	X		**X**			**X**	**X**					**X**			X				X			X
5																X				X				
6	X	X	X					X															X	
7	X	X	X	X	X	X	X	X	X	X	X	X	X		X	X			X	X			X	
8	X	X	X	X	X	X	X	X		X	X	X	X		X	X	X			X				X
9	X	E	X		X				X					E							X			
10	X	B					X			X		X						X					X	
13	X	**X**		**X**		**X**		X		X	**X**	X	X		**X**			X				X		X
14			X	X		X	X												X					
15	X	E		**X**		X																		
21	X			X		X	X						X					X	X			X		
24	X		X																					
25		E	X		X				X					E							X			
26	X			X						X												X		

B- Both Internal and External E- External

Pain, Nose (Includes Pain, Nostrils)

	AUR	HEP	MERC	KALI BIC	ARS	ARUM T	SIL	ARS IOD	BELL	GELS	IOD	MEZ	PHOS	PETR
1												X		
2				**X**										**X**
4			X			X								
5						X								
6	X	X					X		X	X	X		X	
7	X	X	X	X	X						X	X		X
8		X								X	X			
10							X		X					
12	X		X											
13		X	X	X	X		X					X		
14	X			X						X				
15			X											
16								X						
17	X	X			X	X	X	X					X	
19					X	X								
21								X						
24	X								X				X	

Pain, Nose, Root Of

	KALI BIC	STICTA	BAPT	ELAPS	KALI IOD	LACH	PULS	IGN	NAT ARS	PLAT	SANG	ZINC
1	X											
2									X			
4										X		
5		X										
6	X			X			X				X	
7	X		X									
8			X	X		X		X				X
9						X						
10							X					
14	X	X				X						
15								X				
17		X	X		X				X		X	
18		X			X							
19	X				X							
20	X											
24	X			X			X					X
26										X		

Pain, Oesophagus- See also Oesophagitis

	ARS	MEZ	ACON	CARB AC	COCCUL	KALI BIC	MERC C	OX AC	PHOS	SPIG	SANG
1	X										
2									X		
6		X				X		X			
7	X	X	X	X			X		X		**X**
8	X	X	X	X	X	X		X		X	
10										X	
11							X				
15					X						

Pain, Orbit- See also Pain, Eye

	APIS	IGN	KALI BIC	LACH	NAJA	TEREB
7	X			X	X	
8		X				X
14			X			

Pain, Ovaries- See Ovaralgia

Pain, Palms

	SULPH	RHUS T	PHOS	SANG	CALC	PETR
1	X					
4	X					
10		X	X			
11	X					
12		X				
13			X			X
14				X		
15					X	
17	X			X		
24		X				

Pain, Palate

	MEZ	COFF	LACH	NIT AC	NUX V	PHYTO	RAN B
7	X	X				X	
13	X		X	X	X		
17							X

Pain, Pancreas

	IRIS V	ARS	CARB A	CARB V	COLCH	CON	KALI BIC	PHOS	PLAT	PLUM	RHUS T	STANN	THUJA	ZINC
1	X													
4	X													
7	X													
8	X	X	X	X	X	X	X	X	X	X	X	X	X	X

Pain, Parotid Gland

	AUR	MERC	BRY	CARB A	KALI BIC
3					X
6		X			
7	X	X		X	
8	X		X		

Pain, Pelvis- See also Coccygodynia; Pain, Uterus; Ovaralgia

	BELL	AESC	CARB A	COCCUL	CONVAL	HYDROC	KREO	MELILOT	PULS	SEP	USTIL
3		X								X	
6	X		X				X				
8					X			X			X
9						X					
10	X			X							
20									X		

Pain, Penis- See also Pain, Genitalia, Male; Pain, Prepuce

	PARIERA	KREO	BERB V	CANTH	GEUM	MAG M	PHYTO	THUJA
1	X	X				X		
2					X			
3		X			X			
6	X			X			X	X
7	X	X				X		
12							X	
13			X					X
14	X		X	X				

Pain, Perineum

	ARN	CANTH	CARB V	LYC	PHYTO	CAUST	AUR	CALC PH	MELA	MEZ	RHOD	RUTA	SANIC	SEP	THUJA
2									X						
5													X		
6		X			X									X	
7	X	X	X	X	X	**X**	X	X		X					
8															X
13			X	X							X				
24	X											X			

Pain, Periosteum- See also Periostitis

	SYMPH	KALI IOD	MEZ	RUTA	ARN	AUR	AUR M	MANG	MERC	PHYTO	RHUS T	STILL
1								X				
2	X										X	
4	X											
5	X											
6						X	X					
7		X			X				X			
8			X									X
11		X										
12										X		
18	X											
19			X	X								
24	X											
28				X								

Pain, Pharynx

	ARG N	ARS	SANG	ACON	ARUM T	ASAF	CALC PH	CANTH	CARB V	CHLOR	GELS	MEZ	NIT AC	TUB
1		X	X											
4	X													
5					X									
7	X	X	X	X		X	X				X	X	X	
14								X						
17									X	X				X

Pain, Pleura- See also Pleurisy

	BRY	ACON	BAD	ELAPS	FORMICA	GUAIAC	KALI CAR	PNEUMOC	RHAMN C	SULPH
7	X				X		X			X
8	X					X				
11									X	
17			X	X				X		
26	X	X								

Pain, Prepuce- See also Pain, Genitalia, Male; Pain, Penis

	MERC	CALC	COR R	NIT AC	NUX V	SULPH	ACON	ARS	BENZ AC	BERB V	CHAM	CYCL	EUPHR	IGN	LOB I	LYC	MANG	OSMIUM	PULS	RHUS T	SABIN	SIL	THUJA
1		X	X	X			X																
7	**X**			X	X	X								X		X							
13	X	X	X		X	X		X	X	X	X	X	X		X		X	X	X	X	X	X	
14																							X

Pain, Prostate Gland

	KALI BIC	CHIM	ALL C	APIS	CAPS	CAUST	CON	COP	CYCL	KALI CAR	PARIERA	PULS	SULPH															
7	X		X		X		X		X	X																		
13	X							X																				
19		X									X		X															
20	X	X		X		X						X																

Pain, Pylorus

	CAD S	CANTH	LACT V	LOB S	NUX V	ORNITHO																						
1	X																											
2			X	X																								
8		X			X																							
19						X																						

Pain, Rectum (Includes Neuralgia, Rectum)

	NIT AC	ALOE	AESC	IGN	ARS	RAT	NAT M	NUX V	SULPH	CAUST	BELL	CAPS	CARB V	COLLINS	KALI CAR	LYC	CALC	GRAPH	HYDRAST	IRIS V	MERC C	MUR AC	PETR	SEP	THUJA			
1	X	X		X		X			X	X		X	X						X			X						
2															X	X				X								
3	X					X																						
4				X	X	X	X	X																				
5	X													X				X							X			
6	X		X	X	X	X	X	X	X		X	X	X	X	X	X		X	X	X			X		X			
7	X	X	X	X	X		X	X	X	X	X	X	X	X	X	X	X		X		X			X				
8	X						X			X	X																	
9		X	X																									
10	X			X	X			X																				
11	X	X	X	X	X		X		X																			
12		X	X		X																							
13	X	X			X		X	X	X	X		X			X	X	X	X			X	X	X	X				
14	X	X	X	X	X	X															X	X						
15																	X											
18			X																									
19		X	X	X		X					X			X														
21		X				X														X								
23	X		X																									
24	X			X		X		X	X	X			X										X	X	X			
25		X	X																									
27		X																										

Pain, Sacrum- See also Lumbago (AKA Sacralgia)

	AESC	NUX V	AGAR M	BERB V	SEP	ZINC	CALC PH	LACH	LOB I	SABIN	KALI CAR	PHOS	PULS	ACON	AMM M	CHEL	CIMEX	IGN	LITH C	MERC	MUREX	NUX M	POD	RUTA	VER A			
2	**X**		**X**	**X**	X																							
3	X																											
4	X						X			X																		
5								X																				
6	X					X		X												X				X				
7	X	X		X	X	X	X		X	X	X	X	X			X	X	X	X			X	X		X			
8	X																											
9		X							X	X																		
10			X																									
11	X																											
13		X	X	X	**X**	**X**	X	X			**X**	**X**	**X**	X	X		X	X	X	X	X	X	X	X	X			
14		X																			X							
17									X							X												
18															X													
24	X													X														

Pain, Scalp

	KREO	RHUS T	ANT T	ARS	BAR C	BELL	CARB A	CARB V	CAPS	CHINA	COLOC	FERR	KALI BIC	KALI NIT	LITH	NAT SUL	NIT AC	NUX V	PETR	SARS	SEL	SEP	SIL	SOL T A	STAPHYS	SULPH IO	THUJA	
2																								X		X		
5											X		X															
8	X	X																				X						
13	X	X	X	X	X	X	X	X	X	X		X		X	X	X	X	X	X	X	X		X		X		X	

Pain, Scapula

	CAUST	CAMPH	CHINA	PHOS	SULPH	JUG C																						
1	X																											
2						**X**																						
7	X	X	X		X																							
9				X																								
13	X	X	X	X	X																							

Pain, Scapula, Between

	LYC	PHOS	BELL	FERR	PULS	SULPH	AMM C	ARS	BOR	CALC	CHENO	CHIN S	DROS	GLON	HEP	IPEC	LAPIS	NAT CAR	NUX V	PETR	SIL	TAB
1																	X					
4	X	X		X																		
5	X				X						X											
6		X		X		X						X								X		X
7	X	X			X	X	X	X		X			X	X	X	X			X		X	
10	X	X																				
13			X						X									X				
19			X																			

Pain, Scapula, Right

	CHEL	CIC	ASPARA	BRY	COLOC	SEP
1	X					
7		X	X		X	X
8		X				
17				X		
19	X					
21	X					

Pain, Scapula, Under

	CHENO V	CALC	CHEL	GELS	OX AC	SEP
1					X	
2	X					
5						X
6				X		
7	X	X	X			

Pain, Scapula, Under Left

	CUPR AR	CHENO	GELS
9	X		
13		X	X
25	X		

Pain, Scapula, Under Right

	CHEL	JUG C
1	X	X
2	X	
4	X	
5	X	
6	X	
7	X	
10	X	
11	X	
14	X	
16	X	
17	X	
18	X	
21	X	
28	X	

Pain, Scars

	CIC	HYPER	NAT M	SIL	STAPHYS
1		X	X		X
19	X				
21				X	

Pain, Scrotum

	BERB V	CON	SULPH	ACON	ARS	CALC	EUPHR	FERR M	KALI CAR	LACHNAN	MERC	NAT M	NAT SUL	RAN S	SIL	THUJA	ZINC
1			X														
7		X				X							X				
13	X		X	X			X	X	X	X	X	X		X	X	X	X
14	X				X												
24		X															

Pain, Shoulder

	SANG	FERR	GELS	BRY	CON	FERR PH	LED	LOB I	MAG CAR	MERC	NUX V	PHYTO	PULS	RHUS T	VER V
1							X								
2								X							
4	X	X				X			X		X	X			
7	X	X		X	X	X		X	X		X		X		X
9	X														
11			X												
13		X	X	X	X					X			X	X	
14	X		X				X					X			
15										X					X
21		X												X	
25	X														

Pain, Shoulder, Left

	ACON	FERR	SULPH	ARG N	CALC	CHEL	CIST	CONDUR	DIG	NAJA	NUX M	OX AC	ZINC OX
1	X									X			
4												X	
6		X											X
7		X		X	X	X	X	X	X				
8											X		
11	X		X										
21			X										

Pain, Shoulder, Right

	SANG	CHEL	MAG ACR	PHYTO	BERB V	CHENO	FERR	FERR M	LACH	PLECT	PULS N	URT U
2	X									X	X	X
3			X									
4					X							
6			X									
7		X	X			X						
8	X			X			X					
9	X	X										
10	X											
12		X										
13									X			
14				X								
17				X								
19		X						X				
21	X	X										
25	X											

Pain, Sigmoid Flexure

	ARG N	SCROPH
2		X
11	X	

Pain, Skin- See also Hyperaesthesia

	HEP	ACON	AGAR M	ALL C	AMBRA	ARS	BAR C	BELL	CARB V	CHAM	EUPHR	KALI CAR	LACH	LYC	MERC	NIT	PHOS	RHUS T	SEP	SIL	STAPHYS	ZINC
13	X	X	X		X	X	X	X	X		X	X	X	X	X	X	X	X	X	X		X
14	X																				X	
15										X												
17				X																		

Pain, Soles (Includes Soles, Burning)

	SULPH	PULS	CALC	GRAPH	PH AC	SANG	MUR AC	CHAM	LED	PETR	AMBRA	ANT C	CANN I	CANTH	CUPR	LYC	MANG	PHOS	PHYTO	SIL	TART AC	CAUST
1	X																X				X	
2		**X**					**X**			**X**												
3	X				X			X													X	
4	X											X										
5									X													
6	X		X			X																
7	X	X	X	X	X			X						X	X	X	X		X	X		
8	X	**X**	X	X	X		X		X		X				X	X		X		X		**X**
10	X											X						X				
11	X																					
13		X		X	X	X					X											
14	X					X		X	X				X	X					X			
15			X																			
17	X					X							X									
18	X																					
21	X			X			X			X												
24	X																					

Pain, Spermatic Cord- See also Neuralgia, Spermatic Cord

	BERB V	CLEM	OX AC	PULS	SPONG	ARN	STAPHYS	MERC	NUX V	OL AN	SULPH
1				X	X	X	X				
2	X		X							X	
4		**X**	X	X	X						
7	X	X		X	X		X	X	X		X
8	X		X			X					
13	X	X	X	X		X		X	X		X
14	X	X			X					X	
24							X				

Pain, Spermatic Cord, Left

	AMM M	BELL	HAM
7			X
24	X	X	

Pain, Spermatic Cord, Right

	CLEM	STAPHYS
4	X	X
7	X	

Pain, Spinal Cord

	HYPER	ALUM OX	ARN	BELL	BRY	DULC	LACT V
1	X		X	X	X		
2							X
6						X	
7	X						
8		X					

Pain, Spine

	PHOS	CHIN S	BELL	CIMICI	COCCUL	NAT M	ZINC	AGAR M	GELS	HYPER	PH AC	TAR H
1	X						X					
4	X	X	X	X	X	X	X	X			X	X
5									X			
6			X		X	X				X		X
7	X	X	X		X	X	X	X	X	X	X	
8	X	X	X	X	X	X	X	X	X		X	X
15				X								
17	X	X								X		
18				X								
19	X											
21		X										
24	X											

Pain, Spleen

	CHINA	CEANOTH	SULPH	CAPS	ARS	BERB V	NAT M	ARN	CHEL	HYDRAST	RAN B	APIS	BELL	BRY	CARB V	CHIN S	COB	CON	FL AC	GRIND	IGN	JUG R	SULPH AC	NIT AC
1	X	X		X										X										
2		X	X																	X		X		
4	**X**	X	X	**X**		X			X		X									X				
5										X	X													
6	X	X			X		X	X				X	X		X									
7	**X**		X	X	X		X		X	X					X		X	X	X		X		X	
8	X	X				X			X							X		X				X		
9		X				X																		
10	X	X	X	X	X		X	X		X														
11					X																			
13	X		X			X	X	X			X		X			X	X		X		X		X	**X**
17	X																							
26														X										
27												X												

Pain, Sternum, Inside

	DIOSC	OSMIUM	RUTA	AMM C	CAUST	KALI IOD	KALM	KREO	LAC V	PAEONIA	RAN S	STRONT C	SULPH
2		X	**X**	X					X	X	X	X	
6	X	X											
7	X				X	X	X	X					X

Pain, Sternum, Behind- See also Oesophagitis; Pain, Oesophagus

	KALI CAR	RUMEX	SYPH	RAN S	AUR	CACT	CAUST	CHEL	CONDUR	CUPR AC	CUPR	DIOSC	EUP PERF	KALI BIC	LACH	PHOS
1							X									
2				**X**												
4		X														
5		X														
6	X															
7	X		X			X		X		X	X		X		X	X
10			X		X				X							
15														X		
17												X				

Pain, Sternum, Under

	CARB V	ACON	ARS	ASAF	CAUST	CHAM	CURP AC	HEP	PHOS	TEREB
4					X					
6	X						X		X	
7	X	X		X		X		X		X
19			X							

Pain, Stomach- See Gastralgia

Pain, Stump- See also Neuralgia, Stump

	AMM M	SYMPH	ALL C	HYPER	PH AC
1	X	X	X	X	
2	X	X			
3	X		X	X	
4		X			
7					X
8	X				
24		X			

Pain, Surgery, After

	ARN	HYPER	BELLIS	STAPHYS	ALL C	BRY	CROC	NIT AC	NUX V	RHUS T	STICTA	STRONT C	SULPH
4		X											
8					X		X				X		
12	X												
13								X	X				X
14	X	**X**											
16				X									
19	X	X	X	X									X
21		X											
24	X	**X**	X			X				X			
28	X	X											
29[1]	X												
29[2]	X												

29[1] Jeffrey SL, et al. Use of Arnica to relieve pain after carpal-tunnel release surgery. Alternative therapies in Health and Medicine, 2002, Mar-Apr, 8, 2, 66-8.

29[2] Robertson A, et al. Homeopathic Arnica montana for post-tonsillectomy analgesia: a randomised placebo control trial. Homeopathy. 2007 Jan;96(1):17-21.

Pain, Swallowing- See Dysphagia

Pain, Teeth- See Hyperaesthesia, Teeth; Toothache

Pain, Tendon

	RHUS T	ARIST M	CALC PH	MYRICA	RUTA	TET	UPAS
2		X		X		X	X
8	X		X				
11	X						
12	X						
14	X						
17	X				X		

Pain, Testes- See also Pain, Genitalia, Male

	CLEM	HAM	RHOD	IOD	AUR	NUX V	OL AN	PULS	ACON	ARG	BELL	BERB V	CALC	CANTH	CHINA	CON	LYCOP	MERC	NAT CAR	OX AC	PH AC	PLUM	SEP	SIL	SPONG	STAPHYS		
1	X		X	X	X			X					X			X												
2							X													X								
3							X																					
4	X	X																							X			
6														X														
7	**X**	X	X	X	X	X		X	X	X					X	X	X	X	X		X	X	X	X		X		
8		X																										
9				X		X																						
12					X																							
13	X		**X**		X	X	X	X	X	X	X	X			X			X	X	X	X	X	X			X		
14	X	X	X									X		X			X								X			
21		X									X																	
24													X											X				
25				X																								

Pain, Thigh (Includes Arthralgia, Thighs)

	RHUS T	BRY	SULPH	ARN	BERB V	COCCUL	HEP	NUX V	CALC
1						X			
4	X								
5		X							
7	X		X	X		X	X	X	X
8	X	**X**	**X**	X		X	X	X	**X**
9					X				
10	X								
11					X				
13		X		X					
14	X				X			X	
17			X						
24							X		

Pain, Throat- See also Pain, Larynx; Pain, Trachea (Includes Sore Throat)

	HEP	BELL	LACH	ACON	NUX V	MERC	DULC	APIS	ARS	BAR C	PHOS	PHYTO	ARUM T	KALI BIC	SULPH	CAPS	CANTH	CIST	GELS	IGN	LYC	SABAD	BRY	CARB V	KALI CAR	NIT AC	SIL
1	X	X	X	X	X		X	X				X	X	X				X		X		X					
2	**X**	**X**	**X**					**X**	**X**	**X**		**X**		**X**		**X**	**X**	X		**X**	**X**	X			X		
3	**X**	X	X	X						X											X						
4	**X**	**X**	X		**X**	**X**	X	X				**X**	X	**X**		X	X	X	X			X				X	
5													X			X											
6		X	X	X	X	X		X	X		X	X	X	X						X	X		X				X
7	X	**X**	**X**	X	X	X		X	X	X		**X**	X	X	X	X	X	X	X		X		X		X	X	X
8	**X**	**X**	**X**	**X**	**X**	**X**	X	X	X	X	X	X	X	X	X	X	X	X	X	X	X	X	X		X	X	X
9		X		X			X	X		X															X		
10	X	X	X	X	X	X					X				X								X				X
11											X	X															
12		X	X	X		X	X	X		X									X								
13	X	X	X	**X**	X	**X**	X	X	**X**	X	**X**		X	X	X	X	**X**	X	X	X	X	**X**	X		X	X	X
14	**X**	X	X	X	X		X			**X**					X		X		X				X			X	
15	X	X	X	X	X	X	X		X		X			X	X				X	X						X	
16			X										X					X									
17	X	X	X		X		X	X	X	X	X	X	X		X	X	X				X	X			X		
18	X												X														
19	X		X		X		X	X	X		X				X			X				X	X				X
20	X	**X**	X	X		X		X	X			X			X				X		X						
21	X			X		X	X	X	X		X	X	X						X	X		X			X	X	
22	X			X	X		X		X		X							X									
24	X	X	X		**X**				X					X		X	X										
25	X	X	X	X		X	X			X				X											X		
26	X	X	X	X	X	X			X		X				X	X				X			X			X	X
27						X	X			X	X	X															X

Pain, Throat, Left Side

	MERC I R	LACH	BROM	KALI CAR	LACHNAN	NAJA	SEP	USTIL
1	X							
7	X							
8	X		X	X	X		X	X
9		X						
17						X		
21		X						
28	X							

Pain, Throat, Right Side

	BELL	MERC I F	LYC	MERC	PHYTO	ARG N	ARS	DOLICH	HAM	LAC C	NICCOL	SABAD
1	X	X			X							
4					X							
7		X	X	X					X	X		
8	X	X						X			X	X
9				X								
19						X	X					
21	X		X									
22	X											
28		X										

Pain, Tibia (Includes Arthralgia, Tibia)

	DULC	ARG	LACH	MEZ
1			X	
2	X			
3		X		
8	X	X	X	X
9				X
17	X			

Pain, Toe- See also Gout (Includes Arthralgia, Toes)

	CAULO	AGAR M	ASAF	AUR	CARB V	CHINA	COLCH	KALM	RAN S	STAPHYS	ARN	CAUST	SABIN	SULPH
7	X		X		X		X	X	X					
8		X	X	X	X	X		X		X	**X**	**X**	**X**	**X**
13		X		X		X	X		X	X				
21	X													
22	X													

Pain, Toe, Big- See also Gout

	PLUM	SIL	ARN	CIMICI	SABIN
8		X	**X**	**X**	**X**
9	X				
17	X				
21		X			

Pain, Tongue (AKA Glossalgia)

	SEP	BAPT	CALC	ARS	CAUST	CIST	CON	LACH	MUR AC	NAT M	NIT AC	ACON	ARUM T	BELL	CROT H	PHELL	PH AC	PHOS	PHYTO	SABAD	SIL	SULPH
1	X	X			X			X							X							
2																X						
5													X									
6	X			X						X												
7	X		X			X	X	X	X		X	X	X		X		X		X		X	X
8		X	X			X	X		X	X										X		
9								X	X													
10	X			X			X				X								X			
11		X												X								
13	X		X	X	X	X				X	X	X		X		X	X	X			X	X
14																		X				
15		X																				
17																				X		
26			X		X																	

Pain, Tongue, Root Of

	PHYTO	KALI IOD	LACH	CON	KALI BIC	SPIG
1	X					
4	X					
7		X	X			
8				X		
12						X
14	X				X	
17	X					
19	X	X				
20	X					
21			X			
24	X					

Pain, Tongue, Sides Of

	CARB A	SANG
8		X
10	X	

Pain, Tongue, Tip Of

	CARB A	NAT M	ARG N	BAR C	CALC	CARB V	CAUST	CHINA	COLOC	CYCL	GAMBOG	HEP	HYDRAST	HYDR AC	KALI CAR	KALI IOD	LATH	MERC	MERC SU	NAT CAR	PHYTO	SANG	TEUCR	THUJA
1	X																							
6		X																						
7			**X**									X												
8					X																	X		
10	X					X	X						X								X			
13		X						X	X	X	X			X	X	X		X		X			X	
14				X																				X
17																	X		X					

Pain, Tonsils- See also Tonsillitis

	BELL	HEP	LACH	MERC	CALC PH	BAR C	BROM	CAUST	CROT H	GUAIAC	MERC I F	MERC SU	PHYTO	SIL	WYETHIA
1			X												
6		X													
7			X					X	X		X				
8				X											
9	X	X	X	X	X	X				X		X	X		
10	X			X											
14	X	X			X										
17							X							X	X

Pain, Trachea- See also Tracheitis

	BRY	CHINA	MERC C	PHOS	ARUM T	CARB V	CAUST	GELS	LACH	LYC	NAT M	SPONG	STANN	OSMIUM
2	**X**													**X**
3					X									
4				X										
5					X									
7		X	X								X	X		
8		X	X	X		X	X		X	X			X	
13	X	X	X	X		X	X	X	X	X	X	X	X	
15								X						
17	X													

Pain, Umbilicus

	DIOSC	IPEC	BELL	CINA	COLOC	PLAT	PULS	CHAM	COCCUL	CUPR	DULC	KALI BIC	KREO	PLUM	THUJA	VER A
1	X					X					X		X			
3			X													
4	X															
5						X										
6	X		X	X	X	X	X		X	X		X		X		
7	X															
8															X	
9	X	X														
10		X											X		X	
11		X														
12														X		
13												X				
14		X		X				X								
15																X
18											X					
19				X												
24	X				X		X			X						
25	X															
26		X	X		X		X	X	X							X

Pain, Ureter

	TAB	CANTH	BELL	BERB V	TEREB	APIS	ARG N	CHAM	CHEL	COLOC	IPOMOEA	LACH	LYC	SCROPH
1		X			X									
2														X
4		**X**		X										
6	X		X											
7	X	X				X		X	X	X	X		X	
10							X					X		
17	X													
20				X										
21					X									
24	X		X											

Pain, Urethra- See also Dysuria

	CANN S	BERB V	CANTH	CLEM	PULS	SULPH	ARG N	MERC	NAT M	THUJA	STAPHYS	ACON	ASPARA	CAMPH	CANN I	IPEC	KALI BIC	SEP	ANT C	KALI CAR
1	X		X				X										X	X		
6		X				X			X	X										
7			X	X	X	X	X	X	X	X				X		X	X	X		X
8	X			X								X							X	
11	X				X										X					
13	**X**	X	**X**	X	X	X	X	X		X	**X**		X			X		X	**X**	**X**
14	X	X	X		X		X			X	X	X	X	X	X					
18											X									
19	**X**	X		X										X	X					
20		X				X		X	X								X			
24		X		X					X				X			X				
26			X		X	X		X				X								

Pain, Uterus- See Metralgia

Pain, Uvula

	CAPS	HYDRAST	TRIFOLP	TUSSIL	APIS	SANG	SIL
2			X	X			
3			X	X			
4	X						
7		X				X	
8							X
15		X					
18					X		
24	X						

Pain, Vagina- See also Pain, Genitalia, Female (Includes Neuralgia, Vagina)

	SEP	KREO	RHUS T	SULPH	CALC	BELL	LYC	THUJA	KALI CAR	BERB V	CANTH	CHINA	MERC	NUX V	PLAT	PULS	SABIN	AMBRA	ARS	CON	FERR	FERR M	GELS	GRAPH	NAT M	NIT AC	STAPHYS
1		X													X												
6	X		X		X													X									
7	X	X		X	X	X	X	X	X	X	X	X	X		X			X		X		X		X	X	X	X
8	X	X	X	X	X	X	X	X	X		X	X	X	X	X	X	X		X	X	X		X	X	X	X	X
9				X																							
10		X	X			X																					
11								X																			
13	**X**	X	X	X	**X**	X	X	X	**X**	X	X	X	X	X		X					X	X					
14	X		X	X			X			X						X	X						X				
15	X													X					X								
21																	X										

Pain, Veins- See also Phlebitis

	VIP	ARS	HAM	LACH
1	X			
10		X		
13	X		X	X

Pain, Vertebra

	AGAR M	CHIN S	CIMICI	PHOS	OVI G P	SOL T A
2				X	X	X
8		X	X			
9	X					

Pain, Vulva

	AMBRA	CALC	KALI CAR	KREO	OVI G P	RHUS T	COCCUS	CANTH	CENCHR	FERR IOD	GRAPH	MERC	NIT AC	SULPH	THUJA
2					X				X						
3					X										
6		X				X						X			X
7			X												
8	X	X	X	X			**X**			X	X		X	X	
9				X											
10						X									
14	X							X							

Pain, Wounds

	HYPER	CALEND	STAPHYS
1	X		
8	X		
21	X	X	X
24	X		

Pain, Wrist

	VIOL O	EUP PERF	RHOD	RUTA	PROP	ACT SP	HIPPOM	HOMAR	LACH	PLECT
1					X	X				
2			X		X		X	X		X
3	X		X	X	X	X		X		X
7	X	X	X						X	
11	X	X								
13				X					X	
14		X		X			X			
18	X									
19	X									

Pain, Zygoma

	VERBASC	ACON	AUR	SPHING	SPIG
2				X	
4	**X**	X			
14					X
17			X		

Palpitations (Note that only the main remedies are used from 17)

	SPIG	ACON	NAT M	CACT	PULS	CALC	LACH	NUX V	ARS	DIG	LYC	SULPH	PHOS	BELL	FERR	GLON	IGN	AUR	KALI CAR	LIL T	MOSCH	NAJA	SPONG	RHUS T	AMM C	COCCUL	SEP	
1	X	X	X	X	X	X	X	X	X	X	X	X	X	X	X	X	X	X	X	X	X	X		X	X		X	
2					X					X					X	X				X						X		
3	X		X	X	X	X		X		X							X	X			X	X			X			
4	X	X	X	X	X	X	**X**					X								X		X		X				
5	X		X	X	X	X	X	X	X	X	X		X				X		X	X		X			X		X	
6	X	X	X	X	X	X	X	X	X	X	X	X	X	X	X	X	X	X	X	X	X		X	X		X	X	
7	**X**	X	X	X	X	**X**	**X**	**X**	**X**	**X**	**X**	X	**X**	X	X	X		X	X	X		X	**X**	X		X	X	
8	X	X	X	X	X	X	X	X	X	X	X	X	X	X	X	X		X		X	X	X	X	X	X	X	X	
9	**X**	X	X						X		X				X	X							X					
10	X	X			X	X	X	X	X		X	X	X	X	X	X	X	X					X	X	X	X	X	
11	X	X	X	X						X		X		X		X					X				X			
12	X	X		X				X	X			X		X	X		X				X							
13	**X**	**X**	**X**	X	**X**	**X**	X	**X**	**X**	**X**	**X**	**X**	**X**	**X**	X		X	**X**	X		X	X	X	X	**X**	**X**	**X**	
14	**X**	X	X	X			X		X	X	X		X	X	X				X	X		X						
15	X	X		X	X	X	X	X				X	X				X									X		
16				X		X								X		X												
17	X	X	X	X	X	X	X	X	X	X	X		X	X		X	X	X	X	X	X	X	X	X	X	X	X	
18		X															X											
19	X	X	X	X	X	X	X	X	X		X	X	X		X		X	X	X	X	X	X	X	X	X			
21	X	X	X	X	X		X	X		X	X								X	X	X							
23							X			X											X	X	X					
24			X			X						X							X				X					
25	**X**		X		X			X		X						X												
26	X	X	X		X	X		X	X		X	X	X	X	X	X	X	X						X		X	X	
27				X			X		X									X	X									

Palsy (Includes Cerebral Palsy)

	CAUST	AGAR M	PIC AC	PLUM	ANAC	CON	GELS	HYOSC	SIL	CALC PH																		
6			X																									
7					X																							
8	**X**	X	X	X	X	X	X	X	X																			
10			X																									
14	X	X		X		X		X																				
17	X			X			X		X																			
29*		X								**X**																		

29* Mohan GR, et al. A clinical study of the role of homeopathy in cerebral palsy syndrome. Homoeopathic Links, 18, Autumn 2005, 149-152.

Panaritium- See Paronychia

Pancreas, Congestion/Catarrh

	MERC	PULS	BELL	CALC	CARB A	LYC
7	X	X				
8	X	X	X	X	X	X

Pancreas, Diseases Of

	PHOS	IRIS V	BELL	IOD	CARB A	ARS	ATROP S	CALC ARS	CARB V	CHEL	CHION	CON	CYCL	KALI BIC	KALI IOD	LYC	MERC	PANCR	PLUM	POD	SIL	TRIFOL P	URAN N	ZINC
1	X		X								X													
2	X	X			X													X				X		
3		X	X	X																				
4	**X**	**X**	**X**				X										X							
5										X			X											
7		X																						
8	X	X	X	X	X	X		X	X			X		X	X	X			X	X	X		X	X
10	X																							
11				X																				
18	X																							

Pancreas, Fatty

	PHOS	ARS
1	X	
6	X	
7	X	
8	X	X
24	X	

Pancreatitis

	IRIS V	IOD	ATROP	KALI IOD	MERC	CON	PHOS	BELL	CARB A	CARB V	SPONG
2			**X**	**X**	**X**						
5	X					X	X				
7	X	X				X					**X**
8	X	X				X		X	X	X	
9	X										
11	**X**	**X**	**X**		X		X				
14	X							X			
19									X		
21	X	X	X	X	X		X				
23	X	X									
26				X						X	
28	X										

Pannus

	APIS	AUR	CALC	CHIN M	KALI BIC	MERC P	MERC I F	PETR
2	X			X		X		
24		X	X		X		X	X

Pannus, Cornea

	ARG N	AUR	APIS	CALC	EUPHR	MERC I R	GRAPH	HEP	MERC P R	NIT AC	PETR	ALUMEN	ARS	BAR C	BELL	CANN I	CAUST	CHINA	CHIN M	KALI BIC	KALI CAR	MERC P	MERC I F	NAT M	PULS	RHUS T	SULPH
6	X	X	X	X	X	X	X	X	X		X		X		X	X			X	X	X		X	X	X	X	X
7	**X**	X	X	X	X	X	X			X				X													
8	X	**X**	X	X	X	X		X	X	X	X	X					X	X				X					

Papilloma

	THUJA	EUCAL	NIT AC	PH AC
4	X			
8	X	X	X	X
17	X			

Paraesthesia (Includes Tingling, Sensation of)

	ACON	LACH	NAT M	PHOS	SEC	MAG M	NUX V	PLUM	RAPH
4	X								
11	X							X	
13		X		X					
14	X		X		X				X
15	X								
17	X								
13	X		X		X	X			
19		X		X					
21							X		
27	X								

Paralysis- See also Paraplegia; Paresis

	CAUST	GELS	PLUM	CON	COCCUL	PHOS	OP	ACON	RHUS T	ARG N	ARS	LACH	HYOSC	SULPH	BAR C	CURARE	NUX V	BELL	OX AC	CUPR	PIC AC	ARN	OLEAND	ZINC	ALUM	KALI IOD		
1	X	X	X	X			X		X	X	X	X	X	X		X			X		X	X	X	X	X	X		
2	X	**X**	**X**	**X**	**X**	**X**	**X**	**X**	**X**	**X**		X	**X**		**X**	X	**X**	**X**	**X**	**X**	**X**	**X**	X		X	**X**		
3	X	X	X	X	X		X			X		X	X		X									X				
4	**X**	**X**	**X**	X	X	**X**	X	**X**	**X**	X		X	X	X	X					X				X				
5	X	X		X			X								X													
6	X	X	X	X	X	X	X	X	X	X	X		X	X	X	X		X	X	X	X	X		X	X			
7	**X**	**X**	**X**	**X**	X	**X**	X	X	**X**	X	**X**	X	X	**X**	X	X	**X**		X	X	**X**	**X**	X	**X**	X	X		
8	**X**	**X**	X	X	**X**	**X**	X	X	**X**	X	X	**X**	X	**X**	**X**	X	**X**	X	X	**X**	X	**X**	X	X	X	X		
9	X	X	X																X									
10	X	X		X												X			X		X							
11	X	X	X			X				X																		
12		X	X	X	X	X	X				X									X								
13	**X**	X	X	X	**X**	**X**	**X**	X	**X**	X	X	X	X	**X**			**X**	X					**X**	X		X		
14	X	X										X						X										
15		X	X	X	X	X		X			X						X	X										
17	**X**	X	X		X	X	X	X	X		X	X	X	X		X	X	X	X				X			X		
18				X							X																	
19	X	X	X	X	X	X		X		X	X	X				X	X								X			
21			X	X																		X						
23		X	X	X	X											X		X		X	X		X					
24			X																									
26	**X**							X	X					X	X										X			
27	X	X																										

Paralysis Agitans- See also Parkinson's Disease; Trembling

	MERC	PLUM	GELS	HYOSC	ZINC	RHUS T	AUR S	BAR C	BUFO	PHOS	PHYSO	TAR H	LOL T	AGAR M	CAMPH	HELOD	KALI BR	LYC	MAG PH	ZINC CY	ZINC PIC	MANG AC						
1			**X**			X					X			X		X												
2		X	X				X				X		X			X	X	X		X	X							
4	X	X		X																								
6	X					X		X				X						X										
7	X	X	X	X		**X**		X	X	X		X					X		X									
8	X	X	X	X		X		X	X	X	X	X																
9				X																								
10	X	X		X																								
11		X					**X**						**X**	X	X						X	**X**						
13															X													
14							X		X										X									
16	X																											
17										X																		
23																				X								

Paralysis, Anus

	HYOSC	PHOS	BELL	CAUST	LAURO	OP	SULPH	COLOC	LYC	MUR AC	RUTA	ZINC
6	X	X	X									
7	X	X			X					X		
8	X			X	X	X	X	X	X		X	X
10		X		X		X	X					
24			X									

Paralysis, Ascending

	CON	PHOS	HYDR AC	LED	SYPH	PIC AC	SULFON
2	X				X		X
4	X						
8				X			
9	X	X					
10	X						
11		X				X	
13			X				
14	X	X					
17	X	X					
19	X	X					

Paralysis, Arms

	NUX V	CALC	CAUST	COCCUL	DULC	LYC	RHUS T	BELL	ACON	ARN	MERC	PLUM	SEP	AESC	ANT T	CHINA	COLCH	FERR	OP	VER A
1				X																
4												X								
6	X	X	X	X	X	X	X	X	X	X	X		X	X	X	X	X			X
7	X	X	**X**		X	X			X			X							X	
8	X	X	X	X	X	X		X	X	X	X		X	X	X	X	X			X
10	X	X	X	X	X	X	X	X	X	X	X		X							
13	**X**	**X**	X	**X**	X	X	X	**X**				X						X	X	
14							X													
25	X	X	X	X			X											X		

Paralysis, Arm, Left

	RHUS T	ARG N	ARS	LATRO M	NUX V
7	X	X	X		
8	X				X
19				X	

Paralysis, Arm, Right

	TEREB	ARN	NUX V	BAR C	CANN I	CAUST	RHUS T
6	X				X		
7		X	X	X			
8	X	X	X				X
10	X						
13						X	

Paralysis, Auditory Nerve

	CAUST	HYOSC	BELL	PULS	SIL	NUX V	OP	ARN	CALC	CHEL	DULC	GLON	GRAPH	KALI PH	LYC	MERC	NIT AC	PETR	PH AC	PHOS	SEC
1	X																				
7	X	X										X		X							
8	X	X	X	X	X	X		X										X	X	X	
13	X	**X**	**X**	**X**	**X**	X	**X**		X	X	X		X		X	X	X				X

Paralysis, Back

	BERB V	COCCUL	CUPR	NAT M	PHOS	RHUS T
4				X		
6	X					
7			X		X	X
8		X				

Paralysis, Bladder (Includes Paralysis, Bladder, Neck Of)

	CAUST	OP	ARS	CIC	DULC	NUX V	HYOSC	SEC	GELS	RHUS T	BELL	CACT	CANTH	LACH	LAURO	LYC	STAPHYS	ACON	HELL	NAT M	PHOS	PLUM	ZINC	FERR PH
1	X			X																				
2		**X**		X			X	**X**				X												**X**
3		X																						
4	**X**	X				X																	X	
6	X	X	X	X	X	X	X	X	X	X	X		X	X		X	X		X	X	X			
7	**X**	X	**X**	X	**X**	**X**	X	X	**X**	X		X										X		
8	X	X	X	**X**	X	X	X	X	X	**X**	X	X	X	X	X	**X**	**X**	X	X	X	X		X	
9	X	X																						
10						X									X									
13	X	X	X	X	X		X				X		X	X	X			X						
14	X		X					X																
19	**X**	X	X																			X		
25		X																						
26			X		X																			

Paralysis, Bowel

	CARB V	OP
6	X	
24		X

Paralysis, Bulbar

	CARB V	GELS	MANG OX	OP	PLUM
9	X	X		X	X
17			X		

Paralysis, Ciliary

	CAUST	GELS	PARIERA	PARIS	RHUS T
1	X	X			
2				X	
4	X				X
8			X		

Paralysis, Deltoid

	CAUST
7	X
8	X

Paralysis, Deltoid, Right

	CURARE
7	X
10	X

Paralysis, Descending

	STANN	MERC
7	X	
8	X	
14		X

Paralysis, Diaphragm

	ARG N	MORPH	NICOTIN	TAB
6	X		X	
8				X
17		X		

Paralysis, Extensor Muscles

	CURARE	PLUM
19	X	X

Paralysis, Extremities

	CAUST	NUX V	RHUS T	AGAR M	ARN	BELL	CIC	COCC	CROT H	CURARE	GELS	IGN	IPEC	MERC
6	X		X											
8		X				X			X	X			X	X
9	X													
10		X												
14	X										X			
15					X									
17	X													
19				X										
26	X		X				X	X				X		

Paralysis, Extremities, Left Side

	ALUM	CAUST	COCCUL
3	X	X	
6			X

Paralysis, Extremities, Right Side

	BELL	COCCUL
6		X
8	X	

Paralysis, Eye

	GELS	CAUST	EUPHR	NUX V	PHYSO	RHUS T	SENEGA	ARN	CON	KALI IOD	MERC I F	NAT M	PHOS
3	X												
4	X												
7	X	X	X	X	X	X	X	X	X	X	X	X	X
8	X	X	X	X	X	X	X	X		X	X		X
10	X												
14	X				X								
17	X	X	X	X		X	X		X			X	
24	X												

Paralysis, Eyelids- See also Ptosis

	GELS	SEP	SPIG	BELL	COCCUL	NIT AC	PLUM	RHUS T	ZINC	ALUM	ARN	ARG N	CAUST	OP	STRAM	VER A	CANTH	CUPR AC	HYDR AC	HYOSC
3										X			X							
6	X	X	X	X	X	X	X	X	X		X	X		X	X	X	X	X		X
7	X	X	X			X							X			X				
8	X	X	X	X	X	X	X	X	X		X	X		X	X		X	X	X	X
10	X	X	X	X	X		X	X	X		X	X								
13	X	X	X	X	X	X	X	X	X	X				X	X	X			X	
14													X							
15	X																			
19										X										
24	X																			

Paralysis, Facial- See also Bell's Palsy

	CAUST	COCCUL	BAR C	NUX V	ACON	BELL	GRAPH	CAD S	CURARE	OP	RHUS T	AMM PH	KALI CHL	ALL C	ZINC PIC	CUPR	MERC	AUR	PHOS
2	X				X			X	X			X	**X**	X	X				
3	X	X	X		X														
4	**X**		X		X						X								
5	X																		
6	X	X		X		X	X			X							X		
7	X	X						X	X										
8	X	X	X	X		X	X	X		X	X								
9	X										X	X							
10		X	X	X		X	X			X									
12	X		X		X	X													
14	X																		
17	**X**	X	X	**X**			X	**X**	**X**		X	X	**X**	**X**	**X**	X		**X**	**X**
13	X				X				X										
24	X	X															X		
25	X																		
23				X		X	X			X						X			

Paralysis, Facial, Left Side

	ALL C	CAD S	NUX V	CURAR	LACH	SENEG
3						X
7	X					
14	X				X	
17	X	X	X	X		
19		X	X			

Paralysis, Facial, One Sided

	COCCUL	ACON	AGAR M	BELL	CAUST	RHUS T	STAPHYS	SYMPH
1								X
7	X				X			
8				X		X	X	
19	X	X	X					

Paralysis, Facial, Right Side

	CAUST	ARN	PHOS	PLAT	BELL	KALI MUR
3	X					
7		X				X
8					X	
9	X					
14	X					
17	X	X	X			
19	X		X	**X**		

Paralysis, Feet

	PLUM	CHINA	OLEAND	ARS	ZINC	COCCUL	BELL	NUX V	ANGUST	ARN	CAUST	PHOS	RHUS T	SULPH
1					X									
6	X	X	X	X										
7					X	X								
8	X	X	X							X				
10	X	X		X										
13	**X**	**X**	**X**	X	X	X	**X**	**X**	X			X	X	X
19											X			
21	X													

Paralysis, Fingers

	CALC	CUPR	NAT M	PHOS	SEC	SIL	AMBRA	CARB V	CHINA	ACON	ASAR	AUR	CALC PH	COCCUL	CYCL	DIG	EUON	KREO	MENY	MEZ	PLUM	RHUS T	STANN	STAPHYS
6	X	X	X		X	X	X																	
7	X			X										X						X	X			
8	X	X	X		X	X	X																	
10	X	X	X		X	X																		
13	X			X				**X**	X	X	X	X	X		X	X	X	X	X					X
14				X																		X	X	

Paralysis, Forearm

	ACON	AMBRA	ARG	BISM	BOV	KREO	PLUM	PRUN SE	SENEG	STAPHYS	STRONT C
1							X				
8			X								
13	X	X		X	X	X		X	X	X	X

Paralysis, Hands

	SIL	CAUST	ARS	CUPR	AMBRA	NAT M	PLUM	RHUS T	RUTA	ZINC	FERR	SULPH	CHINA	TAB
1										X				
6	X	X	X	X	X	X		X	X		X			
8	X	X	X	X	X	X	X	X	X		X			
10	X	X	X	X		X			X					
13	**X**			X	X		X			**X**		X	**X**	**X**
19		X												
21							X							
26	X	X	X					X				X		

Paralysis, Hand, Left

	SIL	COCCUL
6	X	
7		X
10	X	

Paralysis, Heart

	CARB V	LACH	ACON	CROT H	GELS	PLUM	VER A	ANTIPYR	ARS	CHLOR	ERGOTIN	HYDR AC	JATR U	LOB PUR	MERC CY	NAJA	VIPERA
2								X		X	X		X	X			
6	X											X					
7	X	**X**	X	X	X	X	X										
8	X	X	X	X	X	X	X		X						X	X	X

Paralysis, Infantile

	GELS	LATH	RHUS T	CAUST	SULPH	ACON	AETHUSA	ARN	BELL	HYOSC	MERC	NUX V
2							X					
4	X		X		X							
7	X			X								
8	**X**		X	**X**	X	X		X	X	X	X	X
9		X										
10	<u>**X**</u>											
11		X										
14			X									
16	X	X										

Paralysis, Intestines- See also See Bowel Atony;Bowel Obstruction; Ileus; Obstruction, Intestines

	OP	PLUM	ALUM	ARN	BRY	CARB V	CAUST	COCCUL	OLEAND	PHOS	SULPH	VER A
1									X			
3	X											
4	X	X	X		X							X
7		X		X			X	X			X	
8	X					X				X		
10	X											

Paralysis, Iris

	ARN	ARS	PARIERA
7	X		
8			X
19		X	

Paralysis, Jaw, Lower

	NUX V	ARS	BAR C	CROT H	DULC	LACH	MUR AC	RAN B
6	X							
7	X							
8							X	
17	X	X	X	X	X	X		X

Paralysis, Joints

	ACON	ARN	CROC	LAURO	RHUS T	SULPH
7				X		
13	X	X	X		X	X

Paralysis, Larynx

	GELS	CAUST	HYDR AC	IOD	ACON	ARN	ARS	BAR C	BELL	COCCUL	CUPR	LACH	OP	PLUM
1	X													
4	**X**													
6			X											
7			X	X										
8			X	X										
10		X			X	X	X	X	X	X	X	X	X	X
14	X													
17		X												
23		X												

Paralysis, Legs

	NUX V	COCCUL	RHUS T	PLUM	SULPH	LATH	PHOS	SEC	ARS	DULC	BELL	SIL	AGAR M	ALUM	ARN	BRY	KALI CAR	OP	GELS	MERC	NAT M	VER A	CALC	CANN I	CAUST	CHINA	COLCH	LACH
1				X		X																						
3	X						X						X															
4	X	X	**X**			X				X				X														
6	X	X	X	X	X		X	X	X	X	X	X		X	X	X	X			X		X				X	X	
7	X	X	**X**	X	X		X	X	X	X							X	X	X		X	X	X	X			X	X
8	X	X	X	X	X	X	X	X		X	X	X		X	X	X	X	X	X	X		X				X		
9						X																						
10	X	X	X	X	X	X	X	X		X	X	X	X	X	X	X	X			X	X							
11						X																						
13	**X**	**X**	X	**X**	**X**			X	X		**X**	**X**				X		**X**			X							X
14									X				X											X				
15	X																											
17													X															
19		X							X										X						X			
26	X	X	X		X		X	X							X								X		X			

Paralysis, Leg, Left

	TEREB	ALL C	ARN
6	X		
8			X
10	X		
14		X	

Paralysis, Leg, Right

	CAUST	PLUM	RHUS T
8		X	X
14	X		

Paralysis, Left Sided

	LACH	ART V	CURP AR	NIT AC	NUX V	PHOS	PHYSO	PLUM	SIL	XANTH
1							X			
2			X	X						
5										X
6	X	X						X		
8	**X**								X	
14	**X**									
17					X	X				
19	X									

Paralysis, Limbs

	ARS	DULC	GELS	MERC	NUX V	RHUS T	ARN	COLCH	OP	SANG	VER A	ACON	CAUST
6	X	X	X	X	X	X	X	X	X	X	X		
7	X	X	X	X	X				X		X	**X**	**X**
8	X	X	X	X	X	X	X	X		X			
9						X							
10	X		X	X	X	X	X						
17		X											

Paralysis, Limbs, Extensors

	PLUM	GELS	NUX V	RHOD
8	X	X	X	X
10	X			
17	X			

Paralysis, Limbs, Flexors

	NAT M	PLUM
8	X	
10		X

Paralysis, Limbs, Lower- See Paralysis, Legs

Paralysis, Lungs

	ANT T	LACH	MOSCH	CARB V	OP	PHOS	BAR C	ARS	CAMPH	CHINA	CURARE	GELS	HYDR AC	LYC	LAURO	AUR	CALC	CAUST	CROT H	GRAPH	HYOSC	LOB PUR	MERC CY	NIT AC	NUX V	SENEG	SOLAN
1												X															
2			X			X																X					X
4																					X						
6	X	X	X						X															X			
7	X	X				X						X		X			X										
8	X	X		X	X		X	X	X	X						X				X					X		
10											X																
11	X																										
13	**X**	X		X	X	X	**X**	X		X			X	X	**X**											X	
14	X			X									X														
16		X																					X				
17			X		X														X								
19											X							X									
26	**X**		X																								

Paralysis, Mouth

	ART V	CURARE	STAPHYS
7	X	X	
19			X

Paralysis, Oesophagus

	CAUST	NUX M	ARS	BAR C	BELL	CON	GELS	HYDR AC	LACH	OP	PLUM
1										X	
6								X			
7	X	X						X			
8	X		X	X		X					
11		X					X				
13	X	**X**			X		X		X	X	**X**
14	X			X		X					
26	X		X		X				X		

Paralysis, One Sided- See Hemiplegia

Paralysis, Optic Nerve

	BOV	CON	PHOS	DUBO M	HYOSC	PULS	RHUS T	SEC	SIL
1	X		X	X					
7		X				X			
8	X								
13		X	X		X		X	X	X

Paralysis, Palate

	PLUM	SIL	GELS	LACH
7	X	X		
17	X	X	X	X

Paralysis, Pharynx (Includes Organs of Deglutination, Paralysis Of)

	CAUST	COCCUL	ARS	GELS	BELL	CUPR	LACH	SIL	STRAM	BAR C	CALC	CANTH	CON	IOD	HEP	PLUM
1				X												
4	X															
6		X														
7		X	X						X						X	
8	X	X	X	X	X	X	X	X	X	X	X	X	X	X		X
9	X															
10	X	X		X	X	X		X								
17			X				X									

Paralysis, Progressive

	CAUST	CUPR	CURAR	PHOS	ALUM	ARS	COCCUL	CON	FERR	KALI CAR	LATH	NAT S	NUX V	PIC AC	PLUM
6		X													
7	X	X	X	X					X	X		X	X	X	
8				X											
19	**X**		X		X	X	X	X			x				X

Paralysis, Rectum- See also Weakness, Rectum

	CAUST	HYOSC	OP	TAB	COLOC	LYC	PHOS	RUTA	SULPH	ALUM	ARS	CUPR	GRAPH	IGN	MERC	SEC	SIL	VER A	ZINC	ZINC SUL
2				X																
3				X																
4	X																			
5	X																			
6	X	X	X		X	X	X	X							X	X				X
7				X								X		X						
8	X	X	X		X	X		X	X										X	
10	X		X				X		X											
12																		X		
14																	X			
19										X	X									
24													X							
26		X																		

Paralysis, Right Sided

	CAUST	BAR C	SIL	ARN	ART V	BELL	CHEL	COCCUL	CROT C	CROT H	KALI IOD	OP
1	X											
4	X											
6	X		X	X								
8			X		X	X	X	X		X	X	
9		X										
17	X								X			X
19	X											
25		X										

Paralysis, Senile

	BAR C	CON	KALI CAR	OP
4	X	X		
6	X			
7	X		X	X
8	X			
10	X	X		
12	X			
13	X	X	X	

Paralysis, Shoulder

	AMBRA	CAUST	ARG	CARB V	EUPHORB	FERR IOD	LYC	MAG SUL	MANG	MUR AC	NAT M	NUX V	PULS	SEP	STANN	STAPHYS	SULPH	VALER	VER A
5	X	X				X	X												
13	X				X			X	X	X	X	X	X	X	X	X	X	X	X
17			X	X															
19		X																	

Paralysis, Single Parts (Includes Monoplegia)

	CAUST	AMM C	AMM M	ANAC	ARS	CALC	COCCUL	DULC	KALI PH	OX AC	PLAT
1	X										
4	X										
8	X			X					X		
9							X				
10	X										
11	X										
17	X	X	X		X	X		X		X	X
27	X										

Paralysis, Spastic

	LATH	NUX V	GELS	PLUM	SEC	AGAR M	ARG N	ARN	BELL	BENZ D	CAUST	CUPR	HYPER	HYOSC	MAG PH	MANG	MYGAL	PHOS	PLECT	STRAM	TANACET	TAR H	USTIL	ZINC
2		**X**	X		X					X			X						X					
8	X			X					X							X		X					X	
9			X			X	X				X	X		X	X		X			X	X	X		X
10	X																							
11	X																							
17	X																							
19	X	X																						
21	X			X	X			X																

Paralysis, Sphincters

	GELS	HYOSC	ARN	BELL	CHLOR	ERGOTIN	LAURO	PHOS	RHUS T
2						X			
3	X		X						
6	X	X							
8	X	X		X	X		X	X	X
12	X								

Paralysis, Spinal

	PHOS	PHYSO	ALUM	ARS	CON	GELS	LATH	PLUM	SIL	ACON	ARN	BELL	CALC	CAUST	CINA	COCCUL	GRAPH	NUX V	PIC AC	RHUS T	STANN	WILDBAD
2		X					X												X			X
4	X		X																			
6						X		X		X		X										
7	X			X	X				X													
8	X	**X**	X	X	X	X	X	X	X		X		X	X	X	X	X	X		X	X	
19	X																					
24		X																				

Paralysis, Spinal, Infantile

	GELS	ARS	CAUST	COCCUL	LATH	NUX V	RHUS T	ACON	BELL	ALUM	APIS	ARN	BRY	CINA	CON	DULC	GRAPH	LACH	MERC	NAT SUL	OP	PHOS	PHYSO	PLUM	SIL	STANN	SULPH
8	X	X	X	X	X	X	X			X		X		X	X		X						X	X	X	X	
10	**X**	X	X	X	X	X	X	**X**	**X**		X		X			X		X	X	X	X	X					X

Paralysis, Throat

	GELS	LACH	CAUST	APIS	LAC C	PLUM	ARUM T	ALUM	ARS	KALI PH	OP	POP CAN	PULS
1	X		X	X	X						X		
2												X	
3							X						
6	X												
7	X					X							X
8		X		X									
14	X	X	X		X					X			
19		X	X			X		X	X				

Paralysis, Tongue- See Glossoplegia

Paralysis, Vocal Cord

	CAUST	LACH	ARG N	CANTH	CINA	GRAPH	KALI PH	OX AC	PLUM	SENEG	STRAM
1		X							X		
3		X									
7	X	X			X						X
9			X								
13	X			X		X					
14	X	X					X				
17	X									X	
18	X										
21								X			
25			X								

Paralysis, Vocal Cord, Left Side

	LACH
6	X
7	X

Paralysis, Wrist

	HIPPOM	ACON	ASAR	BISM	BOV	CARB V	KALI CAR	MERC	PETR	PLUM
2	X									
3	X									
7		X								X
13			X	X	X	X	X	X	X	
14	X									

Paranoia

	HYOSC	CANN I	MERC	LACH	METH BL
4	X	X	X		
19	X	X	X		
21	X			X	
23					X

Paraphimosis

	MERC C	COLOC	LACH	MERC	NIT AC	ARN	DIG	NUX V	RHUS T	ACON	APIS	ARS	BELL	CANTH	MAG P AM	SULPH	TEREB	THUJA
2	X	X	X				X	X	X						X			
4				X														
7	X	X	X	X	**X**			X	X									
8		X	X			X				X		X	X					
13	X																	
24	X			X	X	X	X				X			X		X	X	X

Paraplegia- See also Paralysis

	NUX V	COCCUL	ARG N	GELS	SEC	LATH	ARS	PLUM	THALLIUM	CAULO	CON	CUPR	IGN	PHOS	ANHAL	HYPER	KALI TAR	RHUS T	ACON	CAUST	KALI CAR	LAURO	OLEAND	PETIVER	PIC AC	RHUS V	MANG OX	NAT M
2				X		X			X	X					X		X							X	X	X		
4			X			X													X									
6	X	X			X					X			X									X						
7	X	X		X	X		X																					
8	X	X			X																	X						
9	X	X	X	X				X			X	X		X				X		X								
10	X	X	X	X	X					X			X						X									
11	X	X	X	X	X	X	X	X	X		X	X		X		X				X	X					X		
17	**X**	X	**X**	X	X	**X**	**X**	**X**	**X**		X	X	X	X	**X**	**X**	**X**	**X**			X		X		X		**X**	**X**
23			X			X																	X	X				

Parasites- See also Worms

	CINA	ALOE	BERB V	CUPR AC	PERTUSS	SANTON	SPIG	SOLID	TEUCR	VIP
5	X	X	X	X	X		X	X	X	
12						X				
17										X
29*	X									

29* Lopez R. J., et al. Homeopathic Treatment with Cina 30C of Parastism in Rabbits. Gaceta Homeopatica de Caracas, 2002, Jul- Dec, 17-19.

Paresis- See also Paralysis

	PLUM	CON	GELS	IGN	ACON	ANAC	AUR IOD	AUR	AVENA	BOV	CAUST	CIC	CIMICI	DULC	ELAPS	GRIND	GUAIAC	KALI CAR	LAURO	MUR AC	NUX V	PH AC	PHOS	PIC AC	PLUM AC	RHUS T	ZINC PH	
1			X					X											X							X	X	
2							X																					
4					X																							
6				X																								
8	X	X				X				X	X	X		X	X	X	X			X	X	X		X	X			
10	X																	X										
11																							X					
19	X			X																								
23		X	X						X				X															

Paresis, Eye, Muscles Of

	NUX V	ACON	CHEL	GELS	PHOS	PHYSO	RHUS T
8	X	X	X		X		X
11						X	
24	X			X			

Paresis, Tongue

	GELS	BELL
6	X	
10	X	
12		X

Parkinson's Disease- See also Paralysis Agitans; Tremor

	MERC	GELS	ARG N	HYOSC	PLUM	RHUS T	ZINC	AGAR M	MANG	BAR C	KALI BR	PHOS	TAB	ANT C	ANT T	AUR S	CAMPH	HELO	HYOSC	LOLIUM	LYC	ZINC PIC
9		X																				
16	X	X																				
17	X		X	X	X	X	X	X		X	X	X	X	X	X	X	X	X	X	X	X	X
19	X		X	X	X	X	X		X	X	X	X	X									
21	X	X		X		X		X	X													
27	X	X	X		X		X															

Paronychia (Includes Panaritum)

	HEP	SIL	NAT SUL	SULPH	APIS	BUFO	LACH	MERC	NIT AC	BELL	LYC	RHUS T	AMM C	ANTHRAC	GRAPH	ALL C	AMM M	CALC	CAUST	LED	ARS	FL AC						
1			X																									
2		X	X		X	X					X					X												
6	X	X	X	X	X		X	X	X		X	X	X	X	X				X	X	X							
7	**X**	**X**	X	X	X	X	X	X	**X**		X	X	**X**	**X**		X	X	X	X	X		**X**						
8	X	X	X	X	X	X	X	X	X			X	X	X			X	X										
9	X	X					X			X					X													
12	X	X						X		X																		
13	**X**	**X**	X	**X**	X	X	X	X	**X**		X	X			**X**	X	X	X	X	X	**X**	X						
14	X	X	X							X																		
19	**X**	X				X																						
21	X	X								X																		
26	X	X		X																								

Periodontal Disease

	SIL	MERC	PLANTAG	BAPT	CALEND	CARB V	GUNPOW	KALI CAR	PHOS	CALC REN	CAUST	CIST	KREO	MERC C	NIT AC	STAPHYS	SYMPH											
1	X	X	X	X	X		X	X		X			X															
12	X	X				X			X								E											
14	**X**	X			X	X		X								X												
17	X		X	X			X				X	X		X	X													
19			X						X																			

E- External

Parosmia- See Smell, Sense of, Diseases Of

Parotid Glands, Diseases Of

	BROM	MERC	CALC	CON	KALI CAR	PHYTO	RHUS T	AUR	BAR C	BAR M	BELL	CARB A	CROT H	DULC	IGN	IRIS V	JAB	KALI BIC	KALI PH	LACH	LYC	NAT M	PILO	PULS	SIL	SULPH IO		
2	X															X	X						X			X		
7	X	X	X	X	X	X	X	X	X	X	X	X	X	X	X			X		X		X		X	X			
8		X	X	X	X		X												X									
20		X				X																						
24	X																				X							

Parotitis

	CALC	RHUS T	BAR C	BELL	ARS	COCCUL	KALI CAR	LYC	MERC	PHYTO																		
2	X		X			X			X	X																		
4		**X**																										
5	X		X	X																								
8	X	X	X	**X**	X	X	X	X	X	X																		
26	X	X			X		X	X																				

Pediculosis- See also Head Lice

	STAPHYS	LYC	SABAD	PSOR	NAT M	MEZ	CARB AC	LED	SULPH	TUB	ARS	LACH	OLEAND	VINCA
1	**X**	**X**		X			X							
2	**X**		**X**	X	**X**	X		X						
3	**X**	X		X			X							
8	X	X	X			X		X				X	X	X
9	X		E		X					X				
11	X			X		X			X		X			
13			X											
14	X	X												
25	X		E		X					X				
28		X							X					

E- External

Pellagra

	BOV	ARS	PLUM IOD	PHOS	ARG N	LACH	NAT M	SULPH
2			X					
3	X							
4	X	X		X	X			
11	X							
12		X		X		X	X	X
23			X					

Pelvis, Congestion Of

	SEP	APIS	BELL	CHAM	COLLIN	HAM	HYDRAST	POD	PULS	VER V
5	X	X	X	X		X	X	X	X	
6										X
8	X				X					
18	X									

Pelvic Inflammatory Disease- See Salpingitis

Pemphigus

	RHUS T	ARS	CANTH	CAUST	DULC	RAN B	ANAC	CALTH	CARB OX	LACH	MERC	SEP	SULPH	THUJA	LYC	BELL	CHINA	HEP	JUG C	PHOS	RAN S	RAPH	SCROPH	SULPH AC	MERC C
2	**X**			X	X	X	X	X	X					X					X		X	X	X		**X**
4	X					X																			
6	X	X	X	X	X	X				X	X	X	X	X		X	X			X					
7	**X**	X			X		X			X	X	X	X		**X**			X						X	
8	X	X	X	X	X	X	X	X	X	X	X	X	X	X		X	X	X	X	X	X		X	X	
23			X					X	X													X			
26	X	X	X	X											X										

Pericardial Effusion- See also Hydropericardium

	APIS	ARS	DIG	BRY	COLCH	LACH	SULPH	LYC	APOC	ARS IOD	HELL	PSOR	ACON	CANTH	GLON	KALI CAR	KALI IOD	MERC	PHASEOL	SPIG	SPONG	VER A
6						X					X											
7	X	**X**	X	X	X	X	X	**X**	X		X											
8	X		X	X	X					X		X					X				X	X
11	X	X	X	X					X				X					X		X		
16	X			X																		
17		X	X									X		X					X			
19			X			X	X															
21										X												
24							X															
26	X	**X**			X			X							X	X						

Pericarditis (Includes Congestive Pericarditis) (Note that only the main remedies are used from 17)

	SPIG	BRY	ACON	ARS	COLCH	APIS	CACT	DIG	KALI CAR	SULPH	SPONG	ARS IOD	KALI IOD	KALM	PSOR	PULS	VER V	ADONIS	ANT T	ASC T	BELL	IOD	VER A
1	X											X						X					
2					X															X			
3			X										X										
4	**X**	**X**	X	X		**X**	X							X			X						
6	X	X	X	X				X	X	X					X	X	X		X			X	
7	X	X	X	X	X	X	X		X	X	X		X		X							X	X
8	X	X	X	X	X	X	X	X	X	X	X		X	X	X	X	X		X	X	X	X	X
10		X	X	X		X			X	X						X					X		
11	X	X	X	X		X		X				X											
14	X	X			X			X						X									
16							X																
17	X	X	X	X	X	X		X	X	X	X	X	X		X								X
19	X			X			X	X	X	X	X			X				X	X				
21	X	X	X	X							X	X											
23	X			X	X												X	X		X			
26		X	**X**		X											X					X		
28		X																					

Perichondritis

	SIL	CIMICI	BELL	OLEAND	PLUM	RUTA	ASAF	AUR	CHAM	SYPH
2		**X**	**X**	**X**	**X**	**X**			X	
6	X									
17	X						X	X		X

Perimetritis- See also Metritis

	BELL	MERC C	VER V
2	**X**	**X**	X

Periodontal Disease- See also Gums, Diseases Of

	CALEND	KALI CAR	SIL	STAPHYS	AMM C	ARS	AUR	CALC REN	CARB V	CLEM	GUNPOW	MERC	MERC C	MEZ	PLANTAG	SEP	SYMPH	THUJA
1	**X**	X	X					X			X	X			X			X
3		X	X	X									X				X	
5				X	X	X	X		X	X				X		X		

Periosteum, Diseases Of

	KALI IOD	AUR M	NIT AC	RUTA
7	X	**X**	X	
8	X			
11	X			
12	X			
18				X

Periostitis

	MEZ	STILLING	ASAF	HECLA	PH AC	RUTA	MANG AC	SIL	AUR	FERR IOD	MERC	PHOS	PHYTO	SYMPH
1									X					
2		X		X		X				X		X		
3			X											
4	X	X												
6	X				X	X		X						
7	X		X	X	**X**	**X**		X	X	X	X		X	X
8	X	X		X			X							X
12													X	
13			X		X			X			X			
17							X					X		
23	X	X	X	X			X							
24	X	X												

Periostitis, Facial Bones

	AUR	NIT AC	CALC	FL AC	MERC	MEZ	PHOS	RUTA	SIL	STAPHYS	STILL
7	**X**	**X**	X	X	X	X	X	X	X	X	

Periostitis, Skull

	PHOS	KALI IOD	NAT M	PH AC	RUTA
6	X		X		
7	X	X		X	X

Periproctitis

	HEP	KALI CAR	MERC	ARN	ARS	BELL	BERB V	BRY	CON	HYDRAST	IGN	KREO	LACH	LYC	NUX V	OP	PHOS	PULS	RHUS T	SEP	SIL	SULPH AC
6	X	X	X	X	X	X	X	X	X		X	X	X	X	X	X	X	X	X	X	X	X
7	X	X	X							X						X						

Peristalsis, Reduced, Irregular or Reversed

	OP	COLLINS	HEP	VER A	ALL S	ALUM	COCCUL	LYC	PHOS	PLAT	PLUM	RUTA	SEL	STAPHYS
6	X		X	X										
7	X	X						X	X	X	X			
8							X					X	X	X
10			X											
14		X				X								
24	X			X										
28					X									

Peritonitis

	ACON	BRY	BELL	RHUS T	ARS	MERC	APIS	LACH	COLOC	MERC C	LYC	NUX V	CANTH	SULPH	CALC	ARN	CHAM	VER A	OP	TEREB	CHINA
1	X	X	X	X				X										X			
2	**X**	**X**	**X**		**X**				**X**	**X**	**X**		**X**	**X**	**X**		X	X			**X**
3	X	X	X			X															
4	**X**	**X**		**X**	X	**X**	X	X	X	X				X						X	
6	X	X	X	X	X	X	X	X			X	X	X	X	X	X		X	X		
7	X	X	X	X	X	X			X	X	X	X		X	X		X	X	X	X	
8	X	X	X	X	X	X	X	X	X	X	X	X	X	X	X	X	X	X	**X**	X	X
10	X	X	X	X	X		X	X				X		X		X	X				
11	X	X	X	X		X	**X**	X		X	**X**		X								X
13	X	X	X	X					X			X					X				
14	X	X	X				X		X							X					
15	X	X	X	X	X	X			X			X	X								
19		X			X																
21	X	X	X						X	X											
23	X		X				X	X													
24	X	X	X	X	X	X	**X**	X		X		X	X		X	X			X	X	
26	**<u>X</u>**	X	X	X		X		X			X										
28		X																			
29*			X																		

29* Pedalino CMV, et al. Effect of atropa belladonna and echinacea angustifolia in homeopathic dilution on experimental peritonitis. Homeopathy, 2004, 93, 193-198.

Perityphlitis

	LACH	ARS	BELL	CROT H	GINSENG	MERC	THUJA	BRY	DIOSC	ECHIN	HEP	IGN	IRIS T	PLUM	RHUS T
2	**X**	**X**		X									X		
6	X		X		X	X	X								
7				X											
10	X	X	X		X	X	X	X	X	X	X	X		X	X

Pernicious Anaemia- See Anaemia, Pernicious

Perspiration, Abdomen

	AMBRA	ANAC	ARG N	CANTH	DROS	GRAPH	PHOS	PLUM	STAPHYS	THUJA
5	X					X				X
8	X	X	X	X	X		X	X	X	

Perspiration, Absent- See also Skin, Dryness

	ACON	SULPH	GRAPH	PSOR	BELL	BRY	CHAM	COLCH	DULC	LYC	SIL	ALUM	ARN	ARS	IPEC	LACH	PULS	STAPHYS	TEUCR	VIOL OD								
2																X												
3																X												
7	**X**	**X**	X	X	**X**	**X**	**X**	**X**	**X**	**X**	**X**		X	X	X		X	X	X	X								
8		X	X	X	X	X	X	X	X	X	X	X	X				X	X	X	X								
9	X																											
10		X	X																									
18	X			X																								
21												X																
26														X	X													

Perspiration, Axilla

	DULC	KALI CAR	PETR	SEP	SULPH	THUJA	ALL C	BAR C	BRY	CALC	CAPS	CARB A	CEDRON	HEP	HYDRAST	KALM	LACH	NAT M	NIT AC	RHOD	SEL	SQUILLA	ZINC	TELL				
5		X				X									X													
7	X	X	X				X			X			X					X										
8	X		X	X	X	X		X	X		X	X		X		X	X		X	X	X	X	X	X				
10				X																								
14					X																							

Perspiration, Axilla, Offensive

	LYC	NIT AC	PETR	SEP	SIL	OSMIUM	TELL	BOV	CALC AC	HEP	KALI PH	LACH	NUX M	SULPH														
1			X			X		X					X															
2	**X**	**X**					X																					
3	X	X																										
5		X	X	X	X		X				X	X																
7	X	X	X	X	**X**					X																		
9									X																			
13						X																						
14														X														
18				X																								
21	X																											

Perspiration, Back

	CHINA	HEP	ARS	CALC	DULC	GUAIAC	LACH	PETR	PH AC	SEP	SIL	VER A																
5	X	X																										
7	X																											
8	X	X	X	X	X	X	X	X	X	X	X	X																

Perspiration, Bloody

	CROT H	ARN	CALC	LACH	NUX M	NUX V	CHAM	CLEM	COCCUL	LYC
6	X									
7	X	X	X	X	X	X				X
8	X	X	X	X	X	X	X	X	X	

Perspiration, Chest

	LYC	AGAR M	ARG	ARN	CALC	CANTH	CEDRON	CHINA	COCCUL	GLON	GRAPH	HEP	NIT AC	PETR	PH AC	PHOS	SEL	SEP	SIL
7	X		X		X		X			X				X					
8	X	X		X		X		X	X		X	X	X		X	X	X	X	X

Perspiration, Diminished- See Also Perspiration, Absent

	ALUM	APOC
1		X
6	X	

Perspiration, Diseases Of

	CALC	SAMB	FL AC
2	**X**	**X**	**X**
8	X	X	

Perspiration, Excessive/Profuse- See Hyperhidrosis

Perspiration, Face

	BELL	PULS	SIL	CARB V	IGN	MERC	SPONG
7	X	**X**	**X**	X	X	X	X
8	X	X	X	X	X	X	X
18	X						

Perspiration, Feet

	SIL	LYC	CALC	SULPH	NIT AC	BAR C	MAG M	ZINC	SEP	GRAPH	PETR	PULS	THUJA	CARB V	CUPR	LAC AC	NAT M	STAPHYS	VER A	HELL	KALI CAR	MERC
1					X																	
2	**X**	X		**X**	**X**																	
3	X																					
4							X															
5	X	X	X			X						X	X					X	X			
6	X	X	X	X	X	X	X	X	X	X	X	X	X	X		X		X		X	X	
7	**X**	**X**	X	X	X	X	X	X	X	X	X				X	X	X		X			**X**
8	X	X	X	X	X	X	X	X	X	X	X	X	X	X	X		X					
10	X																		X			
11								X														
13	**X**	**X**	**X**	**X**	X	**X**	**X**	X	**X**	X	X	X	X	**X**	X		X	X		**X**	**X**	X
15	X			X																		
17	X															X						
18	X																					
20	X																					
21	X	X	X																			

Perspiration, Feet, Offensive

	SIL	BAR C	GRAPH	NIT AC	CALC	PLUM	SEP	ZINC	TELL	KALI CAR	THUJA	LYC	PETR	PHOS	PSOR	SANIC	CARB V	PULS	RHUS T	SEC
1	X								X											
3	X			X	X														X	
4	X																			
5	X	X	X	X	X	X	X	X	X	X	X	X	X	X	X	X	X	X	X	X
6	X	X	X	X	X	X	X	X		X	X	X	X	X						
7	**X**	**X**	X	X	X	X	X		**X**			X	X		X		X			X
8	X	X	X	X		X	X	X	X						X					
9	X		X					X												
10	X	X														X				
13	**X**	**X**	**X**	X		X	X	X		**X**	**X**			X				X		
17																X				
18	X																			
21	X																			
24					X															
25	X																			

Perspiration, Genitals

	CANTH	MERC	PH AC	SEL	SEP	SULPH	THUJA	AMM C	AUR	BELL	BOV	CON	HEP	HYDRAST	IGN	LYC	MAG M	NUX V	PETR	RHOD	SIL	STAPHYS
5			X	X	X									X								
7	X	X				X	X									X			X			
8	X	X	X	X	X	X	X	X	X	X	X	X	X		X		X	X		X	X	X

Perspiration, Genitals, Offensive

	CINNAB	FL AC	HEP	MERC	NAT M	NIT AC	PETR	SEP	STAPHYS	SULPH	THUJA																	
5	X		X	X		X	X		X		X																	
7		X			X																							
18								X																				
24										X																		
27	X																											

Perspiration, Hands

	NIT AC	SIL	SULPH	CALC	FL AC	NAT M	THUJA	HEP	IGN	PETR	SEP	ZINC	NUX V	ARS	CANTH	CARB V	CIMICI	CON	IOD	IPEC	LED	PHOS	PSOR	PULS	TAB	VER A		
1	X	X	X		X	X																						
2					**X**																							
5	X						X	X			X			X	X		X			X	X	X	X		X	X		
7	X			**X**	X	X			X	X	X	X								X								
8	X	X	X	X			X	X	X	X		X	X			X		X	X		X		X	X				
10																										X		
13	X	X	**X**	**X**		**X**	**X**	X	X	X	X	X	**X**	X	X	X		X	X			X		X	X			
17		X	X														X											
20		X																										

Perspiration, Head

	CALC	SIL	CHAM	MERC	PULS	CHINA	GUAIAC	HEP	RHEUM	SANIC	BELL	GRAPH	LYC	NUX V	PHOS	VER A												
4	X																											
5	X	X	X		X	X	X	X	X	X		X	X	X	X	X												
7	**X**	**X**	**X**	**X**	**X**	X	X	X	X		X		X															
8	X	X	X	X	X	X	X	X	X		X	X		X	X													
9		X																										
10	X	X	X							X						X												
12	X	X																										
17										X																		
18	X																											
19	X																											
20		X		X																								
21	X	X																										
22	X																											
24	X																											
26	X	X	X																									
27		X																										

Perspiration, Head, Offensive

	SIL	BRY	CALC	CHAM	HEP	MERC	MERC C	RHEUM	SEP
5	X	X			X		X		X
7	X	X		X				X	
10						X			
12	X		X						

Perspiration, Neck

	ARS	BELL	KALM	MANG	NIT AC	NUX V	PH AC	RHUS T	SANIC	SIL	STANN	SULPH
8	X	X	X	X	X	X	X	X			X	X
10									X			
17										X		

Perspiration, Night (AKA Night Sweats)

	SIL	CHINA	PHOS	LYC	MERC	STANN	ARS	CALC	SULPH	ACET AC	RHUS T	ARS IOD	HEP	STAPHYS	TUB
1														X	
3										X					X
4	X			X		X			X						
5	X	X	X	X				X							
6	X	X		X	X	X	X		X				X		X
7	X	X	X	X	X	X	X	X	X	X	X		X	X	
8		X	X	X	X	X	X	X	X	X	X		X	X	
10		X	X			X		X			X		X		
11			X												
12									X			X			
14		X						X		X		X			
15			X		X		X								
17	X	X	X				X			X		X		X	X
19				X	X	X									X
20					X										
22			X												
23	X														
24	**X**			X		X					X				
26	X	X			X		X	X			X				
27												X			

Perspiration, Offensive

	MERC	SIL	HEP	SULPH	LYC	STAPHYS	ARN	NIT AC	PETR	RHUS T	BAPT	CARB V	MAG CAR	PSOR	SEP	VER A	ARS	CARB A	CHAM	GRAPH	IPEC	LED	THUJA	BAR C	DULC			
1	X	X				X			X				X							X								
2		**X**				**X**			**X**																			
3		X		X		X			X																			
4	X	X		X																								
5	X	X	X					X						X									X					
6			X	X	X		X			X	X	X		X	X		X	X	X		X	X						
7	X	**X**	X	X	X	X		X		X	X	X	X		X	X		X	X	X	X	X		**X**	**X**			
8	X	X	X	**X**	**X**	X	X	X		**X**		X	X		X	**X**	X	X	X	X	X			X	X			
9				X																								
10	X	X					X																					
11	X		X		X		X	X	X		X			X														
14	X																											
15															X													
17																						X	X					
18	X												X										X					
19								X						X														
21	X		X																									
22			X																									
24											X																	
26					X		X			X		X				X	X											

Perspiraton, Palms

	AGAR M	MERC	PSOR	THUJA	NAJA	NAT M
1	X	X	X	X		
5	X	X	X	X		
17					X	
18						X

Pertussis- See Whooping Cough

Petechiae

	ARS	BRY	RHUS T	SEC	ARN	HYOSC	LACH	PHOS	BELL	NUX V	SIL	STRAM	SULPH AC	BAPT	BERB V	CARB V	CHLOL	CON	HAM	LED	MUR AC	NIT AC	PHELL	PH AC	RUTA	ZINC		
4					X																X							
6	X	X	X	X								X																
7	X	X	X	X		X	X	X																				
8	X	X	X	X	X	X	X	X	X	X	X		X	X	X	X	X		X			X		X	X	X		
13	**X**	**X**	X	X	**X**	X	X	X	**X**	X	X	X	X					X		X			X					

Phantom Limb Pain- See Neuralgia, Stump

Pharyngitis (Note that only the main remedies are used from 17)

	PHYTO	HEP	LACH	NUX V	DULC	KALI BIC	NAT M	BELL	MERC	ACON	ARG N	GELS	GUAIAC	KALI IOD	MERC C	SANG
1	X					X		X					X	X	X	X
2																X
3						X	X						X			
4	X			X												
5					X											
6							X					X				
7	X		X				X									
8	X	X	**X**	**X**	X	X	X	**X**	**X**	X	X			X		X
9		X	X		X			X	X	X			X		X	
17	X	X	X	X	X	X	X	X	X	X	X	X	X	X		X
18		X	X			X					X				X	
19	X	**X**		X	X				X	X	X	X		X	X	
24				X								X				

Pharyngitis, Atrophic

	AESC	SABAL
2		X
17	X	

Pharyngitis, Catarrhal

	ALUM	ARG N	COCCUS	AMM CAU	CALC IOD	KALI BIC	KALI MUR	NAT CAR	SANG N	WYETHIA
1	X	X			X					
8						X	X			
17	X	X	**X**	X				X	X	X

Pharyngitis, Follicular (AKA Clergyman's Sore Throat)

	KALI MUR	PHYTO	SANG N	ALUM	ARUM T	DROS	HEP	HYDRAST	LACH	SEC	AESC	AMBRA	ARG N	ARN	CALC FL	CIST	KALI BIC	KALI IOD	MERC I F	MERC I R	PHOS	TEUCR	WYETHIA
1			X																				
2																X							
4	**X**	X	**X**																				
7	X							X		X													
8	X	X				X	X		X	X	X	X					X	X	X				
14		X																					
17		X	X	X	X	X	X	X	X				X		X					X		X	X
22																					X		
23					X									X									
24	**X**			X																			

Pharyngitis, Left Side

	LACH	MERC I R
9	X	
19	**X**	**X**

Pharyngitis, Right Side

	MERC I F	GUAIAC	LYC	BELL	PHYTO	SANG N
1						X
4		**X**				
17	X					
19	**X**		**X**	X		
24					X	

Pharyngitis, Singers

	ARG
1	X
17	X
18	X

Pharynx, Diseases Of

	MYRICA	SEL
2	X	
17		X

Phimosis

	MERC	NIT AC	SULPH	CANN S	JAC C	ACON	HEP	CINNAB	APIS	BELL	RHUS T	SABIN	SEP	THUJA	HAM	MERC I F	ARN	CALC	CANTH	DIG
1	X	**X**	X		X	X	X	X	X	X						X				
2	**X**	X	X	X	X							X	X		X					
3		**X**			X		X									**X**				
4	X		X																	
6	X			X																
7	X	**X**	X	X			X	X							**X**			X		
8	**X**	X	**X**	X		**X**	X	X		X	X	X	X	X			X	X	X	X
12				X		X				X										
13	X	X	**X**	X	X						X	X	X	X						X
14		X	X			X			X											
21	X				X															
24	X	X	X						X		X			X			X		X	

Phlebitis- See also Pain, Veins

	PULS	HAM	ARN	ACON	LACH	BELL	VIP	APIS	SULPH	ARS	ANT T	BOTHR	BRY	CON	CROT H	FERR PH	HEP	NUX V	PHOS	RHUS T	SIL	VIP RED						
1	X	X					X																					
2	**X**						X	X			X				X													
3		X																										
4		**X**																										
5	X		X		X							X			X							X						
6						X																						
7	**X**	**X**	X					X			X		X	X		X												
8	**X**	X	**X**	X	X			X	X	X				X			X	X	X	X	X							
9	X	B	B	X	X	X						X																
10	X		X	X		X			X	X			X					X		X								
12	X	B		B	X														X									
15	X			X					X								X				X							
16	X	B	X				X									X												
18			X		X	X	X	X														X						
23		X					X																					
25	X	B	B	X	X	X																						

B- Both Internal and External

Phlegmasia Alba Dolens- See also Phlegmasia Dolens (AKA Milk Leg)

	HAM	ARS	BELL	LYC	PULS	RHUS T	BRY	SULPH	LACH	ARN	CALC	SIL	LED	SEP	CHINA	IOD	ANT C	CHAM	KALI CAR	MERC	NUX V							
1	X			X	X				X			X																
3	**X**																											
4	**X**																											
7	X	X	X	X	X	X	**X**	X	**X**	X	X		X					X	X									
8		X	X	X	X	X	X	X			X	X		X	X	X	X			X								
10		X	X		X	X	X	X		X											X							
13	X	X	X	X	X	X	X	X	X	X	X	X	**X**	**X**	**X**	**X**	X	X	X	X	X							
26		X	X	X		X																						

Phlegmasia Dolens- See also Phlegmasia Alba Dolens

	BRY	HAM	PULS	BELL	LYC	SULPH	ACON	LACH	ARN	ARS	BUFO	CALC	NAT SUL	RHUS T	BISM	ALL C	APIS	CROT H	HIPPOZ	KALI CAR	NUX V	SEP	URT U					
2	X	**X**	**X**	X	X	X	**X**	X			X		X		**X**				X				X					
7	**X**	X	X	X	X	X		**X**	X	X	X	X	X	X														
8	X	X	X	X	X	X	X		X	X		X		X		X	X	X		X	X	X						

Phlyctenula

	PULS	BAR C	BUFO	CROT H	EUPHR	GRAPH	MERC	MERC C	MERC D	MERC I R	NAT CAR	SIL	SQUILLA	SYMPH
2					X									
6	X											X		
7			X											
8	X	X		X		X	X	X	X	X	X		X	X
24	X													

Phlyctenular Ophthalmia- See also Keratoconjunctivitis

	BAR C	CROT T	GRAPH	IGN	MERC	MERC C	MERC D	MERC I R	PULS	SQUILLA	SYMPH
2				X							
8	X	X	X		X	X	X	X	X	X	X

Phobia

	ARG N	ANAC	GELS	PHOS	STRAM	AGAR M	ARS	BAR C	BOR	CALC	CALC PH	CANN I	CANTH	CIMICI	LAC C	LACH	LYC	SYPH	MERC	PLAT	PSOR	SIL	SULPH
19	X	X		X	X	X	X	X		X	X	X		X	X	X		X	X	X	X	X	
2'	X	X	X	X	X				X								X						X
25	X		X																				
26													X										

Phosphaturia

	PH AC	MAG PH	CALC PH	PHOS	PTEL	RAPH	SOLID	BELL	FERR	KALI HP	MEDIC
1	X	X				X	X				
2	X		X		X		X				
3	X									X	
5	X	X	X	X	X	X	X		X		X
7	X	X		X	X	X			X		
8	X										
10	X										
11	X							X			
14								X			
18			X								
23	X									X	X
24	X	X		X							

Photophobia

	BELL	EUPHR	ACON	NUX V	CON	ARS	PHOS	MERC	BRY	CALC	GRAPH	IGN	AUR	RHUS T	SULPH	HEP	MERC C	PULS	SIL	NAT SUL	SEP	ALL C	APIS	CALC PH	CAUST	CLEM	CHINA	LYC
1	**X**	X	X	X	X		X	X		X	X	X		X		X	X						X					
2																				X								
3													X	X														
4	X	X	X		X				X	X						X										X		
5	X																											
6	X	X	X	X	X	X		X			X		X	X	X	X		X			X		X			X		
7	**X**	X		**X**	**X**	X	X	X		X	X	X	X	X	**X**	X	X	X		X	X		X	X	X	X	**X**	**X**
8	X	X	X	X	X	X	X	X	X	**X**	X	X		X	X	X		X	X	X	X				X			X
9	X	X	X	X		X			X		X													X				
10	X		X	X								X		X														
11				X									X				X											
12	X	X					X										X											
13	**X**	**X**	**X**	X	X	X	**X**	**X**	**X**	X	**X**	**X**		X	**X**			X	**X**	X	**X**	X	X		X	X	X	X
14	X				X	X	X						X				X		X			X						
15	X	X	X			X			X			X																
17	X	X		X	X	X							X						X			X					X	
18	X		X																									
19	X	X	X		X															X								
20		X	X																									
21	X			X	X				X						X			X				X						
22	X	X	X	X																								
23																									X			
24	X	X	X				X	X		X	X		X				X		X									
25	X	X			X				X															X				
26	**X**		**X**	X		X	X	**X**		X		X			X	X		X										
27	X	X		X		X																		X				

Photopsia- See also Vision, Diseases Of

	ZINC	AUR	BELL	BRY	CAUST	CROC	HYOSC	NAT M	NUX V	PULS	SPIG
2	X										
8	X	X	X	X	X	X	X	X	X	X	X

Photosensitivity- See Ailments from Sun; Hydroa; Photophobia

Phthiriasis

	SABAD	AMM C	ARS	BACILL	CHINA	COCCUL	IOD	LACH	MAG P AR	MEZ	NAT M	OLEAND	PSOR	STAPHYS	SULPH
2	**X**			X		X									
8	X	X	X		X		X	X	X	X	X	X	X	X	X

Phthisis- See Tuberculosis

Physometra

	PH AC	LYC	SANG	BROM	BELL	CALC	MAG CAR	NUX V	SEP	APIS	CHINA	HYOSC	LUNA	NUX M	SULPH	TAR H	ORIGAN
2	**X**	X	X	**X**									X			X	
7	**X**	**X**	X		X	X	X	X	X								X
8	X	X	X	X	X	X	X	X	X	X	X	X		X	X		

Pica- See Craving, Indigestible/Abnormal Articles

Piles- See Haemorrhoids

Pituitary Gland, Diseases Of

	BAR C	CALC	PITUIT
1		X	
27	X		X

Pityriasis

	ARS	GRAPH	LYC	MEZ	FL AC	KALI BR	PHOS	SULPH	KREO	PHYTO
2	**X**	X		**X**	**X**					
7	**X**		X	X		X			**X**	**X**
8		X	X			X	X			
11	X	X		X	X			X		
12	**X**	X	X							
15	X									
21	X									
26	X	X	X				X	X		

Pityriasis Rubra

	THYROID	NAT ARS	ERYTHRIN
1	X		
2	X	**X**	X

Pityriasis Versicolor

	MEZ	TELL	SEP	ARS	CARB AC	SULPH	SULO AC	ALUM	BACILL	CHR AC	COLCH	FL AC	GRAPH	KALI ARS	NIT AC
2	X	**X**	**X**		X		**X**								
8	X		X	X		X									
7	X				X										X
11	X	X		X		X		X			X	X	X	X	

Placenta, Diseases Of

	PHOS
9	X
25	X

Placenta Praevia

	SABIN	CINNAM	ERIG
2			X
8		X	
19	**X**		

Placenta, Retention Of

	PULS	SABIN	SEC	BELL	CANTH	VISC A	ARS	ART V	CAULO	CIMICI	GELS	IPEC	SEP	AGNUS	CROC	GOSS	NUX V	PLAT	PYROG
1		X		X	X	X													X
2	X	X	X		X	X													
4	X																		
7	X		X	X	**X**		X	X	X			X		X			X		
8	X	X	X	X	X	X	X	X	X	X	X	X	X		X	X			
9	X																		
13	X	X	X	X	X					X	X		X						
14		X																	
19	X	X		X															
21	X		X	X														X	
25	X		X																
26	X	X	X	X															
28		X	X																

Plague

	ARS	PHOS	CROT H	IGN	IOD	LACH	NAJA	OPERCUL	TAR C	PYROG	BAD	BAPT	CARB V	CAD S	ELAPS	KALI MUR	TUB AV	VER V	YERSIN
11	X	**X**	X	X	X	X	X	X	X	**X**							X	X	
12	X		X			X	X					X			X				
15													X						
16	X	X		X	X			X	X		X			X		X			X

Plantar Fasciitis- See Fasciitis

Plethora- See Hypervolaemia

Pleurisy (Note that only the main remedies have been used from 17)

	BRY	ACON	SULPH	ARS	ARN	CANTH	HEP	APIS	KALI CAR	BELL	RAN B	KALI IOD	PHOS	SENEG	MERC	SQUILL	ASC T	LYC	CARB V	COLCH	IOD	CARB A	CHINA	NIT AC	BOR	CALC	RHUS T	STANN
1	X		X	X		X	X	X	X	X	**X**			X			X											X
2	**X**	**X**	**X**	**X**		**X**	**X**	**X**	X	X		X		X			X					X	**X**		X			
3	X	X		X	X	X	X							X				X					X				X	
4	**X**	X	X	X	X	**X**	X	X		**X**	X						X	**X**										X
5	X																											
6	X	X	X	X	X	X	X		X	X		X	X	X	X	X		X	X	X	X		X	X		X	X	
7	**X**	**X**	X	X	X	X	X	X	X		X	X			X	**X**	X		X	X	X			X	X			
8	X	X	X	X		X	X	X	X		X	X		X	X	X	X		X	X		X		**X**			X	X
9	X		X			X																						
10		**X**	X	X	X								X		X			X										
11	**X**	**X**	X	X	X		X	X	X	X		X	X	X	X							**X**			X	X		
12	**X**	X		X	X								X								X							
13	X	X											X															
14	X	X	X		X		X				X	X																
15	X	**X**		X	X										X													
16	X	X	X										X															
17	**X**	X	X	X	X	X	X	X	**X**	X	**X**	X	X	X	X	X	X		X	X	X	X	X	X	X	X		X
18	**X**				X	X		X																				
19	X																											
21	X	X	X			X	X			X						X												
23	X				X	X		X			X						X			X								
24	**X**	X	X	X	X	X	X	X	X	X	X	X	X	X	X	X		X			X						X	
26	X	X	X	X	X				X							X		X	X							X	X	
28	X																											

Pleuritis, Senile

	NIT AC
8	X
11	X

Pleurodynia

	ARN	BOR	RAN B	ACON	CIMICI	COLCH
6	X					
7						X
8	X	X	X	X	X	X
12	X		X	X	X	
17	X	X				
23		X	X			

Pleurodynia, Right Side

	CIMICI	BOR	CHEN A
6	X		
8	X	X	X

Plica Polonica

	VINCA	LYC	ANT T	PSOR	SARS	VER A	VIOL T	BOR	BOV	KREO
2	**X**	**X**	X	X	X	X	X	X		
4							X			
7	X		X		X	X				
8	X									
13	X	X		X					X	X

Pneumonia (Includes Bronchopneumonia; Lobar Pneumonia; Pleuropneumonia)

	PHOS	BRY	ACON	ANT T	SULPH	LYC	CHEL	ARS	FERR PH	VER V	BELL	HEP	CARB V	IOD	IPEC	KALI CAR	LACH	RHUS T	SANG	TUB	PULS	HYOSC	KALI IOD	KALI MUR	ARN	GELS	ARS IOD
1	X	X	X	X	X		X			X				X	X					**X**							
2	**X**	**X**	**X**	**X**	**X**	**X**	X	**X**	X	X	X	**X**					X	X	X	X		**X**					**X**
3		X	X		X	X		X	X	X		X	X	X	X		X										
4	**X**	**X**	**X**	**X**	**X**	X	**X**		X	**X**		X		**X**		**X**			**X**	X	X	X		**X**		X	
5	X			X								X											X				
6	X	X	X	X	X	X	X	X	X	X	X		X	X		X	X	X	X		X	X	X	X	X	X	
7	**X**	**X**	**X**	**X**	**X**	**X**	**X**	**X**	**X**	X	X		**X**			X	X	**X**	X		X		**X**	X	X	X	
8	**X**	X	X	**X**	**X**	X	X	X	X	X	X	X	X	X	X	X	X	X	X		X	X	X	X	X	X	X
9		X																									
10	X	X	X	X	X	X					X	X			X					X	X						
11	**X**	**X**	**X**	**X**	**X**		X	**X**	X		X	X			X	X				**X**				X			X
12	**X**	X	X	X	X	X	X	X	X	X			X	X			X	X							X		
14	X	X	**X**	X	X				X				X		X					X							X
15	X	X	X	X						X	X															X	
16	X			X		X				X			X			X											
17	X	X	X	X	X	X	X	X	X	X	X	X	X	X	X	X	X	X	X	X	X	X	X		X	X	X
18	X	X		X				X				X			X												
19	**X**	**X**	**X**	X	**X**	**X**	**X**	**X**	**X**	**X**	**X**		X		**X**	**X**		X			X		X				
21	X	X	X				X				X								X								
23	X	X	X	X	X	X	X		X			X		X			X		X					X			
26	X	X	X	X	X			X			X						X	X			X	X			X		
27	X	X				X																					

Pneumonia, Lobar- See Pneumonia

Pneumonia, Left Sided

	LACH	NAT SUL	SANG	ACON	CALC	CHEL	OX AC	SULPH
5	X	X						
7	X		X					
17	X	X	X	X	X	X	X	X

Pneumonia, Right Sided

	CHEL	PHOS	BROM	CARB A	IOD	KALI CAR	LYC	MERC	BRY	BAR C	BELL	CALC	ELAPS	KALI IOD	SANG
1	X				X										
4	X														
5	X	X				X		X							
6	X														
7					X		X			X					
8			X	X									X	X	
10		X													
17	X	X	X	X		X	X	X	**X**		X	X			X

Pneumonitis

	PHOS	SANG
17	X	
19		X

Pneumothorax

	ACON	ARN	ARS	BRY	STAPHYS
6	X	X	X		X
8		X			
21	X			X	

Podagra- See Gout

Podarthrocace- See Abscess, Ankle Joint

Polio

	LATH	ACON	BELL	BUNGA	GELS	PLUM	ARG N	BRY	CAUST	KALI PH	NUX V	OX AC	RHUS T
3	**X**												
9	X	X				X	X					X	
11	X	X	X	X	X					X			
14		X	X		X						X		X
16	X			X		X			X				
21	**X**	X	X					X					

Polio, Prophylaxis

	LATH
10	X
16	X

Polyarthritis

	CAUST	ANT C	BENZ AC	BRY	CALC	DULC	NAT SUL	PULS	RHOD	RHUS T	RUTA	STELL AQ
5	X	X	X			X	X					X
9	X			X	X			X	X	X	X	

Polycystic Ovary Disease- See Cysts, Ovary

Polymenorrhoea

	CALC	IGN	PLAT	FERR	BOR	CALC PH	CARB V	COCCUL	HELON	PHOS	PHYTO	TRILL P
1		X	X									
6		X	X	X		X		X				X
7		X		X			X	X	X		X	
9					X							
10	X		X								X	X
12	X											
17									X			
18	X					X						
24										X		
25					X							
26	X	X	X	X			X			X		

Polyneuritis

	ARS	PHOS	ACON	ALL C	ARN	BELL	BOV	CARB SUL	CEDRON	CON	GELS	HYPER	MORPH	PLUM	STANN	THALLIUM
4	X	X														
17	X	X	X	X	X	X	X	X	X	X	X	X	X	X	X	X

Polyneuropathy (Includes Diabetic Polyneuropathy)

	AGAR M	CALC	CAUST	GELS	IGN	KALM	MEDO	PHOS	CANN I	CARC	LYC	NAT M	NUX V	PLUM	RHUS T	SULPH	THUJA
11	X		X	X		X			X					X	X	X	
29*		X			X		X	X		X	X	X	X				X

29*Pomposelli R, et al. Observational study of Homeopathic and Conventional therapies in patients with Diabetic Polyneuropathy. Homeopathy. 2009 Jan;98 (1):17-25.

Polyps

	CALC	TEUCR	THUJA	PHOS	SANG	SIL	CON	KALI BIC	LYC	NIT AC	LEM MIN	STAPHYS	AUR	BERB V	CALC PH	CARB A	HEP	HYDRAST	MEDO	MERC	MEZ	SANG N	PSOR
1		X									**X**												
2	**X**	X	**X**	**X**	**X**			**X**		**X**	X			X		X			X			X	**X**
3				X	X																		
5	X		X					X										X					
6	X																						
7	**X**	**X**				X	X		X						X	X							
8	**X**	X	**X**	**X**	X	**X**	X	X	**X**	**X**		**X**	X	X	X		X	X		X	X		
9	X	X	X																				
13	**X**		X	**X**	X	X	**X**		X			**X**	X				X			X	X		
17			X																				
18	X	**X**	X	X	X	X													X			X	
28		X																					

Polyps, Anus

	NIT AC	CALC PH	CINNAB	KALI BR	PHOS
5	X		X		
7	X	**X**		X	X

Polyps, Bladder

	CALC	THUJA	TEUCR	NIT AC	COLIBAC	CON	MEDO	MERC	PHOS	PULS	SANG	SIL	STAPHYS	VISC A
1	X													
5		X	X	X							X			X
7	X													
8	X	X				X		X	X	X		X	X	
18	X	X	X	X	X									
19							X							

Polyps, Cervical

	ARS	CALC	THUJA
1			X
7	X		
21		X	

Polyps, Ear

	CALC	THUJA	MERC	SANG	TEUCR	CALC IOD	HYDRAST	LACH	LYC	KALI SUL	PHOS	SULPH	HEP	TUB	ALUMEN	DULC	KALI BIC	KALI MUR	NIT AC	STAPHYS	TAXUS							
1	X	X	X				X																					
2		**X**		**X**				X	X				**X**	**X**							X							
3							X																					
4		X																										
6	X	X	X	X	X	X									X													
7	**X**	X	X		X		X	X	X	X	X																	
8	X	X	X		X	X						X				X	X			X								
13	**X**											X																
14	X																											
17	X	X	X	X	X	X		X	X	X	X							X	X									
24	X	X	X																									
27				X																								

Polyps, Eye, Canthus

	LYC																											
2	X																											
7	X																											

Polyps, Eyelid, Under

Deleted:

	KALI BIC																											
1	X																											
3	X																											

Polyps, Larynx

	SANG	ARG	ARG N	BERB V	CALC	CALC PH	PHOS																					
1	X																											
5	X	X	X	X	X	X	X																					
7	X																											

Polyps, Nasal

	TEUCR	CALC	SANG	PHOS	LEM MIN	THUJA	ALL C	KALI NIT	SIL	SULPH	KALI BIC	NIT AC	PULS	SANG N	ALUMEN	ARUM M	CAD SUL	CON	LYC	NAT M	SEP	STAPHYS
1	**X**	X	X		X	X		X				X			X							
2																X	X		X			
3	X	X	X	X	**X**	X																
4					X	X																
5	X	X	X	X	X	X	X	X	X		X			X					X	X		
6	X	X	X	X			X	X					X									
7	**X**	X	X	X			X		X	X												
8	X	X	X	X			X		X	X	X	X			X			X		X		X
9	X	X																				
12	X	X	B	X		X					X											
13	X	X	X	X					X												X	X
14	E	X		X						X							X					
17	X	X	X	X	X	X	X	X				X	X	X				X			X	
19	**X**				X					X												
21	X	X	X	X									X									
23	X		X		X									X		X						
24						X																
26		X	X	X																		
28	X																					

B- Both Internal and External E- External

Polyps, Rectum

	PHOS	TEUCR	CALC PH	KALI BR	NIT AC	CALC	CINNAB	MERC C	MILL
1	X	X	X						
2				X					
3	X								
5					X		X		
6	X					X			
7	X		X	X	X				
14	X	**X**						X	X

Polyps, Uterus

	CALC	PHOS	TEUCR	THUJA	CON	CALC PH	BUFO	HYDRAST	LED	LYC	PH AC	PLAT	SEP	SIL	STAPHYS	ARS	AUR	CHINA	EROD	MERC	MEZ	NIT AC	PETR	PULS	SANG
1	**X**		X	X	X																				
2						X													X						
5					X			X																	
7	**X**	**X**	**X**	**X**	X	**X**	X		X	X	X	X	X	X	X	X									
8	X	X	X	X	X			X	X	X	X	X	X	X	X		X			X	X	X	X	X	X
14		X					X																		
16																		X							
18	X																								
19	X	X																							
23			X	X																					

Polyps, Vaginal

	CON	TEUCR	CALC	HYDRAST	PULS	AUR	LED	LYC	MERC	MEZ	NIT AC	PETR	PH AC	PHOS	PLAT	SANG	SEP	SIL	STAPHYS	THUJA
1	X	X																		
5	X			X																
7		X	X		X															
8	X	X	X	X	X	X	X	X	X	X	X	X	X	X	X	X	X	X	X	X

Polyps, Vocal Cord

	BERB V	THUJA
1	X	
8	X	
17		X

Polyuria- See also Urination, Profuse; Urination, Urgent

	NUX V	APIS	CANTH	PH AC	SABAL	ARG N	BERB V	LYC	NAT M	URAN N	ARG	CALC	CAUST	EQUISET	MUREX	PULS	SULPH	THUJA	KALI CAR	LIL T								
1	X			X	X	X			X	X			X	X	X	X		X										
2	**X**																		**X**	**X**								
3						X																						
4		X					X			X	X							X										
5				X		X			X	X					X													
6		X	X					X	X			X					X											
8	X	X	X	X				X					X			X	X											
9	X		X	X	X		X																					
10		X		X				X	X	X	X					X												
11				X	X			X							X			X										
14		X					X																					
15			X																									
16	X																											
17												X																
18	X		X		X	X								X			X											
19		X									X																	
21	X												X						X	X								
24		X										X																
25	X		X		X		X							X														

Pork, Diseases From- See Ailments from Pork
Porrigo Decalvans- See Alopecia Areata
Post- Nasal Drip- See Catarrh, Post Nasal
Posthitis

	MERC	NIT AC	CALC	NAT CAR	NAT SUL	SULPH	THUJA	CANN S	ARN	ARS	CINNAB	COLOC	CON	CROT T	RHUS T													
1	**X**	X	X		X				X		X		X	X	X													
7	X	**X**	X	X								X																
8						X																						
11							X																					
13	X	X	X	X		X		**X**		X																		
14					X		X																					

Pott's Disease- See also Spine, Curvature Of (AKA Pott's Curvature; Malum Pottii)

	CALC	SIL	ASAF	CALC PH	GETTY	HEP	MEZ	PHOS	PH AC	SULPH	PYROG	ACON	ARN	CALC IOD	KALI IOD	HYPER	LYC	MERC	NAT M	PLUM	PSOR	PULS	RHUS T	STICTA	STILL	SULPH
1	X																									
2					X			X			**X**				X									X	X	
4		**X**																								
6	X	**X**	X	X		X	X		X			X	X	X		X	X	X	X	X	X	X	X			X
7	X									X																
8					X																					
12	X		X	X		X	X	X	X	X																
24	X	X																								

Pregnancy- In addition to the following, see also listings under Ailments from Pregnancy; Labour (various); Conception, Failure of; Morning Sickness; Wounds, Incisional

Pregnancy, Albuminuria From

	MERC	APIS	HELON	GELS	APOC	ARS	ARS IOD	CANTH	KALI CAR	KALI MUR	KALM	LYC	PHOS	TEREB
1	X	**X**	X										X	
2				X							X			
3		X												
6				X										
7	X	X	X	X		X	X	X	X	X		X		X
8	X	X	X		X	X	X	X	X	X	X	X	X	X
14	**X**													
23	X		X		X									

Pregnancy, Bladder Disorders From

	PULS	LYC
2	**X**	
7		X

Pregnancy, Breasts Painful From- See also Mastalgia

	CON	SEP
2	**X**	
7		X

Pregnancy, Constipation From

	SEP	NUX V	ALUM	BRY	OP	SULPH	COLLIN	LYC	HYDRAST	PLAT	POD	CALC	CON	GRAPH	KALI CAR	PHYTO	PLUM	VERBASC	ALUMEN	DOLICH
2			X																	
3	X				X															
4	X				X															
5	X	X	X	X			X		X	X	X									
7	**X**	**X**		X	X	X	**X**	X	X	**X**	X	X	X	X	X	X	X	X	**X**	**X**
8	X		X	X		X	X	X	X	X	X	X	X	X	X	X	X	X		
10	X	**X**	X	X	**X**	X		X												
13	X	X					X	X												
14			X																	
15		X		X	**X**	X														
18									X											
21	X	X	X	X		X														

Pregnancy, Cramp, Calves, From- See also Cramp, Calves

	NUX V	VER A	CHAM	CUPR AC	COFF	FERR
8	X	X	X	X	X	X
21	X	X				

Pregnancy, Diarrhoea From

	PULS	CHAM	SULPH	PH AC	LYC	NUX V	ANT C	DULC	PHOS	APIS	CALC	CARB V	CHINA	HYOSC	IRIS V	PETR	RHEUM	SEC	SEP
2	**X**			**X**															
7	X	X	X		X	X	X		X	X			X	X	X	X			X
8	X	X	X	X	X	X	X	X	X	X	X	X	X	X	X	X	X	X	X
10	X	X	X	X	X	X	X	X			X						X	X	
14												X							
21	X	X	X					X											

Pregnancy, Diseases Of

	SEP	NUX V	PULS	BELL	IPEC	NUX M	ACON	CAULO	COCCUL	COLLIN	KALI CAR	SULPH	CIMICI	CALC	CROC	NAT M	PHOS	ALET	ANT T	CAPS	CAUST	CHAM	COFF	CON
2	**X**	**X**		**X**	**X**	X		**X**		**X**	**X**	**X**	**X**		**X**					**X**		**X**		
6							X										X							
7	X	X	**X**	X		X	**X**				X		**X**	**X**		X		**X**	**X**		**X**			
8	X	X	X		X				X	X	X	X				X	X	X	X				X	X
9	X	X	X					X	X															
13	**X**	**X**	**X**	**X**	**X**	X	X		**X**			X			**X**	X	X			X	X	X	**X**	**X**
23	X					X		X		X				**X**										

Pregnancy, Dyspepsia Of- See also Pregnancy, Heartburn, During; Pregnancy, Indigestion From

	PULS	ACON	ARS	CANTH	CON	DIOSC	FERR	IPEC	KREO	LACH	MAG M	NAT M	NUX M	NUX V	PETR	PHOS	SABAD	SEP	SINAP A
2																	X		X
7				X		X													
8	X	X	X		X		X	X	X	X	X	X	X		X	X		X	
10	X													X					

Pregnancy, Dysuria From

	ACON	CANTH	PULS	BELL	LYC	NUX V	APIS	BERB V	CANN S	COCCUL	CUPR AR	EQUISET	HELON	HELL	MERC C	NAT M	PH AC	SULPH	TEREB	UVA
7	X	X	X		X	X										X				
8	X	X	X	X	X	X			X		X	X	X	X	X				X	X
10	X	X	X	X						X							X	X		
22	X	X					X	X												

Pregnancy, Hair, Falling Of, During or After

	NAT M	LYC	CALC	SEP	SULPH	LACH	CHINA	HELL	HEP	MEZ	PHOS	SIL
1	X					X						
3	X			X								
4	**X**											
5	X	X		X								
7	X			X				X		X		
8	X	X	X		X		X				X	
10		X	X		X							
13	X		X		X	X						
26	X	X							X			X

Pregnancy, Heartburn, During- See also Pregnancy, Dyspepsia Of; Pregnancy, Indigestion From

	CAPS	NAT M	NUX V	PULS	ACET AC	APIS	CALC	COLCH	DIOSC	LAC AC	LYC	PHOS	SULPH	TAB	ZINC
2									X						
3				X			X				X				
7	X	X	X			X				X				X	X
8		X			X										
10			X	X											
21	X							X				X	X		

Pregnancy, Incontinence From- See Incontinence, Urinary

Pregnancy, Indigestion From- See also Pregnancy, Heartburn, During; Pregnancy, Dyspepsia Of

	PULS	NUX V	CHINA	SABAD	SINAP A
2	X			X	X
21	X	X	X		

Pregnancy, Insomnia From

	COFF	BELL	ACON	PULS	CHAM	GELS	LYC	NUX V	OP	SULPH	CIMICI	AMBRA	ANAC	ARS	CACT	CHINA	COCCUL	CYPRIP	HYOSC	IGN	KALI BR	MAG PH	MOSCH	RHUS T	SCUT	STAPHYS	STRAM	TAR C
3													X															
7	X	X							X		X										X							
8	X	X	X	X	X	X	X	X	X			X			X	X		X	X	X		X	X	X	X	X	X	X
22	X			X		X		X						X			X											
25	X		X	X	X		X			X																		
26	X	X	X							X																		

Pregnancy, Oedema, From

	APIS	APOC	ARS	DIG	BRY	MERC C	SANIC	SULPH
1						X		
2							X	
3	X				X			X
7	X	X	X	X				
8	X	X	X	X				

Pregnancy, Pain, Back, During

	AESC	BELL	BELLIS	BRY	CAUST	KALI CAR	NUX V	PULS	RHUS T	SARS	SULPH
3	X		X			X					
7										X	
10		X		X	X		X	X	X		X

Pregnancy, Pruritis From

	ARS	GRAPH	LYC	SIL	SULPH
8	X	X	X	X	X
10	X	X	X	X	X

Pregnancy, Ptyalism, From

	MERC	PULS	ACET AC	ARS	BELL	CARB V	EPIPHEG	JAB	IPEC	IRIS V	KALI BIC	KALI IOD	NAT M	SINAP A	SULPH	TRIFOL R	VER A
8	X	X	X		X	X	X	X		X	X	X	X	X	X	X	
21	X	X		X					X								X

Pregnancy, Toothache From

	SEP	NUX V	PULS	CHAM	MAG CAR	BELL	COFF	STAPHYS	CALC	ACON	HYOSC	MERC	NUX V	RHUS T	ALUM	BRY	KREO	RAPH	RAT	TAB
1	X	X	X	X	X	X	X	X	X									X		
2					X										X			X		X
3	X	X	X	X	X		X													
4	X	X			X															
5					X															
6		X	X			X		X	X		X	X	X	X		X				
7	X		X	X	X	X		X	X	X	X								X	X
8	X	X	X	X			X	X	X	X		X	X	X	X		X		X	
10	X	X	X	X		X	X	X				X	X	X		X				
12	X	X	X	X		X	X										X			
21	X																			
26		X	X	X	X	X	X	X	X	X	X									

Pregnancy, Urine, Retention/Suppression Of

	NUX V	PULS	ACON	CAMPH	APIS	APOC	ARS	BELL	CANTH	EUP PUR	HELL	NIT AC	OP	STRAM
3	X	X		X										
6													X	
8	X	X	X	X	X	X	X	X	X	X	X	X		X
21	X	X												
22			X											
26	X	X	X	X										

Pregnancy, Varicose Veins, From

	PULS	HAM	CARB V	LYC	MILL	NUX V	ARN	FL AC	LACH	ARS	CAUST	FERR	GRAPH	CALC FL	ACON	AESC	ALOE	APIS	CARD M	COLLIN	HYDRAST	POD	SULPH	VIB OP	ZINC
1						X		X	X																
3	X					X			X																
5	X	X	X	X	X	X	X	X		X	X	X	X	X		X	X		X	X	X	X		X	
7	X	X	X	X	X	X	X	X			X	X	X												
8	X	X	X	X	X	X	X	X		X	X	X	X		X			X					X		X
9	X																								
10	X	X	X	X		X	X		X	X															
13					X																				
14	X	X	X	X					X					X											
15		E																							
16							X																		
21	X		X	X	X																				
22		B																							

B- Both Internal and External E- External

Premenstrual Syndrome- See also Dysmenorrhoea (AKA PMS, PMT)

	SEP	PULS	NAT M	LACH	CALC	SULPH	CHAM	LYC	MAG CAR	PLAT	BELL	CIMICI	CON	CYCL	FOLLIC	KREO	CAULO	CAUST	COCCUL	CUPR	KALI CAR	NUX M	NUX V	PHOS	SIL	VER A		
5	X	X	X	X						X		X		X	X													
7	X	X	X	X	X		X	X	X	X	X		X			X		X	X	X	X	X		X	X			
8	X	X	X	X	X	X	X	X		X			X						X	X				X	X	X		
13	X	X	X	X	X		X		X	X	X			X		X		X				X				X		
18	X	X	X	**X**	X			X	X				X	X	X													
19	X					X								X		X				X				X				
20		X		X													X											
21	X	X	X	X	X	X		X										X			X		X					
22							X				X																	
23	X	X	X		X	X			X	X		X				X	X				X	X						
24					X																							
25												X																
26	X	X				X	X				X						X		X				X		X	X		
27	**X**	X	X	X	X			X					X															
28	X	X																										
29[1]	X	X	X	X																			X					
29[2]															X													
29[3]	**X**		X						X			X																
29[4]															X													

29[1] Yakir M, et al. Effects of Homeopathic Treatment in Women with Premenstrual Syndrome: a Pilot Study. Brit Hom J, 2001, 90, 148-153.
29[2] Martinez B. Folliculinum: Efficacy in Premenstrual Syndrome. Brit Hom J, April, 1990, 79, 104-105.
29[3] Klein-Laansma CT, et al. Semi-standardised homeopathic treatment of premenstrual syndrome with a limited number of medicines : Feasability study. Homeopathy, 2010, 95, 99, 192-204.
29[4] Danno K, et al. Homeopathic treatment of premenstrual syndrome: a case series. Homeopathy. 2013 Jan; 102 (1):59-65.

Presbyopia- See also Hypermetropia

	PETR	LACH	NAT CAR	CARB A	DROS	LED	SEP	SULPH	ALUM	AMM C	BELL	BRY	CAUST	CON	DUB M	HYOSC	MAG M	MEZ	MOSCH	NAT M	ONOS	PHOS	SPIG					
2	X		X												X						X							
8		X																										
13	**X**	X	X	**X**	**X**	**X**	**X**	**X**	X	X	X	X	X	X		X	X	X	X	X		X	X					

Priapism

	CANTH	PULS	CANN S	PIC AC	CAMPH	NAT CAR	CANN I	NAT M	COLOC	GRAPH	PLAT	CINNAB	NIUX V	OENANTH	PETROS	KALI CAR	MERC	THUJA
1	X			X	X			X			X							
2		X	X	X	X	X				X		X		X	X			
4							X											
6							X											
7	**X**		X	X	X	X									X			
8	**X**	X	X				X		X									
9	X			X									X					
11	X																	
13	**X**	**X**	X			**X**		**X**	**X**	**X**	**X**		X			**X**	**X**	**X**
14	X	X			X							X						
17														X				
21	X																	
23			X	X														
24		X																
27	X																	

Proctalgia- See Pain, Rectum

Proctitis

	SULPH	PHOS	POD	NIT AC	ACON	ALOE	ALUM	BELL	COLCH	NUX V	NAT SUL	CHIM	COLLIN	HEP	HYDRAST	IGN	KALI CAR	LACH	MERC	MUR AC	SABAL
1		X	X	X		X			X							X					
2		**X**	**X**	**X**		X						X	X								X
4							X														
6	X				X			X		X											
7														X	X		X				
8	X	X	X		X			X		X								X			
10							X														
18	X																				
19	X			X							X										
24									X												
26					X														X	X	

Progressive Muscular Atrophy- See Atrophy, Muscular, Progressive

Prolapse, Anal- See also Prolapse, Rectum

	POD	SULPH	IGN	CALC	MERC	GAMBOG	NUX V	ASAR	BELL	RUTA	TROMB	SEP	MEZ	MUR AC	APIS	ARS	BRY	COLCH	COLLIN	LACH	LYC	NIT AC	PHOS	PLUM
1	X																							
2	X	X						X		X	X		X	X								X		X
6	X	X	X	X	X	X	X		X		X										X			
7	**X**	X		**X**		X	X	X	X						**X**				X				X	
8	**X**	X	X	X	**X**	X	X	X	X		X	**X**	X	X	X			X	X	X	X		X	
10		X	**X**		X		X																	
11	X	X	X							X														
12	X	X	**X**	X	X	X	X					X				X	X							
13	X	X	X	X	X	X		X		X	X	X	X	X		X	X	X		X				X
14										X														
23																						X		
24	X	X							X															

Prolapse, Bladder

	CALC	CON	GRAPH	LYC	PYRUS	POD	THUJA
2					X		
5						X	
13	X	X	X	X			X

Prolapse, Bowel

	IGN	POD
12		X
15	X	

Prolapse, Disc, Intervertebral

	RHUS T	COLOC	ACON	ANT T	ARN	BERB V	BRY	CALC	CALC FL	CIMICI	HYPER	LYC	SULPH	THUJA
14	X	X	X	X		X	X			X				
17	X													
21					X									
29*	**X**	X						X	X		X	X	X	X

29* Gundimeda RM. Herniated Lumbar Disc. Homoeopathic Links, Winter, 2008, 21, 217-220.

Prolapse, Iris

	PHYSO	ALUM	ANT S A	ATROP	HEP
2	X		X		
7	X	X		X	X

Prolapse, Rectum- See also Prolapse, Anus

	IGN	POD	MERC	SULPH	RUTA	NUX V	SEP	CALC	MUR AC	GRAPH	NAT M	LACH	LYC	BELL	FERR	HAM	INDIG	SIL	FERR PH
1	X	X		X	X				X					**X**					
2	X	**X**		X	X				**X**						X		X		**X**
3	X	X				X	X												X
4	X	X	X													X			
5	X												X						
6	X	X	X	X	X	X		X	X	X	X			X	X		X	X	
7	X	X	X		X	X	X	X		X	X	X						X	
8	**X**	**X**	X	X	X	**X**	X	X	X	X	X	X	X		X	X	X	X	
10			X																
12	X																		
13	**X**	**X**	**X**	**X**			**X**	X		X	X	**X**	**X**						
14	X	X			X		X												
15	X		X	**X**		X													
18							X												
19	X	X			X														
22					X														
24			X						X	X									
26	**X**		X	X		**X**	X	X								X			

Prolapse, Urethral

	ALOE
2	X
7	X

Prolapse, Uterus

	SEP	BELL	NUX V	POD	LIL T	HELON	SEC	STANN	AUR	ARG	MUREX	PULS	ALET	PLAT	CALC	KREO	PALLAD	CON	NUX M	KALI CAR	RHUS T	SULPH	AESC	ALOE	CARB A	FERR IOD	MERC
1	X	X		X	X	X	X	X	X	X	X	X	X					X		X			X	X			
2			X	X			X	X		X	**X**	X	X				X		X			X	X	X		X	
3	X		X	X																	X			X			
4	**X**	X					X							X		X										X	
5				X	X																						
6	X	X		X											X		X	X									X
7	**X**	X	X	X	X	**X**	X	X	**X**	**X**	X	X	X	**X**	**X**	X	**X**	X	X	X	**X**	X	X	X	X	X	
8	**X**	X	**X**	**X**	X	X	X	X	X	X	X	X	X		X	**X**	X	X	X	X	X	**X**	X		X		X
9			X	X																							
10	X	X	**X**				X	X	X					X	X	X			X								X
11								X																			
13	**X**	X	**X**	X	X		X	X	**X**	X	X	**X**		X	X	X	X	X	X	**X**	X				X	X	X
14	X	X			X	X					X		X														
15	X																										
17	X				X	X																					
19					X	**X**							X														
21	X	X	X		X							X															
23	X					X				X																	
26	**X**	**X**	**X**				X	X	X					**X**								X			X		
28	X																										

Prolapse, Vagina

	SEP	MERC	FERR	KREO	NUX M	NUX V	OCIMUM	POD	STANN	AGNUS	AUR	FERR AC	FERR IOD	FILIX	GRANAT	HELON	STAPHYS	STRAM	SULPH	SULPH AC	VER A
1								X													
2						X	X		X								X			X	
3	X									X											
5								X													
6	X	X																			
7	X	X	X	X	X																
8	X	X	X	X	X	X	X		X		X	X	X	X	X	X		X	X		X
10		X																			
14	X																				

Prosopalgia- See Neuralgia, Facial

Prostate, Diseases Of

	THUJA	SULPH	APIS	BAR C	CALC	CON	STAPHYS	AGNUS	CHIM	COP	DIG	NUX V	PARIERA	SABAL	AESC	ALOE	CAUST	FERR PIC	LYC	PULS	SEL							
1			X																									
2	**X**						**X**							X	X	X		X										
3								X				X																
6	X	X																										
7	X	X	**X**	X	**X**	**X**			X	X	X						X											
8	X	X	X	X	X	X	X	X	X	X	X				X	X	X	X	X	X	X							
11				X																								
14													X															
18		X										X	X	X														
19	X	X	X	X	X	X	X	X	X	X	X	X	X	X					X	X	X							
24	X	X	X	X	X	X	X	X	X	X	X	X	X	X	X	X	X	X	X	X	X							

Prostate, Hypertrophy, Benign

	SABAL	CON	BAR C	THUJA	CHIM	DIG	FERR PIC	IOD	LYC	APIS	SULPH	CALC	PULS	STAPHYS	NIT AC	PERIERA	SEL	SOLID	AUR M	CANN I	COP	MERC	PHOS	SEP	ARG N	HYDRANG		
1	X	**X**	X	X		X		X						X		X		X		X			X					
2	**X**		X			X		**X**								X		**X**							**X**			
3	X	X		X	X		X			X										X						X		
4	**X**	**X**		X	X	X	**X**		X																			
6		X	X	X		X		X	X	X	X	X	X	X	X		X				X	X	X	X				
7		**X**	X	X		X		X	X	X	X	**X**	**X**		X				X			X						
8		X	X	X	X						X		X		X				X	X		X						
9	X					X																						
10		X	X																									
11	**X**		X	**X**	**X**		**X**		**X**									**X**								**X**		
12		X	X	X			X			X	X	X	X				X						X	X				
13								X																				
14		X	X		X	X								X		X												
16	X				X		X														X							
17		X																										
18	X	X	X	X	X				X		X								X									
19	X	X	X	X	X	X			X	X		X		X		X	X				X			X				
21	X		X	X			X	X																	X			
23			X				X																					
24	X	X	X		X					X			X	X			X											
25	X					X																						
26											X				X													
27	X											X																
28	X			X																								

Prostate, Hypertrophy, Benign, Senile

	BAR C	CON	FERR PIC	ALOE	COP	DIG	LYC
1	X						
7				X		X	
8		**X**			X		
11	X						X
24	X	X	**X**				

Prostatitis

	PULS	THUJA	CHIM	SABAL	APIS	BELL	CAUST	CUB	LYC	NIT AC	PETR	SULPH	ACON	CON	COP	HIPPOM	MERC D	SEL	AGNUS	CYCL	HEP	NUX V	SALIX N	SIL	COLCH
1		X				X							X												
2	**X**		X		X		X	X	X		X			X	X	X	X	X		X			X		**X**
4				**X**		X		X					X												
5		X	X	X										X											
6	X					X				X	X	X													
7	**X**	X	X					X	X	X	X						X				X			X	
8	X	X	X				X				X		X				X								
9		X												X											
11			X																						
12						X																			
13	X	X			X		X		X						X	X		X	X	X	X				
14	X		X																						
18				X								X										X			
19	X	X	X		X					X		X			X				X			X			
20	X		X		X		X		X																
21	X	X		X																					
23			X	X				X								X		X					X		
24				X																					
26	X	X								X		X												X	

Prostatorrhoea

	SEL	AGNUS	PULS	STAPHYS	THUJA	ZINC	SEP	SULPH	NAT CAR	PH AC	SIL	SPIG	TAB	ANAC	HEP
2	X		X			X		X				X	X		
7	X	X	X	X	X	X	X			X	X				
8		X							X						
13	**X**		X	X	X	X	**X**	**X**	X	X	X	X	X	**X**	**X**
24	X	X		X	X										

Prurigo- See also Pruritis

	SULPH	CARB V	RUMEX	MERC	ANTHROK	MEZ	RHUS T	ACON	AMBRA	ARS	CAUST	GRAPH	HOANG	IGN
1					X									
2			X		X								X	
4							X							
7		**X**	X	**X**	X				X			X		X
8	X	X	X			X	X		X	X	X	X		
12	**X**	X		X		X	X	X		X	X			X
18						X								
23	X		X										X	
26	X	X		X				X						

Prurigo Contagiosa (AKA Prairie Itch)

	RUMEX	LED	APIS	RHUS T
6	**X**	X		X
8	X	X	X	

Pruritis- See also Prurigo; Urticaria (Includes Itch)

	SULPH	RHUS T	ARS	DOLICH	GRAPH	MERC	MEZ	PSOR	APIS	AGAR M	NAT M	CROT T	HEP	SEP	PULS	CAUST	OLEAND	STAPHYS	ALUM	CALAD	CALC	DULC	IGN	LYC	PETR	CHEL	SIL	
1	X	X	X	X	X		X	X	X	X	X	X	X		X			X	X		X	X			X		X	
2	**X**		X	X				**X**		X				X														
3	X							X		X		X		X			X		X									
4	**X**	X		X	**X**		X						X				X			X	X							
5		X	X	X	X	X	X		X					X			X	X										
6	X	X	X	X	X	X	X	X	X		X	X	X					X			X		X	X				
7	**X**	**X**	X	X	**X**	X	X	X	**X**		**X**	X	X			X					X			X		**X**	X	
8	X		X	X	X	X	X	X			X	X	X		X	X	X	X	X	X	X		X	X	X	X	X	
9	X	X				X			X		X			X		X		X		X								
10	**X**	X	X			**X**	X	X	X	X	X		X		X							X	X	X	X			
11	X						X																					
12	X	X	X						X	X																		
13	**X**	**X**	X	X	X	**X**	X	X		X	X	X		X	**X**	X	X	X		X	X	X	X	X	X	X	**X**	
14	X	X	X			X				X			X			X	X		X	X		X				X		
15	**X**	X	X		X	X			X				X	X	X	X						X	X					
17										X																		
18	X	X		X	X	X		X	X	X		X						X							X		X	
19	**X**	X	**X**	X	X	X	**X**	X	**X**	X	X	X		X	X		X		X						X	X		
20	X	X	X		X							X		X														
21		X	X				X															X						
23				X			X												X	X								
24	X	X																										
25	X		X			X		X							X													
29[1]	X			X	X				X		X																	
29[2]		X						X								X							X					
29[3]				X																								

29[1] Cavalcanti A.M.S et al. Effects of homeopathic treatment on pruritis of haemodialysis patients: a randomised placebo-controlled double-blind trial. Homeopathy, 2003, 92, 177-181.
29[2] Schlappack O. Homeopathic treatment of radiation induced itching in breast cancer patients. A prospective observational study. Homeopathy, 2004, 93, 210-215.
29[3] de Paula Coelho C, et al. Therapeutic and pathogenetic animal models for Dolichos pruriens. Homeopathy, 2006, 95, 136-143.

Pruritis, Anus

	SULPH	TEUCR	CINA	IGN	NIT AC	NUX V	SEP	GRAPH	ALOE	CARB V	ACON	ALUM	ARS	FERR	MERC	PHOS	RAT	CAUST	LYC
2		**X**														X			
3	X			X					X								X		
4	**X**																		
5				X		X	X		X			X							
6	X	**X**		X						X	X			X	X				
7	X	X	X		**X**	**X**	X	**X**		**X**			X	X		X	X	X	
8	X	X	X	X	X		X	X	X	X	X		X	X	X		X	X	X
9	X	X	X																
10			X			X					X								
11	X	X	X																
12	X		X	X	X								X						X
13	**X**	**X**	X	**X**	X	X	X	X	X	**X**		X		X	X	X		**X**	**X**
14	X		X		X	X			X		X								
15	X			X									X						
16			X																
17		X																	
18																	X		
19							X												
21	X	X	X	X	X							X							
22	X					X		X				X							
24	X					X		X								X			
25	X	X	X																
26	X				X		X								X				
27	X	X	X																

Pruritis, Ankles

	BERB V	BOR	CALC	KALI CAR	LED	LYC	NAT M	RAN B	SEL
5					X				
8							X		
13	X	X	X	X		X		X	X

Pruritis, Axilla

	CARB V	ELAPS	ANAC	JUG R	PHOS	SULPH
3		X		X		
7	X					X
13	X	X			X	
19			X			

Pruritis, Breast

	CAUST	CON	DULC	ORIGAN	SIL	SULPH
5				X		
6						X
7	X		X		X	
24		X				

Pruritis, Coccyx

	BOV	GRAPH
5	X	
8		X
14	X	

Pruritis, Ears

	PHOS	AGAR M	TELL	BAR C	NUX V	SEP	SIL	SULPH	ALUM	AMM C	ARUNDO	BOR	CAPS	HEP	MERC	PSOR	SPIG
6	X		X		X							X	X		X	X	
7	X	X		X		X	X	X						X			
8	X	X		X	X	X		X	X	X							X
13	X	X	X	X		X	X	X	X	X				X			X
17			X														
18											X						
19		X															
20							X										
21					B						X						
24	X		X									X	X		X	X	

B- Both Internal and External

Pruritis, Elbow

	PSOR	SEP
7		X
25	**X**	

Pruritis, Eyes

	ALL C	AMBROS	MERC	SULPH	CALC	PULS	ZINC	ALUM	ANT C	APIS	BELL	BRY	CAUST	KALI BIC	MUR AC	NAT M	NUX V	PHOS	RAN B	RHUS T	SIL	AGAR M	PHELL
5	X																						
7	X		X	X	X	X	X		X					X	X	X				X			
8			X	X	X	X					X	X	X				X				X		
12			X												X	X	X	X					
13	X		X	**X**	X		X	X	X	X	X	X	X	X				X	X		X	**X**	**X**
14		X					X																
15																				X			
17		X																					
19		X				X				X									X				
21								X															
24	X																						
27		X																					

Pruritis, Face

	RHUS T	GELS	APIS	SULPH	BELL	NAT M	NAT SUL	SEP	AGNUS	ARS	CALC
7	X	X	**X**	**X**		X	X	X		**X**	
8		X									
13	X	X			X	X	X	X	**X**		**X**
14	X				X						
19	X		X	X							

Pruritis, Feet

	SULPH	LACH	SEP	LED	SEL	ANT S A	BELL	BERB V	BISM	BOV	CALC	CALC SUL	CAUST	CHAM	COCCUL	DULC	IGN	HYDROC	LITH C	MAGNOL	MEZ	RHUS T	ZINC
7	X	X	X			X									X								
8				**X**															X				
13		X	X		**X**		X	X	X	X	X		X	X		X	X					X	X
14	X											X						X		X			
19																					X		

Pruritis, Fingers

	AGAR M	SULPH	SEL	ANAG	APIS	BOR	CON	LACH	NAT CAR	NAT SUL	NUX V	OX AC	PLAT	PRUN S	PULS	RAN B	RHUS T
5	X		X	X		X											
6	X																
7		**X**															
8					X					X							
13	X	X	X				X	X	X		X	X	X	X	X	X	
19																	X

Pruritis, Fingers, Between

	SULPH	PH AC	PSOR
7	**X**	X	X

Pruritis, Genitals

	SULPH	AMBRA	COLLIN	KREO	NAT SUL	SEP	CALC	CALAD	CARB V	CON	CROT T	HELON	LIL T	MERC	NAT M	NIT AC	STAPHYS	CAUST	DOLICH	KALI BR	LYC	MAG M	PETR	PLAT	RHUS T	SIL	TAR H	URT U
1	X	X	X	X	X		X	X				X	X	X														X
5		X				X		X			X	X				X	X		X					X	X			X
6	X		X	X		X				X					X													
7	X	X	X	X	X	X	**X**		X	X	X	X	X	X	X	X	X	X	X	X	X	X	X	X		X	X	
8			X						X				X							X								
10	X																											
13	X	X			X	X	X		X	X				X	X	X		X			X	X	X			X		
14	X			X	X			X																	X		X	
18																	X											
19											X																	
27	X																											

Pruritis, Genitals, Female (Includes Pruritis, Pudenda)

	CALC	KREO	SIL	CARB V	NAT M	SEP	AMBRA	CON	ARS	CALAD	COFF	CROT T	KALI CAR	LAC C	LYC	STAPHYS	SULPH	TAR H	ZINC	PETR
6				X				X									X			
8	X	X	X	X	X	X	X	X	X	X	X	X	X	X	X	X	X	X	X	
10	X	X	X																	
13	X	X	**X**	**X**	**X**	**X**	**X**	**X**	X	X	X	X	X	X	X	X	X	X	X	**X**
20	X	X																		
26	X		X	X	X	X		X					X		X		X			
27		X																		

Pruritis, Groin

	CALEND	GRAPH	RHUS T
19		X	X
22	E		

E- External

Pruritis, Hands

	SEP	ZINC	AGAR M	ANAG	ANT S A	APIS	BERB V	MEZ	PETR	PH AC	PIX	PSOR	RHUS T
5			X										
7	X				X				X	X		X	
8		X									X		
10	X												
13		X					X						
19				X		X		X					X

Pruritis, Hands, Posterior Aspect Of

	BOV	CAMPH	SULPH
4	X		
7		X	X

Pruritis, Joints

	AETHUSA	KREO	SEP	SPIG	URT U
7				X	
8		X			
10			X		
14	X				
21					X

Pruritis, Joints, Flexures Of

	PSOR	GRAPH	MEZ	RHUS T	SEP	SULPH
19		X	X	X	X	X
25	**X**					

Pruritis, Knees

	PSOR	SULPH	ARS	COB	LYC	MANG	SEP
5			X				X
7	X	**X**				X	
13				X	X		
25	**X**						

Pruritis, Neck

	CRAT	GRAPH
5	X	
19		X

Pruritis, Nipples

	AGAR M	HEP	PETR	SEP	SULPH
5	X				
6					X
7	X	X	X	X	
8	X				

Pruritis, Nose

	CINA	ARG N	ARUNDO	AGAR M	CARB V	SPIG	CHEL	MERC	NUX V	SABAD	SAMB	TEUCR
3						X						
5	X					X						
6	X	X										
7	X				X		X		X			
8		X		X				X				
12	X											
13	X	X		**X**	**X**		X	X	X		X	
14	X											
16	X		X									
17	X	X	X							X	X	X
18			X									X
19			X							X		
24		X										

Pruritis, Palms

	SULPH	AMBRA	ANAC	ANAG	BERB V	CARB V	GRANAT	HEP	KALI CAR	LYC	NAT M	RAN B	SEL	SIL	SPIG
5										X			X		
13	X	X	X		X	X		X	X		X	X		X	X
17							X								
19	X			X											

Pruritis, Penis

	HEP	IGN	KALI BIC	NAT SUL	SULPH
7	X	X	X	X	**X**
8	X				
13	X	X	X	X	

Pruritis, Perineum

	NAT SUL	PETR	AGNUS	CARB V	CHEL	FL AC	NUPH	NUX V	SULPH	TARAX
7	X	X		X	X		X			
9									X	
13	X	X	X			X		X		X

Pruritis, Prepuce

	CINNAB	CON	ACON	IGN	ALOE	EUPHORB	MERC	NIT AC	RHUS T	SARS	SEP	VIOL T
1	**X**	X		X		X			X	X		X
7	**X**	X		X			X	X			X	
8		X	X		X							
24			X									

Pruritis, Pudenda- See Pruritis, Genitals, Female

Pruritis, Rectum

	NIT AC	SULPH	AESC	ALOE	AMBRA	BOR	BOV	CALC	CALC PH	CARB V	CHIN S	CIC	FERR	GRAN	GRAPH	NUX V	PH AC	PHOS	RHUS T	SABAD	SEP	SIL	SPIG
13	X	X			X	X	X	X			X	X	X	X		X	X	X	X		X	X	X
19		X	X	X					X	X					X					X			
21	X																						

Pruritis, Scalp

	OLEAND	ARS	SULPH	VINCA	GRAPH	MEZ	STAPHYS	AGAR M	AMM M	BOV	CLEM	FL AC	KALI CAR	LYC	MERC	PHOS	SIL	RHOD	RHUS T	RUTA	SEP
1	X	X						X													
5				X		X				X	X										
6	X																				
8			X		X				X			X	X	X			X				
13	**X**	X	X	X	**X**	**X**	**X**	X	X	X	X	X	X	X	X	X	X	**X**	**X**	**X**	**X**
14	X	X	X	X												X					
21	X	X	X												X						
25							X														

Pruritis, Scrotum

	NIT AC	SULPH	PETR	AMBRA	CAUST	CIST	COCCUL	CROT T	GRAPH	LYC	NAT M	RHOD	RHUS T
7	X	X			X	X	X		X	X	X	X	X
8	X	X	X	X	X		X	X	X	X			
13	X	X	**X**		X	X					X	X	X
14				X									
19								X					
21				X									
26	X	X	X										

Pruritis, Senile

	BAR C	AMBRA	ARS	CALC PH	CON	COP	CROT T	DOLICH	FL AC	MEZ	SEL	SULPH
4								X				
5	X	X							X		X	
8	X		X	X	X	X	X			X		X

Pruritis, Thigh

	ANAC	CALC	CUBEB	KALI IOD	NAT SUL	SULPH
7		X		X		X
8			X			
10					X	
19	X					

Pruritis, Toes

	AGAR M	STAPHYS	CLEM	GRAPH	JATR	NAT SUL	NUX V	PAEONIA	SIL	SULPH	ZINC
6	X										
7											X
8									X		
13	**X**	**X**	X	X	X	X	X	X		X	

Pruritis, Urethra

	CANTH	PETROS	PETR
1		X	
6		X	
8	X		X
13	X		
21	X		

Pruritis, Vaginal

	CALAD	CALC	CANTH	HYDROC	KALI BIC	KREO	LYC	SEP	NIT AC	ALUMEN	AMBRA	ARS	AUR M	COFF	CON	ELAPS	FERR IOD	GRAPH	GRIND	HELON	LACH	SIL	SULPH					
1	**X**							X												X								
2	X																	X	X									
3											X																	
4						X																						
6							X	X							X								X					
7		X	X			X	X		**X**				X				X											
8	**X**		X	X	X					X						X					X							
10		X			X							X																
14	X			X																		X						
15		X																										
21														X														

Pruritis, Vulva

	KREO	AMBRA	SEP	SULPH	CALAD	CALC	PLAT	ALUM	CANTH	CARB V	COFF	COLLIN	CON	GRAPH	HELON	HYDRAST	LIL T	NIT AC	TAR H									
1	X		X		**X**			X						X	X													
2		X					X					X			X		X											
3		X																										
4	X		X			X																						
6		X	X	X	**X**	X	X		X	X		X	X						X									
8	X	X	X	X		X	X		X	X	X	X	X	X		X		X	X									
9	X		X	X			X																					
10	X					X		X																				
11	X																											
14	X	X	X	X	X				X								X											
18	X	X		X							X			X	X	X		X										
19	X																											
21		X	X	X	X	X		X		X	X		X				X											
23		X					X									X			X									
25																		X										

Pseudofolliculitis Barbae- See Barber's Itch

Psoriasis- See also Dermatitis

	ARS	SEP	SULPH	PETR	ARS I	GRAPH	KALI ARS	PHOS	LYC	BOR	NIT AC	CALC	IRIS V	PHYTO	THYROID	PSOR	RHUS T	CARB AC	CLEM	COR R	MERC	TELL	BERB V	CHR AC
1	X				X		X								X					X				E
2	**X**	X		**X**		**X**	X	X		X			X		**X**			X		X			X	**X**
3			X							X					X									
4	**X**	X								X					X							X	**X**	
5	X	X			X	X	X	X				X							X					
6	X	X	X	X				X			X	X	X			X	X		X	X	X	X		
7	**X**	**X**	X	X	**X**	X		X	**X**		X	X	X	**X**			X	X			X			
8	**X**	**X**		X	**X**	X	X	X	X	X	X	X	X	X		X	X	X	X	X		X		X
9	X		**X**	X						X						X								
11		X		X	X		X		X					X										
12	**X**		X	X					X		X		X					X			X			
14			X							X														
15	X					X																		
17			X																					
19	**X**	<u>**X**</u>	**X**	**X**	X	**X**	X	X	X	X	X	X	X	X	X	X	X				X	X		
21	X		X	X		X	X																	
23							X																X	
25	X		**X**	X												X								
26		X	X	X				X	X		X	X					X							
27		X			X						X			X					X					
29*		X	X					X	X			X												

E- External

29* Witt CM, et al. Homeopathic treatment of patients with psoriasis--a prospective observational study with 2 years follow-up. J Eur Acad Dermatol Venereol. 2009 May; 23 (5):538-43.

Psoriasis, Ears, Behind

	GRAPH
19	**X**
21	X

Psoriasis, Elbows

	IRIS V	KALI SUL	MANG AC	MANG	MEDO	PHOS
19	X	X		X	X	X
27			X			

Psoriasis, Eyebrows

	PHOS
19	**X**

Psoriasis, Fingers (Includes Psoriasis, Fingers, Between)

	ANAG	LYC	MEDO	TEUCR
5	X	X		X
19			X	

Psoriasis, Genitals

	NIT AC	PETR	GRAPH	CROT T	RAD BR	SEP	SULPH	THUJA
5	X	X		X				
19	X	X	**X**		X	X	X	X

Psoriasis, Hands, Dorsum

	GRAPH	ARS	RHUS T	LYC	MALAND	PETR	PHOS	SARS
5	X	X	X	X	X	X	X	
19	**X**	X	X					X

Psoriasis, Head

	GRAPH	ARS IOD	BAR C	CIC	FL AC	KREO	LYC	OLEAND	SEP	STAPHYS	VIOL T
5	X		X	X	X	X	X	X	X	X	X
7		X									
19	**X**										

Psoriasis, Knees

	IRIS V	ARS	CHEL	MANG AC	MANG	PHOS
5	X		X			
19	X	X			X	X
27				X		

Psoriasis, Limbs, Lower

	PHOS	KALI ARS	MERC	SEP	THUJA
5	X	X			
19	X		X	X	X

Psoriasis, Limbs, Upper

	KALI ARS	IRIS V	KALI SUL	RAD BR	RHUS T	SEP	SIL
5	X	X	X		X		X
19	X			X		X	

Psoriasis, Palms

	PETR	SEL	PHOS	LYC	MEDO	MEZ	CALC	COR R	CROT H	GRAPH	HEP	MERC	SEP
1	X	X				X		X					
2		X			X		X		X				
5	X												
1[illegible]	X			X						X	X		
19	X	X	**X**		X	X						X	
26	X		X	X									X

Psoriasis, Scalp

	GRAPH	CLEM	IRIS V	LYC	MEZ	NAT M	SIL	STAPHYS	SULPH
19	**X**		X	X	X	X	X	X	X
27		X							

Psoriasis, Soles

	PHOS	COR R	SULPH
1		X	
19	**X**		X

Psoriasis, Tongue

	MUR AC	SEP
1	X	
2	X	
11		X

Pterygium

	RAT	ZINC	SULPH	AMM BR	ARS	CHIM	LACH	NUX M	SPIG	ARG N	CALC	GUAREA	PSOR	FORMICA	KRAM	STAPHYS	TELL	ZINC SUL										
2	**X**			X		X			X			X																
4	**X**	X																										
6	X	X	X		X	X	X	X	X	X	X		X															
7	X		X	X	X		X	X						X														
8	X	X	X	X	X	X	X	X	X	X	X		X			X	X											
9	X	X	X																									
16	X	X																										
21	X	**X**																										
23												X			X													
24		X																X										
28	X	X																										

Ptomaine Poisoning- See Food Poisoning

Ptosis

	GELS	SEP	CAUST	ALUM	PLUM	RHUS T	SPIG	CURARE	KALM	NUX V	ZINC	CON	COCCUL	EUPHR	HYOSC	MERC P	NUX M	BELL	GRAPH	GUAREA	MERC	MORPH	OP	SPONG	VER A	VIOL T		
1	X	X	X	X		X		X	X				X															
2	X	X	X			X		X	X		X	X		X		X	X		X	X					X			
3	X		X	X					X					X														
4	X	X	X	X	X	X			X	X																		
5		X																										
6	X	X	X	X	X	X				X	X		X		X		X											
7	**X**		**X**				**X**			X			X			X	X			X				X	X			
8	X	X	X	X	X	X	X		X	X	X	X		X	X	X					X							
9	X				X																							
10	**X**	X			X																							
11	X	X	X								X	X										X						
12	X						X											X										
13		X					X				X							X	X		X	X	X	X		**X**		
15	X																											
17	X	X	X	X	X	X	X	X		X																		
18			X					X																				
19	**X**							X				X																
20	X																											
21	X																											
22	X																											
23	X																											
24	X			X	X										X								X					
25	X																											
27	X	X		X																								
28	X																											

Ptyalism

	MERC	IPEC	IRIS V	NIT AC	HELL	IOD	SULPH AC	JAB	NAT M	ALL S	BAR C	BELL	COLCH	DIG	HEP	LOB I	MERC C	NUX V	PHYTO	VER A								
1	X	X	X	X	X	X	X	X	X	X	X		X			X	X											
2	**X**	X	**X**	**X**		**X**		**X**		X				X					X	X								
3			X							X	X																	
4	X				X							X																
5		X	X											X														
6	X	X		X	X		X											X	X									
7	**X**	X	X	**X**	X	**X**	X	X	X		X			X					X	X								
8	X	X	X	X	X	X	X	X	X		X	X	X		X			X										
9	X	X																										
10	X			X											X													
11	X		X																									
12	X																X											
13	X	X	X	X	X	X	X		X			X	X	X	X	X	X	X	X	X								
14	X		X																									
15	X						X											X		X								
17	X	X														X	X											
18	X	X											X															
19	X															X												
20	X	X																										
21	X	X	X	X						X																		
22	X	X	X																									
23				X		X																						
24	X																											
25	X																											
26	X	X		X	X				X			X			X													
27	X							X																				

Ptyalism, from Pregnancy- See Pregnancy, Ptyalism From

Puerperal Fever

	ACON	BELL	BRY	ARS	HYOSC	PULS	RHUS T	VER V	KALI CAR	MERC	OP	CHAM	COLCH	PYROG	ARN	LACH	SEC	NUX V	STRAM									
2	**X**		X			X								**X**														
3									X					**X**														
6		X																										
7	X	**X**	**X**	**X**	X	X	X	**X**	X	X	X	X	X		X	X	X											
8	X	X	X	X	X	X	X	X	X	X	X	X	X		X	X	X	X										
12	**X**	**X**	X	X	X			X		X	X								**X**									
13	**X**	**X**	**X**	X	X	**X**	**X**	X	X	X	X	**X**	**X**		X	X	X	X	X									
21	X																											
26	**X**	X	X	X	X		X																					

Pulmonary Oedema- See Oedema, Lungs
Pulse, Fast- See Tachycardia
Pulse, Missed Beats- See Arrhythmia
Pulse, Slow- See Bradycardia
Pulse, Thready

	COLCH	CARB V	AMM C	CAPS	CARB AC	CHINA	CUPR	HELL	JATR	LATRO M	LAURO	MERC	PHOS	SEC	VER A
3	X														
8	**X**	X		X	X		X	X			X	X	X	X	X
11		X													
12						X									
14	X														
17	X		X						X	X					

Purpura

	LACH	CROT H	HAM	PHOS	SULPH AC	ARN	ARS	SEC	ACON	PH AC	RHUS V	BELL	BRY	CARB V	CHLOL	LED	RHUS T	MERC
2	**X**	**X**	**X**	**X**	X	**X**	**X**	X	**X**	**X**	**X**			X	X			**X**
4			X															
5	X			X														
6	X	X	X	X	X	X	X	X					X			X		
7	X													X				
8	X	X	X	X	X	X	X	X			X	X	X		X	X	X	
11			X															
12					X	X			X			X					X	
17	X	X		X														
18					X													
21	X	X																
23										X								

Purpura Haemorrhagica- See Idiopathic Thrombocytic Purpura
Purpura Miliaris

	ACON	COFF	BELL	AMM C	AMM M	APIS	ARN	DULC	SULPH	SULPH AC
8	X	X	X	X	X	X	X	X	X	X
13	X	X	X							

Pyaemia

	LACH	ARN	ARS	CHIN S	ECHIN	RHUS T	CALEND	CROT H	PHOS	SIL	MERC	PYROG
2	**X**	**X**	**X**	**X**	**X**	**X**		X			**X**	**X**
4		**X**			X							
6									X			
7	**X**		X						X			
8	X	X	X	X		X	X	X				
16		B			B							
17	X									X		
24	X	X	X							X		
26							X					

B- Both Internal and External

Pyelitis

	STIG	ARS	APIS	CANTH	CAPS	CUPR AR	JUNI V	MERC C	PETR	PHOS	PULS	SEP	TEREB	TRIT R	UROTROP	UVA
2	X	**X**														
3																X
6				X				X	X	X	X	X				
17			X			X							X			
23	X				X		X							X	X	

Pylorus, Diseases Of

	NUX V	PHOS	SIL	CHINA	HEP	ACET AC	ANANTH	ATROP	BAR C	BRY	CANTH	CONDUR	CON	LACH	LOB DOR	LYC	MERC	SEP	SPIG	TUSSIL	URAN N
2	**X**	**X**	**X**	**X**	**X**										X	X	X	X		X	
8	X		X			X	X	X	X		X	X	X						X		X
13	X	X												X							

Pyothorax

	HEP	ARS	SIL
6		X	
7	**X**		X

Pyrosis- See Heartburn
Pyrosis (Waterbrash) of Pregnancy- See Pregnancy, Heartburn Of
Pyorrhoea- See Periodontal Disease
Pyrexia- See Fever

Pyuria

	BRY	SIL
2	**X**	
18		X

Quinsy (AKA Abscess, Peritonsillar)

	BAR C	SIL	HEP	LACH	ACON	LYC	MERC	MERC I R	BELL	PHYTO	PSOR	ARS	GUAIAC
1								X					
2	**X**		X	X	**X**	X		X			X		
3	X	X			X		X		X	X			
8	X												
12	X		X	X	X	X		X				X	X
14	X			X		X							
15		X	X				X		X			X	
16	X												
17	X	X	X	X						X	X		X
19	X	X											
24	X	X	X	X	X	X	X	X	X	X	X		
25	X						X						
27	X	X											

Quinsy, Prophylaxis

	BAR C	BELL	MERC	PSOR
10	X			
15		X	X	
16	X			X

Rabies- See also Hydrophobia

	STRAM	LYSS	BELL	LACH	CANTH	HYOSC	XANTH	SCUT
2				X				
3	X	X	X					
6	X	X	X	X	X	X		
8	X	X	X	X	X	X	X	X
10		X						
11	**X**	**X**	X	X	X	**X**	**X**	
12	X		X	X	X			X
16	X	X	X		X	X	**X**	
17	X	X						
21	**X**	X	**X**	X				

Rabies, Prophylaxis

	BELL	LYSS
12	<u>**X**</u>	
16		X
21	X	X

Rachitis- See Rickets

Ranula

	THUJA	MERC	AMBRA	CALC	NIT AC	FL AC	STAPHYS	BELL	LAC C	MEZ	NAT M	SACCH	AM BENZ	APIS	CANTH	CHR OX	LYSS	PLUM	THLASPI
1	**X**	X	X	**X**													X		
2	X	**X**	X	X	X		X		X		X	X	X			X			X
3	X	X				X													
6	X	X	X	X	X	X		X		X				X					
7	**X**	X	**X**	X	X					X					X			X	
8	X		X	X	X	X		X											
13	**X**	X	X	X	X		**X**		X		X	X							
26	X	**X**			X														

Rash- See Erythena; Exanthema

Raynaud's Disease- See also Acrocyanosis; Circulation, Peripheral, Poor

	SEC	AGAR M	CARB V	ARS	FERR PH	PULS	ARN	BACILL	BELL	CACT	ECHIN	EUPHORB	HAM	HEP	LACH	NAT M	PHOS	RHUS T	SEP	SIL	SULPH AC	TUB
2	X				X			X														
11	X		X	X							X	X			X						X	
17									X													
18	X	X	X			X	X						X			X	X					X
21	X		X	X	X	X				X												
27		X												X				X	X	X		
28	X	X																				

Recuperation, Failure Of

	CHINA	PSOR	SIL	SULPH	CARB V	COCCUL	NUX V	CALC	HEP	KREO	PH AC	ALL C	ARS	CALC PH	CHIN ARS	COCA	COFF	CUPR AR	EUCAL	KALI BR	NAT M	NUPH	PULS
2		X	X	X											X				X	X		X	
7	X	X	X	X		X	X	X	X	X		X				X	X	X	X	X		X	
8	X	X	X	X		X	X	X	X	X		X			X	X	X	X					
9	X				X		X				X												
10	X	X	X	X		X	X	X		X			X										X
11														X									
12	X	X	X	X							X												
14					X																		
17		X			X																		
18	X																				X		
21														X									
24	X																						
25	X										X		X										
26	X					X			X												X		
28					X																		X

Rectal Fistula- See Fistula, Rectal

Rectal Prolapse- See Prolapse, Rectum

Rectal Stricture- See Stricture, Rectum

Rectum, Diseases Of

	CAPS	GRAPH	HYDRAST	NIT AC	SULPH	ACET AC	COLLIN	IRIS V	KISSING	PYRUS	RUTA
2	X	X	X	X	X			X	X	X	X
8						X	X				

Rectum, Dryness Of

	ALUM	AESC	NAT M	CAUST
6	X			
8		X		X
14	X		X	
17	X			
21		X	X	
24	X			
25		X		

Reflux, Oesophageal (Includes Regurgitation, Oesophageal)

	PHOS	BRY	IGN	AETHUSA	AMBRA	AMM M	CANTH	CARB AC	CHINA	FERR	HEP	IPEC	LYC	LYCOP	MAG M	NIT AC	NUX V	POD	PULS	SANG	SULPH
4	X																				
6	X																				
8	X	X	X	X	X	X	X	X	X	X	X	X	X	X	X	X		X	X		X
10		X																			
19																	X			X	

Reiter's Syndrome

	MEDO	NUX V	SULPH
19	X		
21			X
29*		X	

29* Gupta R, et al. Reiter's disease treated with Nux Vomica. Homeopathy, 2006, 95, 103-104.

Renal Failure- See Kidney Failure

Respiration, Diseases Of

	BROM	PHYTO	ATROP	BEN N	TUB
2	X	X	X	X	
19					X

Respiration, Arrested- See also Asphyxia (Includes Respiration, Interrupted/Stoppage)

	CINA	ARS	CUPR	OP	SAMB	VER A	BELL	CACT	CAUST	CIC	KALI CAR	LACH	MERC C	NUX M	NUX V	SIL	SULPH	NIT AC
7	**X**	X	X			X		X	X	X	X	X	X	X				**X**
8												X					X	
13	X	X	X	X	X	X	X		X	X	X		X		X	X	X	
17	X	X	X	X		X		X						X				
18					X													
26	X	X	X	X	X		X								X	X		

Respiratory Failure

	ANT T	ANT ARS	ASPIDO	BRY	CACT	CAMPH	CARB V	CAUST	COLCH	CUPR	LAURO	NUX M	OP	VER A
11	X	X	X				X				X			
17	X			X	X	X		X	X	X		X	X	X
22	X													

Restlessness

	RHUS T	ACON	ARS	CHAM	BELL	NUX V	PHOS	MERC	PULS	STRAM	APIS	CIMICI	LACH	CANTH	CINA	VER A	CALC	COLOC	HYOSC	SULPH	CAUST	IOD	TAR H	COFF	IPEC	LYC	BRY
1	X	X	X	X		X	X				X		X	X	X	X	X			X		X					
4	X	X	X		**X**		X	X	X	X	X	X				X						X	**X**			X	
5	**X**	X	X	X	X	X	X		X	X		X	X	X	X		X	X	X		X	X	X		X		
6	X	X	X	X	X	X	X	X	X	X	X	X	X	X	X	X	X	X	X	X	X			X		X	X
7	X	X	X	X	X	X	X		X	X	X		X			X	X			X			X	X		X	
8	X	X	X	X	X	X			X	X	X			X	X	X	X	X	X	X						X	X
9	X	X	X	X	X					X		X		X	X					X			X		X		
10	X	X	X	X	X	X	X	X	X		X	X	X								X	X		X	X		
11	X	X	X		X																						
12	X	X	X		X			X				X	X						X					X			X
13	**X**	**X**	**X**	**X**	**X**	**X**	**X**	**X**	**X**	**X**	X		**X**	X	X	X	**X**	**X**	**X**	**X**	X	X			X	X	**X**
14	X	X	X	X	X		X							X				X			X						
15	X	X		X		X	X	X	X	X		X						X							X		X
16	X		X	X	X																						
17	X	X	X	X							X	X											X				
18						X																					
19	X	X	X	X	X										X			X	X			X					
20	X	X			X		X							X													
21	X	X	X	X															X				X	X			
22	X	X	X		X																X						
24	X	X	X	X				X								X										X	
25	X	X	X	X	X			X	X	X	X	X			X		X			X					X		
26		X	X	X		X										X								X			
27	X	X	X					X					X								X						

Restlessness, Feet

	ZINC	ARS
6	X	
7	X	X
8	X	
9	X	
10	X	
13	X	X
16	X	
17	X	

Restlessness, Hands

	TAR H	FERR IOD	KALI BIC	ZINC
7	X			
8	X			
17		X		
18				X
19			X	

Restlessness, Legs

	ZINC	ARS	RHUS T	SEP	CARB V	CAUST	GRAPH	KALI CAR	LACH	LYC	MAG CAR	MOSCH	PHOS	TAR H
6	X													
7	X	X	X		X		X		X		X	X	X	
8		X								X				
13	X	X	X	X	X	X	X	X	X	X	X	X		
16		X												
17				X										
18	X													
19	**X**		X			X								X
21	X	X		X				X					X	X
27	X													
28	X													

Restlessness, Limbs

	RHUS T	NUX V	TAR H	ZINC	ARS	CHEL
7	**X**	**X**	**X**	**X**		
8						X
14	X					
16					X	

Retina, Detachment Of

	GELS	AUR	ARN	NAPHTHA	APIS	DIG	JAB	NAT SAL
1	X	X	X	X	X			
2	X			X				
3		X	X	X	X			
4	X							
7	X	X						
14	X	X	X	X		X		
21	X		X		**X**			
23		X					X	X

Retina, Haemorrhage- See Haemorrhage, Retina

Retinitis

	GELS	BELL	PHOS	PULS	SULPH	ARS	AUR	BRY	CROT H	DUBO M	LACH	ACON	AMM C	APIS	ARN	ASAF	AUR M	AUR M N	BENZ D	CACT	CAUST	CHINA	KALI IOD	MERC C	MERC	NUX V	SAL AC	SEC
1			X	X				X	X	X	X			X										X				
2			X																X									
3							X			X																		
4		X																										
6	X	X	X	X	X	X		X	X		X	X	X		X		X			X		X	X		X	X		X
7	X	X		X		X										X												
8					X																							
14							X																					
19																					X						X	
23																		X										
24	**X**				X																							

Retina, Scotomata

	ARS	CARB S	GLON	MERC	TAB
7	X			X	
17		X			X
18			X		

Retina, Vein, Occlusion Of

	ARN	HAM
21	**X**	X

Retinitis Albuminurica

	MERC C	APIS	ARS	GELS	KALM	PHOS	PLUM	AUR	COLCH	HEP	NAT SIL	PH AC	SPIG	ZINC
1	**X**	X	X	X							X			
4	X					X								
6	X	X						X						
7	X				X									
8	X	X	X	X	X	X	X		X	X		X	X	X
24							X							

Retinitis Pigmentosa

	PHOS	NUX V
4	X	
21	X	X

Rhagades

	CALC	PETR	SULPH	RHUS T	HEP	LYC	SARS	SEP	GRAPH	MERC	NAT M	ALUM	LACH	NIT AC	SIL	ARN	AUR	CHAM	CYCL	PULS	ZINC	MANG
1			X								X											
2	X				X	X	X					X										
6		X																				
7	X	X	X	X	X	X	X	X	X	X	X			X	X							
8	**X**	**X**	**X**	**X**	X	X		X		X	X	X	X	X	X	X	X		X	X	X	
13	**X**	X	X	**X**	**X**	**X**	**X**	**X**		X	X	X	X	X		X	X	X	X	X	X	**X**
14							X															
23									X													
24									X				X									
26	X	X	X	X				X	X	X					X			X				

Rhagades, Feet

	HEP	SARS
7	X	X
8	X	

Rhagades, Hands

	RHUS T	SULPH	CALC	HEP	MERC	CALEND	GRAPH	PETR	SARS	AESC	ALUMEN	ANANTH	ANT C	ARN	CHAM	LYC	MAG CAR	SASSAF	SEP
7	**X**	**X**	X	X	X	**X**	**X**	**X**	**X**	X		X		X		X	X		
8	X	X	X	X	X						X		X		X			X	X

Rhagades, Lips

	IGN	MERC	SULPH	ARN	ARS	CAPS	CHAM	CONDUR	NAT M	PULS
8	X	X	X	X	X	X	X	X	X	X
26	X	X	X							

Rhagades, Nose

	SIL	MERC
8	X	
26	X	X

Rheumatic Carditis

	CACT	KALM	RHUS T	SPIG	ARS	AUR	BRY	LITH C	COLCH	PHOS	ARN	ACON	AMM C	ANT T	BELL	CALC	DIG	FERR	GUIAIAC	KALI CAR	MAGN GR	NUX V	PULS	SABAD	THYROID
1	X	X							X												X				X
3						X																			
4	**X**											X					X								
7	**X**	X	**X**	**X**	X			**X**		X										X					
10		X		X	X	X	X			X					X	X							X		
13							X				**X**											X		X	
14	X																								
17	X	X	X	X			X		X										X						
19	X		X		X	X		X					X	X				X							

Rheumatic Fever

	ACON	BRY	RHUS T	MERC	BELL	PULS	ARN	CIMICI	COLCH	CACT	NUX V	SULPH	CHAM	CHINA	DULC	VER V	AUR IOD	KALI MUR	NAT SAL	RHAMN C	SAL AC	STELL AQ
1							X															
2												**X**										
3	X															X						
4	X																					
7	X	X	X		X		X		X	X	X											
8					X			X							X			X				
10	**X**	X	X	X	X	X	X						X	X								
11	**X**	**X**	**X**	**X**		X	**X**		X			**X**					X		X	X	X	X
12	**X**	X	X		X			X														
14	X	X	X					X		X												
15	X	X	X	X		X		X		X	X		X									
16									X													
17									X							X						
21	X	X		X		X									X							
26	**X**	X	X	X	X	X					X			X								

Rheumatic Gout- See Gout

Rheumatic Heart- See Rheumatic Carditis

Rheumatism- See also Arthritis, Polyarthritis, and Pain by location for all of the following entries

	RHUS T	BRY	LED	PULS	COLCH	DULC	CAUST	RHOD	ACON	ARN	KALM	BELL	CHAM	GUAIAC	SULPH	CALC	KALI BIC	PHYTO	CIMICI	NUX V	MERC	LYC	CALC PH	CHINA	COLOC	KALI SUL	SANG	SIL
1	X		X	X	X	X		X			X			X				X				X						
2	X	**X**	**X**	X	**X**	**X**	X	**X**		**X**	**X**	X	X	X		**X**	**X**	**X**				**X**	**X**	X	X	X	X	X
3	X	X	X	X	X	X	X			X	X	X	X		X	X	X					X	X					X
4	**X**	**X**	**X**	**X**	X	X	**X**	X	X	X	**X**	X		**X**	X	**X**	X	X	X		X		X		X	X		X
5	X	X	X	X	X	X	X	X						X		X	X	X	X	X		X	X	X	X	X		X
6	X	X	X	X	X	X	X	X	X	X	X	X	X	X	X	X		X	X	X	X	X		X	X	X	X	X
7	X	**X**	X	X	X	X	X	X	X	X	X	X	X	X	X	X	X	X			X	X	X			X	X	
8	**X**	**X**	X	**X**	X	**X**	X	**X**	X	**X**	X	X	X	X	**X**	**X**	X	X	X	**X**	X	**X**	X	X	X	X	X	X
9	X	X			X										X												X	
10	**X**	**X**	X	X	X	X	X		X	X	X	X	X	X	X	X	X	X	X	X	X	X	X			X	X	X
11			X				X			X				X	X													
12	X	X	X		X	X	X	X	X	X		X			X		X	X	X		X				X			
13	**X**	**X**	X	X	X	X	**X**	X	**X**	**X**		**X**	**X**		X					**X**	**X**			**X**			X	X
14	X	X	X				X		X		X	X	X						X									
15	X	X		X	X	X			X	X		X	X		X				X	X	X			X				
17	X	X	X											X					X									
18	X	X	X			X		X	X		X		X				X			X					X			
19	**X**										X																	
21	X	X		X	X	X	X	X	X												X							
23	X	X	X	X	X	X		X	X		X		X	X			X	X	X	X			X	X		X	X	
24				X																					X			
25	**X**	X		X			X	X																				
26	X	X		X	X				X	X		X	X							X				X				

Rheumatism, Ankle

	ABROT	CAUST	RUTA	ACT S	BRY	LAC C	LED	LYC	MERC	NAT SUL	PULS	RAD BR	RHUS T	SEP	STICTA	SULPH	ZINC
1															X		
6									X								
7						X											
8		X	X		X			X		X			X	X		X	X
10											X						
11	X																
12											X						
14				X													
19	X	X	X				X					X					

Rheumatism, Arms

	GUAIAC	KALM	PHYTO	SANG	BRY	CACT	COLCH	FERR	MERC	RAN B	RHUS T	VIOL O
7	X	X	X	X	X	X	X	X	X	X	X	X
10		X	X									
11	X											

Rheumatism, Back

	NUX V	RHUS T	CIMICI	ARN	ARS	AUR	BRY	CALC FL	CALC PH	COLCH	CORNUS	HEP	MERC	RAD BR	RAN B	RHOD	RUTA	SULPH	VER V
7	X	X	X				X			X	X	X				X			
10		X																	
12			X																
15	X		X															X	X
19						X		X	X					X	X		X		
26	X	X		X	X								X						

Rheumatism, Chest

	ARN	ARS	AUR	MERC	NUX V	RAN B	RHUS T
19			X			X	
26	X	X		X	X		X

Rheumatism, Coccyx- See Coccydynia

Rheumatism, Elbow

	COLOC	KALI BIC	CAUST	COLCH	GUAIAC	HYDRAST	LACH	LAC AC	LYC	SAL AC
1							X			X
5	X	X	X		X				X	
7	X	X		X		X				
19								X		

Rheumatism, Feet

	LED	RUTA	CAUST	NIT AC	PHYTO	RHOD	ACT S	AUR	CALC	CIMICI	GUAIAC	HEP	MANG AC	MERC	PULS	RHUS T	SABIN
5	X	X	X	X	X	X		X			X	X		X		X	X
6	X	X								X							
7				X	X	X											
9									X								
10	X														X		
14													X				
19	X	X	X				X										

Rheumatism, Fingers

	CAULO	CAUST	LYC	ACT S	AMM PH	ARS	BRY	CALC	CALC FL	CARB S	COLCH	KALI BIC	LACH	NAT M	PHYTO	RAN B	RUTA	TEUCR
6	X				X													
8			X												X			
13											X	X	X					X
14				X						X								
19	X	X							X					X		X	X	
26		X	X			X	X	X										

Rheumatism, Hands and Fingers

	ACT S	CALC	CAULO	CLEM	GUAIAC	LYC	PULS	RHUS T	ANAC	ARS	BENZ AC	BRY	CALC HP	CAUST	COLCH	DIG	FERR	LACH	PHYTO	POLYG A	RAD BR	RUTA	SARS	STAPHYS	VIOL O	ZINC
5	X		X	X	X		X	X	X						X	X			X				X	X		
7				X			X	X									X									
8						X																				
9		X																								
11					X																					
13																		X								X
14	X																									
18	X		X																	X					X	
19	X										X										X	X				
25													X													
26		X				X				X		X		X												

Rheumatism, Heel

	ARAN D	CHEL	PHYTO	RHOD	VAL
5	X	X	X		X
7				X	

Rheumatism, Hip

	LED	PHYTO	LYC	RHUS T	RUTA	ABROT	ALL S	ARS	AUR	BELL	BERB V	CARB V	CARB S	CAUST	COLCH	COLOC	KALM	LAC C	MEDO	MERC	NUX V	PHOS	SULPH	VAL
5	X	X	X	X			X						X	X	X		X		X			X		X
6	X	X																						
7		X																X						
9					X																			
19	X					X			X		X													
25					X																			
26			X	X				X		X		X				X				X	X		X	

Rheumatism, Jaw

	CAUST
9	X
25	X

Rheumatism, Knee

	BRY	CAUST	BERB V	LED	PULS	BENZ AC	CALC	LACH	LYC	PHYTO	RHUS T	RUTA	SAL AC	STICTA	ABROT	AGAR M	CALC PH	CHINA	CLEM	GUAIAC	KALI CAR	KALI IOD	LAC C	LAC AC	MEDO	RAD BR	SULPH	THUJA
1								X					X	X														
5	X		X	X		X	X		X		X			X		X	X		X	X	X				X			
6				X																								
7	**X**	**X**	X					X		X			X										X					
8																												X
9												X																
10					X																							
12					X																							
14	X																											
17																						X						
19		X	X	X	X	X				X					X									X		X		
25												X																
26	X	X					X		X		X							X									X	

Rheumatism, Left Sided

	LACH	OX AC
1		X
6	X	

Rheumatism, Legs

	KALM	CARB S	CLEM	LITH C	NIT AC	PHYTO	SULPH	ZINC
7	X	X	X	X	X	X		X
10	X							
19							X	

Rheumatism, Limbs

	ARS
6	X
7	X

Rheumatism, Lumbar- See also Lumbago

	ANT C	ARG	ARN	BERB V	BRY	CALC	PHYTO	RUTA	SULPH
7	X			X	X		X	X	
8						X			
19		X	X						
25									X

Rheumatism, Neck (Includes Rheumatism. Neck, Nape Of)

	CIMICI	CAUST	NUX V	COLCH	LYC	PULS	ANGUST	ARS	BELL	BRY	CALC	CALC FL	CALC PH	CUPR	KALI CAR	LACHN	MERC	PHOS	RAN B	RHUS T	SULPH	VER V
1	X																					
5	X		X	X	X						X			X		X		X		X		
7	X		X	X		X																
9		X																				
15			X																		X	X
19	X						X					X	X						X			
25		X																				
26		X			X	X		X	X	X					X		X					

Rheumatism, Right Sided

	APIS	BELL	BENZ AC	LYC
6				X
19	X	X	X	

Rheumatism, Shoulders

	BRY	MERC	SANG	CAUST	FERR	FERR PH	MAG CAR	MAG M	PHYTO	RHOD
5			X		X	X				X
6			X							
7	X	X	X	X		X				X
8							X	X		
10					X				X	
13							X	X		
15	X	X								
19									X	
26	X	X		X						

Rheumatism, Small Joints

	CAULO	LITH C	ACT S	COLCH	GUIAIAC	LED	ANT C	BENZ AC	CALC	DIG	KALI BIC	KALI IOD	KALM	LYC	MANG AC	RHOD	RUTA	STELL	STICTA	VIOL O	ZINC
1	X	X										X		X							
4	X	X	X	X		X		X					X			X	X			X	
5	X	X	X		X	X	X				X				X			X			
6										X									X		X
7			X																		
9									X												
10				X																	
19	X	X			X																
26	X																				

Rheumatism, Spine

	CIMICI	RUTA	ANGUST	ARG	BRY	CALC	CALC PH	FERR	KALI IOD	MEDO	NUX V	RAD BR	RHOD	RHUS T	SANG
5	X	X			X	X	X	X	X	X	X		X	X	X
19	X	X	X	X								X			

Rheumatism, Toes

	BENZ AC	CAULO	CAUST	LYC	ACON	BRY	CALC	COLOC	LITH C	NUX V	PHOS	PHYTO	PLAT	RHOD	STICTA	SULPH
5	X	X	X	X				X	X		X	X	X	X	X	
19	X	X														
26			X	X	X	X	X			X						X

Rheumatism, Vertebra

	CIMICI	ANGUST
1	X	
19		X

Rheumatism, Vertebra, Cervical

	CHIN S	CIMICI	LACHN
17	X		
18		X	X

Rheumatism, Wrist

	ACT S	CAULO	GUAIAC	KALI BIC	LACH	RUTA	RHUS T	ABROT	ANT C	BOV	BRACH	BRY	CALC	CALC HP	COLCH	KALI NIT	KALM	LAC AC	OX AC	PULS	RHOD	SABIN	STICTA	VIOL O				
1																							X					
5		X	X	X			X		X							X	X		X	X	X	X						
6		X			X	X																						
7	X		X	X	X						X				X													
8	X	X				X	X			X		X												X				
9	X												X															
11								X																				
13				X	X																							
14	X																											
19	X		X			X												X										
25														X														

Rheumatoid Arthritis

	RHUS T	CAUST	BRY	CALC	PULS	RHOD	CIMICI	LED	ACT S	ARN	RUTA	ABROT	CAULO	GUAIAC	ACON	ARS	COLCH	DULC	KALI CAR	MEDO	NAT M	SAL AC	SULPH	THUJA				
1		X																		X				X				
2																						X						
8		X							X																			
9	**X**	X	X	X	X	X					X																	
11	**X**	**X**	**X**	X	X	X	**X**	**X**	X	X		**X**	**X**	**X**	X			X		X								
14	X	X	X				X		X								X											
19	**X**	**X**	X	X	X	X	X	X		X	X	X	X	X		X	X	X	X		X	X	X					
27	X		X					X							X				X									
29*	X	X	X	X	X	X				X	X					X					X		X	X				

29* Gibson R.G, et al. Homoeopathic Therapy in Rheumatoid Arthritis: Evaluation by Double Blind Clinical Therapeutic Trial. Br J Clin Pharmac, 1980, 9, 453-459.

Rhinitis- See also Hay Fever

	ALL C	ARS	NUX V	AMM C	ARS I	CARB V	DULC	EUPHR	HEP	KALI BIC	KALI IOD	LEM MIN	PULS	SABAD	SANG													
1												X																
5	X	X		X	X		X	X	X	X	X		X	X														
7									X	X																		
9	X																											
10			**X**			X	X																					
11				X																								
14			X																									
17	X	X	X	X	X	X	X	X	X	X	X	X	X	X	X													
18															X													
21		X			X	X					X		X	X	X													
23		X			X							X																
24	X	X						X		X																		

Rhinitis, Atrophic

	LEM MIN	ALUM	AUR	BAR M	KALI BIC	LYC	MERC C	MEZ	NAT ARS	SABAL	SEP	STICTA	SULPH															
2	X				X					X																		
4	X																											
17	X	X	X	X		X	X	X	X		X	X	X															

Rhinorrhoea- See Coryza; Catarrh, Nasal

Rickets- See also Bones, Curvature Of

	CALC	SIL	CALC PH	PHOS	PH AC	SULPH	FL AC	KALI IOD	LYC	MERC	PINUS S	SANIC	THER	ALUM	ANGUST	ASAF	BAR C	BELL	CALC FL	FERR PH	MEZ	NAT M	STAPHYS	THUJA	TUB	ARS		
1	X	X	**X**				X										X		X						X			
2	X	**X**	**X**	**X**				X		X		X	X											X		**X**		
3	X	X	X		**X**															X					X			
4	X	**X**		X		X																						
6	X	X	X	X	X		X	X	X	X			X	X	X			X			X	X	X					
8	X	X	X	X	X	X	X	X	X	X	X		X		X	X	X	X	X		X		X	X				
9	X	X																										
10	X	X	X			X						X		X								X						
11											X																	
12	X	X	X	X	X	X										X												
13											X																	
14	X		X																									
15	X	**X**			X																							
16	X	X	X																									
17	X		X									X																
23	X	X	X		X															X								
24	X		X	X																								
26	X	X		X		X	X		X																			

Ringworm- See also Crusta Serpiginosa; Favus; Tinea

	SEP	BACILL	SULPH	TELL	CALC	ARS	DULC	RHUS T	GRAPH	HELL	PHYTO	TUB	APIS	CHR AC	HEP	MEZ
1	X	**<u>X</u>**	X	X	X								X			
2	**X**	**X**	**X**	**X**	**X**	**X**					X			X		X
3	X	**X**	X	**X**	X		X	X	X	X	E				X	
4	X			X												
6	X	X														
8	X				X	X	X			X	X					
9	X	X				X						X				
10	**<u>X</u>**		**X**		X			**X**	X						X	
11	X	X		X					X					X		X
12	X		X		X											
13	X			X			X	X		X						
14	X	**X**	X	X									X			
15	**X**		X		X	X		X								
19	**<u>X</u>**	**X**			X		X					**X**				
20	**X**		X	X	X	X	X		X							
21	X		X	X												
28		X														

E- External

Ringworm, Scalp

	DULC	CALC	ARS	HEP	RAD BR	RHUS T	STAPHYS
10		X	X	X		X	X
14	X						
19	X				X		
20	X	X					

Risus Sardonicus- See also Spasm, Face; Tetanus

	BELL	HYOSC	RAN S	STRAM	VER A	ACON	ALUM	ASAF	BOV	CALC	CIC	CON	CROC	CUPR	NAT M	PHOS	PLAT	SEP	ZINC	ANAC	CAUST	COLCH	HYDR AC	NUX M	NUX V	OENANTH	SOL N	STRYCH
6	X	X	X	X	X	X	X	X	X	X	X	X	X	X	X	X	X	X	X	X		X		X				
7	X	X		X	X																X							
8	X	X	X	X	X	X	X	X	X	X	X	X	X	X	X	X	X	X	X						X			
13	X		X																								X	
17																												X
19	X	X																								X		
24																							X					

Rodent Ulcer- See Basal Cell Carcinoma

Roseola

	ACON	BELL	PULS	BRY	ARS	HYOSC	MERC	PHOS	RHUS T	SULPH	ANTIPYR	CALC	CAUST	COP	CORNUS	CUBEB	LYC	NIT AC	NUX V	PHYTO	STRAM
2	**X**	**X**									X					X					
6					X	X		X	X												X
7	**X**	X	**X**	**X**	X	X	X	X							X						
8	**X**	X	X	X			X		X	X		X	X	X			X	X	X		
21		X	X																	X	
26	X	X	X							X											

Roundworms- See Trichinosis
Rubella- See Measles, German
Rupia

	ARS	KALI IOD	NIT AC	GRAPH	SYPH	CALC	CLEM	HEP	MERC	SEP	SIL	SULPH	THUJA	ALUM	BOV	CAUST	MERC I F	NAT M	NAT SUL	PETR	PHYTO	RHUS T	SARS	STAPHYS	THYROID
2		**X**																							X
6			X				X		X			X	X										X		
7	**X**	X	X	X	X	X		X	X									X							
8	**X**	**X**	**X**	X	**X**	X	X	X		X	X	X	X	X	X	X	X		X		X	X		X	
26	X			X						X	X									X					

Salivary Glands, Diseases Of

	COLCH	MERC	MERC CY	MERC I F	SIL
6	X				
8			X	X	X
10		X			

Salivation, Deficient- See also Tongue, Dryness; Xerostomia

	NUX M	ARS	BELL	BRY	CAPS	IOD	MERC P	VER V
4						X		
7	X							X
8							X	
21	X	X	X	X	X			

Salivation, Profuse- See Ptytalism
Salpingitis (Includes Pelvic Inflammatory Disease)

	ACON	APIS	BELL	COLOC	EUPION	FERR PH	LACH	MAG PH	MERC C	MERC	SULPH
9	X		X			X		X			X
21	X	X	X	X					X		
27		X		X	X		X			X	

Sarcocele

	AUR	CON	MERC I R	PULS
1	X			
6		X		
7	X		X	X
8		X	X	

Sarcoidosis

	BERYL	AQ MAR	ASAR	CRESOL	HIPP AC	HYDRAST	PARATHY	MANDRA	THUJA
17	X	X	X	X	X	X	X	X	
28	X								X

Sarcoma- See also Cancer, Scirrhus Form

	BAR C	CROT H	THUJA	CALC	CALC FL	GELS	LAPIS	NIT AC	SIL	STAPHYS	SULPH
1	X	X				X				X	
4			X								
7	X	X									
8	X	X					X				
24			X		X				X		
26				X				X			X

Satyriasis- See Sexual Desire, Increased, Male

Scabies

	SULPH	CARB V	MERC	HEP	PSOR	SEP	CAUST	ANTHROK	ARS	LACH	CALC	SEL	CROT T	DULC	LYC	NAT CAR	RHUS T	SULPH AC	VER A
1		X						X		X									
2	**X**	X			**X**		X	X				X							
3	X	X	X	X	X			X									X		
6	X	X	X	X	X	X	X		X									X	
7	**X**	X	X	X	**X**	X	X	X	X	X	X			X	X	X			
8	**X**	X	**X**	X	X	X	X		X	X			X		X		X	X	X
10	X	X	X	X		X	X				X								
11	X			X	X	X		X					X						
13	**X**	**X**	X			**X**	X		X	X		**X**		X		X			X
15	B		X	X															
21	X																		
26	X		X	X		X	X				X								
28					X														

B- Both Internal and External

Scarlet Fever (AKA Scarlatina)

	BELL	APIS	ACON	RHUS T	AILANTH	ARS	MUR AC	AMM C	ARUM T	LACH	SULPH	BRY	PHOS	GELS	TEREB	MERC	STRAM	CARB AC	NIT AC	ZINC	CARB V	HYOSC	CALC	HEP	CUPR AC	CUPR	OP	VER V
1	**X**	X		X	X																							
2	**X**	**X**	**X**	**X**	**X**	**X**	**X**	X	**X**	**X**		**X**			**X**		X	X						**X**				
3	X																											
4	**X**	X	X	**X**	**X**	X	X	**X**	X	**X**	X	**X**		**X**		X				**X**								
5	X	X			X		X		X				X	X														
6	X	X	X	X	X	X	X	X	X	X	X	X	X	X	X	X	X	X	X	X	X	X	X	X		X	X	X
7	**X**	**X**	**X**	**X**	**X**	**X**	X	**X**	**X**	X	X	X	X	X	X	X	X	**X**	**X**	X	X	X	**X**		X	X	X	X
8	X	X	X	X	X	X	X	X	X	X	X	X	X	X	X	X	X	X	X	X	X	X	X	X	X	X	X	X
10	X		X																									
12	**X**	X	X		X	X	X	X		X	X		X	X	X		X	X	X		X	X			X		X	X
13	**X**	X	X	X	X	X	X	X	X	X	X	X	X	X	X	**X**	X		X			X	X	X	X			
14	**X**	X	**X**	X							X	X																
15	**X**			**X**	X	X	X			X				X		**X**											X	X
16	X	X		X	X	X	X	X	X	X	X		X		X		X			X					X	X		
17	X									X	X								X		X			X				
18	X	X							X																			
19	X		X																									
21	X																											
22	X																											
23	X	X	X	X	X	X	X	X	X									X				X						
24													X															
25	X		X			X					X																	
26	X	X	X	X		X		X			X	X	X							X	X		X			X		

Scarlet Fever, Prophylaxis

	BELL	AILANTH	BAR C	EUCAL	PHYTO	SCARLET	SULPH
14	X					X	
16	X	X	X	X	X		X
21	X						

Scarletina- See Scarlet Fever

Scars- See also Cicatrix; Keloid

	GRAPH	CALEND	CAUST	THIO	SIL	FL AC	IOD	LACH	PHYTO	CALC FL	CARB A	HYPER	KALI IOD	SARR	THUJA
1	X		X	X	X	X		X	X	X			X	X	
2				X		**X**	X		**X**			X			
3			X												
5	X	E	X		X					X					
6	X													X	X
7	X	X				X	X	X			X		X		
8	X		X			X	X	X			X	X			
10	X														
12													X		
16	X	X	X												
18	X													X	X
19		X	X	X											
21	X			X	X										
24	X	X													
27				X											
28		X		X	X										

E - External

Schizophrenia

	LACH	STRAM	TAR H	SULPH	ANAC	BELL	HYOSC	NUX V	PULS	THUJA
21	X	X	X		X	X	X			X
29*	X	X	X	**X**				X	X	

29* Balachandran VA. Homoeopathic Management of Schizophrenia. CCRH Quarterly Bulletin, 18, 1&2, 1996, 15-18.

School Phobia

	ARG N	GELS	LYC
25	**X**	X	X

Sciatica

	ARS	GNAPH	RHUS T	NUX V	RUTA	CHAM	COLOC	LYC	PHYTO	PLUM	ACON	BRY	IGN	KALI IOD	ARN	GELS	MAG PH	AMM M	LACH	SULPH	CARB S	COFF	HYPER	PULS	VISC A	BELL		
1	X	X	X		X	X	**X**	X	X	X		X													X			
2	**X**	**X**	**X**		**X**	X	**X**	**X**		X			X	X			X	X	X	X	X	X	X		X			
3		**X**		X					X			X				X					X		X					
4	**X**	**X**	**X**	**X**	X	X		X	X	X	**X**	X		**X**	X	X	X	X		X		X		**X**	X	**X**		
5		X					X																					
6	X	X	X	X	X	X	X	X		X	X	X	X		X				X	X		X		X				
7	X	X	**X**	**X**	X	X		X	X			X	X	X	X	**X**	**X**		X	X	X	X	**X**	X		X		
8	X	X	X	X	X			X	X	X	X	X		X	X	X						X	X		X			
9	X	X	X	X	X					X				X	X													
10	X			X		X					X	X	X		X					X						X		
11	X	X	X		X	X	X	X	X	X			X	X			X	X								X		
12	X	X	X				X	X	X		X						X							X				
13		X						X	X										X									
14	X	X	X		X	X					X										X				X			
15	X		X	X		X					X		X			X												
16	X																											
17	**X**				**X**	**X**				X	X		X	**X**	**X**	X			X	**X**	X	X	**X**	**X**		X		
18				X																								
19				**X**					X	X		X							X									
21	X	X	X													X	X	X										
23		X					X						X								X				X			
25	X	X	X	X														X	X									
27	X						X										X	X										

Sciatica, Left Side

	KALI BIC	RHUS T	AMM M	COLOC	IRIS V	CARB S	STILL	BELL	CAUST	CIMICI	LACH	KALI IOD	NUX V	ARS	CALC	CAPS	CHAM	EUP PUR	KALI CAR	MEDO	SULPH	TELL	THUJA					
1				X			X							X														
3	X	X																										
4	X																											
6							X	X	X																			
7	X			X	X						X																	
8	X		X	**X**	X					X							X	X	X			X						
9			X			X					X																	
10		**X**													X													
13	X																											
14								X	X																			
17			**X**		**X**								**X**															
18	X																											
19	X	**X**								X		**X**				X				X	X		X					
21						X																						
25						X																						

Sciatica, Right Side

	COLOC	DIOSC	MAG PH	TELL	LYC	GNAPH	PHYTO	COLCH	LACH	BELL	BRY	KALI CAR	POD	RHUS T	SEP	VISC A	CHIN S	CIMICI	GINSENG	INDIGO	KALI IOD	KALI PH	LAC C	NAT M	STAPHYS	VALER		
1	X		X					X																				
3	X	X	X		X																	X						
4	**X**							X																				
6		X		X			X														X							
7		X							X								X											
8		X	X						X											X				X				
9	**X**		X																									
10	**X**																											
12																		X							X			
13				X																								
14		X																					X					
17	**X**	**X**	**X**	**X**	**X**	**X**	**X**				**X**		**X**	**X**	**X**	**X**												
19	X	X	**X**	X	X	X				**X**		**X**							X							X		
21	X	X			X																							
25	X																											

Scirrhus- See also Cancer, Scirrhus Form; Sarcoma

	CARB A	BROM	CON	LAPIS	SIL	ACET AC	APIS	ARG N	ARN	ARS IOD	AST R	BELL	BUFO	CALC	CALEND	CARB AC	CONDUR	GALIUM	HYDRAST	MERC AU	MUR AC	NIT AC	NUX V	SEP	STAPHYS	SULPH		
2				X																								
4	**X**		X																									
6														X														
7	X	X			X			X			X		X															
8	X	X	X	X	X	X			X	X		X			X	X	X	X	X	X	X	X	X	X	X	X		
24							X																					

Scirrhus, Breast- See Cancer, Breast
Scirrhus, Pylorus- See Cancer, Pylorus
Scirrhus, Tongue- See Cancer, Tongue
Scirrhus, Uterus- See Cancer, Uterus
Scleritis

	SULPH	THUJA	ACON	KALM	MERC	COCCUL	ERYNG A	PULS	SIL	SPIG																		
6	X	X	X	X	X	X		X	X	X																		
7		X		X																								
8	X						X																					
21		X	**X**																									
26	X				X																							

Scleroderma- See also Lichen; Skin Thick/Hard

	ARS	RAN B	ANT C	GRAPH	SEP	ALUM	ELAEIS	DULC	HYDROC	LYC	RHUS T	SIL	THYROID	CALC	CROT T	IOD	KALI BIC	KALM	LACH	PETR	SARS	THUJA
1		X	X						X				X									
2							X						X					X				
4	X	X	X																			
5	X	X	X	X	X			X		X	X	X		X					X			
7		X														X	X					
13	X	X	X	X	X			X		X	X	X										X
18	X								X													
19				X	X	X									X					X	X	
23							X															
25	X																					
27						X																

Scleroma Natorum

	LACH	ANTHRAC	BRY	GRAPH	GUAIAC	HYDROC	PHOS	SIL	SOL N	STILL
1	X									
8	X	X	X	X	X	X	X	X	X	X

Sclerosis

	PLUM	ARG N	CARB V	HELOD	LACH	LED	SEC	ARS	BAR M	CUPR	HYOSC H	LATH	MERC PH	OX AC
8	**X**													
10									X					
11	X	X	**X**	**X**	**X**	**X**	**X**	X						
17		X												
23		X								X	X	X	X	X
24	**X**													

Sclerosis, Amyotrophic Lateral

	LATH	ARG N	BAR M	CURARE	CUPR
4	X	X			
8					X
10			X		
11	X	X			
17	X				
19				X	

Sclerosis, Brain

	PLUM	AGAR M	ARG N	BAR C	OX AC	VER A
1	X				X	
7	X					
8	X	X		X		X
11			X			
17	X					

Sclerosis, Lateral- See Sclerosis, Amyotrophic Lateral

Sclerosis, Optic Disc

	PLUM
8	X
24	X

Sclerosis, Optic Nerve

	STRYCH N	CARB S	PHOS
2	X		
3	X	X	X

Sclerosis, Spinal Cord

	ARG N	BAR C	BAR M	NUX V	PLUM
7				X	
8		X			X
10			X		
11	X				

Sclerosis, Spine

	OX AC
1	X
3	X

Sclerosis, Testes

	RHOD	IOD	AGNUS	CLEM	AUR	CON	BROM	CALC	CINNAB	COP	MERC	SULPH	SIL	ARG N	ARN	BAR M	CALC FL	CARB A	KALI IOD	MERC I R	NUX V	OX AC	PULS	SPONG	VIOL O
2			X				X															X			
7	**X**	X				**X**		X	X	X	X	X	**X**			X	X	X	X	X			X		X
8	X	X	X	**X**	X	X	X	X	X					X	X										
13	**X**	**X**	X	**X**	**X**					X	X	X									X			X	

Scoliosis

	SIL	ARN	CALC	CALC FL	CALC PH	FERR IOD	PH AC	PHOS	PULS	SULPH
2						X				
8					X			X		
12	X	E	X				X		X	X
19	X			X						

E- External

Scorbutus- See Vitamin C Deficiency Symptoms

Scrofula- See also Tuberculosis

	CALC	HEP	SULPH	AUR	SIL	ASAF	MERC	MEZ	CON	GRAPH	IOD	KALI BIC	KALI IOD	LYC	ALNUS	BAR C	BROM	CALC PH	CAUST	CHIM	DULC	NAT CAR	ARS	ARS IOD	BAD	BAR M	CIST	THER
2	X	X		X				X	X	X	X	X	X		X		X		X	X	X	X			X	X	X	
4	**X**	X	X		**X**		**X**			**X**					X	X	X	X	X									
7	**X**	**X**	**X**	**X**	**X**	X	**X**	X	**X**	X	**X**	**X**	X	**X**		X	X	X		X	X	X	**X**	**X**	**X**	**X**	**X**	X
8	X	X	X	X		X						X	**X**	X						X								**X**
10			**X**																									
13	X	X	X	X	X	X	X	X	X					X		X					X	X	X					
17																		X										
23	X	X		X	X	X		X			X				X				X					X				
24	X																											

Scrofulosis- See Tuberculosis

Scurvy- See Vitamin C Deficiency Symptoms.

Seasickness- See also Motion Sickness

	PETR	COCCUL	TAB	NUX V	APOMOR	THER	GLON	SEP	STAPHYS	ARS	COLCH	KREO	BOR	HYOSC	OP	SANIC	CARB AC	CHLOR	CUCURB	FERR	KALI BIC	PULS	SIL	SULPH	VER A
1	**X**	X	X		X	X			X		X		X									X			
2	**X**	**X**	X	X	X	X	X		X	X		X	X			X			X						
3	X	X	X											X											
4	**X**	**X**	X		**X**	X	X		X																
5									X																
6	X	X		X	X			X			X		X		X							X			
7	**X**	**X**	X	**X**		X	X	X				X					X	X			X				
8	**X**	X	X	X	**X**	X	X	X	X	X	X			X		X		X		X			X	X	
9	X	X	X	X	X																				
10	X	X	**X**	X			**X**			X					X										X
12	**X**	X	X	X								X													X
13	**X**	**X**	X			X		X			X			X	X					X	X		X		
14		X																							
15	**X**	X		X								X													
16	X	X	X	X		X																			
17	X		X			X																			
19		X																							
23	X	X	X													X	X		X						
26		**X**						X		**X**														X	
28	X	X	X																						

Seasickness, Prophylaxis

	NUX V	COCCUL	PETR
10	X		
12	X	X	**X**
15	X	X	

Seborrhoea

	NAT M	MERC	THUJA	LYC	VINCA	GRAPH	SEP	SULPH	IOD	CALC	HYDRAST	MEZ	PHOS	RAPH	SARS
2	**X**				**X**		X		**X**		X			X	X
6	X	X			X	X				X			X		
8	X			X	X		X	X	X	X	X	X	X		X
9	X		X	X											
11	X														
12		X				X	X	X				X			
13	X	X	X												
18	X		X	**X**											
19			X					X							
21	X	X				X									
23														X	
25	X														

Senility

	BAR C	CON	AGNUS	ALOE	ALUM	ANAC	ARS	CARB V	FERR PIC	FL AC	PH AC	SUMBUL	THIO
14	X					X							
16	X	X			X		X	X					X
17												X	
21									X				
23		X	X	X						X	X		
27	X												

Sepsis- See also Blood Poisoning; Septicaemia

	LACH	ARS	ARN	CARB V	CROT H	ECHIN	PYROG	RHUS T	APIS	ARS IOD	BAPT	BELL	BRY	IOD	LYC	MERC C	MUR AC	PHOS	VER V
16	X		X			X		X						X					
19					X														
24	X	X	X	X		X		X		X						X			
27																	X		
29[1]	**X**	X		X	X		X		X		X	X	X		X			X	
29[2]		X					X												X

29[1] Frass M, et al. Adjunctive homeopathic treatment in patients with severe sepsis: a randomised, double-blind, placebo-controlled trial in an intensive care unit. Homeopathy, 2005, 94, 10-16.
29[2] Teixeira MZ, et al. Homeopathic practice in Intensive Care Units: objective semiology, symptom selection and a series of sepsis cases. Homeopathy. 2008, Oct, 97, 4, 206-13.

Sepsis, Prophylaxis

	RHUS T
24	**X**

Septicaemia- See also Blood Poisoning; Sepsis

	LACH	ECHIN	RHUS T	ARS	BAPT	ARN	CARB V	PYROG	CROT H	SIL	ANTHRAC	GUNPOW	CARB AC	AMM C	ARS IOD	BRY	CHINA	PHOS	SEC	TAR C
1	X	X	X	X	X	X	X	X			X	X		X						X
2		X						X												
3	X	X	X	X	X			**X**						X						
4	**X**	**X**	**X**	X	X	**X**		X					**X**		X					
5		X							X											
7	**X**			**X**		X	**X**		X		X								X	
8	X		X	X		X	X		X	X			X			X	X	X	X	
10	X	X		X		X			**X**	X										
11	X																			
12			X	X	X		X													
14			X				X													
16	X	X	X	X	X		X	X				X								
17	X	X	X		X	X			X	X		X								
18								X												
19					X											X				
23		X						X												X
24	X	X	X	X	X	X	X			X	X				X		X	X		

Serous Membranes, Diseases Of

	BRY	CIMICI	APIS	HELL
7	**X**	X	X	X
18	X			

Sexual Desire, Female, Decreased

	NAT M	SEP	FERR	BERB V	CAUST	CON	HELON	ONOSM	PETR	AGNUS	BAR C	GRAPH	IGN	KALI BR	LYC	PH AC	PHOS	SIL
1						X		X										
2								X										
3																	X	
5	X	X	X		X		X		X	X	X				X	X	X	
7	X		**X**	X			X							X				
8	X	X	X	X			X		X		X			X	X			X
9		X																
10		X																
13	X		X	X	X	X			X									
14				X				X				X	X					
21	X	X			X	X				X						X		
25	X												X					X
27												X						

Sexual Desire, Female, Increased

	CANTH	PLAT	MUREX	MOSCH	PHOS	NUX V	VER A	BELL	HYOSC	MERC	STRAM	TAR H	GRAT	CALC PH	CANN I	COFF	LIL T	ORIGAN	SABIN	SULPH	PULS
3					X																
7	X	X	X	X	X	X	X	X	X	X	X	X		X	X	X	X	X	X	X	
8	X	X	X	X	X	X	X	X	X	X	X	X	X	X	X	X	X	X	X	X	
9	X	X	X			X											X				
10			X																		
11		X		X																	
13	**X**	**X**	X	X	**X**	**X**	**X**	**X**		X	X		**X**			X					**X**
14	X		X	X	X							X			X						X
18			X	X										X							
19																			X		
20	X																				
21		X							X				X								
23	X	X	X	X								X						X			
26	X	X			X	X	X	X	X	X	X									X	

Sexual Desire, Male, Decreased

	LYC	GRAPH	ONOS	AGNUS	BAR C	IGN	NAT M	NUPH	STAPHYS	ARG N	CHINA	CON	FERR	KALI BIC	KALI BR	KALI CAR	KALI IOD	MAR CAR	PH AC	SIL	SULPH
1			X					X													
2			X																		
3	X								X		X						X				
5	X	X				X	X			X				X	X	X					
7	X			X	X	X	X	X	X				X			X	X	X		X	
8			X	X	X	X		X	X	X			X	X	X			X	X		X
11					X							X									
12																			X		
13	X	X					X				X									X	X
14		X	X	X																	
17												X									
21	X	X																			

Sexual Desire, Male, Increased

	CANTH	PHOS	PIC AC	NUX V	LYC	CHINA	HYOSC	MERC	NAT M	PLAT	VER A	AUR	BELL	CALC	CANN I	CARB V	FL AC	LYSS	PHOS	PULS	SALIX N	SEL	STRAM
2	X														X		X	X			X		
3		X																					
7	**X**		X														X	X	X				X
8	X	X	X												X				X				X
11	X																						
13	**X**	**X**		**X**	X	**X**	**X**	**X**	**X**	**X**	**X**	X	X	X		X				X			
14	X	X																		X		X	
21		X	X	X	X																	X	
23	X		X																		X		
26	X	X		X	X	X	X	X	X	X	X	X	X	X		X							

Shingles- See Herpes Zoster

Shock

	ARN	OP	VER A	ACON	CARB V	CAMPH	GELS	ARS	CUPR	DIG	LACH	CHAM	CHINA	HYPER	NAT M	NUX M	NUX V	PHOS	SULPH
1	X	X		X	X	X		X					X	X					
3	X	X	X		X					X		X		X			X	X	
5	X					X					X								
6		X																	
7	X	**X**	**X**	X	X	**X**	X	**X**	X	**X**	**X**	X	X		X	X		X	
8	X	X	X	X	X	X	X	X	X	X	X	X	X	X	X	X	X	X	**X**
9	X		X																
10		X		X	X														
13	**X**			X					X						X		X		X
14	X																		
15							X												
17	X	X	X		X	X	X	X											
18	X																		
20	**X**		X						X										
21	X	X	X	X	X														
22	**X**																		
24	X		X	X		X	X	X								X			
25	X																		
27	X																		
28	X			X															

Shock, Anaphylactic

	APIS	ARS	CARB AC	HIST	KALI IOD	SER EQ	URT U
5	X	X		X	X	X	X
17	X						
19			X				

Shock, Haemorrhagic

	CARB V	CHINA	ARN	VER A
4	**X**	X		
17	X	X	X	X

Shock, Surgical

	VER A	CARB V	CAMPH	OP	HYPER	STRONT C	ACON	ALL C	AMM M	ARN	ARS	DIG	HELL	NUX V	PHOS	PULS	PYROG	RHUS T	STAPHYS
1	X	X	X	X	X	X	X	X	X	X			X	X	X	X	X	X	X
4	**X**	**X**	**X**	**X**	X						X	X							
5	X	X																	
10		X																	
14	**X**	X				X													
16	X																		
17			X																

Shoulder, Diseases Of

	FERR	PHYTO	SANG	SANIC	VER V	WILDBAD
2	X		X	X		X
8		X			X	

Shoulder, Frozen

	AGAR M	BRY	COLOC	FERR	KALM	RHUS T	RUTA	SANG	THIO
5	X		X		X				
27		X		X		X	X	X	X

Singers' Hoarseness- See Voice, Hoarseness, From Singing

Singultus- See Hiccough

Sinusitis- See also Neuralgia, Face; Prosopalgia

	KALI BIC	SIL	HEP	HYDRAST	KALI IOD	STICTA	PULS	NAT M	THUJA	AUR	BELL	CINNAB	EUPHR	PHOS	SANG N	SEP
1	X	X							X	X						
2		X						X	X							
3	X	X		X		X							X		X	X
4				**X**												
5	X	X	X	X	X	X	X	X	X	X	X	X	X	X	X	
9	X	X														
12													X			
14	X		X		X		X									
17			X	X	X	X										
18	X		X	X	X	X						X			X	
19	**X**	X	X	X	X	X			X	X	X	X		X		
20	**X**	X	X				X									
21	X	X	X				X				X					
22	X															
24								X								
27	X															
29[1]		X					X	X								**X**
29[2]		X			X									X		

29[1] Witt CM, et al. Homeopathic treatment of patients with chronic sinusitis: A prospective observational study with 8 years follow-up. BMC Ear, Nose and Throat Disorders 2009, July 27, 9-7.
29[2] Nayak C, et al. Homeopathy in chronic sinusitis: a prospective multi-centric observational study. Homeopathy. 2012 Apr; 101 (2) :84-91

Sinusitis, Frontal

	KALI IOD	STICTA	BELL	CUPR	KALI BIC	MERC	NAT M	SIL	BRY	EUPHR	LACH	LYC	ANT C	ASAF	AUR M	CALC	HEP	IOD	NAPHTH	PULS	SABAD	SANG	SPIG	VERBASC	VERBENA	VINCA
6	X		X		X		X		X	X	X	X														
7	X			X		X										X									X	
8	X			X	X		X	X				X	X						X			X		X		X
9																					X					
14	X	X			X		X	X		X																
17	X	X						X						X	X		X	X								
18	X	X									X															
19		X				**X**			X														X			
21			X																	X						
24	X		X	X					X																	

Sjogren's Syndrome

	EUPHR	FL AC	NAT M	NUX M	PETR	SIL
19				X		
27	X	X	X		X	X

Skin, Congestion Of

	BERB V	DULC	FUM	NAT M	PSOR	RHUS V	SAPO	VIOL T																				
5	X		X			X	X	X																				
7		X		X	X																							

Skin, Cracking of- See Cracking, Skin
Skin, Discoloration of- See Discoloration, of Skin
Skin, Diseases Of

	SULPH	GRAPH	HEP	PSOR	CALC	PETR	DULC	SEP	ARS	CON	LYC	SEL	AETHIOP	ANAG	ARS IOD	CAUST	ICTHYOL	IGN	KALI ARS	NAT M	RHUS T	STAPHYS	THUJA	SPONG				
1			X																									
2	**X**	X	**X**	X	X	**X**				X		**X**	X	X			X	X	X									
3																								**X**				
5		X	X	X	X	X	X	X			X									X		X						
6										X										X								
7	X	X	X	X	X	X	X	X			X				X	X												
8	**X**	X		X	X		**X**	X		X	X		X			X						X						
10	X	X	X	**X**		X		X	X																			
12	X								X																			
15	X								X																			
16				X																								
17	X	X										X																
18																							X					
23	X		X				X							X	X		X		X		X		X					
24	X	X																										
26	X				X													X			X							
27	**X**	**X**	X																									
28	X																											

Skin, Dryness- See also Perspiration, Absent

	ACON	ARS	BELL	SULPH	LYC	PHOS	GRAPH	PETR	ALUM	NAT CAR	SEP	CALC	NAT M	PLUM	APIS	KALI IOD	SEC	IOD	NIT AC	THYROID	KALI CAR	NUX M	SIL
1	X	X	X	X				X	X				X		X		X						
2										**X**				**X**		**X**							
4	X	X		X				X			X		X	X									
5		X			X	X	X	X	X	X	X												X
6	X	X			X	X					X			X		X			X		X	X	
7	**X**	**X**	X	X	X	**X**		**X**	X	X	X	X	X	X	X				X		X	**X**	X
8		X		X	X	X	X			X		X					X						
9	X	X	X		X															X			
10	X	X		X			X		X				X	X									
11			X					X	X								X			X		X	
12	X	X				X												X					
13	X	X	**X**	**X**	X	**X**	**X**			**X**	X	**X**	**X**			X	**X**	X	X		**X**		**X**
14	X	X	X					X										X					
15	X	X	X				X					X											
17	X							X	X						X								
18	X				X										X								
19	X	X				X	X	X	X		X	X			X								
20	X			X			X																
21	X	X	X	X					X														
22			X																				
24	X	X	X	X	X	X	X									X		X		X			
25	X	X	X		X															X			
27	X		X																X				

Skin, Flabby- See Skin, Turgor, Diminished

Skin, Foreign Body Lodged Within

	SIL	HEP	LED
14	X	X	
19	X	X	
21	X		
22			X

Skin, Oily/Greasy- See Seborrhoea

Skin, Peeling Of

	MEZ	GRAPH	HELL	PHOS	SEP	SIL
1	X		X			
2						
5		X			X	X
8	X			X		
13	X	X	X	X	X	X

Skin, Thick/Hard- See also Lichen; Scleroderma

	ARS	GRAPH	HYDROC	RHUS T	ANT C	CIST	CROT T	DULC	LYC	RAN B	SEP	SIL	THUJA	THYROID
9	X													
10		X		X										
11			X											
13	X	X		X	X			X	X	X	X	X	X	
14			X			X								X
19							X							

Skin, Turgor, Diminished

	ABROT	VER A	ARS	SARS	SEP	CALC	CUPR	LYC	SEC	ANT C	ARG N	BOR	BOV	CAMPH	CAPS	CON	IOD	KREO	MEZ	NAT M	SULPH
1	X	X				X		X	X		X										
4	X																				
5	X	X	X	X	X		X	X	X	X		X				X		X	X		
6		X	X																	X	
7	X	X		X	X	X	X	X				X		X	X	X		X	X	X	X
8	X	X					X						X								
9	X										X										
10	X	X	X		X				X					X							X
11				X																	
13		X		X	X	**X**	X	X	X	X			X		X		X				
14			X	X													X				
15						X															
18			X		X																

Skin, Wrinkled- See Skin, Turgor, Diminished

Sleep Apnoea

	GRIND	CARB A	LACH	OP	AMM C	ANT T	ARUM T	BAD	BRY	CAD	CARB V	GRIND SQ	GRAPH	GUAIAC	NUX M	PSOR
1	X															
7	X													X		
8	X	**X**	X	X	X	X	X	X	X	X	X	X	X		X	X
9	X															
10			X													
11				X												

Sleep, Disorders Of

	BELL	CARB V	HYOSC	IGN	LYC	NUX V	OP	PHOS	RHUS T	SULPH	CALC	CHINA	MAG ARC	CINNAB	GELS	MORPH
2	**X**	**X**	**X**	**X**	**X**	**X**	**X**	**X**	**X**	**X**	X	X	X	**X**	**X**	**X**
8	X	X	X	X	X	X	X	X	X	X	X	X	X			

Sleep, Excessive- See Stupor

Sleep, Loss of, Ailments From- See Ailments, Sleep, Loss Of

Sleep Walking- See Somnambulism

Sleeplessness- See also Insomnia

	ACON	BELL	NUX V	COFF	CHAM	SULPH	PULS	IGN	OP	ARS	CALC	HYOSC	LACH	CHINA	BRY	PHOS	GELS	LYC	SEP	AMBRA	CIMCI	KREO	MEZ	CAMPH	CINA	MERC	PASS	
1	X	X	X	X	X	X		X	X	X		X	X				X			X							X	
2	**X**			X							X													X			X	
3		X		X	X		X	X	X						X					X	X							
4			**X**			**X**	X			X	X				X					X	X							
6	X	X	X	X	X	X	X	X	X	X	X	X	X	X		X	X	X	X		X	X	X	X	X	X		
7	X	**X**	**X**	**X**	**X**	**X**		X	**X**		X	X	X	X		X	X	X	X			X	X	X	X			
8	X	X	**X**	X	X	**X**	**X**	**X**	X	**X**	**X**	X	X	**X**	X	X	X	**X**	X	X	X	X		X	X	**X**	X	
10	X	X	X	X	X	X	X	X	X	X	X	X		X	X	X	X			X		X	X			X		
11	X	X							X				X								X		X					
12	X	X	X	X	X	X	X	X		X			X			X	X	X	X			X					**X**	
13	X	**X**	X	**X**	X	X	**X**	X	X	**X**	**X**	X	X	**X**	**X**	**X**		X	**X**	X		X	X	**X**	**X**	X	X	
14	X	X	X	X			X	X				X																
15	X	X	X	X	X		X	X	X	X	X	X		X	X		X				X				X			
17	X	X			X																							
18													X															
24	X		X			X																	X					
26	X	X	X	X	X	X	X		X	X	X	X	X	X	X	X		X	X							X		

Smallpox

	ANT T	VARIOL	SARAC	BELL	BRY	THUJA	ARS	RHUS T	BAPT	CROT H	SULPH	MERC	APIS	PHOS	HYDRAST	ACON	LACH	MALAND	VACCIN	VER V	HAM	GELS	ANAC	CARB AC				
1	X	**X**	X	X	X	X				X		X		X			X	X		X	X							
2	**X**	X	X	X				X	X	**X**			X	X			X	X	X		**X**		X	**X**				
3	X	**X**	X	X	X	X	X	X		X	X			X			X		X			X	X					
4	**X**	**X**	X	X	**X**	**X**	**X**	X	X	X	X		X		**X**	X	X		X	X	X	X	X					
6	X	X	X	X	X	X	X	X	X		X	X	X	X	X			X	X									
7	**X**	X	X	X	X	X	**X**	**X**	**X**	X	X	X	X		X									X				
8	X	X	X	X	X	X	X	X	X	X	X	X	X	X	X	X				X	X	X	X	X				
10	X	**X**		X	X	X	X					X				X		X										
12	**X**	X	X	X		X	X		X	X	X	X	X	X		X	X		X	X								
15	X		X	X	X		X	X	X			X			X	X				X		X						
16	X	X	X			X																						
17	X																											
23	X	X	X															X										
26		**X**		X	X			X			**X**																	

Smallpox Pitting, Prophylaxis

	HYDRAST	THUJA	ANT T	CERATO	GLYCERIN	KALI CY	MALAND	VACCIN	VARIOL
15	X	X		X	X				
16	X	X	X			X	X	X	X

Smallpox, Prophylaxis

	VARIOL	ANT T	MALAND	THUJA	VACCIN	CIMICI	HYDRAST	KALI CY	SULPH
1			X						
10	X								
12	X	X		X	X	X			X
16	X	X	X	X	X		X	X	

Smell, Sense Of, Diseases Of- See also Anosmia (Includes Parosmia)

	CALC	ANAC	BELL	GRAPH	KALI BIC	SANG	PULS	SULPH	AUR	CARB AC	DIOSC	NUX V	PARIS	PHOS	SEP	ZINC M	ACON	LACT V	MAG M
2	**X**	X	**X**	**X**	**X**	**X**	**X**	X	**X**	**X**	**X**				X	X	**X**	**X**	**X**
6	X	X		X								X							
8	X	X	X	X	X	X	X	X	X			X	X	X					
12							X												
17	X	X	X		X	X							X	X	X	X			
21		X	X	X	X	X		X		X	X								
24	X																		

Sneezing

	ALL C	GELS	ARS	NAT M	SABAD	ACON	ARS IOD	NUX V	CYCL	HEP	MERC	EUPHR	IPEC	RHUS T	SQUILL	BELL	KALI IOD	EUP PER	AGAR M	ARUM T	CINA	KALI CAR	PHOS	SENEGA	SULPH			
1		X	X		X		X			X		X		X	X			X		X								
2																								X				
3						X			X	X									X									
4	X		X		**X**	X	X		X		X		X	X			X											
5	X			X	X		X	X	X				X											X				
6	X	X	X			X			X							X	X						X		X			
7	X	X		X				X				X			X			**X**			X							
8	<u>**X**</u>	X	**X**	X	**X**	X	X	X	X	X	X	X		X	X	X	X	X	X	X		X	X	X	X			
9	X	X	X		X	X							X									X						
10		X		X							X			X														
11	X			X	X		X		X	X			X		X													
12						X			X		X		X															
13	X	X		X	X			X	X	X	X	X		X		X		X	X		X	X	X		X			
14	X	X	X	**X**		X	X					X			X			X										
15		X	X								X																	
16					X		X																					
17	X	X	X	X	X		X	X		X		X	X	X	X		X		X	X	X	X	X	X				
18	X					X		X																				
19	X	X	X	X	X			X				X					X		X	X	X			X	X			
20			X	X				X		X			X															
21		X	X	X	X	X	X	X			X				X	X												
22	X	X	X	X		X		X			X																	
24	X	X	X	X		X	X									X	X			X			X		X			
25	X	X	X			X																X						
26							X			X				X							X							
28	X				X			X																				

Snoring

	OP	HYOSC	BELL	STRAM	NUX V	HIPPOZ	LAURO	PLUM	CHAM	CHINA	SULPH	CAMPH	IGN	LEM MIN	LYC	RHEUM	RHUS T	HEP
1	X	X				X		X						X				
2	X															X		
3						X								X				
4		X																
6	X	X	X	X	X			X			X							
7	**X**		**X**	X	X		X		X			X					X	
8	**X**	X	X	X	X		X	X		X			X		X		X	
10	X																	
11	X																	
13	**X**	X	X	**X**	X		X		**X**	**X**	**X**	X	X		X	X		**X**
14	X																	
15	X	X																
17	X		X			X												
19	X																	
21	X																	

Somnambulism

	SIL	KALI BR	PHOS	ART V	NAT M	ZINC	BRY	KALI PH	ACON	ANAC	SPONG	OP	IGN	KALM	STRAM
1				X	X								X		
2	X	**X**	X	**X**	X	X								X	
3	X	X		X	X										
5	X	X	X				X	X	X	X	X				X
6			X		X										
7	X		**X**	X		X	X						X		
8	X		X	X	X		X		X	X	X	X			X
9		X						X							
11						X									
12						X									
13	**X**		**X**		X	X	**X**		X	X	X	**X**		X	
14	X	X						X							
18		X						X							
21	X														
23		X		X											

Sordes

	BAPT	HYOSC	MUR AC	RHUS T
11			X	X
12		X		
24	X			

Sore Throat- See Pain, Throat

Spasms

	CUPR	HYOSC	BELL	NUX V	OP	CAUST	CINA	CHAM	IGN	COCCUL	MOSCH	STRAM	CAMPH	CIC	IPEC	SULPH	CIMICI	LACH	GELS	PLAT	PLUM	SEC	AMBRA	ARS	COFF	CON	LAURO	SIL
1	X																											
2	X						X	X		X			X						X	X								
3			X																									
4	X															X												
5	**X**		X								X						X						X					
6	X	X		X	**X**	X	X		X	X	X	X		X		X	X		X	X	X	X		X			X	X
8	**X**	**X**	**X**	**X**	**X**	**X**	**X**	**X**	**X**	X	X	X	**X**	X	X	X	X	**X**	X	X	**X**	X		X	X	X	X	**X**
9	X	X										X						X										
10	X	X	X																									
11	X	X																										
12				X																								
13	**X**	**X**	**X**	**X**	X	X	X	**X**	**X**	**X**	**X**	**X**	**X**	**X**	**X**	**X**		X		X	**X**	X	**X**	**X**	**X**	**X**	**X**	X
14		X		X																								
15																			X							X		
16	X	X	X		X	X	X	X	X			X			X										X			
17		X	X																									
18	X																						X					
19				X																								
21	X				X	X																						
23													X															
24			X																									
25	**X**																											
26	X	X	X	X		X	X	X	X	X	X			X	X							X						
27	X																X											

Spasm, Abdomen- See also Colic, Abdomen

	IGN	NUX V	CUPR	BELL	CALC	COCCUL	IPEC	MOSCH	PULS	VER A	ARS	CAMPH	KALI BR	KREO	LYC	MAG M	PLUM	STANN	STRAM	SULPH	TAB	VAL						
5			X																									
6								X					X															
7		X		X	X																X							
8	X	X		X		X	X	X		X	X					X		X	X	X		X						
10		X							X					X														
12									X			X																
15	X									X																		
18	X																X											
19			X																									
24			X		X										X													
26	X	X				X	X																					

Spasm, Anus

	COLCH	PLUM	NAT M	BELL	NIT AC	NUX V	OP	CAMPH	FL AC	FORMICA	IGN	LACH	LYC
4		X											
5		X	X			X							
6	X		X		X								
7	X	X			X	X	X	X	X	X	X	X	X
8		X	X	X			X						
11	X												
13	X												
24				X									

Spasm, Arms

	AGAR M	BELL	SEC	BRY	CUPR	JATR	LYC	MENY	NAT M	PHOS	PLAT	SIL	SULPH	VER A
6	X													
8	X													
10	X													
13		**X**	**X**	X	X	X	X	X	X	X	X	X	X	X
14	X													
17	X													

Spasm, Artery

	CUPR AR	GLON	SEC
5	X		X
14		X	

Spasm, Back

	CIMICI	HYDR AC	IGN	LACH	MAG PH	NUX V	PHYSO
5	X						
7				X		X	X
19			X				
24		X					
27					X		

Spasm, Bladder (AKA Cystospasm)

	BELL	ASAF	CANTH	CAMPH	COLCH	NUX V	SEP	CAPS	GELS	OP	PH AC	PRUN S	PULS	SARS	TEREB
5												X			
6	X				X	X				X					
7	X		X						X						
8		X	X	X	X		X	X	X		X		X	X	X
12				X		X									
13		X	X				X	X		X	X	X		X	X
15	X														
21				X											
24					X										
26	X	X				X	X						X		

Spasm, Bladder, Neck Of

	BELL	CAMPH	HYOSC	NUX V	PULS	APIS	ARN	CANN S	MAG PH	UVA
5	X		X	X	X					
8			X		X				X	
10		X								
12		X								
13							X			
19	X			X		X		X		X

Spasm, Chest

	CUPR	MOSCH	STRAM	ARS	CINA	IPEC	BELL	COLCH	HYOSC	KALI CAR	NUX V	PHOS	ACON	AUR	CIC	LACH	LAURO	PULS	SAMB	COCCUS	FERR	MERC	SULPH	VER A
6			X							X					X									
7	X	X	X	X		X	X	X	X								X							
8	X	X	X	X		X	X				X	X	X	X				X						
10				X	X																			
13	**X**	**X**	**X**	X	**X**	X	X	**X**	**X**	**X**	**X**	**X**				X	X	X	X	**X**	**X**	**X**	**X**	**X**
14	X																							
16					X																			
17	X	X																						
19		X												X		X								
24															X									
26						X							X						X					

Spasm, Ciliary- See also Spasm, Eye

	PHYSO	AGAR M	ESERIN	HYOSCIN	JAB
1	X	X			
2	X		X	X	X
8	X				

Spasm, Clonic

	CIC	HYOSC	AGAR M	ARS	CAMPH	CANTH	CHAM	COCCUL	COFF	CUPR	IGN	IPEC	LAURO	MOSCH	NUX M	NUX V	OP	PLUM	SQUILLA	SEC	SEP	STANN	TANACET
13	X	X	X	X	X	X	X	X	X	X	X	X	X	X	X	X	X	X	X	X	X	X	X
17		X																					
23	X																						
24			X																				

Spasm, Diaphragm

	CIC	CUPR	BELL	CHEL	COCCUL	GELS	LED	MOSCH	SEC	STANN
1					X					
6							X			
7	X	X	X	X		X		X		
8	X	X								
13										X
17									X	

Spasm, Epiglottis

	STRAM	CHLOL	MEDO
1		X	
6	X		
7	X		
10			X

Spasm, Extensor Muscles

	CINA	IPEC
6	X	
8		X

Spasm, Extremities

	CUPR	ARN	CIC	IGN	LAURO	LYC
5	X					
6					X	X
8	X			X		
9	X	X				
17			X			

Spasm, Eye- See also Spasm, Ciliary

	BELL	HYOSC	CIC	ACON	AGAR M	CANTH	CHAM	CROC	CUPR	HEP	MAG CAR	MERC	NAT M	PHYSO	RUTA	SIL	STAPHYS	STRAM	VIOL O
5	X	X	X		X				X					X					
6	X																		
8	X	X					X	X		X		X	X		X	X	X		
9											X								
13	X			X		X													X
14			X																
24		X																X	

Spasm, Eyelids (AKA Nictitatio)

	HYOSC	NAT M	BELL	AGAR M	ALUM	CUPR	NUX V	RHUS T
5			X					
7		X					X	
8	X	X		X	X		X	
10								X
13	X	X	X		X	X		
18						X		
24	X	X		X				X
26	X		X					

Spasm, Eyes and Eyelids

	AGAR M
1	X
4	X

Spasm, Face

	BELL	STRAM	OP	CUPR	IGN	HYOSC	ANAC	ARN	CHAM	HYPER	MERC	NIT AC	NUX V	PLUM	SIL
6	X	X	X		X	X	X	X		X	X		X	X	X
8	**X**	X	X		X	**X**	X	X		X	X		X		X
10	X	X	X						X						
13												X			
17	X	X		X	X							X		X	
19				X											
21				X											
26	X	X	X						X						

Spasm, Fingers

	CUPR	ARN	ARS	NAT M	STANN	CALC	CANN S	LYC	CHEL	COCCUL	COFF	CUPR AR	DROS	FERR	HELL	MAG PH	NIT	NUX V	PHOS	SEC	STAPHYS	SULPH	TAB
5		X		X	X				X			X				X							
8			X																				
9	X																						
10	X																						
13		X	X	X	X	**X**	**X**	**X**		X	X		X	X	X		X	X	X	X	X	X	X
14	X																						
26	X																						

Spasm, Flexor Muscles

	CUPR
6	X
8	X

Spasm, Gastric

	ABIES N	AGAR M	ANAC	ASAF	IGN	IPEC	LYC	NUX V
5	X		X	X	X	X	X	X
8		X						

Spasm, Glottis- See also Spasm, Throat (Includes Globus Hystericus)

	BELL	CUPR	IGN	GELS	ACON	ASAF	MOSCH	IPEC	SAMB	VER A	CHLOR	LACH	BROM	MEPH	PLUM	SPONG	ARS	CHEL	CHLOR	COR R	IOD	MAG M
1		X								X			X						X			
4				X																		
5	X		X	X			X					X		X								
6	X	X	X	X		X	X	X	X	X	X	X	X	X	X	X	X			X	X	
7	**X**	X	**X**	X		**X**	**X**	X	X	X	X	**X**	X	X	X	X	X	X	X	X	X	X
8	X	**X**	X	X	X		X	X	X	X	**X**	X	X	X	X	X	X	X		X	X	
9			X			X																
11		X																				
12	X	X		X	X			X	X							X						
13					X										X							**X**
17	X				X	X			X									X	X			
19			X																			
23						X	X				X								X			
26	X	X			**X**			X		X												

Spasm, Hands

	AMBRA	ANAC	BELL	CALC	CANN S	COLOC	CUPR	CYCL	GELS	GRAPH	KALI BIC	MAG PH	NAT M	NAT PH	SULPH AC
5		X						X	X			X		X	
13	X		X	X	X	X				X	X		X		X
14							X								

Spasm, Jaw

	CUPR	HYDR AC	CAUST
11	X		
14	X	X	
21			X
24		X	

Spasm, Larynx (Includes Laryngismus, Laryngismus Stridulus)

	BROM	SAMB	CUPR	GELS	BELL	MEPH	MOSCH	SPONG	CHLOR	IOD	ACON	COR R	IGN	IPEC	LACH	ARS	CHEL	HYOSC	PHOS	PHYTO	SIL	STRAM
1	X		X						X													
2	X	X	X			X	X	X	X						X		X			X		
4		X		**X**																		
5	X	X	X	X	X	X	X	X				X	X	X	X	X						
7	X		X	X						X								X	X		X	X
8	**X**	**X**	**X**	X	X	X	X	X	**X**	**X**	X	X	X	X	X	X	X	X	X	X	X	X
12											X											
14					X																	
17	X	X	X	X	X	X	X	X	X	X	X	X	X	X	X	X	X		X	X	X	
18		X				X		X														X
19	X						X			X												
23												X										
26		X			X						X		X	X				X				

Spasm, Legs

	BELL	CAULO	CINA	COCCUL	CUPR AC	CUPR	EUPH C	HELL	IPEC
7				X	X	X		X	X
8		X	X				X		
21	X								

Spasm, Limbs

	CUPR	BELL	NUX V	BUFO	CAUST	CIC	CUPR AC	HYOSC	IGN	LACH	MERC	MOSCH	PLUM	STRAM	VALER	VER A	VER V
5															X		
6		X							X								
7	X	X	**X**	X	X	X	X	X		X	X	X	X	X		X	X
21	X																
24	X																

Spasm, Lungs- See also Asthma

	CUPR	IPEC	ARG N	IGN	MOSCH	OP	PULS	SAMB	SEP
6			X						
8		X				X			
19	X							X	
26	X	X		X	X		X		X

Spasm, Neck

	CIC	MEDO	AGAR M	CANN I	CIMICI	COD	HYOSC	IGN	LYSS	MAG PH	PALLAD	PHYTO	RAN B	SIL
1		X												
4	X													
7	X	X	X	X		X			X		X	X	X	
8							X			X				X
19					X			X						
24	X													

Spasm, Oesophagus

	CIC	BELL	STRAM	HYOSC	LAURO	VER V	NAJA	LACH	ALUMEN	BAR C	PHOS	ACON	ARS	CALC	PLAT	ASAF	HYDR AC	IGN	LYSS	ZINC	CON
1	X				X																
2			X			**X**				X		**X**								X	
4	X																				
5							X								X	X		X			
6		X	X	X			X												X		
7		X		X	**X**	X	X	X	X				X	X			X				
8	X	X	X	X	X	X	X	**X**	X		X		**X**					X			
11	X			X		X			X	X											
13		**X**	**X**		X			X			X			**X**	**X**		X			X	**X**
14	X									X	X										
18			X													X					
23	X											X							X		
26		X		X																	

Spasm, One Sided- See also Convulsions, One Sided

	BELL
6	X
8	X

Spasm, Pharynx- See also Spasm, Throat

	BELL	AGAR M	CALC	HYOSC	NUX V	STRAM	CHAM	KALI IOD	CAUST	COCCUL	GELS	HYDR AC	IGN	LACH	MAG CAR	SANG N	SULPH
7	X		X		X	X	**X**	**X**			X	X					X
8	X	X	X	X		X			X								
17		X														X	
26	X			X	X					X			X	X	X		

Spasm, Rectum

	NUX M	SIL	AMBRA	ARS	CAUST	CHINA	GRAPH	IGN	KALI BIC	PHOS	PLAT	PLUM	SARS
1	X	X				X			X				X
5	X		X				X	X			X		
7					X					X		X	
8				X									
14		X											

Spasm, Single Muscle Sets

	CROC	IGN
6	X	
10		X

Spasm, Stomach- See also Cramp, Stomach; Vomiting

	COCCUL	IGN	NUX V	ANAC	ASAF	BELL	BISM	CARB V	CHAM	CHINA	COLLIN	COLOC	CON	CUPR	IOD	IPEC	MERC C	PLAT	PULS	SEC	VER V
1																		X			
5				X	X		X									X					
7	X												X	X							X
8	X										X				X						
10																				X	
12			X																		
14						X															
15	X	X	X					X	X	X									X		
17																	X				
18		X																			
21												X									

Spasm, Tetanic- See also Tetanus

	MOSCH	NUX V	ARS	CHAM	ABSINTH	CAMPH	CHIN S	CIC	CINA	COCCUL	CON	CUPR	GELS	HYDR AC	IPEC	NUX M	OENANTH	SOL C	STRYCHN
4	**X**																		
6	X		X				X												
14								X											
17	X	X	X	X	X	X				X	X		X	X			X	X	
19		X																	X
26	X	X		X					X			X			X	X			

Spasm, Throat- See also Spasm, Glottis

	BELL	CUPR	STRAM	MERC C	LACH	IGN	ASAF	GELS	HYOSC	NUX V	CANTH	LAURO	MAG M	MOSCH
1		X	X				X					X	X	X
4				**X**		**X**	**X**							X
5	X	X	X		X	X			X		X			
6					X									
7	X	X	X	X	X			X	X	X				
8							X	X					X	
9	X													
10	X													
13		X								**X**		X		
15			X					X	X					
17	X			X										
18	X			X		X								
19		X			X									
21			X											
24											X			

Spasm, Toe, Great

	CUPR AC	SULPH
1	X	
4		X

Spasm, Toes

	CUPR	ANGUST	ARS	ASAF	CALC	CAUST	CHAM	CIMIC	CUPR AC	FERR	HYOSC	LYC	MOSCH	NUX V	PH AC	PLAT	SEC	STRAM	TAR H	VER A
5		X	X	X	X	X	X	X		X	X	X	X	X	X	X	X	X	X	X
7	X								X											
9	X																			
10	X																			
14	X																			
26	X																			

Spasm, Tongue

	RUTA	AGAR M	SEC	STRAM
1	X	X		X
8			X	
13	X			

Spasm, Tonic

	BELL	CIC	ALUM	AMBRA	ANG	ANT T	CAMPH	CHAM	COCCUL	COLOC	CON	HYOSC	IGN	IPEC	LAURO	LYC	MOSCH	NUX M	NUX V	OP	PETR	PLAT	SEC	SEP	SOL N	STRAM	TAB	VER A
13	**X**	**X**	**X**	**X**	**X**	**X**	**X**	**X**	**X**	**X**	**X**	**X**	**X**	**X**	**X**	**X**	**X**	**X**	**X**	**X**	**X**	**X**	**X**	**X**	**X**	**X**	**X**	**X**
17	X																											
23		X																										

Spasm, Trachea

	AMYL N	ARS	CHLOR	CUPR	GELS	IGN	MOSCH	SPONG
1			X					
7	X	X				X	X	X
8				X				
15					X			

Spasm, Urethra

	NUX V	CAMPH	ACON	BELL	CANTH	CIC	CLEM	COCCUL	COFF	GELS	IGN	PULS	SABAL
1							X						
2	X												
8	X	X	X	X	X	X		X	X	X	X	X	
9		X											
21													X

Spasm, Uterus

	MAG M	CAULO	CHINA	PLAT	CIMICI	COCCUL	CON	GELS	IGN	AMBRA	BELL	BOR	CACT	CHAM	CIC	COLOC	COP	CUPR AR	DIOSC	SEP	TAR H	VER A
1	X																					
4	X	X						X														
5	X	X		X	X					X		X		X		X						X
6	X	X																				
7	X			X			X	X	X		X										X	
8		X	X			X							X				X	X				
10	X	X	X																			
15			X																			
16					X																	
26	X			X		X	X		X						X					X		

Spasm, Vocal Cords

	CHLOR	IPEC
1	X	
7	X	X

Spasticity- See Motion, Involuntary

Speech, Disorders Of- See also Aphasia; Aphonia; Stammering; Stuttering

	CAUST	LACH	NUX V	STRAM	HYOSC	BELL	LYC	CUPR	GELS	CHAM	KALI BR	COCCUL	CON	MERC	MUR AC	OP	PLUM
1	X	X	X	X	X		X	X	X	X	X	X	X	X			
2			**X**				**X**			**X**	**X**						
4		X															
6	X	X	X	X	X	X		X				X			X	X	X
7	X	X	X	X	X	X		X	X			X		X		X	X
8	X	X	X	X	X	X	X			X	X		X	X			X
9	X	X		X													
10	X								X				X		X		
12						X											
13	**X**	X	X	**X**	X	**X**	X	X		X		X	X		X	X	X
14	X																
15					X										X		
17	X		X	X				X								X	
19	X													X			
21		X			X				X								
25							X		X		X						

Sperm, Diminished or Absent- See Azospermia

Spinal Cord, Diseases Of

	FORMICA	ZINC	ANG	APIS	CALC	DULC	KALI PH	PHOS	PIC AC	STRAM
7	**X**	**X**		X	X		X	X		
8			X			X				X
11									X	

Spinal Cord, Degeneration Of

	PIC AC	ARS	AUR M	BAR M	PHOS	PLUM	AGAR M	ALUM	ALUM SIL	ARG N	AUR	CARB S	KALI PH	MAG PH	NAJA	OX AC	PHYSO	STRYCH P	TNT
10	X																		
11	X																		
17	X	**X**	**X**	**X**	**X**	**X**	X	X	X	X	X	X	X	X	X	X	X	X	X

Spine, Curvature Of- See also Pott's Disease

	CALC	CALC PH	SIL	SULPH	CALC FL	PH AC	RHUS T	FERR IOD	LYC	PLUM	PULS	PHOS	ASAF	CARB V	HECLA	KALI IOD	MERC	THUJA
1	X	X	X	X												X		X
2				X				X			X	**X**						
3						X												
4		X																
6	X																	
7	**X**	X	**X**	**X**			X	X						X				
8	X	X	X	X	X		X		X	X								
10		X																
13	X		X	X			X		X	X	X							
14	X	X																
15	X																	
19			X		**X**													
23		X																
27	X	X				X							X		X		X	

Spine, Diseases Of

	PHOS	ALUM	CALC	IGN	NUX V	PLUM	RHUS T	SIL	ZINC	AMM C	ANAC	ARS	BELL	DOLICH	FORMICA	HEP	GUAIAC	LYC	MERC	OLEAND	PARIS	PHYSO	SABAD
2			X			X	X		X		X				X		X			X	X		
3	X		X			X		X		X						X		X					
6	X			X																			
7	X	X		X	X		X	X						X					X				X
8					X				X				X									X	
10	X	X										X											

Sphincters, Atony

	ALOE	APOC	ARS IOD	CAUST	GELS	OXYTROP	PHOS	PLANTAG	SEP
2						X			
8	X	X	X	X			X	X	X
12					X				

Sphincters, Urinary, Atony- See also Incontinence, Urinary

	PLANTAG	FERR	GELS
6	X		
8	X	X	
12			X

Spina Bifida

	CALC	SIL	CALC PH	ARS	LYC	PSOR	SULPH	BRY
1	X	X						
2			**X**			X		**X**
6	X	X	X	X	X		X	
7	X	X				X		
8	X			X	X		X	

Spleen, Congestion- See also Splenomegaly

	ARAN D	CHINA	CEANOTH	BRY	CARD M	CHEL	CHIN S	HELIANTH	NAT M	VER V
1	X			X						
2	X									X
5	X	X	X		X	X		X		
7		X					X			
10		X							X	
28			X							

Spleen, Diseases Of

	CEANOTH	CHINA	BRY	CAPS	SULPH AC	AGAR M	AGNUS	ANAC	ARN	ASAF	BERB V	CARD M	CHIN S	CITRUS L	DULC	EUCAL	IGN	NAT M	NAT SUL	PSOR	PULS	RHUS T	SUCCIN	VER A	URT U
1	X	X	X	X																			X		
2	**X**	X			X	**X**	X				X	X				X			X	X			X	X	**X**
4	**X**	**X**		X					X				X												
6		X	X		X			X		X					X		X				X	X			
7														X				X							
8	X	X	X	X	X	X	X	X	X	X	X		X	X	X	X	X	X	X	X	X	X		X	
10	X	X																							
17												X													
19	X																								

Spleen, Enlargement Of- See Splenomegaly

Spleen, Fatty

	PHOS
7	X
24	X

Splenitis (Includes Lienitis)

	CINA	ACON	ARN	ARS	BRY	CEANOTH	NUX V	SULPH	NAT M	ARAN D	CAPS	IOD	AGAR M	APIS	ASAR	CHIN S	CITRUS L	CON	CUPR	DAPHNE	IGN	LACH	NAT CAR	RAN B				
1					X																	X						
2																	X			X								
7	X		X		X	X	X		X	X				X														
8	**X**	X	**X**	**X**	X	X	X	X	**X**	X	X	X	X		X	X		X			X		X	X				
10				X				X																				
13	**X**	X	X	X			X	X				X							X									
14						X																						
23						X																						
26	X	X	X	X	X		X	X			X																	

Splenomegaly

	CEANOTH	CHINA	ARS	NAT M	FERR	CAPS	FERR ARS	CARB V	CHIN S	SULPH	ARAN D	IOD	PH AC	AGNUS	ARS	FERR IOD	GRIND	IGN	LACH	PHOS	RHUS T	RUTA	QUER G S					
1	**X**	X		X		X	X	X			X					X												
2				**X**			X		X					X		X				X								
3	X				X	X	X		X		X						X						**X**					
4	X	X		X	X	**X**			X		X						X											
5			X		X		X					X				X				X								
6	X	X	X	X	X			X		X			X		X			X	X		X	X						
7	X	**X**	X	X	X				X	X		X						X	X	X								
8	X	X	X	X	X			X	X	X	X	X	X	X			X		X		X	X						
9	X	X		X																								
10	X	X	X			X				X					X													
11			X										X															
12	X		X																									
13		X	X			X						X		X				X				X						
14	X	X	X																									
17	X						X																					
18		X																										
19		X																										
21	X			X																								
23	X						X	X															X					
26		X	X	X	X	X		X		X			X		X						X							
28	X																											

Spondylitis

	CALC FL	NAT M	PHOS	ACT S	ASAF	BELL	CALC ARS	CALC	CALC IOD	CALC PH	CAULO	CAUST	FL AC	GNAPH	HEP	HYPER	IOD	KALI MUR	LED	LACHN	MAG PH	MEDO	MEZ	RHOD	RHUS T	SIL	SULPH	
1	X			X				X			X	X	X	X					X			X		X				
3	X																	X		X	X							
8		**X**	**X**		X	X	X		X	X					X		X						X			X	X	
17																X									X			

Spondylosis, Cervical- See also Neuralgia, Cervico-Brachial; Pain, Neck; Stiffness, Neck

	ACON	AGAR M	ARG N	BRY	CALC FL	CIC	CIMICI	PIC AC	RHUS T
11	X			X					
14						X	X		
17									X
21		X	X					X	
29*					X				

29* Mohan GR, et al, Cervical Spondylosis- a Clinical Study. Brit Hom J, July 1996, 85, 131-133.

Spotted Fever

	AMM C	CIMICI	BRY	EUP PERF	SIL	VER V
1		X				
2	X			X		
6			X		X	X
7	X	X		X	X	
15			X			X
17	X					

Sprains- See also Dislocation; Weakness, Ligaments

	RHUS T	RUTA	ARN	LED	BELLIS	BRY	CALC	AGNUS	NAT CAR	NAT M	STRONT C	AMM C	SIL	AMM M	CARB A	NUX V	PETR	PHOS	PULS	SULPH
1	X	X	X		X															
2	**X**	**X**	**X**					X			X	X		X			X	X		
3	X	X	X	X	E		X													
4	**X**	**X**			X															
5	X	X	**B**	**B**				X	X	X	X		X							
7	**X**	**X**	**X**			X		X				X								
8	X	X	B			X	X	X		X			X		X	X	X	X	X	X
9	X	X	B	X	X	X	X													
10	**<u>X</u>**	X	B				X							X	X					
12	B	B	B																	
13	X	X	X			X	X	X	X	X		X	X	X	X	X	X	X	X	X
14	X	X	**<u>X</u>**	X			X		X											
15	X		X		X															
16		X	X	X	X				X	X	X		X							
17		X																		
18	X	X	X																	
19	**X**	X	**X**	X	X	**X**	X			X	X								X	X
20	**<u>X</u>**																			
21	X	X	**<u>X</u>**	X		X			X											
22	X	X	X	X		X														
23											X									
24	**<u>X</u>**	X			X															
25	B	X	B	B	**X**	X	X													
26	X	X				X						X				X				
28				X																

B- Both Internal and External E- External

Sprain, Achilles Tendon

	KREO	PREDNIS	RHUS T
19	X	X	
22			X

Sprain, Ankle

	LED	RUTA	ARN	RHUS T	STRONT C	NAT CAR	BRY	CALC	CAUST	ARG	CALC FL	NAT M	NAT SUL	SIL	SULPH
1		X													
2					X										
4		**B**													
5						X					X	X		X	
7	**X**	X	**X**	**X**	X										
8	X														
14	X		X	X		X				X					
16	X														
17					X										
18													X		
19	**X**	X	**X**	**X**	**X**		**X**	**X**	**X**						X
20	X														
21		X	X	X											
22	X														
24		**B**													

B- Both Internal and External

Sprain, Easy- See also Dislocation, Easy

	CALC	NAT M	CARB A	LED	NAT CAR	PETR
7			X			X
8			X			
9		X				
18					X	
19	X	X		X		
25	X					

Sprain, Neck

	RHUS T
3	X
19	**X**

Sprain, Shoulder

	RHUS T	SULPH	FERR M	RAN B
19	**X**	**X**	X	X

Sprain, Wrist

	RUTA	ARN	BRY	CALC	CAUST	AMM C	LED	BOV	RHOD	RHUS T	VERBASC	AMBRA	CIST	HEP	HIPPOM	NAT M	NUX V	PHYTO	PULS	SULPH
1	X																			
4	**X**																			
13	X	**X**	**X**	X	X	X		**X**	**X**		**X**	X	X	X			X		X	X
14	X														X			X		
19		X	X	**X**	**X**		X			**X**						X				
22	X						X													
24	**B**																			
26						X														

B- Both Internal and External

Spurs, Bone- See Exostoses

Squint- See Strabismus

Staphyloma

	APIS	LYC	CALC	NIT AC	SULPH	EUPHR	ILEX	ALUM	ANT S A	BELL	CAUST	HEP	MERC	PULS	SENEG	THUJA
1	X						X				X					
2						X	X									
6	X	X	X	X	X	X				X		X	X	X	X	
7	X	X		X				X	X							X
8	**X**	X	X		X	X	X									
26	**X**	X	X	X	X											

Status Epilepticus- See also Epilepsy

	OENANTH
2	X
17	X

Steatoma- See Cysts, Sebaceous

Steatorrhoea

	MERC	DIG	CHEL	PHOS	CHINA	IOD	POD	SULPH	CALC	ACON	ARS	CHAM	HEP	LACH	MYRICA	PH AC	THUJA
8				X		X		X			X						X
10	X	X	X					X	X	X							
11	X		X												X		
12	X			X		X							X				
13	X	X	X		X	X	X	X	X	X	X	X	X	X		X	X
14	X	X	X	X	X		X					X					
15							X		X								
17		X															
19		X		X	X									X	X		
20	X																
21																X	
24	X																
27		X															

Stenosis

	CIC	MERC	NUX V	RHUS T	AGAR M	BAR C	BELL	BRY	CALC PH	CAMPH	CANTH	COCCUL	CONDUR	LAURO	MEZ	NAT M	PHOS	PULS	SPONG
7	**X**	**X**	**X**	**X**	X		X	X		X	X	X			X	X	X	X	X
8						X			X				X	X					

Stenosis, Mitral Valve

	CALC	SIL	SULPH	LAURO	NAT CAR	SABIN	THUJA	CARB A	CARB V	CAUST	FL AC	GRAPH	HEP	LYC	MERC	NIT AC	PHOS	PLAT	PULS	RHUS T	SEC	STAPHYS	STRY ARS	STRY PH
2					X	X													X					
7				X																				
8		X	X		X										X						X			
9						X																		
11	X	X					X	X		X	X	X	X	X		X						X		
12							X																	
13	X		X																					
17				X																			X	X
26	X	X	X						X								X	X		X				

Stenosis, Oesophagus

	CONDUR	BELL	BRY	CIC	FL AC	GELS	HYOSC	LYSS	NAJA	OX AC	VER A
6	X	X	X	X	X	X	X	X	X	X	X
8	X										

Stenosis, Pulmonary

	ASPIDO
11	X
14	**X**

Sterility (Male or Female)- See also Impotence; Weakness, Genital Organs

	CON	AGNUS	NAT CAR	PHOS	NAT M	PLAT	IOD	BOR	ALET	AUR	CALC	CAULO	SULPH AC	AMM C
1		X	X	X		X			X	X		X		
2	**X**	X	X	X	**X**		**X**	**X**	X			X	X	
3		X	X	X		X	X			X	X			
6	X				X									
8	X	X	X	X	X	X		X			X		X	
10	X													
13														**X**

Sterility, Female- See also Conception, Failure Of

	SEP	CON	BOR	PHOS	NAT M	ALET	IOD	CALC	AUR	FERR	NAT CAR	SIL	AGNUS	CANN S	SULPH	BAR M	CANTH	CAUST	HELON	IGN	MERC	MILL	NUX M	AUR M N	GRAPH	HYOSC	SULPH AC
1						X																					
3	**X**	X	X			X																		**X**			
4																			X								
6	X																	X									
7	X		X	X	**X**		X	X		X	X	X				X	X						X				
8		X	X	**X**	X	X	X	X	X	X	X		X	X	X	X	X		X		X	X	X				
9	X	X	X	X	X		X		X			X															
13	**X**	**X**	X	**X**	X			**X**		X	X		**X**	**X**	**X**			X			X	X			**X**	**X**	**X**
21	X	X																									
23						X														X							
25	X	X	X	X	X		X		X			X								X							
29*	X																										

29* Williamson AV, et al. A Trial of Sepia 200. Brit Hom J, 1995, 84, 1, 14-20.

Sterility, Male- See Azospermia; Impotence

Stiffness

	RHUS T	BRY	PHYTO	ANAC	ANGUST	ARS	BELL	CAUST	CIMICI	COFF	MOSCH	RUTA	SANG	STRAM
5									X					
6			X								X			
8	X	X		X		X	X			X	X		X	X
9	X	X										X		
10	X		X				X			X			X	X
11		X			X									
13				X										
14	X													
17	X													
18	X													
19	X		X		X			X	X			X		
21	X							X						
24						X								
27	X													

Stiffness, Ankles

	SULPH	CHEL	PETR	RHUS T	RUTA	SEP	BRY	CARB A	CAUST	COLOC	DROS	LYC	PULS	SIL
6			X											
7	**X**	X	X	X		X				X				
9				X	X		X						X	
13	X	X			X	X		X	X		X	X		X

Stiffness, Arm

	NUX V	CHAM	AGAR M	AMM C	AMM M	CANTH	CAPS	HAM	HYOSC	KALI CAR	LYC	MENY	MERC SU	NAT CAR	PETR	PHYTO	PLAT	RHUS T	SARS	SEP
7	X							X												
8									X											
13	**X**	**X**	X	X	X	X	X			X	X	X	X	X	X		X	X	X	X
14																X				

Stiffness, Back- See also Stiffness, Spine

	RHUS T	BRY	BELL	BERB V	CAUST	CIMICI	GINSENG	LACHN	LED	PETR	SEP	STRYCHN
1								X				
5						X						
7	X			X						X		
8	X	X	X	X					X		X	
10			X									
11		X										
13					X				X	X	X	
14	X	X	X	X	X	X		X				X
15	X	X				X						
17							X					X
19	X				X		X					
21	X											

Stiffness, Back, Lower- See also Stiffness, Sacrum

	AESC	BENZ AC	BRY	CARB A	PHOS	RHUS T	SEP	SULPH
7		X	X	X			X	
19	X							
21						X		
24								X
26					X			

Stiffness, Chest

	ALL C	AUR	RHUS T
8	X		
19		X	X

Stiffness, Elbow

	BRY	PULS	SEP	ALUM	ANG	ASAF	BELL	CALC	KALI CAR	LACH	PHOS	RHUS T	RUTA	SPIG	SULPH	ZINC
7			X					X								
9	X	X										X	X			
13	X	X	X	X	X	X	X		X	X	X			X	X	X

Stiffness, Extremities

	CALC PH	MAG PH	PHYTO
5		X	
6			X
11	X		

Stiffness, Eyelids

	KALM	APIS	ALUM OX	CAUST	GELS	NUX M	VER A
4	X			X	X		
7	**X**	**X**				X	X
8	X		X				

Stiffness, Eyes, Motion Of

	KALM	NAT M	CALC	ONOS	PHOS	RHUS T
6		X				
8	X		X		X	X
12	X					
24		X		X		

Stiffness, Feet

	APIS	ARS	DROS	STICTA	SEP	AMBRA	CALC	CAPS	CHEL	FERR	GRAPH	IGN	KALI BIC	KALI CAR	LACH	LAURO	LED	PETR	RAN B	RHUS T	RUTA	SEC	SULPH	SULPH AC	ZINC
5			X																						
6		X																							
7	X			X			X			X				X								X			
8		X		X																					
13			X		**X**	X		X	X		X	X	X		X	X	X	X	X	X			X	X	X
14	X																				X				
21	X																								

Stiffness, Fingers

	AMYL N	CARB A	CAULO	RHUS T
1			X	X
7	X	X	X	
8	X			
13		X		X

Stiffness, Hands

	STICTA	ASAF	CALC	CARB A	CHAM	COLOC	CUPR	FERR	HYOSC	KREO	MERC	RUTA
7	X		X	X		X	X	X				
8	X											
13		X			X				X	X	X	
14												X

Stiffness, Hip

	RHUS T	BELL	ACON	AGAR M	ANANTH	BAR C	BRY	EUPHR	HELL	PULS	RHEUM	RUTA	STAPHYS
8	X	X			X								
9	X						X			X		X	
13	X	X	X			X		X	X		X		X
17				X									
25	X												

Stiffness, Jaw

	BELL	CAUST	MEZ	ANG	GELS	LACH	LYC	LYSS	MERC	MERC C	RHUS T
6		X	X	X			X				
7		X	X		X	X			X	X	X
8	X							X			
24	X										

Stiffness, Joints- See also Rheumatism; Rheumatoid Arthritis; Synovitis

	RHUS T	CAUST	BRY	COLCH	LYC	PETR	COCCUL	COLOC	RUTA	CAPS	ABROT	CIMICI	FORMICA	LED	NAT M	PULS	SIL	STAPHYS	TRIOST	CARB A	SEP
1	X		X	X														X			
2																			X		
4		X																			
5													X		X		X				
6					X																
7		**X**			X	X	X			X			X	X	X						
8	X			X		X		X											X		
9	X		X						X		X					X					
10	X	X															X				
11	X		X								X										
12		X										X									
13	X	X	X	X	**X**	**X**	X	X	X	**X**						X		X		**X**	**X**
14				X				X													
15														X							
16			X																		
19	X	X					X		X			X									
21	X																				

Stiffness, Knee

	BRY	PETR	CAUST	NAT SUL	NUX V	SULPH	LED	ARS	COLOC	LACH	LYC	NIT AC	PHOS	PULS	RHUS T	SEP	AMM M	GRAPH										
4					X																							
5			X	X																								
6				X				X																				
7		X	X	X		**X**	X		X	X	X	X		X		X												
8		X			X								X															
9	X													X	X													
11	X																											
13	**X**	X			X	**X**	**X**	X	X	X	X	X	X		X	X	**X**	**X**										
14	X	X	X																									

Stiffness, Legs

	RHUS T	NUX V	CON	FERR	BERB V	BRY	CIC	HYDR AC	PHYSO	ACON	ARG N	AUR	CARB S	COCCUL	GINSENG	HYOSC	LAC C	LATH	MAG PH	PETR	PULS	SARS	SPONG	TRIOST	ZINC			
6		X																										
7	**X**	X		X	X	X	X	X											X	X			X					
8		X		X	X		X	X	X			X		X	X	X								X				
10		X	X																		X							
13	X			X		X				X												X			X			
14			X								X						X											
16			X																									
18	X																											
21	X																	X										
24									X																			
25													X															

Stiffness, Limbs

	RHUS T	NUX V	BELL	ARS	CHINA	MERC	OLEAND	PETR	SULPH	ACON	ARN	BRY	CAUST	CHAM	LITH C	OX AC	PLUM	VER A	CAPS	CHEL	PLAT	TEREB	THUJA					
6				X		X	X									X												
7	X			X	X	X		X					X							**X**								
8	X	X	X	X			X			X					X	X		X										
9	X	X																										
10					X	X	X																					
12																	X											
13	**X**	X	**X**					**X**	**X**	X	X	X	X	X	X		X	X	**X**		**X**	**X**	**X**					
15					X							X		X														
24			X																									
25		X																										
26									X		X																	

Stiffness, Neck (Includes Stiffness, Cervical; Stiffness, Nape; Stiffness, Occiput)

	BELL	BRY	CIMICI	ACON	CAUST	RHUS T	DULC	LACHN	NAT CAR	CHEL	LACH	LYC	ARS	CALC	CALC PH	MERC I R	ZINC	AGAR M	BAR C	HELL	KALI CAR
1				X	X			X													
2		**X**	**X**	**X**			**X**	X		**X**					X						
3	X	X	X	X		X	X	X													
4	X																				
5						X				X											
6	X	X	X			X		X	X		X	X	X								
7	**X**		X		**X**	X	X	X	X	X	**X**		X	X	X		X	**X**	**X**	X	X
8	X	X	X	X	X	X		X	X		X	X	X	X	X	X	X	X	X	X	
9	X	X																			
11	X	X	X	X	X		X	X								X	X				
12	X			X			X														
13	**X**	**X**			X	**X**	**X**		X		X	**X**	X	X			X	X	X	**X**	**X**
14	X	X	X		X	X	X	X		X						X					
15		X		X		X															
17							X									X					
18			X					X													
19			**X**		X	X									X						
20							X														
21	X		X	X	X																
24	X								X												
25	X		X	X	X			X													
26	X	X		X	X							X		X							X
27		X				X															

Stiffness, Os Uteri

	GELS	BELL	ACON	CIMICI	CAULO	LOB I	VER V
6	X						
7							X
13	X	X	X	X	X	X	
25	X	X					

Stiffness, Sacrum- See also Stiffness, Back, Lower

	LACH	ACON	AMM M	APIS	BAR C	BERB V	BRY	LAURO	LED	LYC	MEPH	PRUN S	PULS	RHEUM	RHUS T	SIL	SULPH	THUJA
8	X			X														
13	X	X	X		X	X	X	X	X	X	X	X	X	X	X	X	X	X

Stiffness, Shoulders

	PETR	HAM	INDIUM	KALI BIC	LYC	SANG	SPIG
6	X						
7	X	X	X		X		
13				X			
20							X
27						X	

Stiffness, Shoulder, Left

	NAT CAR
6	X
24	X

Stiffness, Spine- See also Stiffness, Back

	PHYSO	CALC FL	CIMICI	AGAR M	ARS	BELL	CALC PH	GRAPH	PHYTO
3	X			X					
5								X	
6			X						
8					X				
19		**X**					X		X
24	X					X			

Stiffness, Tendons

	RHUS T	CAUST
1		X
5	X	
9	X	

Stiffness, Throat

	CAUST	MERC I R	RHUS T
8	X		
14		X	
17			X

Stiffness, Toes

	GRAPH	APIS	COLOC	SIL	SULPH
7		**X**	X		
8	X				
13	**X**			X	X

Stiffness, Tongue

	COLCH	BOR	EUPHR	LACH	NAT M	ARS	CARB V	LYC	SEP	BERB V	CON	HELL	HYDR AC	LAC C	MERC	MERC C	MERC I R	NICCOL	NUX M	PHOS
5														X						
6	X	X	X		X	X	X		X											X
8	X	X	X	X	X			X											X	
10	X			X		X			X											
13	**X**	X	X	X	X		X	X		X	X	X	X		X	X		X		
17																	X			

Stiffness, Vertebra- See Stiffness, Spine

Stiffness, Wrist

	CHEL	RHUS T	RUTA	SEP	BELL	BRY	KALI CAR	LYC	MERC	NAT SUL	PHYTO	PULS	SABIN	STAPHYS	SULPH
7	X			X											
9		X	X			X						X			
13	X	X		X	**X**		X	X	X	X			X	X	X
14			X								X				

Still-Birth, Tendency To- See Abortion, Threatened

Stings- See Bites and Stings, Effects Of

Stomacace- See also Aphthae

	MERC	STAPHYS	NUX V	SULPH	CAPS	CARB V	HELL	ARS	BOR	DULC	HEP	NAT M	NIT AC
6	X	X	X	X			X	X			X		X
8		X	X										
13	**X**	X	X	X	**X**	**X**	**X**	X	X	X	X	X	X
26	**X**	X		X	X	X			X	X		X	

Stomach, Congestion (Includes Stomach, Catarrh)

	NUX V	ALUM	ANT C	ANT T	ARS	BRY	CHAM	CHEL	CHINA	COCA	COLOC	COP	DIG	GELS	HYDR AC	IGN	IPEC	ISIR V	KALI BIC	LYC	MERC	MEZ	POD	PULS	RHUS T	STAPHYS	SULPH	VER A
5	X															X				X						X		
7	X	X	X	X	X	X	X	X	X	X	X	X	X	X	X		X	X	X		X	X	X	X	X		X	X

Stomach, Diseases Of

	PULS	ANT C	NUX V	ARS	PHOS	BRY	CARB V	LYC	CHINA	HYDRAST	ROBIN	VER A	ASAF	CHAM	CUPR	IPEC	KALI CAR	ANT T	CALC	COFF	DORYPH	HEP	LAC C	NAT M	SULPH			
2		**X**		**X**			**X**			X	X				X		**X**				X		X					
6			X																									
7	**X**	**X**	**X**	**X**	X	**X**	X	X	X	X	X	**X**	**X**	X			X	X		X	X	X	X	X				
9	X		X		X			X																				
10	X	X	X	X	X	X	X		X							X			X			X			X			
13	**X**	X	**X**	**X**	**X**	**X**		**X**	X		X	**X**	X	**X**	**X**	**X**		X	X	X				X	X			
14		X																										
15	X									X																		
26	X	X																										

Stomatitis

	MERC	BOR	NIT AC	KALI CHL	ARS	HEP	MUR AC	HYDRAST	SULPH	ARUM T	CHINA	BAPT	CAPS	SULPH AC	LACH	ACON	APIS	BELL	NAT M	CANTH	MERC C	NUX V	PHOS	STAPHYS	CARB V			
1		X			X	X				X			X					X	X		X							
2	X			X					X			X	X						**X**						X			
3	X		X			X				X																		
4			X	**X**				**X**		X		X																
5		X	X	X	X	X	X				X			X						X	X		X					
6	X	X			X	X			X			X		X										X				
7	X						X	X					X											X				
8	X	X	X		X	X	X	X	**X**	X	X	**X**	X	X	X		X		X	X	X	X	X	X	**X**			
9		X	X				X								X		X											
10	X	X							X		X											X						
12	X		X	X		X			X		X																	
13	**X**														X	X		**X**		X		X						
14																	X											
15		X			X		X	X			X					X		X					X					
17			X	X	X		X								X													
18	X	X																										
23		X		X				X		X				X		X												
24	X																											

Stomatitis, Ulcerative

	SULPH AC	MERC	MUR AC	SULO AC	ALUMEN	ARS	BENZ AC	HEP	KALI IOD	KALI MUR	LACH	MERC C	NIT AC	PHOS	PHYTO	THUJA												
1		X	X					X				X		X														
2				X																								
7				X						X																		
8	X	X	X		X	X	X		X		X		X		X	X												
18	X																											
24	X																											

Stool, Bloody- See also Haemorrhage, Bowel; Haemorrhage, Intestinal/Rectal (Includes Stools, Black; Malaena)

	MERC	**MERC C**	**ARS**	**SULPH**	**BAPT**	**PHOS**	**CANTH**	**COLOC**	**NUX V**	**RHUS T**	**CARB V**	**ARN**	**CAPS**	**COLCH**	**IPEC**	**NIT AC**	**PULS**	**HAM**	**ARG N**	**DULC**	**KALI BIC**	**LACH**	**NAT M**	**PLUM**				
1		X																				X						
2																		X										
4			X				X																					
5		X				X																						
6	X		X	X	X		X	X	X		X		X	X	X	X		X			X		X	X				
7	**X**	**X**	X		X	**X**	**X**	**X**	**X**	X		**X**	**X**	**X**	x	X	X	**X**	X		X	X		X				
8	X		X	X	X	X		X	X	X	X	X	X	X	X	X	X	X	X	X			X	X				
9		X																										
10	X	X	X	X		X		X	X	X	X			X	X		X											
11	X	X			X		X	X			X	X	X	X			X											
12	X	X													X													
13	**X**	**X**	X	**X**	X	**X**	X	X	X	**X**	X	X	X	X	**X**	**X**	**X**		X	X	X	X	X	X				
14	X	X	X	X	X					X	X	X	X					X										
15	X			X	X	X	X									X												
16										X																		
18	X	X																		X								
19		X	X	X		X			X	X	X	X				X					X		X					
21	X	X			X																							
22			X																									
24	X		X	X			X												X			X						
26	X		X	X				X	X						X					X								
28	X																											

Strabismus (Includes Squint)

	GELS	BELL	HYOSC	CIC	CYCL	ALUM	SPIG	STRAM	CINA	JAB	SULPH	AGAR M	ZINC	SEP	TAB	APIS	CALC	KALI IOD	MAG PH	MORPH	NAT M	NUX V	PLUM	SEC				
1	**X**		X		X		X											X	X									
2	X			X	X	X	X	X	X	X			X		X					X		X		X				
3	X	X				X			X																			
4	X						X									X												
5			X	X	X																							
6	X	X	X	X	X	X	X	X	X	X	X	X		X			X											
7	X	**X**	**X**	X			X		X				X															
8	X	X	X	X	X	X	X	X	X	X	X	X	X	X	X		X	X	X			X	X					
9	X																											
10						X																						
11	X	X	X	X	X			X		X			X							X								
12	X	X	X				X	X	X		X																	
13		**X**	**X**		X	**X**	X	X								X								X				
14	**X**		X	X							X																	
15	X	X						X																				
17		X		X	X	X		X				X									X							
19				X																								
21	**X**					X																						
24	X	X	X	X	X		X	X	X	X	X	X		X	X								X					
25	X																											
26		X	X			X																						
27		X		X	X																X							

Strain, Eyes- See also Ailments from Reading; Vision, Weakness

	RUTA	NAT M	ONOS	GELS	ARN	CALC	EUPHR	LED	PHOS	PHYSO	APIS	AUR	CIMICI	GRAPH	RHUS T													
1	X																											
2		X								X																		
4	X		X																									
6	X														X													
8	X		X						X	X		X		X														
9	X	X		X		X	X	X					X															
10	X										X																	
11			X																									
12				X	X																							
14	X																											
18	X																											
19	X		X																									
21	X	X			X				X																			
22	X																											
25	X	X		X		X	X	X																				
26	X																											
27	X																											
28	X																											

Strain, Muscular

	RHUS T	ARN	CALC	BRY	RUTA	AGNUS	CALC FL	CARB A	LED	SIL	BELLIS	COCCUL	LYC	NAT CAR	NAT M	NUX V	PULS	SULPH
1	X	X																
2			X				X			X			X					
3			X	X							X	X					X	X
4	X																	
5		B			X	X	X		X	X				X	X			
7			X					X										
8	**X**	**X**	X			X	X	X								X		
9	X	B	X	X	X				X		X							
10	X	X	X															
13	X	X	X	X	X	X		X		X		X	X	X	X	X	X	X
14	<u>**X**</u>	<u>**X**</u>																
15	X			X														
20	<u>**X**</u>																	
21	X	<u>**X**</u>		X	X				X									
22	X	X																
27	<u>**X**</u>				X													

B- Both Internal and External

Strain, Tendon

	RHUS T	RUTA	CON
4		X	
7			X
14	<u>**X**</u>		
24		X	

Strangury- See Dysuria
Strangulated Hernia- See Hernia
Strangury, Bladder- See Tenesmus, Bladder
Stress- See also Anxiety

	IGN	AUR	CHAM	HYOSC	NUX V	VER A	NAT M
3	X	X			X		**X**
4				X	X	X	
5	X			X		X	
19	X	X					
21	X						
29[1]			X				
29[2]			X				

29[1] Reis LS, et al. Matricaria chamomilla CH12 decreases handling stress in Nelore calves. J Vet Sci, 2006, Jan, 7, 2, 189-92.
29[2] Pinto SA, et al. An animal model for the study of Chamomilla in stress and depression: pilot study. Homeopathy. 2008 Jul;97 (3):141-4.
Stretch Marks- See Striae

Striae

	CALC FL	AESC	CALEND	GRAPH
5	X	E	E	E
21	X			

E- External

Stricture

	THIO	CHIM	MEDO	PULM	PRUN S	RHUS T	SYPH	TEREB
1	X							
2	X	X	X	X	X	X	X	X

Stricture, Oesophagus

	NAJA	BAPT	ARS	BELL	ALUMEN	CAJUPUT	CIC	CONDUR	KALI CAR	LYSS	PHOS	PLUM	BAR C	CARB V	GELS	MERC C
2	**X**	X			X	X	X					X			**X**	**X**
6								X								
7	X	**X**	**X**	X					X	X			**X**			
8	**X**	X	X	**X**	X		X		X	X	X	X		**X**		
9						X										
10								X								
14											X					

Stricture, Rectum

	ALOE	THIO	BELL	BOR	CANN S	HYDRAST	NITAC	PLUM	RUTA	SYPH	TAB
1		X				X	X		X		
2		X								X	X
7	X			X							
8	X				X			X			
11			X								

Stricture, Urethra

	CLEM	PULS	SIL	PETR	ACON	CANTH	IOD	MERC	SULPH	CAMPH	ARG N	BELL	DULC	NIT AC	NUX V	AGAR M	BERB V	CANN S	COFF	CON	DIG	ERIG	KALI IOD	NAT M	OP	RHUS T	STRAM	THUJA
1	X		X																						X		X	
2	**X**		X	X	**X**					**X**																		
3	X																											
6	X	X		X		X			X				X								X					X		
7	X	**X**	X	X		X	X	X	X		X			X			X	X		X			X	X				
8	X	X	X	X	X	X	X	X	X	X	X	X	X	X	X	X	X	X	X	X	X	X	X	X	X	X	X	X
11		X																										
12	X	X					X								X	X												
13	**X**			**X**							X	X	X															
14		X																										
19	**X**																											
21			X		X	X		X		X																		
24	X	X	X		X		X	X	X			X		X	X				X			X						X

Stroke- See also Hemiplegia (AKA Apoplexy)

	ARN	ACON	OP	BELL	NUX V	LACH	BAR C	LAURO	GLON	GELS	PHOS	HYOSC	IPEC	ANAC	COCCUL	PULS	VER V	AST R	CAUST	CUPR	NAT M	NUX M	PLUM	RHUS T	STRAM	COFF	CROT T	LYC
1	X	X	X	X	X	X		X	X	X						X												
2	**X**	**X**	**X**	**X**	**X**	X	X		X					X			X	X	X			X			X	X	X	
3	X	X	**X**			X	X	**X**				X								X								
4	X	X	**X**	**X**	X			**X**	X			X																
6	X	X	X		X	X	X							X					X	X			X		X			
7	**X**	**X**	**X**	**X**	**X**	**X**	X	X	**X**	X	X	X	X	**X**	X		X	X				X	X		X		X	
8	**X**	X	**X**	**X**	**X**	X	**X**	X	X	X	X	X	X	X	X	X	X	X	X	X		X	X	X	X	X	X	X
9	X	X	X	X	X		X	X	X	X	X							X					X	X				
10	X	X	X	X			X									X			X									
11	X	X	X	X	X	X		X			X						X											
12		**X**		X	**X**		X				X				X									X				
13	**X**	**X**	**X**	X	X	**X**	**X**	**X**	X		X	**X**	**X**	X		**X**						X	X	X		**X**		**X**
14	X		**X**	X		X													X									
15	X	**X**	**X**	X	X	X																						
16	X	X	X	X	X	X			X	X																		
17	**X**	**X**	X	**X**		**X**	X	**X**	**X**	**X**	X	X	**X**		**X**	X	**X**	X		X		X		X		X	**X**	X
19						X																						
21	X	X	X		X		X	X		X		X																
23		X	X		X		X																					
24	X																											
25	X	X	X	X	X		X	X	X		X																	
26	X	X	X	**X**	X	X	X		X	X	X	X	X		X	X	X			X					X			X
27	**X**	X		X	X	X	X			X			X	X	X													
28				X																								

Stroke, Prophylaxis

	ARN	OP	CACT	CARB V	GLON	NUX V
9	X	X		X		
16	X		X			X
25	X	X			X	

Strophulus

	CHAM	ANT C	CALC	CANTH	PULS	SULPH
12	**X**	X	X	X	X	X

Struma- See Goiter

Stupor (Includes Drowsiness; Sleepiness; Somnolence; Sopor)

	OP	ANT T	BELL	GELS	NUX M	APIS	BAPT	ARN	HYOSC	RHUS T	LACH	BRY	PH AC	HELL	SULPH	NUX V	AETHUSA	CAMPH	CHAM	PHOS	PULS	LYC	MUR AC	ZINC	CAUST	NAT M
1							X	X	X						X		X			X	X				X	X
2	X														X									X		
3													X				X				X					
5					X																					
6	X	X	X	X	X	X	X	X	X	X	X	X	X	X	X		X	X	X	X	X	X	X		X	X
7	X	**X**	**X**	X	**X**	X	**X**	X	X	X	**X**	X	**X**	X	X	**X**		X		X	X	X	X		**X**	**X**
8	X	X	X		X	X			X		X	X	X		X	X		X	X	X	X	X	X	X	X	X
9	X	X		X	X	X										X										
10	X	X	X	X			X	X	X	X	X	X		X	X				X	X			X			
11	X	X		X	X	X	X		X	X		X	X	X			X	X						X		
12	X			X						X													X			
13	**X**	X	**X**	X	X	X		**X**	**X**	X	X	X	**X**	X	X	X	X	X	X	X	X	X	X	X	X	X
14	X	X	X	X	X	X	X			X	X															
15	X	X	X	X			X	X	X		X	X	X	X		X			X							
16		X	X	X							X								X							
17	X	X		X	X	X	X	X	X	X			X	X			X	X		X				X		
18		X			X	X																				
19	X	X	X				**X**	X		X												X				
20			X													X										
21	X				X		X	X									X									
22		X	X									X														
24	X		X	X	X	X	X	X		X				X								X		X		
25	X			X		X																				
26	X	X	X						X		X	X			X	X		X	X		X					
27	X	X		X		X																				

Stammering (Includes Stuttering)

	STRAM	CAUST	HYOSC	CUPR	BOV	BELL	MERC	NAT CAR	EUPHR	PLAT	SULPH	BUFO	LACH	SEC	ARS	ACON	AGAR M	CANN S	CIC	KALI BR	LYC	NUX V	OP	PHOS	VER A	ZINC	CANN I	SEL
1	**X**	X	X		X			X				X	X			X			X	X	X				X			
2	**X**	X	**X**		X			X				X		X				X	X		X			X			X	X
3	X	X	X		X	X	X	X	X	X	X		X						X									
5			X																	X								
6	X			X		X								X	X						X		X		X			
7	X	X		X		X	X	X		X	X		X							X		X		X				
8	X	X			X	X	X	X	X	X		X		X		X											X	X
9	X		X	X											X		X									X		
10		X				X	X		X	X	X																	
13	**X**	X	X		**X**	X	X	X	**X**		X	X	X	X		X						X	X		X			
14	X	X		X	X													X										
15	X			X																								
17	X	X		X	X													X					X	X				
19		X																										
21	X		X	X			X										X					X				X		
25	X		X	X											**X**		X									X		
26		X				X	X		X	X																		

Stye- See also Chalazion (AKA Hordeolum)

	PULS	STAPHYS	HEP	SULPH	GRAPH	SIL	THUJA	LYC	SEP	CALC	PH AC	ACON	AMM C	APIS	CON	FERR	MERC	NAT M	PHOS	PIC AC	RHUS T	SENEG	STANN	URAN N	BRY	CANTH	CAUST	ZIZIA
1	X	X	X																									
2	**X**	**X**	X						X											X		X	X	X				X
3	**X**	X	X			X	X																					
4	**X**	X						X																				
5	X	X			X	X	X		X						X			X										
6	**X**	X	X	X															X	X								
7	**X**	**X**			X	X	X				X			X														
8	**X**	**X**		**X**	X	X	X	X	X	X	X		X		X	X	X	X	X	X	X	X	X	X	X	X	X	X
9	X				X																							
10	**X**		X	X		X																						
12	**X**	**X**		X						X		X																
13	X	X		X	X			X	X		X		X		X	X	X		X		X		X		X			
14	**X**	X						X						X														
15	X		X									X																
16	X	X																										
17																								X				
18		X																										
20	**X**	X	X		X									X														
21	**X**	X																										
24	**X**	X	X	X	X		X	X		X	X		X			X	X	X			X	X				X	X	
25	**X**	X	X	X						X		X																
26	**X**	X				X	X		X																			
27		X																										
28			X																									

Stye, Left Side

	LYC	PULS	STAPHYS	COLCH	ELAPS	URAN N
6	X	X	X	X		
8	X	X	X			X
13					X	

Stye, Lower Lid

	RHUS T	PHOS	GRAPH	PULS	SENEG	SENNA	STAPHYS
6	X	X				X	X
8	X	X	X	X	X		
13	X						

Stye, Lower Lid, Left

	HYPER
8	X
13	X

Stye, Right Side

	CALC	CANTH	NAT M
6	X	X	X
8	X	X	X

Stye, Upper Lid

	FERR	PH AC	ALUM	CAUST	MERC	PULS	SULPH	AMM C	STAPHYS	URAN N
6	X	X	X	X	X		X			
8	X	**X**	X	X	X	X	X	X	X	X
13	X					X				

Subsultus Tendinum- See Twitch, Tendons

Sudamena- See also Milaria (AKA Miliaria crystallina)

	BRY	AMM C	ARS	BELL	LACH	PH AC	RHUS T	SULPH AC	VAL
8	**X**	X	X	X	X	X	X	X	X

Sunburn- See also Burns

	SOL	BELL	ACON	CANTH	APIS	GELS	GLON	LACH	NAT M	OP	PHYSAL	RHUS T
1	**X**	X	X			X	X	X	X	X		
2	X											
5		X		X	X							X
14				X								
19		X	X									
21	X											
28											X	

Sunstroke– See also Ailments from Sun; Headache, Sun from (Includes Heat Exhaustion; Heatstroke)

	GLON	BELL	GELS	LACH	NAT CAR	ACON	CAMPH	BRY	VER V	AMYL N	OP	NAT M	CARB V	CUPR	STRAM	ANT C	THERID	CACT	AGAR M	ANAC	ARN	ARS	MELILOT	SANG	SIL	SOL	VER A
1	X	X		X							X									X							
2	**X**		X				X		X	X	X	X			X	X		**X**								X	
3	X	X	**X**	X			X			X	X	**X**					X								X		
4	**X**	**X**	X	X	**X**	X																					
5	**X**	**X**	**X**	X				X																X			
6	**X**	X	**X**	X	X	X	X	X	X	X	X		X		X	X			X	X		X					
7	**X**		X	X		X			X	X	X	X			X							X					
8	X	X	X	X	X	X	X	X	X	X	X	X	X			X	X	X	X		X				X		
10	X	X	X	X	X	X						X	X								X		X				
12	X	X				X	X																				
14	**X**			X	X		X		X															X			
15		X				X		X																			
16	**X**																										
17	X	X			X				X						X		X										
18	X	X		X	X	X		X	X														X				
19	X	X	X	X	X	X							X	X												X	
20	**X**	**X**												X													X
21	X	X						X						X													
22	X	X												X													X
23	X				X		X																				
24							X																				
25	X	X	X		X					X																	
26	**X**	X				X		X																			

Sunstroke, Prophylaxis

	ACON	ILEX P
15	X	
16		X

Suppuration

	HEP	SIL	CALEND	MERC	ARS	CHINA	SULPH	ARN	BUFO	CALC S	LACH	MYRIST	RHUS T	STAPHYS
2	X	X	X		X			X	X			X		
8	**X**	**X**	X	X		X	**X**	X	X		X		X	X
9	X	X			X						X			
10	X			X										
11	X													
12	X	X			X	X								
16	X	X	E	X								X		
17										X				
18	**X**													
19	X		X											X
21	X													
23	X	X								X				
24	X	X	B	X		X	X						X	

B- Both Internal and External E- External

Surgery, Effects Of- See Ailments from Surgery

Surgical Shock- See Shock, Surgical

Swallowing, Difficult- See Dysphagia

Swelling- For all entries here see also site-specific Oedema

Swelling, Achilles Tendon

	KALI BIC	SEP
7		X
14	X	

Swelling, Ankle

	APIS	ASAF	ARG	ARS	LACH	MANG	STANN
1	X		X				
2	**X**						
7	X	X			X		
8						X	
9					X		
10	X			X			
13		X				X	**X**
14			X				
21	X			X			

Swelling, Arm

	ARS	BELL	BRY	RHUS T	SULPH	ACON	ALUM	ANT C	APIS	BAR C	CROT H	DULC	LACH	MERC	SEP	SIL
7	X								X				X			
13	**X**	**X**	**X**	**X**	**X**	X	X	X		X	X	X		X	X	X

Swelling, Bones

	MERC	ASAF	AUR	CALC	FL AC	SIL	GUAIAC	LYC	PH AC	PHOS	STAPHYS	SULPH	KALI IOD	NIT AC	PULS	RUTA	CLEM	DAPHNE	HECLA	LAC AC	MEZ	PHYTO	RHUS T
6				X	X		X		X	X			X								X		
7	X	X	X	X	X	**X**	X	X	X	X	X	X	X	X	X	X				X		X	
8	X	X	X	X		X	X	X	X	X	X	X		X	X	X	X	X					X
10	X	X	X		X																		
14	X																						
24	X																		X				
26	X	X	X	X	X	X		X			X	X											

Swelling, Bones, Skull

	AUR FL	AUR	AUR M	CALC PH	SIL
6	X		X		
10				X	
13		X			X

Swelling, Breast- See also Milk Fever (Includes Breast, Engorgement)

	BELL	BRY	CON	PHYTO	PULS	CALC	APIS	CHAM	PHOS	ARN	LAC C	AST R	CLEM	HEP	RHUS T	SIL	SULPH
1	X																
3								X		X							
5	X			X			X										
6	X	X	X	X			X		X						X		
7	X	X	X	X	X			X		X	X	X	X				X
8	X	X				X		X	X	X				X		X	
9	X	X	X	X	X	X					X						
10	X	X	X		X										X		
13	X	X	X	X	X	X		X	X				X	X		X	X
14											X	X					
17			X														
18	X	X					X										
21		X	X		X	X											
24	X	X		X			X		X								
25					X												
27						X											

Swelling, Cheek

	BELL	CHAM	ARN	KALI CAR	MERC	NUX V	PULS	BRY	SEP	SULPH	ARS	AUR	CARB V	CAUST	HEP	LACH	KALI IOD	SPONG	STANN									
1				X																								
8	**X**	**X**	**X**		X	X	X	**X**	**X**	**X**	X	X	X	X	X	X												
12	X	X																										
13	X	**X**	X	**X**	X	X	X	X	X		X	X	X	X			**X**	**X**	**X**									
14				X																								
26	**X**	X	X		X	X	X			X					X	X												

Swelling, Ear

	CALC	CIST	KREO	NAT M	PULS	SEP	TELL	ACON	ALUM	ANAC	ANT C	APIS	BAR C	BELL	CALC PH	CAPS	CAUST	KALI CAR	LACH	MERC	NIT	PSOR	RHUS T	SIL	SPONG	ZINC		
7	X			X																								
8		X	X			X									X	X			X									
13	X	X	X	X	X	X	X	**X**	X	X	X	X		X			X	X			X	X	X	X	X	X		
14													X							X								
22					X																							
24							X																					

Swelling, Eyelids

	APIS	ARG N	KALI CAR	RHUS T	BELL	EUPHR	GRAPH	MERC	NIT AC	ACON	ARS	DIG	KALI IOD	AM BEN	CHAM	HEP	NAPHTH	PSOR	PULS	NAT CAR								
1																	X											
3	X			X																								
4																	X											
5	X					X					X																	
6	X	X		X				X				X			X	X												
7		**X**		**X**	X	X	X	**X**	X	X		X						X	X	**X**								
8	X		X				X		**X**					X														
9					X		X			X																		
10	X	X	X												X													
11	X													X														
12	X								X																			
13																		X										
14	X				X	X	X	X		X	X								X									
17													X															
18		X																										
19	X		X										X															
20	X																											
21	X																											
24	X		X	X	X							X	X			X												
25			X																									
27	X	X				X					X																	

Swelling, Eyes, Around

	ARS	EUPHR	APIS	ARG N	KALI CAR	RHUS T	ACON	CHLOR	DULC	GELS	GRAPH	MERC C	PETROS	PHOS	STRAM													
1						X							X															
8	X		X	X										X														
13	X				X	X	X								X													
14	X	X	X	X	X						X	X																
19								X																				
21		X							X	X																		
22		X																										

Swelling, Genitals

	ARS	LYC	MERC	AMM C	CANTH	KALI BIC	AMBRA	APIS	ARN	ASAF	CALAD	CALC	COCCUS	DIG	FERR IOD	HELON	KREO	LIL T	MEPH	NIT AC	PLUM	POD	PULS	RHUS T	SEP	THUJA		
1				X																								
6	X		X																									
7	X	X	X	X	X		X	X	X	X		X		X	X	X	X	X		X		X	X	X	X	X		
8		X				X																						
13	X	X	X		X	X					X		X						X		X							

Swelling, Glands

	BELL	BAR C	IOD	MERC	SIL	SULPH	BROM	CALC	GRAPH	MERC C	CIST	CON	KALI IOD	NIT AC	SPONG	CARB A	HEP	LYC	AUR	RHUS T	ARS	CALC IOD	DULC	PHOS				
1	X		X				X		X		X		X		X	X						X						
2	**X**	**X**			**X**			**X**	X		X		**X**	**X**			**X**				**X**	**X**						
3										X										X								
4	**X**		**X**	**X**	X	X	**X**		X	**X**		X										X						
6	X	X			X	X						X		X		X												
7	**X**	**X**	**X**	**X**	**X**	X	X	**X**	X	X	X	**X**	**X**	X	**X**			X	X	**X**			X	X				
8				X																								
10	X	X	X	X			X																					
11										X																		
12	X			X	X	X		X	X	X								X	X					X				
13	**X**	**X**	**X**	**X**	**X**	**X**	X	**X**	**X**		X	**X**		**X**	**X**	**X**	X	**X**	X	**X**	X		**X**	**X**				
14	X	X	X										X			X	X											
15				X		X																						
21		X																										
22											X																	
24	X		X		X		X								X													
25		X																										
26		X				X		X									X	X	X		X		X					

Swelling, Glands, Axillary

	BELL	CARB A	HEP	AST R	CON	LYC	MERC	PHOS	SIL	SULPH	RHUS T	CALC	CLEM	IOD	ARS IOD	KALI CAR	NAT SUL	NIT AC	PHYTO	SEP	AUR	ANANTH						
1	X																											
4		X																										
6											X								X									
7		X	X		X	X	X	X	X		X		X	X		X	X	X		X								
8	X	**X**	X	**X**	**X**	**X**	**X**	**X**	**X**	**X**	X	**X**	**X**	**X**	X	X	X	X		X	**X**	**X**						
9	X																											
10	X		X	X	X	X	X		X	X		X			X													
11								X																				
12										X																		
14			X	X																								
15	X																											
21																			X									
24		X																										

Swelling, Glands, Cervical

	MERC	CALC	BAR C	BELL	SIL	SULPH	BROM	IOD	PULS	DULC	HEP	LYC	LACH	NIT AC	ARUM T	BAR M	CARB V	HELL	KALI CAR	KALI MUR	PHOS	RHUS T	STAPHYS	AUR	CHAM	MERC C		
1													X															
4	X	X	X			X	**X**													X						**X**		
5								X																				
6	X	X	X	X		X	X	X	X		X										X	X	X	X				
7	**X**	**X**		X	**X**	X		**X**	X	X	X	X	X	X	**X**	X	X	X	X	X			X					
8	**X**	**X**	**X**	**X**	**X**	X	**X**	**X**	X	X		**X**	**X**	X	**X**	**X**	**X**	X	**X**		X		X	**X**	X	X		
9	X		X																									
10	**X**	**X**		X	X	X			X	X	X	X										X						
11																					X							
12	X																											
13	**X**	**X**	X	**X**	X	**X**	X	**X**	X	**X**	X	**X**	X	**X**			**X**	X	**X**		X	X	X		**X**			
14			X	X			X				X																	
15	X			X																								
17					X																							
18	X	X													X													
19		X	X		X		X																					
21	X	X														X				X								
22	X																											
24	X	X				X			X											X		X		X		X		
25	X		X																									
26	X													X				X							X			
27					X																							

Swelling, Glands, Cervical, Left

	BAD	GRAPH	LITH C	LYC	MERC I R
4					X
7	X	X	X	X	

Swelling, Glands, Inguinal

	MERC	HEP	CLEM	GRAPH	SIL	CALC	DULC	NIT AC	THUJA	ARS	BELL	IOD	RHUS T	SULPH	BAD	CROT H	CUPR	SPONG	CARB A	STAPHYS
1				X	X	X														
5			X																	
6	X															X				
7	**X**	**X**		X				X					X				X			
8	X	**X**	**X**	X	X		**X**	X	X	**X**		**X**		X	**X**	X	X	X	**X**	
10	X	X	X	X	X	X	X		X		X			X						
11					X								X							
13	**X**	X	X	X	X	**X**	X	**X**	**X**	X	X	**X**	X	X	X			X		**X**
14	X	X																		
15											X									

Swelling, Glands, Lymphatic

	CON	BAR C	CALC	CARB V	SEP	BAR IOD	CALC FL	CALC PH	CARB S	GELS	GRAPH	HEP	IOD	MERC C	PHYTO
1							X			X					
6	X														
7	X		X	X					X						
8	X	**X**		X	**X**	X					X				
9		X													
11														X	
17													X		
18			X					X				X			
25															X

Swelling, Glands, Mesenteric

	CALC	CON	IOD	ARS	BAR C	CALC FL	LAPIS	ABROT	ANTHRAC	CALC IOD	CALC PH	CARB A	GRAPH	GRAT	HEP	MERC C	OLENAD	OL JEC A	PHOS	SACCH	SIL	STAPHYS	SULPH					
1	X					X	X							X														
4	X					X	X																					
6																	X											
7	X	X	X		X							X						X										
8	**X**	X	X	X	**X**			X	X	X	X		X		X				X		X	X	X					
10		X																										
11																X												
12			X																									
13	**X**	X	X	**X**																X								
15	X																											

Swelling, Glands, Parotid

	BROM	RHUS T	MERC	PHYTO	ARS	AUR	BELL	CHAM	DULC	KALI BIC	LACH	SIL	ARN	BAR C	CALC	CARB A	CARB V	CIST	COCCUL	CON	CROT H	HEP	KALI CAR	KALI MAN	LYC	MERC D	MERC I R	
1	X																											
4	**X**	X	**X**																									
6	X	X								X													X					
7		X		X		X		X	X	X	X	X		X		X			X	X	X							
8	X		X	X	X	X		X			X	X			X			X				X		X	X	X	X	
10		X					X										X											
20			X	X																								
24	X																											
26					X				X				X															
27							X																					

Swelling, Glands, Salivary- See also Swelling, Glands, Sub-Maxillary

	BAR M	BELL	CALC	MERC	MERC I F	MUR AC	THUJA	ACET AC	ANANTH	CANTH	CARB V	IOD	KALI MUR	KALM	LAC C	MERC D	PHYTO	PSOR	STAPHYS									
1			X														X											
4						X																						
6				X			X					X																
7				**X**	X	X																						
8	X	X	X					X	X	X			X	X	X	X		X	X									
10		X									X																	
12					X																							
13	X						X																					

Swelling, Glands, Sub-Maxillary- See also Swelling, Glands, Salivary

	MERC	SIL	BAR C	CALC	PHYTO	CHAM	ARUM T	AUR	BAR M	COCCUL	MERC I R	SPONG	BROM	CHIN ARS	GRAPH	IOD	KALI IOD	PETR	ANTHRAC	ARS	CHINA	KALI CAR	MUR AC	PSOR	ZINC			
1					X											X							X					
4	**X**																											
6		X	X				X																					
7	X	X	X	X		X	X	X	X	X	X	X	X	X	X		X		X	X		X	X		X			
8	X	**X**	<u>**X**</u>	<u>**X**</u>	X	**X**	X	X	<u>**X**</u>	<u>**X**</u>		X	**X**	**X**	**X**	**X**	**X**	**X**	X	X	<u>**X**</u>	X		X	X			
10								X																				
14											X	X																
17				X							X							X						X				
20	X				X																							
21	X				X																							
24		X																										
26						X																						

Swelling, Gums

	MERC	LACH	NAT M	NUX V	BELL	CHINA	SULPH	CHAM	HEP	NIT AC	STAPHYS	CALC	CARB V	PHOS	ACON	APIS	CAUST	KALI CAR	KREO	MUR AC	RHUS T	GRAPH	MERC C	PLUM				
1	X	X																X										
3	X			X	X						X								X									
4	X																											
6	X	X	X	X	X	X	X	X	X	X	X	X	X	X	X		X			X	X							
7	X	**X**	**X**			**X**				X	X	X				X						X	**X**	**X**				
8		X	X	X	X	X	X	X	X			X	X	X	X		X				X							
9		X														X				X								
10	<u>**X**</u>	X	X	X	X		X		X	X			X		X				X									
11	X																											
12								X																				
13	**X**	X		**X**	X	X	**X**	X	X	X	X	X		**X**			X	X		X		**X**	X	X				
14	X																	X										
15	X							X																				
21			X													X			X									
26	X		X	X	X	X	X		X	X	X		X								X							

Swelling, Face

	BELL	ARS	MERC	APIS	OP	CANTH	HEP	LYC	STRAM	CARB V	LACH	NAT M	NUX V	PHOS	PULS	RHUS T	SPIG	BAR C
4	X	X																
5	X																	
6			X				X				X				X			
7	X	**X**	**X**	**X**	X	X		**X**	X	X		X	X	X		X		
8			X			X		X	X			X	X		X	X		
10	X	X					X											
11		X		X	X													X
12	X			X														
13	**X**	**X**	**X**		X	**X**	**X**	X	**X**	X	X	X	X			X		**X**
14	X	X		X	X					X	X			X				
15	X	X	X	X											X			
26	X													X				

Swelling, Feet

	APIS	PULS	ARS	BRY	LED	LYC	FERR	CHINA	PHOS	DIG	HYOSC	SULPH	CAUST	SEP	BELL	CALC	COCCUL	COLCH	EUP PERF	KALI CAR	MERC	NAT M	NUX V	PETR	PHYTO	SABAD	ZINC
1						X																					
4					X																						
6	X	X	X	X			X	X	X	X				X									X				
7	X	**X**		**X**		**X**	X			X	X		X				X				X	X		X	X		
8	X		**X**		X		X		X		X	X				X			X							X	X
10		X	X																								
13	X	X	**X**	**X**	**X**	**X**		**X**	**X**	X	X	X	**X**	**X**	X	X	X	X	X	X	X	X	X	X		X	X
14	X			X	X	X												X							X		
15	X	X													X												
21	X																										
26							X	X				X								X							

Swelling, Fingers

	RHUS T	LYC	MAG CAR	THUJA
13	**X**	**X**	**X**	**X**
21	X			

Swelling, Hands

	PHOS	BRY	LACH	APIS	BELL	HEP	ARS	CALC	LYC	RHUS T	ARG N	COCCUL	FERR PH	STANN
2		**X**		X							**X**		**X**	
6	X													
7	X	X	X	**X**		X	X	X	X	X				
8	X		X											
13	X	**X**	X		**X**	**X**	X	X	X	X		**X**		**X**
15					X									

Swelling, Heel

	ARAN D	PETR
5	X	
7		X

Swelling, Ileo-Caecum

	PLUM	HEP	LACH	GINSENG	MERC	RHUS T
10	X	X	X	X	X	X
16	X					
24	X	X	X			

Swelling, Jaw

	HECLA	PHOS	SIL	BRY	MAG P AR
1	X			X	X
7		X	X		
8			X		
14	X	X			

Swelling, Joints

	LED	BRY	RHUS T	APIS	BELL	ARN	COLCH	SULPH	PULS	ACT S	CALC	MANG	CAUST	GUAIAC	IOD	KALI IOD	MERC	RHOD
1							X			X					X			
4	X			X					X				X			X		
5	X	X		X		X										X		
7	**X**		X					X			**X**			X				
8	X	X	X	X	**X**				X	**X**	X	X		X	X		X	
10					X	X											X	
11		X	X				X											
12								X										
13	X							**X**				**X**						**X**
14	X	X	X		X								X					
15	X	X				X												
18	X		X	X		X												
19	**X**			X			**X**		X									
21	X	X	X	X	X													
22	X	X	X															
25					X													
27	X	X																

Swelling, Knee

	CALC	APIS	BRY	KALI IOD	SULPH	IOD	PULS	BENZ AC	COCCUL	HEP	LED	LYC	SIL	LACH	MERC	SARS	RHUS T
3	X			X													
4		**X**		X		X											
6				X													
7	**X**	X	**X**	X	X	X	X							X		X	**X**
8		X						X		X	X	X					
12					X												
13	**X**		**X**		X	**X**	**X**		**X**	**X**	**X**	**X**	**X**	X	X	X	
14	X	X	X					X	X								
21								X									
26					X		X						X		X		

Swelling, Labia

	ARS	KREO	AMBRA	APIS	EUPION	MERC	MERC AC	POD	PULS	SEP	SULPH
3			X								
5				X							
8						X				X	X
11		X									
13							X	X			
14	X	X			X						
15	X										
27									X		

Swelling, Larynx

	ARN	IOD	LACH	SIL	SPONG
7		X	X		
8				X	X
9	X				

Swelling, Legs

	BRY	COLCH	PULS	AGAV A	KALI CAR	LACH	NUX V	ACON	CALC	LED	LYC	MERC	APIS	ARN	BAR M	BERB V	BOR	CROT H	DULC	GRAPH	LATH	NAT CAR	RHOD	RUTA	SIL	STRONT B	SULPH	XANTHO
1																					X							
2																										X		
6				X									X															X
7					X										X	X												
8	X			X		X	X											X										
13	**X**	**X**	**X**		X	X	X	**X**	**X**	**X**	**X**	**X**		X			X		X	X		X	X	X	X		X	
14		X																										
15			X																									

Swelling, Limbs

	DIG	ACET AC	AGAV A	APIS	ARN	BAR C	CANTH	MERC SU	SEP	VIP
6	X									
7	X			X	X	X		X		
8		X					X		X	X
11			X							

Swelling, Lip

	BELL	APIS	HEP	MERC	MERC C	SULPH	AUR	SIL	BRY	ARS	ARUM T	CALC	CARB A	CARB V	KALI CAR	KALM	LACH	LYC	NAT CAR	NIT AC	PULS	STAPHYS
2			X																			
6										X												
7	X			X	X			X			X		X	X	X	X			X	X	X	
8	**X**	X	X	X	X	X	X	X	X								X					X
9		X																				
10																		X				
13	**X**		X	X	X	**X**	X	X	**X**	X	X	X	X	X	X	X	X	X	X	X	X	X
14	X	X	X		X																	
19		X																				
21		X																				
26	**X**			X		X	X					X										

Swelling, Lip, Upper

	BAR C	KALI CAR	NIT AC	PSOR	RHUS V	SIL	SULPH
3			X		X	X	
8	X			X			
9		X					
11	X						
12							X
14	X						
17	X						

Swelling, Liver- See Hepatomegaly

Swelling, Lymph Nodes

	BELL	BAR C	GRAPH	IOD	MERC	ABROT	ARS IOD	BAR IOD	CALC	CARB V	CON	FERR ARS	HEP	KALI IOD	PHYTO	SEP	SIL	THIO
2				X														X
4	X		X						X									
5					X	X	X					X						
8		X	X					X		X	X					X		
9	X																	
17		X		X														
19	X																	
20					X								X					
21														X			X	
25															X			

Swelling, Lymph Nodes, Cervical- See also Cervical Lymphoma; Swelling, Lymph Nodes

	ARS	GRAPH	PHOS	APIS	BACILL	BAR C	BAR IOD	CALEND	CARB A	CON	IOD	LAPIS	MERC	SCROPH	SEC	SIL	TUB
3					X	X		E					X			X	
4		X															
7	X		X												X		
8	X	X	X	X													
11	X						X				X	X		X			
19	X								X	X							X

E- External

Swelling, Mouth (Includes Swelling, Mouth, Interior)

	MERC	BELL	CAUST	KALI MUR	NIT AC	ACON	AMM C	CANTH	CIST	DULC	HYDRAST	LACH	MERC C	NUX V	PARIS	SEP	VER A
7	**X**		X	**X**	**X**						X						
8		X							X								
11													X				
13	X	X	X			X	X	X				X		X	X	X	X
26	X									X							

Swelling, Neck (Includes Swelling, Neck, Nape)

	BELL	MERC	PHOS	ARS	SIL	IOD	SPONG	AESC	AILANTH	APIS	BRY	CALC	CAUST	CIC	CON	CROC	CROT H	KALI BIC	KALI IOD	LACH	LYC	MERC C	NUX V	PULS
7	**X**	X		X	X		**X**			X										X				
8	X	X	X					X	X			X					X	X	X					
10					X																			
13	**X**	X	X	X		**X**							X	X	X	X					X	X	X	X
24			X																					
26	X										X													

Swelling, Nipples

	LACH	AUR SUL	CHAM	LYC	MERC
7	X		X		
13	X			X	X
14		X			

Swelling, Nose

	CALC	MERC	SULPH	HEP	PHOS	AUR	BELL	PULS	RHUS T	SEP	KALI IOD	ARN	ARS	ZINC	CARB A	APIS	BRY
1	X	X						X									
2										X							
6	X	X	X	X	X	X	X	X	X		X						
7	X		**X**	X	**X**				X	X		X	**X**			**X**	
8	**X**		**X**	**X**	X	X	**X**	X	X	X		X	X	X	X		X
10		X															
12	X		X											X			
13	**X**	**X**	**X**	X	**X**	**X**	**X**	X	X	**X**	X	**X**	X	**X**	X		**X**
14	X	X				X										X	
15		X															
18											X						
24	X	X	X	X	X			X			X						
26	X			X	X	X	X		X						X		

Swelling, Ovaries

	GRAPH	APIS	BUFO	IOD	KALI BR	KALI IOD	LACH	LIL T	PALLAD	ALUM	ARS	AUR M	BELL	BROM	BRY	CARB A	COLOC	CON	CUBEB	HAM	MEDO	STAPHYS
5	X	X	X		X	X	X	X	X	X	X			X			X				X	
6															X							
7	X		X	X	X		X	X				X				X		X				
8						X			X				X						X	X		X
13	X	X		X																		

Swelling, Ovary, Left

	GRAPH	LACH	BROM	AMM BR	AMM C	ATROP S	CARB AC	HAM	KALI BR	LIL T
4	X									
6		X								
7		X	X	X		X	X	X	X	X
8	X				X					
13	X	X								
18			X							

Swelling, Ovary, Right

	PALLAD	APIS	IOD	LACH	MAG M
4	X		X		
7	X	X		X	X
13	X				

Swelling, Palate

	BAR C	BELL	CALC	MERC	PHYTO	SIL	SULPH	NUX V	APIS	BAPT	BAR M	CARB A	CHINA	COFF	CROT T	MERC CY	NAT SUL	PARIS	PHOS	SENEG
7	X		X	X	X		X					X				X				
8	X		X							X										
13	X	X	X	X		X	X	**X**			X		X	X	X		X	X		X
14					X															
15		X							X											
26		X																	X	
27						X														

Swelling, Penis

	CINNAB	MILL	CANN S	DIG	ARN	ARS	CANTH	KREO	LED	MERC	MERC C	SIL	RHUS T
1		X		X									
4				X									
6		X				X							
7	X	X	X	X	X		X	X	X		X	X	**X**
8	X	X	X							X		X	
13	X	X	X		**X**		X	X	X	X			
14	X					X					X		
27	X												

Swelling, Pharynx

	AESC	BROM	DROS	HEP	KALI BIC	PULS	SANG
6							X
7		X		X	X		
8	X		X			X	

Swelling, Prepuce

	MERC	RHUS T	CALAD	CINNAB	GRAPH	COR R	NAT CAR	THUJA	SULPH	ACON	APIS	ARN	CANN S	CAPS	JAC CAR	NIT AC	OL SAN	PH AC	SIL	VIOL T
1	X	X	X		X															
7	X	X	X	**X**	X	X	X	X			X			X						
8	X	X								X		X								
11																	X			
13	**X**	**X**	**X**	**X**	X	X	X	X	**X**				X		X	X			X	X
14																		X		

Swelling, Pylorus

	CON	CONDUR
10	X	X
24	X	

Swelling, Rectum

	CURARE	AESC	CAMPH	COLLIN	LACH
7	X	X	X	X	X
8	X				

Swelling, Scrotum- See also Hydrocele

	DIG	RHUS T	ARN	APIS	ARG	BROM	CANTH	CARB V	CHEL	CLEM	FL AC	GRAPH	JAC C	LACH	NAT M	PH AC	PLUM	PULS	SACCH	SEP
1	X																			
4	X																			
7		X							X		X			X	X					
8				X																
13		X	**X**			X	X	X		X		X	X			X	X	X	X	X
14					X															

Swelling, Spermatic Cord

	ARN	CHINA	KALI CAR	BERB V	CALC	PHOS	PULS	SARS	SPONG	KALI BIC	PH AC
1	X	X					X				
7		X	X	X	X	X		X	X	X	
8	X	X	X	X	X	X	X	X	X		X
13	X										
24	X	X	X								

Swelling, Supraorbital Foramen

	KALI CAR	APIS
7	**X**	X

Swelling, Testes- See also Hydrocele

	PULS	AUR	CLEM	CON	IOD	KALI CAR	SPONG	AGNUS	NUX V	RHOD	BROM	GRAPH	HAM	MERC	ARN	APIS	BAR M	BELL	CALC PH	COP	MERC C	MILL	NIT AC	PH AC	PLUM	SULPH	DIG	NAT CAR
1	X	X		X		X					X	X	X			X						X						
3		X						X											X									
4	X		X				X																					
6	X								X																			
7	X		X	X	X	X				X	X	X		X	X		X	X	X	X	X		X		X			
8		X	X		X	X	X				X		X	X										X				
9					X																							
10	X			X					X					X												X		
13	**X**	**X**	**X**	**X**	**X**	X	**X**	**X**	**X**	**X**					**X**	X	X			X		X	X	X	X	X	**X**	**X**
14		X	X				X	X		X											X							
21	X												X					X										
24				X		X																						
25					X							X																

Swelling, Teste, Left

	BROM	MERC	CON	POD	PULS	RHOD
13	X	X	X	X		X
25					X	

Swelling, Teste, Right

	ARG	AUR	AUR S	CLEM
1			X	
13	X	X		X

Swelling, Throat- See also Pharyngitis

	APIS	MERC	MERC C	KALI BIC	BELL	LACH	SANG	AILANTH	AMM C	AMM M	ARS	CALC	CINNAB	FERR PH	NAT M	NUX V	SEP	WYETHIA	HEP	KALI MAN	PHYTO	SENEGA
1	X			X																		
4	X	X	X	X							X											
6								X														
7	X	**X**			**X**	**X**		X			X	X			X	X	X		**X**		**X**	
8	X	X		X			**X**		X	X			X							**X**		
9														X								
10	X				X																	
12	X	X																				
13					X	X			X	X		X	X		X	X	X					**X**
14	X			X														X				
15	X																					
17			X			X	X															
18			X																			
19																		X				
21	X	X																				
22	X																					
24	X		X																			
25		X												X								

Swelling, Toes

	CARB V	LED	SULPH	GRAPH	ARN	CARB A	PAEONIA	THUJA	ACT S	AMM C	BAR C	COLOC	DAPHNE	MERC	NAT C	PH AC	PLAT	SABIN	ZINC
7	X											X							
8		X	X	X															
13	**X**	**X**	**X**	X	**X**	**X**	**X**	**X**		X	X		X	X	X	X	X	X	X
14									X										

Swelling, Tongue- See also Glossitis

	MERC	APIS	LACH	CON	DULC	ARS	BELL	LYC	HELL	ACON	BAPT	CANTH	PLUM	STRAM	CALC	GLON	HYDRAST	IOD	MERC C	MUR AC	NAT M	OX AC	PHOS	SIL				
1		X	X	X	X				X						X													
3	X																					X						
5	X	X			X		X			X		X									X		X					
6	X	X											X	X														
7	X	X	X	X	X	X		X	X		X	X	X				X	X	X		X		X					
8	X				X	X		X						X		X		X										
9																				X								
10	X		X	X		X				X	X						X							X				
11			X				X													X								
13	X	X	X	X	X	X	**X**	X	**X**	X		X	X	X	X	X			X			X		X				
14		X		X			X																					
15											X																	
18	X																											
19								X																				
20	X																											
22		X																										
24	X		X																									

Swelling, Tongue, Root Of

	ARS	MERC																										
5	X																											
15		X																										

Swelling, Tonsils (Includes Tonsils, Enlarged)

	BAR C	BELL	CALC PH	LACH	MERC	CALC	PHYTO	KALI MUR	SULPH	HEP	BAR M	KALI BIC	LYC	NIT AC	AMM C	APIS	CALC IOD	MERC C	PHOS	CHAM	ACON	SIL	STAPHYS	BAPT
1	**X**	X	X		X			X			X						X	X						
4	X		**X**	X	X			X				X	X		X		X							
6	X	X				X					X			X		X	X							
7	**X**	X		X		X	X	X	**X**	X		X	X	X		X		X	X	**X**		X		**X**
8	X				X	X			X	X			X	X			X							
9	X		X				X																	
10		X	X	X	X					X	X		X							X			X	
12							X		X						X			X						
13	**X**	**X**		X	X	X	X		X	**X**			X	X	X			X	X	X			X	
14		X	X			X	X	X				X									X	X		
15	X	X				X																		X
17			X		X		X					X			X				X				X	
18	X			X																				
19	X	X									X					X			X					
21					X		X														X			
22	X	X	X					X								X								
24	X	X	X	X				X			X	X		X										
25	X	X	X	X																				
26	X	X		X	X	X			X	X											X	X		

Swelling, Tonsils, Right Side

	BELL	APIS	BAR C
4	X		
9	X		X
19		X	

Swelling, Urethra

	ARG N	COP	HYPER	LED	MERC C	MERC	MITCH	NIT AC	RHUS T	THUJA
7	X		X			X	X			
8										X
11					X					
13		X		X				X	X	

Swelling, Uterus- See also Metritis

	AUR M	CARB A	IOD	AGNUS	LACH	LIL T	NUX V	AESC	ARS	BELL	CANTH	CIMICI	CON	FRAX	KREO	MUREX	PLAT	SEC	SEP	TAR H								
1		X						X																				
4												X							X									
5			X	X	X	X														X								
6		X																										
7			X	X	X	X			X						X													
8	X						X			X							X											
10		X																										
13			X				X				X							X										
14	X															X												
21	X													X														
24													X															

Swelling, Uvula

	APIS	MERC C	NUX V	BELL	IOD	PHOS	KALI IOD	COFF	KALI BIC	LACH	MERC	MUR AC	SIL	BAR M	CARB V	RHUS T	SENEG											
1	X	X		X								X																
3		X																										
4		X										X																
6	X				X		X						X															
7	**X**				X		X	X	**X**		X	X			X	X												
8	X		X			X	X		X					X		X												
10			X	X						X	X																	
11		X																										
13			**X**	X	X	X		X			X			X	X		**X**											
14	X	X	X						X																			
15				X																								
17					X	X																						
19	X					X				X																		
21	X																											
24		X											X															
26								X		X																		
27													X															

Swelling, Vagina

	KREO	AGAR M	NUX V	NIT AC	CANN S	FERR IOD	IOD	MERC
1	X							
5	X	X	X	X			X	
6	X							
7	X	X		**X**		X		
8		X	X		X			
10	X							
13								X
15			X					

Swelling, Vocal Cords

	CARB V	HAM	KALI BIC	PHOS
6	X		X	X
7		X		

Swelling, Vulva

	AMBRA	SEP	CALC	CANTH	COFF	MERC	NUX V	THUJA
6			X					
8	X	X						
9				X				
14	X							
21		X			X	X	X	X

Syncope- See also Fainting

	ACON	NUX V	CHINA	ARS	DIG	VER A	CARB V	CHAM	PH AC	SULPH	IGN	MOSCH	PHOS	TRILL P	AMM C	CALC	CANTH	CUPR	KALI PH	LACH	SUMBUL	FERR	LINARIA	THYROID
1	X																							
8	X	X	X		X		X	X	X	X		X	X		X			X	X	X				
10															X									
11	X	X	X	X	X	X								X							X			
12				X																				
13		X				X		X	X	X														
14	X																							
17	**X**	**X**	**X**	X	X	X	**X**	**X**	**X**	X	**X**	**X**	**X**	**X**		X	X		X	X	X	**X**	**X**	**X**
19					X																			
24																	X							
26	X	X	X	X		X	X				X					X		X						

Synovitis (Includes Synovitis, Joints)

	BRY	APIS	PULS	LED	SIL	MERC	CALC	RHUS T	BELL	CAUST	IOD	PHYTO	CALC FL	FERR PH	KALI CAR	LYC	SEP	SULPH	ANT T	CIMICI	COLCH	RUTA	SABIN	STELL M	STICTA			
1				X	X						X																	
2		**X**	**X**		**X**														X									
4	**X**	**X**	X	**X**		**X**	X		X	X																		
5	X		X	X										X									X					
6																									X			
7	**X**	**X**	X	X	X	X	X	X	X	X	X	**X**		X	X	X	X	X										
8	X	X	X	X	X	X	X	X	X	X	X	X			X	X	X	X		X	X	X						
9	X	X											X															
11																								X				
12								X																				
14		X											X															
18	X																											
23	X	X																										
24	X																											

Synovitis, Knee

	APIS	LED	SULPH	BRY	CALC	PULS	RHUS T	RUTA	SIL																			
1	X		X	X	X	X	X	X																				
4	**X**	**X**	**X**																									
8	X	X							X																			

Syphilis

	MERC	AUR	KALI IOD	NIT AC	MERC C	ASAF	KALI BIC	THUJA	HEP	MEZ	STILL	SYPH	CARB A	FL AC	CINNAB	LACH	PHYTO	ARS	AUR M	KREO	MERC D	PH AC	SARS	SULPH	SIL	CAUST		
1	**X**	X	X	X	X		X	X			X	X		X	X	X				X	X							
2	**X**	**X**	**X**	**X**	**X**	X	**X**	**X**	X	**X**	**X**	X	X	**X**	X	X	**X**			X		X	X			X		
3	**X**	X	X	X	X	**X**			X	X			X		X	X			X		X							
4	**X**	X	**X**	X	X	X	X	**X**	**X**		X		**X**		X		X	**X**	X		X				X			
6	X	X	X	X	X	X	X	X	X	X	X		X	X		X	X	X	X	X		X	X	X	X	X		
7	**X**	**X**	**X**	**X**	X	X	X	X	X	X	X	**X**	**X**	X			**X**	X	X	X	X	X	X	X	X	**X**		
8	X	X	X	X	X	X	**X**	X	X	X	X	X	X	X	X	X	X	X	X	X	X	X	X	**X**	X	X		
11	X	**X**	**X**	**X**	X		X	X		X	X	X		X	X					X								
12	X	X	X	X	X		X	X										X				X		X				
13	**X**	X		X		X	X		X	X				X			X						X					
14	**X**	X	X	X	X							X			X	X					X							
17	X	X	X	X	X	X			X			X				X		X	X			X		X	X			
23			X	X	X	X				X	X	X	X										X					
24	X	X				X																						
26		X																										

Syphilis, Bones

	AUR	PHYTO	KALI IOD	MERC	PH AC																							
7	X	X	**X**	**X**	X																							
8	X																											
23		X																										

Tabes Dorsalis- See Paralysis

	PHOS	ALUM	ARG N	CAUST	SULPH	ARS	NUX V	CALC	SEC	BELL	NUX M	PHYSO	PLUM	ONOS	AESC	COCCUL	FL AC	GELS	PH AC	PIC AC	RHUS T	SIL	STRAM	ZINC	CON			
1						X																						
6	X	X	X	X	X	X	X	X	X	X	X	X	X		X	X		X		X	X	X	X					
8	X	X	X	X	X		X		X	X	X	X	X	X	X		X				X		X	X				
12	X	X	X			X																						
17	**X**	**X**	**X**	X	X	X	X	X		X	X	X	X	**X**		X	X	X	X	X		X		X	**X**			
26	X			**X**	**X**		X	**X**	**X**										X									

Tabes Mesenterica- See Tuberculosis, Mesenteric Glands

Tachycardia

	ACON	ARS	BELL	FERR PH	VER V	PYROG	DIG	CRAT	GELS	GLON	IOD	PHOS	RHUS T	ANT T	BRY	CACT	LYCOP	AUR	MUR AC	ABIES N	HYOSC	LATRO M	NUX V	STROPH	SULPH	THYROID	LACH	ZINC
1	X		X	X	X	X		X	X					X		X								X		X		
2						X																						
3								X												X								
4		X			X			X			X				X	X	X				X			X				
5																				X								
6	X	X	X	X	X		X		X			X		X					X		X		X		X			X
7	**X**	**X**	**X**	**X**					X	**X**	X	X	**X**		X	X	X	**X**	X		X		X		X			**X**
8	**X**	**X**	**X**	X	X				X	**X**	X	X	X	X				X			X	X	X		X			X
9		X							X		X									X						X		
10	X	X	X			X							X		X		X	X				X						
11	X		X	X		X		X				X		X	X	X	X		X			X		X				
12	X	X			X							X	X						X									
13		X					X												**X**									
14	X	X	X	X										X		X				X						X		
15	X	X	X		X		**X**		X			X			X	X												
16	X		X	X	X		X			X							X				X							
17	X	X	X	X	X	X	X	X	X	X	X	X	X	X	X			X		X		X	X	X	X			X
18	X				X	X				X	X																	
19		X		X	X												X							X				
21			X	X		X	X															X						
22			X	X		X																						
23								X																				
24	X	X	X	X									X					X					X		X	X		
25	X										X															X		
26										X																		
27	X	X						X																				
29*							X																					

29* Varshney JP, et al. Atrial paroxysmal tachycardia in dogs and its management with homeopathic Digitalis--two case reports. Homeopathy, 2007, Oct; 96, (4):270-2.

Tachypnoea

	ACON	BRY	BELL	SAMB	ARS	IPEC	ANT T	CHAM	FERR PH	OP	CUPR	GELS	AMBRA	CARB V	CEDRON	HELL	HEP	HYDR AC	LED	LYC	MUR AC	PHOS	PULS	RHUS T	SPONG	VER V	ASAF	CHEL
1			X	X			X																					
4									X																			
6	X				X				X	X			X	X							X		X					
7	**X**	X	X	X	X	X	**X**	X		X		**X**			X		X	X		X		X		X				**X**
8	X	X		X	X	X			X	X	X		X		X			X	X		X					X		
10	X	X						X																				
11	X		X				X																					
12	X	X																										
13	X	X	**X**	**X**	X	X					**X**	X		X		X	X		X	X		X	X	X	X		**X**	
14	X					X																						
15		X	X	X				X								X									X	X		
24	X																											

Taenia- See Worms, Tape
Tapeworms- See Worms, Tape
Tartar, Accumulation Of

	CALC REN	FRAG	SIL MAR
2	X		X
3	X	X	

Taste, Diseases Of- See also Ageusia (Includes Bad Taste in Mouth)

	PULS	NUX V	MERC	BRY	SEP	CHINA	SULPH	ARN	CALC	LYC	ACON	CHAM	CHEL	NAT M	CARB V	ARS	RHUS T	BELL	ANT C	CUPR	SIL	VER A	COCCUL	HEP	POD	RHEUM		
1	X	X	X	X		X	X			X	X			X	X		X			X		X	X					
2	**X**	**X**	**X**			**X**	**X**	**X**	**X**	**X**			**X**	**X**				**X**							X	**X**		
6	X	X		X	X	X	X	X		X		X		X		X	X	X	X	X					X			
7	X	X	X	X	X	X	X	X	X	X	X	X	X	X	X	X	X	X	X	X	X	X	X	X	X	X		
8	X	X	X	X	X	X	X	X	X	X	X	X		X	X	X	X	X	X	X	X	X	X	X		X		
9		X		X	X				X					X	X													
10	X	X	X	X	X	X	X				X	X	X		X	X			X		X			X	X			
11	X	X	X	X				X		X			X				X	X										
12	X		X								X		X															
13	X	X	X	X	X	X	X	X	X	X	X	X		X	X	X	X	X	X		X	X	X	X		X		
14	X							X	X				X	X						X								
15	X	X	X	X		X	X	X		X		X			X	X					X	X			X			
17		X			X						X																	
18			X	X	X	X							X															
19			X			X					X																	
20	X	X	X										X															
21	X	X	X		X				X			X																
22	X											X																
24	X				X		X			X					X					X			X					
25		X		X	X				X																			
26	X	X		X			X	X	X			X				X	X		X		X	X		X				
27											X																	

Tear Duct, Blocked

	NAT M	MERC I F	RHUS T
1	X		X
6	X		
8	X	X	
28	X		

Teeth, Diseases Of- See also Caries, Dental (Includes Teeth, Crumbling; Teeth, Microfractures)

	CALC	CHAM	FL AC	STAPHYS	MERC	MEZ	ACON	ANT C	BACILL	CALC FL	COFF	EUPHORB	KREO	LACH	MAG CAR	MAG PH	PHOS	PHOS HY	PLANTAG	PULS	SPIG
2					**X**	**X**			X			X						X			
5																	X				
9	X	X	X	X																X	
19	X	X	X	X			X	X		X	X		X	X	X	X			X		X

Teeth, Falling Of (Includes Teeth, Loose)

	MERC	CAUST	PHOS	CARB V	AMM C	BRY	NIT AC	RHUS T	SULPH	HYOSC	ARS	CHAM	CHINA	HEP	NUX V	STAPHYS	ARN	IGN	CARB A	NAT M	NUX M	PULS	SEC	ZINC				
1			X		X																							
5		X					X												X									
6	X	X	X	X	X	X	X	X	X	X	X	X	X	X	X	X	X	X		X	X	X						
7	**X**	X	X	**X**	X	X	X	X	X	**X**				X	X	X			X	X			X	**X**				
8	X	X	X	X		X		X	X	X	X	X	X	X	X	X	X	X		X	X	X						
10											X																	
12												X																
13	**X**	X	X	X	X	X	X	X	X	X	X	X	X	X	X	X	X	X	X		X	X	**X**					
15				X																								
19	X	X	X		X	X		X	X				X											X				
21	X						X																					

Teeth, Loose- See Teeth, Falling

Teething (Includes Dentition, Diseases Of)

	CHAM	CALC	KREO	ACON	BELL	CALC PH	POD	SIL	IGN	MERC	COFF	COLOC	NUX V	PHYTO	RHEUM	ZINC	BOR	BRY	CUPR	SULPH	ARS	STAPHYS	CINA	GELS	MAG PH	ANT C	MAG M	
1	**X**	X	X			X						X		X	X	X												
2	**X**	**X**	**X**	**X**		**X**	X	**X**	X							X	X	X	X			X	X	X	X			
3	X		X	X	X	X										X									X			
4	**X**	**X**	**X**		X	**X**					X					X												
5	X		X				X							X			X										X	
6	X	X	X	X	X		X	X	X	X	X				X	X			X					X		X		
7	**X**	**X**	X	**X**	X	X	X	**X**	X	X	X	X	X	X	**X**	X	**X**	X	X	X	**X**	X	X	X	X	X	**X**	
8	X	X	X	X	X	X	X	X	X	X	X	X	X	X	X	X	X	X	X	X	X	**X**	X	X	X	X	X	
9	X	X		X	X		X			X		X	X		X							X			X			
10	X	X	X	X	X	X			X		X									X								
11		X				X																						
12	X	X	X	X	X		X	X		X	X	X	X					X		X	X			X				
13	**X**	**X**	X					X	**X**						**X**				X									
14	X		X	X			X																					
16	X																				X							
17	**X**	X	X		X	X	X																X					
18	X						X							X			X											
19	**X**	X	X		X	X		X	X					X				X		X		X				**X**		
20	**X**		X						X																			
21	X		X	X						X		X	X				X											
22	X	X			X	X		X																				
23	X		X											X														
24	X	X																										
25	X	X		X	X							X	X															
26	X	X		X	X			X	X	X	X		X					X	X	X	X		X				X	
28	X																											

Teething, Wisdom Teeth

	CHEIR	STAPHYS
2	X	
3	X	
5	X	X

Telangiectasia- See Naevi, Vascular

Tendons and Ligaments, Diseases Of- See also Weakness

	RHUS T	RUTA	ACON	BRY
7	**X**	X		X
9	X	X		
12	X			
14			X	
18	X	X		
21		X		

Tendon, Achilles, Diseases Of

	MUR AC	RHUS T	ZINC	CIMICI	KALI BIC	HEDEOM	MANG	RHAMN C	RUTA	TELL
2	X									
5	X					X		X		X
8							X			
9	X	X	X							
13			X							
14		X		X	X				X	
18		X								

Tendon, Pain- See Pain, Tendon

Tendon, Rupture

	RUTA
8	X
24	X

Tendonitis

	RHUS T	RUTA	BRY	PHYTO	ANT C	ARN	BELLIS	CAUST	KALM	SANG	STICTA
2					X						
12	X										
18	X										
19	X	X	X	X				X	X	X	X
20	**X**										
1	X	X									
22	X										
24		X									
27	X	X	X	X		X	X				

Tendonitis, Shoulder

	RHUS T	ANAC	CALC PH	PHYTO	RHOD	RUTA	SANG
5	X	X	X	X	X	X	
18	X						
19	X						X

Tenesmus

	MERC C	MERC	NUX V	SULPH	ALOE	CAPS	CANTH	ACON	IPEC	BELL	ARS	COLOC	IGN	POD	NIT AC	COLCH	RHEUM	APIS	ARN	CAUST	KALI BIC	LIL T	RHUS T	HEP	SIL
1	X		X	X	X	X				X		X	X	X		X									
2	**X**		**X**	**X**	X					**X**			**X**	**X**										**X**	**X**
3	X																								
4	**X**	X	X	X		X	X	X							X	X						X			
6		X	X	X	X	X	X	X	X	X								X			X				
7	X	X	X	X		X	X			X		X	X	X	X	**X**	X	X		X	X		X		X
8		X			**X**	X					X														
9	X						X		X													X			
10	X	X		X				X			X											X			
11	X	X			X		X	X	X		X							X	X		X				
12			X		X							X													
13	X	**X**	X	X	X	**X**		X		X	X		X				**X**		X	X			X	X	
14	X	X			X	X	X	X	X						X				X	X					
18	X	X	X	X					X					X											
19	X		X																						
24	X														X										
25												X													
26		X	X	X					X		X						X						X		
27												X													

Tenesmus, Urinary

	CANTH	MERC C	TEREB	PULS	PLUM	NUX V	ACON	BELL	CAPS	SARS	ALUM	ALOE	ARN	CHIM	HYOSC	LYC	PRUN S	RHUS T	SIL	STAPHYS	COLCH
1			X			X				X											
4	X	**X**	X					X													
6	X	X	X	X					X		X	X	X	X	X	X	X			X	
7	**X**	X	**X**	X	**X**													X	X		
8									X		X	X			X	X					
9			X																		
10		X																			
11	X		X	X	X			X		X											
12		X																			
13	X			X	X	X	X		X	X			X				X	X	X		**X**
14	X	X		X			X														
18						X															
19	X					X		X												X	
24				X	X		X							X							

Tennis Elbow (AKA Lateral Epicondylitis)

	RUTA	ARN	BELLIS	BRY	RHUS T
14		X			
19	X				
20	X				
22	X				
27	X	X	X	X	X

Testes, Diseases Of

	BELL	ACON	CON	AUR	BAR M	BROM	CLEM	PULS	RHUS T
2	**X**	**X**	**X**	X	X				X
8	X	X	X	X	X	X	X	X	X
12	X							X	
24						X			

Testes, Sclerosis- See Sclerosis, Testes

Testes, Retraction

	CANTH	CLEM	OL AN	NUX V	PLUM	PULS	COLOC	BAR C	BELL	BERB V	CALC	EUPHR	MENY	RHOD	STRAM	THUJA	ZINC
2			X														
3			X														
4	X	X				X											
7	X	X		X	X						X				X		
8	X	X				X	**X**	X									
13			X	X	X				X	X		X	X	X		X	X

Testes, Undescended

	AUR	AUR M	AUR M N	CLEM	RHOD
1			X		
3	X	X	X		
6	X				
14		X		X	X
16	X				
21	X			X	

Testes, Undeveloped

	AUR	BAR C
2	X	
3	X	
7		X

Testicular Atrophy- See Atrophy, Testicular

Tetanus- See also Risus Sardonicus (Includes Tetanus Neonatorum)

	HYPER	CIC	NUX V	HYDR AC	ACON	ANGUST	BELL	PASS	CAMPH	PHYSO	LED	ARN	STRAM	OP	IGN	ARS	RHUS T	STRYCHN	MAG PH	MOSCH	LAURO	PHYTO	IPEC
1	X	X	X	X	X	X	X	**X**	X	X			X			X			X				
2	X	X		**X**	**X**	X		X	X	X	X		X					X			X	X	X
3	**X**	X	**X**	**X**			X	**X**			**X**								**X**				
4	X	**X**	**X**	**X**	X	X		X		**X**			**X**						X				
6	X	X	X	X	X	X	X		X	X	X	X	X	X	X	X	X			X	X	X	
7	**X**	**X**	**X**	X		X	X		X	X	X	X		X	X	X	X		X	X	X	X	X
8	**X**	X	X	X	X	X		X	X			X	**X**	X	X	X	X			X		X	
10	X										X												
12			X	X	X		X					X						X					
13	X	X				**X**	**X**		**X**					**X**	X		X			**X**	X		**X**
14	**X**	X	X					X			**X**												
15			X		X		X					X		X	X		X						
16	X	X	X	X		X	X					X						X					
17				X														X					
21	X	X			X																		
23	X			X				X		X													
24		X	X		X	X	X			X		X	X	X		X		X					
26		X			X	X	X		X						X								

Tetanus, Prophylaxis

	HYPER	LED	ACON	ANGUST	ARN	ASAF	BELL	CALEND	CANTH	CARB V	CIC	GRAPH	KREO	PETR	RHUS T	SIL	STRAM	URT U	VER V									
10	X	X																										
14		X																										
16	X	X	X	X	X	X	X	X	X	X	X	X	X	X	X	X	X	X	X									
21	X																											
24	X	X																										

Tetany

	NUX V	CIC	OP	MAG PH	MOSCH	STRYCHN	ARS	CUPR	ACON	ANGUST	ARN	BELL	CALC	CAMPH	CHIN S	GELS	HYDR AC	IPEC	LAURO	PHYTO	PLAT	SOL N	STRAM	HYPER	THER			
2									X																			
5	X			X	X			**X**	X				X			X					X	X	X					
6			X																									
7	**X**	**X**	**X**	X	X		X			X	X	X		X	X	X	X	X	X	X				**X**	**X**			
8	X	X	X		X	X	**X**			X	X			X	X		X	X	X	X	X	X	X					
11	X	X		X		X		X				X	X															
19	X					X																						

Tetters- See Skin, Diseases Of

Thirst

	ARS	BRY	ACON	BELL	PHOS	MERC	VER A	SULPH	CHAM	NAT M	CHINA	CANTH	ANT C	ANT T	OP	RHUS T	STRAM	DULC	EUP PERF	NUX V	ARN	CALC	SIL	HEP	LACH			
1	X							X				X																
2	**X**	**X**	**X**	**X**				**X**		X	**X**	**X**		**X**			**X**	**X**	X		**X**							
3	X	X	X		X					X						X		X										
4	X	X					X		X			X																
5	X	X	X	X	X	X	X		X	X	X	X	X	X		X			X				X		X			
6	X	X	X	X	X	X	X	X	X	X	X	X	X	X	X	X	X		X	X	X	X		X	X			
7	**X**	**X**	**X**	X	**X**	**X**	**X**	**X**	**X**	**X**	**X**		X	X		X	**X**	X	X	X	X	**X**	**X**	X	X			
8	X	X	X	X	X	X	X	X	X	X	X		X	X			X			X		X	X	X				
9	X	X	X	X						X												X						
10	X	X	X	X	X	X	X	X	X	X	X		X							X				X				
11	X	X	X	X		X	X	X		X		X			X				X									
12	X	X	X	X			X				X			X	X	X												
13	X	X	X	X		X	X		X	X	X		X		X		X	X		X		X		X				
14	X	X	X	X	X			X		X					X						X		X					
15	X	X	X	X		X	X	X	X		X		X		X		X			X			X					
16	X	X		X	X				X																			
17	X	X	X			X	X		X					X		X												
18	X	X	X	X	X	X				X			X			X					X							
19	X	X	X	X	X			X			X																	
20		X	X		X		X	X																				
21	X	X	X	X	X	X						X						X										
22	X	X	X		X	X			X										X									
24	X	X	X			X	X		X		X	X			X										X			
25	X	X	X					X																				
26	X	X																X										
27	X	X	X		X																				X			

Thirst, Absence Of (AKA Adipsia)

	PULS	APIS	GELS	BELL	IPEC	CHINA	CAPS	CYCL	ANT C	ARS	CAMPH	LYC	NUX M	NUX V	SABAD	SEP	ARG N	AGNUS	ANT T	BAPT	FERR	HYDR AC	KALI CAR	MENY	SAMB N	SARS	TAB	
2	X							**X**																				
3				X																								
4	X	X					X																					
5	X	X	X		X			X	X				X		X				X									
6	X	X	X			X	X			X	X		X			X			X	X			X	X				
7	X	**X**		X		**X**	X	X	X		X	X					**X**	X			X		X					
8	X	X		X						X		X				X						X				X	X	
9	X	X	X		X									X														
10	X	X	X	X		X								X														
11	X	X	X	X	X																							
13	X	X	X	X	X	X	X	X		X	X	X	X		X	X	X	X		X	X	X		X	X	X	X	
14	X	X	X	X										X														
15	X																											
16			X																									
17	X	X	X	X	X										X										X			
18	X	X	X		X																							
19	X	X		X																								
20	X		X																									
21	X	X	X																									
22	X	X	X	X																								
24	X	X																										
25	X	X		X																								
26	X				X				X																			
27	X	X	X																									

Throat, Diseases Of

	ACON	AESC	ARG N	IOD	MERC C	NAT CAR	PHOS	PSOR	ALUM	ASAF	BELL	CAUST	CENCHR	GENT	GUAIAC	MERC I F	PHYTO	RAT	SULPH	THEV	TRFOL P	VIP						
1																			X									
2	**X**	**X**	**X**	**X**	**X**	**X**	**X**	**X**	X			X	X	X	X			X		X	X							
4										X																		
8																						X						
10											X																	
16																	X											
17																X												

Throat, Dryness

	BELL	ACON	PHOS	ALUM	MERC	CAUST	PHYTO	PULS	LACH	CIST	GELS	BRY	SULPH	CALC	HYOSC	SENEG	ARS	IPEC	NUX M	NIT AC	SANG	STRAM	WYETHIA	COLCH	LYC	SABAD		
1	X		X	X					X	X						X					X							
4	X			X	X			X		X	X												X					
5				X																						X		
6	X	X	X	X	X	X	X	X	X				X	X	X		X		X		X	X	X					
7	X	X	**X**	X	**X**	X	X		**X**	X	X			X	X		X	X	**X**	X		X		**X**	X	**X**		
8	X	X	X		X		X	X				X	X	X		X				X								
9	X	X	X								X									X								
10	X							X	X			X																
11	X																											
12	X	X																										
13	**X**	**X**	**X**	X	**X**	X	X	X	X	X	X	**X**	**X**	X	X	**X**	X	X	**X**	X	X	X		X	**X**	X		
14		X					X					X	X				X						X					
15	X					X					X				X			X										
17	X		X	X		X	X	X	X	X		X		X	X			X			X	X						
18	X						X																					
19										X			X										X	X	X			
20	X																											
21		X	X	X		X																						
24	X		X	X	X	X		X								X												
25		X	X		X						X																	

Thrombophlebitis

	LACH	PULS	ACETAN	ARN	CROT H	HAM	SIL
17	X	X	X		X		X
21	X	X		X		X	

Thrombocytopaenia

	CROT H	LACH	PHOS
21	X		X
28		X	

Thrombosis- See also Coronary Thrombosis

	BOTHR	ARN	LACH	APIS	ACON	BELL	MERC	NAT SUL	PHOS	SEC
1	X		X	X				X		
2										X
4		X								
7			X	X			X	X		
8									X	X
9	X	X	X		X	X				
14	**X**	X	X	X			X		X	
16		X			X	X				
17		X								
21	X		X							
28	X									

Thrombosis, Arterial, Thigh

	APIS
14	X

Thrombosis, Deep Vein

	BOTHR	CASC	HAM	LACH
21	X		X	X
27		X		

Thrush

	ALUM	BOR	CAULO	HAM	HELON	KREO	MERC	PULS	THUJA
5			X						
6									X
18					X				
21							X		
27	X	X		X		X		X	

Thrush, Oral

	BOR	MERC	ARS	SULPH	BRY	CAPS	CHAM	HEP	HYDRAST	KALI BR	LACH	NAT M	NIT AC	NUX V	STAPHYS	SULPH AC
3	X	X		X												X
4	X															
6		X	X							X	X				X	
8	X	X	X	X	X	X		X	X	X	X	X	X		X	X
10		X	X	X	X									X		
12	**X**	X	X	X	X	X								X		
15	E	X	X				X						X			
17	X															
20	**X**	X		X			X		X							
21	X	X	X									X				
24								X								

E- External

Thyroid Gland, Diseases Of- See also Exophthalmic Goitre; Goitre; Hyperthyroidism; Hypothyroidism

	BROM	CALC	FUCUS	LYCOP	SPONG	THYROID
1		X				
5						X
8	X				X	
19				X		
27			X			

Thyroiditis

	ACON	APIS	AUR	BAR IOD	BELL	CALC	CALC IOD	CON	FERR PH	GELS	LACH	LYC	NAT M	PHYTO	SPONG	THYROID
5															X	
16	X													X		X
19		X	X	X	X	X	X	X	X	X	X	X	X			

Tic- See also Twitching

	AGAR M	CINA	ACON	ARG N	CARC	CAUST	CEDRON	CIMICI	GELS	HYOSC	HYPOTH	IGN	LYC	MAG PH	MYGALE	PLAT	SPIG	STAPHYS	STRAM	TANACET	TAR H	ZINC
1	X						X									X	X					
5	X	X			X			X			X	X	X					X				
9	X	X		X		X			X	X				X	X				X	X	X	X
14	X		X																			
19	X																					

Tic Convulsif

	HYOSC	AGAR M	ANANTH	ARG N	BELL	LAURO	LYC	MERC	SEP	TAR H	ZINC
2		X	X								
8	X				X			X			
17	X			X		X	X		X	X	X

Tic Doloureux- See Trigeminal Neuralgia

Tinea Capitis- See also Tinea Favosa

	PSOR	ARS	SULPH	CALC	MERC	MEZ	SEP	GRAPH	SIL	DULC	LYC	BAR C	RHUS T	STAPHYS	VIOL T	BROM	HEP	NAT M	PETR	VINCA	CARB A	OLEAND	BAR M	CIC	IRIS V	KREO	PHOS	PHYTO
2	X					X																	X					
4	X																											
6	X	X	X	X	X	X	X	X	X	X		X	X	X	X	X	X		X								X	
7	**X**	**X**	**X**	**X**	**X**	**X**	X	**X**	X	**X**	**X**	X	X		**X**			X	X	X				X	X	X		X
8	X	X	X	X	X	X		X		X	X			X	X	X	X	X		X	X	X	X		X		X	X
13		**X**	**X**	**X**	X		X	**X**	X		X	**X**	**X**	**X**		X	X	X	X	X	**X**	**X**		X		X		
19							**X**																					
24	X																											
26		X	X	X	X	X	X		X	X	X																	

Tinea Cilliaris

	MAG M	THUJA
1	X	
7	X	X
8	X	X

Tinea Circinata- See Ringworm

Tinea Corporis- See Herpes Circinatus

Tinea Faciei

	DULC	PSOR	SULPH	SEP	ARS	BAR C	CALC	CIC	CYCL	MERC	SARS	VIOL T
2		X										
7		X	X									
13	X		X		X	X	X	X	X	X	X	X
19	X			**X**								

Tinea Favosa- See also Tinea Capitus

	SEP	JUG R	BAR C	CALC	CIC	GRAPH	HEP	LAPPA	LYC	OLEAND	PHYTO	RHUS T	STAPHYS	SULPH	VINCA	ZINC
4		X														
8	X	X	X	X	X	X	X	X	X	X	X	X	X	X	X	X
19	**X**															

Tinea Furfuracea- See Pityriasis Versicolor

Tinea Pedis (AKA Athlete's Foot)

	SULPH	SEP	BACILL	CALEND	LYC	SIL
5					X	
13	X					
14			X			
18	X					
19		**X**				X
22				E		

E- External

Tinea Versicolor- See Pityriasis Versicolor

Tingling- See Paraesthesia

Tinnitus (Includes Tinnitus Aurium)

	CHINA	BELL	CAUST	SAL AC	SULPH	GRAPH	NUX V	SIL	ACON	CALC	CHIN S	LACH	PULS	LYC	AUR	BAR M	CARB S	DULC	GLON	HYOSC	NAT M	NAT SAL	PHOS	SANG	PETR
1	X			X		X	X				X				X	X		X		X					X
2	X											X				X								X	
4				X																			X		
5	X	X		X		X		X			X						X								
6	X	X	X		X	X	X	X	X	X		X		X	X	X			X	X	X		X		X
7	X	X	X		X	X	X	X	X	X	X		X	X				X	X	X	X		X		
8	X	**X**	**X**	X	**X**	**X**	X	**X**	X	**X**		**X**	**X**	X	X		X	X	X	X	**X**	X	X	X	**X**
9	**X**	X	X	X	X			X		X		X			X		X			X		X		X	
10	X	X			X		X	X					X			X									
11	X																								
12		X					X				X									X		X			
13	X	X	X		X	X	X	X	X	X		X	X	X	X			X	X	X	X			X	X
14	X		X			X		X						X		X	X								
15	X	X			X		X		X				X						X						
17	X	X	X	X	X	X	X	X	X	X	X		X	X	X	X	X	X	X		X	X	X	X	X
18	X			X																					
19			X	X							**X**											X	X		
21	X			X							X			X			X								
22	X								X									X							
23									X										X						
24	X	X	X			X	X		X	X	X	X				X					X	X			X
25	**X**	X	X	**X**	X					X		X			X		X							X	
26	X	X	X		X	X	X		X			X	X					X					X		
27								X		X	X			X								X		X	
28				X	X																				

Titubation- See also Locomotor Ataxia

	ACET AC	ARS	HYOSIN
16	X		
17		X	X

Tobacco Heart- See also Ailments from Tobacco

	CONVAL	KALM	PHOS	STROPH	NUX V	TAB	ACON	ARS	CACT	DIG	IGN	SARO	SPONG	STAPHYS	VER A
1			X												
4	X	X			X	X								X	
7			X		X		X						X		
9								X							
10				X											
11				X											
17	X	X		X					X	X	X	X			X
19	X	X	X			X									

Toe-Nails, Diseases Of

	AMYG P	CAUST	GRAPH	THUJA
2	X			
7		X	X	X

Toe-Nails, Ingrowing

	SIL	MAG P AU	TEUCR	NAT M	PHOS	GRAPH	CAUST	COLCH	KALI CAR	SULPH	THUJA	ARN	HEP	HYDRAST	KALI MUR	MAG PH	NIT AC	STAPHYS
1	X						X											
2		**X**	X												X		X	X
3		X												E				
6	X	X	X	X	X	X		X	X									
7	**X**			X	X	X	X				X							
8	X	**X**	X	X	X	X		X	X									
9	X		X													X		
10	X									X		E						
13	X		X							X								
14	**X**												X					
21		X									X							

E- External

Tongue, Cracked

	LACH	ARS	ARUM T	BAPT	BELL	BRY	CHAM	KALI BIC	NIT AC	NUX V	PHOS	PLUM	RHUS T	SULPH														
8		X	X	X		X		X	X		X		X	X														
9	X																											
10	X			X								X																
11	X																											
12		X																										
13	X	X			X	X	X	X		X	X	X	X	X														
15							X			X																		
17	X		X																									
19									X																			
21					X																							
24	X																											

Tongue, Diseases Of

	ANT C	BRY	HYDRAST	SULPH	AESC	ANT T	ARS	ARUM T	BELL	CANTH	CARB A	CAUST	DULC	GELS	LYC	MUR AC	NAT M	NUX V	PULS	RAN S	RHUS T	ACON	MANC	MERC	POD	SEMP		
2	**X**	**X**	**X**	**X**	**X**	**X**	**X**	**X**	**X**	**X**	**X**	**X**	**X**	**X**	**X**	**X**	**X**	**X**	**X**	**X**	**X**	X	X		X	X		
8	X	X	X	X	X	X	X	X	X	X	X	X	X	X	X	X	X	X	X	X	X	X	X	X	X	X		
21	X	X	X	X																				X				

Tongue, Dry- See also Xerostomia

	BRY	RHUS T	ARS	KALI BIC	LACH	BELL	APIS	BAPT	MUR AC	PHOS	VER A	ACON	LYC	NUX V	PHYTO	PLUM	NUX M	ARG N	CHAM	GELS	NAT M	NIT AC	PSOR	DULC	PULS	VER V		
1		X			X				X				X															
5		X	X	X	X	X	X			X	X	X	X		X													
6	X	X	X	X	X	X		X	X	X	X		X	X	X		X	X			X	X	X		X			
7		**X**	X	X	X	X	X			X	X			X	X	X	**X**	X			X		X	X	**X**	**X**		
8		X	X						X																			
9	X								X											X								
10	X		X		X			X							X	X						X						
11	X			X		X																						
13	**X**	X	**X**	X	X	X	X	X		X	**X**	X	X	X		X	X	X		X	X	X	X	**X**				
14	X	X	X				X					X																
15	X	X	X	X		X	X	X	X	X				X												X		
16	X																											
17	X			X								X																
19	X							X																				
22	X																											
24		X	X		X											X												
25	X																			X								

Tongue, Inflammation- See Glossitis

Tongue, Mapped

	NAT M	ANT C	ARS	LACH	LYC	NIT AC	PH AC	RAN S	TARAX
8	X	X	X		X	X	X	X	X
10	X			X					
17	X								
18	X								

Tongue, Paralysis- See Paralysis, Tongue
Tongue, Ulceration- See Ulceration, Tongue
Tonsillitis

	BAR C	BELL	HEP	MERC	LACH	PHYTO	APIS	SIL	ACON	IGN	LAC C	CALC PH	LYC	BAR M	GUAIAC	KALI MUR	BAR IOD	MERC I F	THUJA	MERC I R	SULPH	CANTH
1	X	X	X	X	X	X	X	X	X	X		X	X	X			X	X	X	X		
2	**X**	X										**X**		X	X			X			X	
3	**X**	**X**	X	X	X	X					X	X	X						X			
4	**X**	**X**	**X**	**X**		**X**	**X**			**X**		**X**			**X**	**X**	X					
5	X	X		X	X	X	X		X		X			X		X	X		X			X
6	X	X	X	X	X	X	X	X		X			X	X							X	
7	**X**	**X**		**X**	**X**	X	X	X	X		**X**		X	X				X				
8	X	X	X	X	X	X		X	X	X	X	X	X	X	X	X	X	X	X	X	X	X
9										X												
10	X	X	X	X	X			X	X	X		X	X	X							X	
11	X																					
12					X	X																
13	X	**X**			X					X												**X**
14	X	X	X	X	X	X	X	X	X				X			X						
16	X	X	X	X																		
17	X		X		X			X	X		X				X			X	X	X		X
18		X		X	X	X	X										X	X		X		
19		**X**	**X**	**X**																		
21			X				X				X											
22	X	**X**	X	X			X					X				X						
23	X	X				X					X		X		X	X				X		
24	**X**	X	X	X		X	X	X	X	**X**					X		X		X		X	
25			X	X								X										
26	X	X	X	X	X			X	X													
27	X	**X**	**X**		X			**X**			X											

Tonsillitis, Left Side

	LACH	MERC I R	APIS	CUPR	SABAD	SIL
5	X	X				
7		X	X			
8	X			X		X
9	X					
10	X					
17					X	
18		X				
19	**X**	**X**				
21	X					
24		X				
25	X					
28		X				

Tonsillitis, Right Side

	BELL	MER I F	BAR C	MERC	PHYTO	GUAIAC	LYC	BAR M	COCC C	GELS	MERC CY	RHUS T
1				X								
4	X		X									
5		X					X					
7	X			X						X		
8	X											X
9	X		X									
10	X		X					X				
14	X				X							
17		X				X			X		X	
18		X										
19	X	**X**										
21	X			X	X		X					
24	X		X		X							
25	X		X									
28		X										

Toothache (Includes Odontalgia)

	CHAM	MERC	STAPHYS	BELL	PLANTAG	PULS	COFF	ACON	BRY	ARN	SPIG	CALC	KREO	ANT C	SIL	ARS	NUX V	SULPH	CHINA	HYOSC	PHOS	IGN	LACH	RHUS T	SEP	MAG CAR	MAG PH	HEP
1	X	X	X	X	E	X	X			X	X	X	X	X	X				X	X	X		X		X	X		
2	**X**	**X**	**X**		**X**	**X**	X	X	**X**		**X**	**X**	**X**					X		X		X			**X**	**X**	X	
3	X	X		X	**X**	X	X	X	X	X	X		X			X	X			X				X			X	
4	**X**	**X**	X	X	**X**		**X**			**X**	**X**											X						
5	X		X																							X	X	
6	X	X	X	X	X	X	X	X	X	X		X		X	X	X	X	X	X	X	X	X	X	X	X			X
7	**X**	X	**X**	X	X	X	X	X	X			X	X	X		X		X	X		X		X		**X**		X	
8	**X**	**X**	**X**	**X**	X	**X**	X	X	**X**	X	X	**X**	X	X	**X**	X	**X**	**X**	**X**	**X**	**X**	X	X	**X**	X	X		X
9	X		X	X	B		X	X		X			X	X	X								X				X	
10	X	**X**	X	X	**X**	X	X		X	X	X	X	X	X	X	X	X	X	X	X	X	X	X	X				X
11	X						X																					
12	X	X	X	X	X	X		X	X					X	X	X	X				X							
13	X	X	X	X		X	X	X	X		X	X		X	X	X	X	X	X	X	X	X	X	X		X		X
14	X	X		X	X			X	X		X	X		X														
15	X	X		X		X		X			X					X	X	X							X			
17	X		X			X																						
18	X			X		X		X		X						X												
19	**X**	**X**	**X**	X	X	X	**X**	X	**X**	X	X	X	X	X	X		X	X	X		X	X	X	X	X	X	X	**X**
21	X	X	X	X	B	X	X		X	X		X	X													X	X	
23													X															
24					X	X																						
25	X	X	X	X	B		X	X		X			X		X													
26	**X**	X	X	X		X	X	X	X		X	X		X	X	X	X	X	X	X		X		X				X
28	X																											
29*										X																		

B- Both Internal and External E- External

29* Albertini H, et al. Homeopathic treatment of the dental neuralgia by Arnica and Hypericum. Journal of the American Institute of Homeopathy, 1985, 3, 126-129.

Tophi- See also Gout

	LYC	STAPHYS	ASAF	AUR	BUFO	CALC	DIG	FL AC	GRAPH	KALI IOD	LED	LITH C	MEZ	PH AC	PHOS	RUTA	SABIN	SIL	SULPH
6	X	X	X	X				X					X	X	X	X	X	X	X
8	X				X					X									
13		X				X	X		X		X								
17												X							

Tormina- See also Pain, Abdomen

	ERIG	FL AC
6	X	
8		X

Torticollis (AKA Wry Neck)

	LACHNAN	NUX V	LYC	CAUST	PHOS	RHUS T	BELL	CAULO	CIMICI	COLCH	CUPR	LACH	SULPH
2	X												
4		X											
5	X	X	X	X	X	X		X	X		X		
6	X	X						X					
7	X	X	X			X	X			X	X	X	X
8	X	X	X		X	X	X			X			X
9				X					X				
17			X		X							X	
19				**X**									

Torticollis, Right Sided

	AUR M	BELL	CUPR	LACHNAN
6		X		
7	X		X	
9				X

Tourette's Syndrome

	ANAC	BELL	CIC	CUPR	HYOSC	RHUS T
19	X	X		X	X	X
28			X			

Toxaemia

	CROT H	LACH	NUX V	SULPH
10	X			
24		X		
28			X	X

Toxicity

	NUX V	PHOS	AQ MAR	BAPT	GUNPOW	LACH	PSOR	URT U	VERIN
1					X				
3				X					X
4							X		
5								X	
9	X								
17			X						
19	X	X				X			
25		X							

Trachea, Diseases Of

	CARB A	LACH	PHOS	STANN	APIS	ARS	BROM	CAPS	CARB AC	CARB V	KALI CAR	NUX V	SIL	SULPH
2	**X**	**X**	**X**	X	**X**	**X**	**X**	**X**	**X**	**X**	**X**	**X**	**X**	**X**
9		X	X	X										
17	X													

Tracheitis (Note here that only the main remedies are used from 17)

	HEP	SPONG	ACON	BRY	BELL	ANT T	BROM	CAUST	KALI BIC	MERC	RUMEX	IOD	CARB V	HYOSC	IPEC	LACH	PHOS	MANG	SAMB	ARS	CON	DROS	PULS	STANN
1				X																				
6										X														
7	X	X	X			X	X						X											
8	X				X	X	X										X				X		X	
9				X						X	X			X		X								
12	X	X	X			X	X		X			X								X				
13	X	X	X	X	**X**							**X**	X		X			**X**	**X**	X		X		
14								X																
15	X	X	X		X			X	X					X	X	X	X				X			
17	X	X	X		X	X	X	X	X	X	X	X	X					X	X				X	X
18				X							X			X								X		
19															X									
21				X				X	X		X					X	X							X
23	X	X																						
24										X														

Trachoma

	ACON	APIS	CHIN M	CUPR SUL	MERC P	SEP	ARS	ALUMEN	AUR	CALC	CAUST	EUPHR	KALI BIC	MERC C	MERC I R	SULPH	THUJA	GRAPH
2			X	X	X													
3				X	X													
4						X												
7	X	X	X				**X**	X					X	X	X	X		**X**
8			X		X	X			X	X	X	X			X		X	
14	X	**X**												X				
24	X			X		X	X	X	X	X	X	X	X			X	X	

Trauma- See also Injury; Wounds

	ARN	BELLIS	HYPER	SULPH AC	RHUS T	CON	PULS	RUTA	BRY	ACON	ALL C	CARB V	CAUST	CIC	CUPR	EUPH PIL	GLON	HEP	LAC AC	MILL	NAT SUL	OP	SYMPH					
2		X		X							X					X	X											
6	X		X	X	X	X	X																					
8	X		X		X																							
9	X	X																										
14	X																											
16	X																											
17	X	X	X	X		X								X	X						X	X						
18	**X**																											
19	***X***	**X**	X	X			X	X	**X**	X		X						X		X			X					
27	**X**				X			X					X						X									
29[1]	X																											
29[2]	X																											

29[1] Gibson J, et al. Double Blind Trial of Arnica in Acute Trauma Patients. Communications of the British Homoeopathy Research Group, 1991, Mar, 21, 34-41.

29[2] Chakrabarty J, et al. Cytogenetical effects of sonication in mice and their modulations by actinomycin D and a homeopathic drug Arnica 30. Indian J of Exp Biol, 2001, Dec, 39, (12), 1235-42.

Trauma, Surgical- See Ailments from, Surgery

Trembling- See Tremors

Tremors- See also Paralysis Agitans; Motion, Involuntary, generally and specifically (Includes Jerking; Trembling)

	GELS	MERC	ARG N	AGAR M	IGN	PHOS	OP	ZINC	PLUM	ARS	CON	BELL	CAUST	HYOSC	RHUS T	LACH	CALC	COCCUL	STRAM	ANT T	CIC	NIT AC	CHINA	NUX V	PLAT	IOD	SULPH	TAB
1	**X**		X	X	X	X		X	X	X	X				X	X											X	
2	**X**	**X**		**X**	**X**														**X**	**X**								
4			X					X	X																	X		
5	X	X	X		X	X	X	X	X	X	X		X	X	X	X	X	X				X	X		X			X
6	X	X	X	X	X	X	X	X	X	X		X	X	X	X	X	X	X	X	X	X	X	X	X	X	X	X	
7	X	X	**X**	X		X	**X**		X	**X**	X	X	X		X	**X**	X	**X**	X		X	**X**			X			X
8		X						X	X		X		X		X		X	X	X		X	X		X	X		X	
9	X		X	X	X	X		X		X	X			X										X				X
10	X	X					X				X	X	X										X					
11			X			X		X							X					X								
13		**X**		X	X	**X**	**X**	X	**X**	**X**	X	**X**	X	X	X	X	X	**X**	**X**	X	**X**	X	X	X	X	**X**	**X**	**X**
14	X		X	X	X									X							X							
15							X			X	X	X		X						X								
16		X					X							X									X					
17	X	X	X	X	X	X	X	X	X	X	X	X	X	X	X	X		X		X			X	X		X		
18	X		X	X																						X		
19	X		X			X						X	X								X							
20		X																										
21	X	X	X	X	X	X		X				X							X								X	
22	X	X																										
24	X	X																										
25																								X				X
26					X		X																					
27	X	X	X						X							X												

Tremor, Arm (Includes Arm, Jerking)

	OP	IOD	PHOS	CIC	CUPR	RHUS T	SPIG	SIL
6	X							
7	X	X	X	X		X	X	
8	X							
13	**X**	**X**	**X**				X	**X**
16	X							
19				X	X			

Tremor, Epigastrium

	CIMICI	ARG N	ARS	CROT H
7		X	X	X
8	X			

Tremor, Eyelids

	IOD	VER A	BELL	CIC	AGAR M	AMBRA	CALC	CARB V	MERC	OP	PHOS	PHYSO	PLAT
5					X	X						X	
7	X	X	**X**	**X**							X		
13	X	X						X	X	X			X
27							X						

Tremor, Extremities

	LACH	BUFO	CAMPH	MERC	OP
8	X		X		
14		X		X	
15	X				X

Tremor, Face (Includes, Face, Jerking)

	OP	AMBRA	AGAR M	BELL	CAD S	COCCUL	HYOSC	LAURO	SEP	STRAM	THYROID
1											X
6	X					X		X	X		
13	**X**	**X**									
14			X								
17					X						
19				X			X			X	

Tremor, Feet

	ZINC	PLAT	HYOSC	STRAM	BAR C	BOV	CAMPH	COFF	CON	IP	LYC	NICCOL	OL AN	PULS	SARS	TAB	TAR H	VER A
4	X																	
6			X											X				
7			X															
11	X																	
13	X	**X**		**X**	X	X		X		X	X	X	X		X	X		X
17									X									
21																	X	
24							X											

Tremor, Fingers (Includes Fingers, Jerking)

	CIC	GLON	MERC	CIMICI	BRY	CINA	COCCUL	IOD	NIT AC	OLENAD	RHUS T
1				X							
4	X										
7	X	X	X				X				
13		X			X			X	X	X	X
14	X					X					
21			X								

Tremor, Hand (Includes Hand, Jerking)

	MERC	PHOS	PLUM	HYOSC	SULPH	ZINC	ARG N	ARS	CIC	COCCUL	GELS	AMM C	CAUST	CHINA	COFF	PLAT	AGAR M	ANT T	IOD	LACH	NUX V
1										X	X										
4		X					X														
5	X	X	X				X				X		X	X			X	**X**	X		
6	X			X		X	X		X		X				X					X	
7	**X**	X	X	X	X	X		X		X	X			X	X	X					
8				X	X	X		X	X												
10												X									
13	X	**X**	X	**X**	**X**	**X**		X	X	X		X	X	X	X	X	**X**	X	**X**	**X**	**X**
14	X								X												
15																X					
17	X				X							X									
19	**X**	X	X				X	X		X			X								X
24			X																		

Tremor, Head

	PLUM	MYGAL	OP	SIL	TAR H
6		X	X		X
7				X	
8	X				
24	X				

Tremor, Jaw

	AGAR M	CAD S	CARB V	COCCUL	PHOS
5	X			X	X
7	X				
13			X		
14		X			

Tremor, Knees

	ANAC	ALUM	LED	OLEAND	RUTA	ACON	BELL	CAMPH	CHEL	DIOSC	LACH	LAURO	NUX V	PULS	RHUS T	VERBASC
5	X	X	X						X							
7		X						X								
8															X	
10				X												
13	**X**		X	X	**X**	X	X				X	X	X	X		X
17										X						

Tremor, Legs (Includes Legs, Jerking)

	ARG N	KALI CAR	NUX V	IGN	AGAR M	GELS	NAT CAR	NAT M	OP	SEP	SULPH	TAR H	ZINC	IPEC	LACH	PULS	RUTA
6												X					
7		X	X		X	X	X	X					X		**X**		
8	X		X								X						
9	X		X														
13		X		**X**			X	X	X	X	X			**X**		**X**	**X**
16									X								
19	X																
21		X		X	X	X				X		X	X				

Tremor, Left Side

	RHUS T	TAR H
6		X
17	X	

Tremor, Limbs (Includes Limbs, Jerking)

	STRAM	NUX V	SULPH	ARS	COCCUL	APIS	ZINC	HYOSC	CIC	LYC	BELL	GELS	SEC	ARG N	CAUST	CUPR	AMYL N	ANT T	IGN	MAG PH	MERC	OP	PHOS	PULS	PHYSO	PLUM
1			X	X				X		X							X									
4			X		X		X						X													
6	X	X	X	X	X	X	X	X			X		X	X									X			
7	X	**X**	X	X	**X**	X		X	X	X		X		**X**	**X**	X			X	X	X	X	X	X		**X**
8	X	X	**X**	X		X	X	X	**X**	**X**			X		X	**X**		X	X			X			**X**	
9		X																								
10	X	X									X										X					
11									X																	
12				X																						
14												X								X						
15	X				X	X					X													X		
17												X					X	X								
19	X																									
27							X																			

Tremor, Lips

	STRAM	ARG N	SULPH	AGAR M	ALOE	ARN	BELL	LACH	RAN S
5	X	X		X			X		
7	X	X	X			X			
13	X		X		X			X	X

Tremor, Mouth

	MERC
1	X
7	X

Tremor, Senile

	AGAR M	AMBRA	ARG N	ARS	BAR C	CAUST	GELS	PHOS	PLUM
5		X	X	X	X	X	X	X	X
8	X								

Tremor, Stomach

	CALC	HAM	IGN	IOD	NUX V
5	X			X	X
7		X	X		

Tremor, Tongue

	LACH	GELS	MERC	ABSINTH	AGAR M	APIS	ARS	BELL	CAMPH	HYOSC	IGN	LYC	STRAM	BAPT	CANTH	HELL	HYDRAST	MERC C	PLUM	SEC	TAR H
1			X	X																	
5	X	X	X		X																
6	X				X			X			X	X							X		
7	X	X							X	X	X				X	X		X			
8	X	X		X		X	X	X		X		X	X							X	
9	X					X															
10	X	X					X										X				
15													X	X							
17	X		X																		
19		X																			
21		X	X																		X
24									X												

Trichiasis

	BOR	PULS	APIS	GRAPH	ACON	BELL	BOV	CIST	NAT M	SEP	TELL	THUJA
1	X	X		X								
2	X			X							X	
3	X	X										
6	X			X	X				X	X		X
7			X		**X**							
13	X	X	X	X		X	X	X				
27	X											

Trichinosis (AKA Roundworms)

	CINA	SANTIN	BELL	CHINA	SABAD	STANN	SULPH	TEUCR	APIS	CALC	DIG	FERR	MERC	NUX V	SIL	SPIG	TEREB	VER A
3								X										
4		X																
6			X	X	X	X	X		X								X	
7	X		X	X	X	X	X	X	X	X	X	X	X	X	X	X		X
8	X	X	X	X	X		X	X		X	X	X	X	X	X	X	X	X
12	X																	
15	X	X				X												
29*	X	X																

29* Sukul NC, et al. Reduction in the number of infective Trichinella spiralis larvae in mice by use of homeopathic drugs. Forsch Komplementarmed Klass Naturheilkd, 2005, Aug, 12, 4.

Trichomonas Infection

	BOV	CARB V	CINNAB	MERC	NIT AC
5			X		
21	X	X		X	X

Tricuspid Valve, Insufficiency

	LITH C	SPONG	BELL	HYOSC	KALI CAR	LACH	PULS	VISC A
6	X			X	X	X	X	
8	X	X						
11								X
17		X						

Tricuspid Valve, Regurgitation

	APOC	ADONIS
1	X	
11		X
17	X	
19	X	

Trigeminal Neuralgia- See also Neuralgia, Facial

	GELS	AGAR M	AUR	CHAM	CHINA	CHIN S	NAT M	PRUN S	RAN B	SPIG	STAPHYS	STRAM	ZINC PH
1		X											
2	X												
17	X	X	X	X	X	X	X	X	X	X	X	X	X

Trigeminal Neuralgia, Left

	ACON	CEDRON	COLOC	KALI IOD	NUX V	SEP	VERBASC
17	X	X	X	X	X	X	X

Trigeminal Neuralgia, Right

	ARS	BELL	CALC	CAUST	CHEL	LYC	MAG PH	MEZ	PHOS	PLAT	SANG	STANN
17	X	X	X	X	X	X	X	X	X	X	X	X

Triplopia

	BELL	SEC	HYOSC
7	X		
8	X	X	
12			X
17	X	X	

Trismus- See also Lockjaw; Spasm, Jaw; Tetanus

	CIC	HYDR AC	BELL	IGN	NUX V	STRAM	ACON	ANGUST	CAMPH	CAUST	HYOSC	LACH	LAURO	MERC	OP	PHOS	PLAT	PLUM	VER A	HYPER	BRY	CARB OX	CON	CUPR	GELS	LINUM U	RHUS T	SIL
2	X					X																X	X			X		
3																										X		
4	X	X		X																X								
6		X				X	X										X											
7			X	X	X		X	X	X	X	X	X	X	X	X	X		X	X		X			X	X			
8	X	X	X	X	X	X	X	X	X	X	X	X	X	X	X	X	X	X	X	**X**				X			X	X
11	X																											
13	X	X	X	X	X	X		X	X	X	X	X	X	X	X	X	X	X	X		X				X		X	X
23																						X	X					
24	X	X	X		X																							

Tuberculosis, Abdominal

	CALC	ARS	PHOS	PULS	BAR C	CALC PH	CARB V	CHINA	HEP	MERC	NIT AC	PH AC	PLUM	SULPH
6	X													
8	X	X	X	X	X	X	X	X	X	X	X	X	X	X
10	X													
11	X	X	X	X										
24	X	X	X	X	X	X	X	X	X	X	X	X	X	X

Tuberculosis, Bone (AKA White Swelling)

	CALC	DROS	PHOS	SULPH	APIS	ARG N	BRY	CALC IOD	CIST	DIG	HECLA	MERC	MERC I F	SEP	SYMPH
2				X											
8	X				X	X			X	X	X				
10		**X**	X					X				X		X	X
15	X			X			X						X		
24	X		X												

Tuberculosis, Glands

	CALC	IOD	CALC IOD	DROS	MERC I F	SULPH	AMM M	BAR C	BROM	KALI IOD	PHOS	PHYTO	SIL	THYROID	TUB
10	X	X	X	**X**		X		X	X		X		X		X
12	X	X			X	X	X			X		X			
24	X	X	X		X									X	

Tuberculosis, Joints

	ARS	BELL	CALC	COLOC	PHOS	SIL	CALC PH	CHINA	HEP	IOD	KALI C	LACH	LYC	MERC	RHUS T	STRAM	SULPH	ACON	CARB V	KALI IOD								
8	X	X	X	X	X	X	X	X		X	X	X	X	X	X	X	X			X								
12	X	X	X	X	X	X			X									X										
24	X	X	X	X		X	X	X	X	X	X	X	X	X	X	X	X		X									

Tuberculosis, Intestinal

	CALC	ARS	PHOS	PULS	TUB	APIS	APOC	ARG N	ARN	BAPT	BRY	BAR C	CALC PH	CARB V	CARB S	CHEL	CHINA	FERR	HEP	LYC	MERC	NIT AC	PH AC	PLUM	SULPH			
6	X	X	X	X				X			X	X	X	X			X	X	X		X	X	X	X	X			
7															X													
8	X																											
11	X	**X**	**X**	**X**	X	X	X		X	X						X				X								

Tuberculosis, Laryngeal

	DROS	SPONG	PHOS	CARB V	ARS	CAUST	HEP	LACH	MANG	SULPH	ARG	CALC	IOD	KALI IOD	NIT AC	SIL	ARG N	KALI BIC	KREO	NAT SEL	SABAL	SEL						
1																					**X**							
2									X											X								
4	X	X			X																							
6			X	X	X			X		X			X	X	X	X	X											
7	X	**X**	X	X	X	X	X	X	X		X		X	X	X			X	X			X						
8	X	X	X	X	X	X	X	X	X	X	X	X	X	X	X	X		X	X			X						
13	**X**	**X**	X	**X**		**X**	X		X	X		X																
17	X		X	X																								
23	X																X			X								
24	X	X																										
26	X	X	X		X	X	X	X		X	X	X				X												

Tuberculosis, Mesenteric Glands

	IOD	CALC HP	SULPH	ARS	BAR C	MERC C	PLUM	ARS I	AUR	BAPT	BELL	CALC	CALC IOD	CHAM	CHINA	KREO	NIT AC	NUX V	OL JEC A	PETR	PHOS	PLUM AC	PYROG	SACCH	TUB			
1																					X							
2	**X**	**X**				**X**	**X**			X										X			X	X				
7	X				X			X	X										X									
8	**X**		X													X												
11		X																							X			
12	X	X	X	X																		X						
15			X	X	X						X	X		X	X		X	X										
24													X															

Tuberculosis, Pulmonary (Includes Scrofulosis & Phthisis) (Note that only the main remedies are used from 17)

	PHOS	CALC	SULPH	LYC	SIL	ARS IOD	ARS	KALI CAR	CALC PH	HEP	IOD	SPONG	TUB	BRY	DROS	NIT AC	STANN	DULC	ACON	CARB A	BAPT	FERR	KREO	PULS	SANG	SEP
1	**<u>X</u>**		X	X	X	X			X		X		X							X						
2	**X**	**X**	**X**	**X**		**X**		**X**	**X**	**X**	**X**	X	X	**X**	**X**		**X**		**X**		**X**		**X**			
3	X	X	X	X	X		X		X								X			X	X					
4	**<u>X</u>**	**X**	**X**	**X**	**X**	X	**X**	**X**	X		X			**X**	**X**	**X**	X	**X**			X	X			**X**	X
6	X	X	X	X	X	X	X	X	X	X	X	X	X	X		X	X	X	X		X	X			X	X
7	**X**	**X**	**X**	**X**	**X**	X	X	**X**	X	**X**	X	**X**	**X**		X	X	**X**	X	**X**	X		X	X	X	X	**X**
8	**<u>X</u>**	**X**	**X**	**X**	**X**	X	X	X	**X**	**X**	X	X		X	X	**X**	X	**X**	X	X	X	X	X	**X**		X
9		X											X													
10	X	X	X	X	X				X	X		X														
11	X																									
12	**X**	**X**	**X**	X	X	**X**	**<u>X</u>**			X	**X**			X	X				X			**X**	X	X		X
13	X	X	X	X	X		X	X		X	X	X				X		X		X			X		X	X
14	**<u>X</u>**					X														X						
15		X													X											
16	X							X	X				X													
17	X	X	X	X	X	X	X	X	X	X	X	X	X	X		X	X	X		X	X	X	X	X	X	X
21		X					X																			
23	X	X	X		X	X						X								X	X	X	X		X	
24			X	X	X	X	X	X					X	X	X	X	X	**X**						X	X	
26	X	X	X	X	X			X		X		X		X	X	X								X		
27	X	X											X											X		

Tuberculosis, Testes

	AUR	CALC	MERC I R	SIL	SPONG	SULPH	TEUCR S
1	X	X	X	X	X	X	
2							X

Tuberculosis, Trachea

	CARB V	DROS	MANG	CALC	CAUST	HEP	NIT AC	PHOS	ARS	ARS IOD	CALC IOD	CARB A	CHINA	CIST	COLOC	CON	IOD	KALI AC	KREO	LED	LYC	SEL	SULPH IO	THERID
7												X												
8	X	X	X	X	X	X	X	X		X	X			X					X	X		X	X	X
13	**X**	**X**	**X**	X	X	X	X	X	**X**				X		X	X	X	X			X			

Tumors

	CON	THUJA	ARS	BAR C	CALC	HYDRAST	KALI IOD	LAPIS	PHOS	APIS	ARN	AUR	CALC FL	CARB A	PHYTO
1	X	X		X	X	X	X	X	X		X		X	X	
2	X	X		**X**	**X**		X	X	X	X	X	X			X
4			**X**												
5		X													
7										X					
8	X	X	X	X	X	X	X	X	X	X	X	X		X	X
12	X	X	**X**		X	X		X	X			X		X	
14	X	X											X		
16	X						X								
24			X	X									X		X
29*		X				X									

29* ES S, et al. Effect of Homeopathic Medicines on Transplanted Tumors in Mice. Asian Pacific J Cancer Prev, 2007, 8, 390-394.

Tumor, Abdomen

	CON	GRAPH	CALC FL	KALI CAR	NAT CAR	THUJA	TUB
3	X	X	X	X		X	X
7	X	X					
13					X		

Tumor, Axilla

	TELL
2	X
3	X

Tumor, Bone- See Osteoma

Tumor, Brain (Includes Cancer, Brain)

	CALC	KALI IOD	BAR C	CALC PH	CON	MERC I F	PLUM	CALC FL	LACH	PHOS	THUJA	TUB	ARS	BELL	CROC	SIL												
1	X	X		X		X	X	X			X	X																
2							X																					
3				X	X	X		X				X																
4			X																									
6	X			X		X			X	X			X	X		X												
7									X	X					X													
8	X	X							X	X	X		X	X	X	X												
11	X	X	X		X		X																					
14	X			X	X	X		X			X	X																
16			X																									
17		X	X		X		X																					
21	X	X																										

Tumor, Breast- See also Cancer, Breast (AKA Breast Lumps) (Includes Fibrocystic Breast Disease)

	CON	PHYTO	SIL	CALC	HYDRAST	CHIM	SCROPH	CARB A	BELL	BROM	CALC IOD	IOD	PHOS	SULPH	BRY	ARN	ARS IOD	BAR IOD	CALC	CHAM	GRAPH	LACH	LAPIS	LYC	MERC I F	MUREX	PLUM IOD	SANG
1	X	X			X		X							X														
2						X	X			X	X						X								X			**X**
3	X	X			X																							
4	**X**	**X**	X	**X**	**X**											X		X								X	X	
5	X	X		X				X		X													X					
6		X	X										X	X														
7	**X**							**X**									X					X						
8						X			X											X								
9	X	E	X																									
14				X		X																						
16							X																					
18	X	X		X								X																
21	X	X							X						X						X							
23	X										X														X			
24	X	X	X	X	X	X	X	X		X	X	X	X	X		X		X	X		X	X	X	X		X	X	
25	X	E	X												**X**													
26	X		X						X			X	X						X	X				X				
27	X																											

E- External

Tumor, Cystic

	APIS	APOC	ARS	BAR C	BROM	CALC	HEP	SIL																				
7	X			X	X	X	X																					
8	X	X	X					X																				

Tumor, Erectile

	PHOS	LYC	NIT AC	ARN	ARS	CARB A	CARB V	COCCUS	KREO	LACH	PLAT	PULS	SEP	SIL	SULPH	THUJA
7	X	X	X													
8	**X**	X	X	X	X	X	X	X	X	X	X	X	X	X	X	X

Tumor, Eye

	THUJA	STAPHYS	BENZ AC	ARN	ARS	BELL	BRY	CALC	CAUST	CHAM	CON	HEP	KALM	LYC	MERC	NUX V	PHOS	RHUS T	SEP	SIL	SULPH	ZINC
2	**X**	**X**	**X**																			X
8	X	X		X	X	X	X	X	X	X	X	X	X	X	X	X	X	X	X	X	X	
24	X																					

Tumor, Eyelid

	CALC	GRAPH	HEP	PULS	STAPHYS	THUJA	ZINC	MAG CAR	NIT AC	SIL	TEUCR
1	X						X				
2											X
3							X				
6	X	X			X	X				X	
7	X		X			X			X		
8		X	X	X	X			X			
24				X							

Tumor, Fatty

	AGAR M	AMM M	BAR C	PHYTO	THUJA	URIC AC
1		X				
2	X				X	X
4			X	X		

Tumor, Fibroid, Uterine

	CALC	CALC IOD	LACH	TRILL P	SIL	AUR M	CON	FRAX	LAPIS	SEP	PHOS	PULS	PLAT	SABIN	THUJA	USTIL	AUR M N	SEC	APIS	CALC FL	KALI IOD	STAPHYS	THLASPI
1			X	X				X	X			X	X								X		
2					**X**				X							X		**X**			X		X
3	X	X		X				X	X		X	X	X	X	X		**X**				X	X	X
5	X		X	X			X			X			X	X	X		X	X		X		X	
7	**X**		X	X	X		X									X			X				
8	X		X	X	X		X						X		X	X		X	X			X	
9		**X**	X			**X**				X													
14				X				X	X			X											
18	X				X	X	X	X	X	X	X				X		X			X			
19	X										**X**			X		X							
21		X	X	X	X	X		X			X												X
23		X																					
25		**X**	X			**X**				X													
29*	X	X			X		X			X		**X**		X					X	X			

29* Popov AV. Homoeopathy in the Treatment of Patients with Fibromyoma of the Uterus. Brit Hom J, October 1992, 81, 164-167.

Tumor, Genital, Female- See also Tumor, Ovary; Tumor, Uterus

	LYC	CALC	CARB V	NIT AC	ARN	BELL	CARB A	CHAM	CON	GRAPH	KALM	KREO	MERC	NUX V	PHOS	PULS	SEP	STAPHYS	SULPH	THUJA
7	**X**	X	X	X											X					
8	X	X	X	X	X	X	X	X	X	X	X	X	X	X		X	X	X	X	X

Tumor, Glands

	CON	IOD	ARS BR	BAR C	BRY	FERR IOD	LAPIS	PHYTO	SIL	SULPH
4	**X**									
8	X	X		X	X		X	X	X	X
23			X			X				
24		X								

Tumor, Head

	HEP	SIL	ARS	CALC	CHEL	GRAPH	MERC	PETR	PHOS	RHUS T	SEP	STAPHYS
8	X	X	X	X	X	X	X	X	X	X	X	X
26	X	X										

Tumor, Jaw

	HECLA	PLUM	THUJA
2	X	X	**X**
3	X	X	

Tumor, Lip

	CON	STAPHYS	ACET AC	ARS	CARB V	CONDUR	PHOS	SIL	SULPH
1	X	X			X	X	X	X	X
3	X	X							
7	X								
8	X								
14			X	X					

Tumor, Mouth

	LYC	BELL	CALC	CHAM	CHINA	MERC	NIT AC	NUX V	PHOS	PULS	SEP	SULPH	ZINC
7	X												
8	X	X	X	X	X	X	X	X	X	X	X	X	X

Tumor, Neck

	BAR C	PHOS	ARS	ARS IOD	CALC	CALC PH	CAUST	MERC	NIT AC	SULPH
1	X	X								
3	X									
8		X	X	X	X	X	X	X	X	X

Tumor, Nipple

	CARB A
1	X
7	X

Tumor, Nose

	AUR	CALC	CARB A	CAUST	HECLA	KALM	MERC	NAT CAR	NAT M	PH AC	PULS	SULPH	THUJA
7			X		X							X	
8	X	X		X		X	X	X	X	X	X		X

Tumor, Ovary- See also Tumor, Genital, Female

	APIS	ARS	CALC	COLOC	POD	LYC	BAR IOD	GRAPH	LYC	PLAT	SEC	ALUMEN	APOC	BAR M	BOV	CANTH	CARB A	CHINA	CON	IOD	KALI BR	LIL T	OOPHOR	PALLAD	PLUM	RHUS T	STRAM
1												X												X			
2	**X**				X			X			**X**												X			X	
3									X																		
4							X								X												
5																			X								
6	X	X	X	X	X	X		X								X		X		X		X			X		X
7	**X**	X	X	X		**X**				X				X													
8	X	X	X	X	X				X	X			X				X				X						
14	X																										
24							X																				

Tumor, Ovary, Right

	POD	APIS	FL AC
6	X		
7		X	
8	X		X

Tumor, Placenta- See Tumor, Trophoblastic

Tumor, Pylorus

	HYDRAST	CONDUR
4	X	
8		X
24	X	

Tumor, Sebaceous- See also Cysts, Sebaceous

	AGAR M	BAR C	BELL	GRAPH	HEP	KALI CAR	SIL	THUJA
2	X							X
7	X	**X**	X	X	X	X	X	

Tumor, Stomach

	HYDRAST	ANT T	ARS IOD	ART V	CONDUR	HEP	KALI BIC	KREO	LAPIS	SULPH
4	X									
8		X	X	X	X	X	X	X	X	X
24	X									

Tumor, Tarsal

	STAPHYS	CALC	GRAPH	SEP	THUJA	ZINC
2	X					X
6	X					
8	X	X	X	X	X	

Tumor, Thyroid

	CALC IOD	IOD
7		X
19	X	

Tumor, Tongue

	ANTHRAC	CARB A	CIC	MERC	MEZ	THUJA
3	X	X		X		X
7			X		X	

Tumor, Tongue, Under- See Ranula

Tumor, Trophoblastic (AKA Tumor, Placenta)

	CANTH	PULS	SABIN	SEC
1			X	X
21	X	X		

Tumor, Urethra/Ureter

	ANIL	LACH
3	X	
13		X

Tumor, Uterus- See also Tumor, Fibroid, Uterus; Tumor, Genital, Female

	APIS	CON	AUR M	AUR M N	CALC	FRAX	LAPIS	SEP	TEREB	BUFO	CALC PH	LYC	NIT AC	PHOS	SABAD	SANG	SANIC	SIL	STAPHYS	TAR H	TEUCR	THUJA	TRILL P					
1				X																								
2			X			X									X		X											
3							X																					
5		X																										
6	X	X			X						X	X	X	X		X		X	X		X	X						
7					X				**X**																			
8	X																			X								
9								X																				
14			X			X				X																		
16		X		X																			X					
24	X						X																					
25								X																				

Twitch- See also Tremor (Includes Tic)

	BELL	HYOSC	ARAG M	ZINC	CUPR	IGN	GELS	STRAM	TAR H	OP	CAUST	CHAM	LYC	NUX V	VER A	ABSINTH	AMBRA	ANT T	ASAF	AST R	BUFO	CINA	IOD	LACH	LAURO	SEC	SULPH	TER
1	X	X	X	X		X	X					X													X	X		
4	X	**X**	X	X															X									
5		X			**X**				X																			
6		X		X							X		X															X
7	**X**	**X**	**X**	X		X	X	X		X			X	X	X		X	X	X			X	X	X	X			
8	**X**	**X**	**X**	**X**	**X**	X	X	**X**	X	**X**	X	X	X	X	X		X	X		X	X		X			X	X	X
9	X	X		X	X			X				X		X										X				
10	X																	X										
11	X	X		X																								
12	X						X																					
13	X	X			X	X		X			X	X	X				X		X		X	X	X	X	X	**X**	**X**	
14			**X**		X	X			X	X						X					X	X						
15	X	X			X		X			X					X													
17	X	X	X	X					X						X	X				X								
18			X																									
19	X	X	**X**	**X**	X	X			X		X			X		X				X								
21	X	X	X		X	X	X	X																			X	
24	X																											X
25				X																								

Twitch, Abdomen

	AGAR M	RHUS T	ARS	CALC	CROC	GUAIAC																						
7	**X**			X																								
8					X																							
13	X	**X**	X			X																						

Twitch, Arms (Includes Twitch, Forearms)

	OP	ASAF	MERC	ANT T	BELL	CAUST	CIC	CUPR	KALI CAR	LYC	THUJA
6	X				X		X				
7	X	X	X	X		X			X	X	
8		X	X								
13	X	**X**	X	X	X	X	X	X	X	X	**X**
19								X			
24	X										

Twitch, Back

	ANGUST	AGAR M	MYGAL
6	X		X
8	X		
11	X		
19		X	

Twitch, Extremities

	CIC	CUPR	NAT M	OP	RHUS T
1		X	X		
8	X				X
26				X	

Twitch, Eye

	AGAR M	IGN	PHYSO	STANN	CHAM	HYOSC	CINA	GLON	MEZ	RAT	AMM M	ANAC	APIS	BRY	CIC	CROT T	GELS	IOD	LACH	MAG PH	NICCOL	PETR	PULS	RAPH	RHUS T	SEL	VER A
1	X			X					X											X				X			
4	**X**					**X**																	X				
6		X	X				X								X												
7	X	X		X				X				X						X	X								
8	X					X																					X
11			X																								
13	**X**			X	**X**			X	X	**X**	X		X			X					X	X			X	X	
14	X																X										
16					X																						
19	X	X																									
20														X													
21	X																										
24	X		X				X																				

Twitch, Eyelids

	AGAR M	CHAM	CROC	NUX V	SPIG	SULPH	BELL	CALC	CARB V	CAUST	CODEIN	CROT T	CUPR	IPEC	KALI BIC	KREO	MAG PH	PLAT	PULS	RHEUM	CIC	PHYSO						
1	X																											
6							X													X								
7	X	X	X	X		X						X		X			X				**X**	**X**						
8	X	X	X	X	X	X	X	X	X	X	X				X	X												
9																	X	X										
10		X											X															
12		X																										
13	X	X	X	X	X	X		X	X	X		X		X	X	X		X	X	X								
14	X																											
15		X																										
18													X															
19	**X**																											
21	X										X								X									
24					X																							

Twitch, Face

	CHAM	AGAR M	OP	HYOSC	IGN	BELL	CINA	LYC	MEZ	MYGAL	OENANTH	SPIG	ABSINTH	AMBRA	ARS	LAURO	MENY	MERC	PHOS	SEL	STRAM	VER V	IPEC					
1							X																					
5		X															X											
6			X	X		X	X	X	X	X		X									X	X						
7	X	X	X	X				X	X						X	X		X		X								
8		X	X	X	X						X	X		X		X												
9					X					X																		
10	X			X																								
11			X								X																	
12	X											X																
13	**X**	X	**X**	X	**X**	X		X	X					X	X		X	X	X	X			**X**					
14	X	X	X										X															
15	X					X															X							
16	X			X																								
17										X	X		X									X						
19		**X**			X														X									
21					X																							
24							X																					

Twitch, Feet

	ZINC	HYOSC	IOD	KALI CAR	MAG CAR	NAT SUL
6	X					
7	X			X		
8	X		X		X	X
9	X					
19		X				
25	X					

Twitch, Fingers

	CUPR	RHEUM	CINA	MERC	CIC	ACON	CIMICI	ANAC	BRY	CHAM	COCCUL	CROT T	IGN	KALI BR	KALI CAR	LYC	MAG CAR	NAT CAR	OX AC	PHOS	RHUS T	SULPH
6		X																				
7	X	X	X	X		X	X				X											
8		X						X						X			X					
13	X		X	X	**X**				X	X		X	X		X	X		X	X	X	X	X
26	X																					

Twitch, Hands

	STANN	CUPR	HYOSC	NAT SUL	OP	AGAR M	BELL	CARB AC	CIC	COCCUL	COFF	CON	KALI BR	LYSS	MEPH	NAT CAR	RHEUM	STRAM	SULPH	VIOL T	ZINC
1	X																				
6								X	X												
7	X	X	X		X					X	X							X			
8				X								X	X	X						X	X
13	X	X		X			X								X	X	X		X		
19			X			X															
24					X																

Twitch, Head

	OP	CIC	GELS	LAURO
6	X	X		
8			X	X
24	X			

Twitch, Jaw

	BELL	CUPR	KALI MUR	PHOS
7	X			X
8			X	
11		X		

Twitch, Legs

	MERC	SEP	TAR H	ZINC	AGAR M	AMYL N	ASAF	CHEL	CODEIN	CUPR	HELL	MERC C	OP	PHOS	VALER
6			X												
7								X	X	X	X		X		
8	X					X	X					X			X
14	X														
17		X													
21		X	X	X	X									X	
27				X											

Twitch, Limbs

	BELL	OP	CHAM	CUPR	NUX V	HYOSC	RHUS T	STRAM	CHINA	CIC	LYC	NAT M	ZINC	CINA
6	X			X							X			
7	**X**	**X**	X	X	X	**X**	**X**	**X**	X	X	X	X		**X**
8		X	X	X	X	X	X	X	X	X		X		
10			X											
11		X												
15					X									
20	X													
21	X												X	
25													X	

Twitch, Lips

	RHEUM	SQUILLA	AGAR M	BELL	CARB V	CHAM	GRAPH	IGN	OL AN	OP	SULPH	ZINC
1									X			
6	X	X		X	X	X						
7	X						X				X	X
8										X		
9								X				
14			X									
24		X										

Twitch, Mouth

	OP	IGN	BRY	MOSCH
6	X	X		
7	**X**	X		X
8	X			
10		X		
20			X	
24	X			

Twitch, Right Sided

	PHOS	SEP	ZINC
6			X
8		X	
21	X		

Twitch, Shoulder

	LYC	FL AC	SULPH
7	X		
13	X	X	X

Twitch, Single Muscle

	IGN	ACON	COCCUL	CROC	HYOSC	LYC	MERC	PHOS	STRAM	ZINC
4				X						
6	X					X		X		
8		X	X		X		X		X	X
10	X									

Twitch, Tendons (Includes Subsultus Tendinum)

	HYOSC	RHUS T	SEC	ZINC	BELL	CON	IOD	KALI CAR	MEZ	PULS
4	X									
6	X	X	X	X						
8	**X**			X						
13	**X**	**X**	X		**X**	**X**	**X**	**X**	**X**	**X**
17	X									

Twitch, Thigh

	KALI CAR	NAT M
7		X
8	X	

Twitch, Toes

	ACON	CIMICI	AGAR M
7	X	X	
19			X

Tympanic Membrane, Inflammation (AKA Myringitis)

	ACON	BELL	CALC IOD	HEP	TUB AV
8			X		
9		X			
17	X			X	
18					X

Tympanic Membrane, Injury

	TELL
8	X
19	X

Tympanic Membrane, Perforation

	SIL	CAPS	PULS	KALI BIC	HEP	MERC	AUR	CALC	TELL	ARN	HYDRAST	KALI PH	TUB
1	X				X								
3					X								
4	X	X											
6	X		X				X						
7	X	X	X	**X**		**X**		X	X		X	X	
8	X	X											
14	X		X		X	X				X			
17	X	X		X			X	X	X				X
24	X	X	X										
28				X									

Tympanic Membrane, Rupture

	ACON	CAPS
8		X
21	X	

Tympanic Membrane, Thickening Of

	GRAPH	MEZ	TELL
1		X	
7	X		
8	X		X
19		X	

Tympanic Membrane, Ulceration

	CALC	IOD	KALI BIC	KALI PH	MERC D	PULS
8	X	X	X	X	X	
24						X

Tympanitis- See also Otitis Interna

	ECHIN	COLCH	LACH	MERC C	METH BL	OENAND	URAN N	ZINC
1	X				X	X		
4	X							
6		X						
11			X					X
12				X				
17							X	

Tympany- See Distension, Abdomen

Typhlitis

	PLUM	BELL	COLCH	LACH	MERC	RHUS T	THUJA	CARD M	GINSENG	HEP	LYC	ARS	BRY	CROT H	DIOSC	OP	PLAT	RHAM C
2	X		X					X										X
6	X	X	X	X	X	X	X		X	X	X	X					X	
7	X	X	X	X	X	X	X	X			X			X		X		
8	X	X	X	X	X	X	X	X	X	X	X		X	X	X	X	X	X
10	X	X		X	X	X	X		X	X		X	X		X			

Typhoid Fever (Includes Enteric Fever)

	ARS	BAPT	BRY	RHUS T	HYOSC	MUR AC	PH AC	PHOS	BELL	LACH	ARN	GELS	TEREB	NIT AC	OP	STRAM	CALC	CARB V	SULPH	AGAR M	ARUM T	APIS	HAM	HELL	LYC	PYROG	VER A
1	X	X	X	X	X	X	X	X	X	X	X	X	X		X	X	X		X		X						
2	**X**	**X**	**X**	**X**	**X**		**X**	**X**	X	**X**			**X**				X			**X**	X		**X**	X	X	**X**	X
3	X	X	X	X	X	X		X	X					X					X		X					**X**	
4	**X**	**X**	**X**	**X**	**X**		**X**			**X**	**X**	**X**			X												
6	X	X	X	X	X	X	X	X	X	X	X	X	X	X	X	X	X	X	X	X	X	X	X	X	X		X
7	**X**	**X**	**X**	**X**	**X**	**X**	**X**	X	**X**	**X**	**X**	**X**	**X**	**X**	**X**	**X**	**X**	**X**	**X**	**X**	X	**X**	X	X	**X**		**X**
8	X	X	X	X	X	X	X	X	X	X	X	X	X	X	X	X	X	X	X	X	X	X	X	X	X		X
10	X	X	**X**	X		X	X			**X**	X	**X**						X								X	
11	**X**	**X**	**X**	**X**	X	**X**	**X**	X	X	**X**	**X**	X	X	X	X	X	**X**					X	X	**X**	X	**X**	
12	**X**	**X**	X			X		**X**	X	X			X	X	X			X									X
14	X	**X**		X				X											X								
15	X	X	**X**	X	X	X		X	X			X		X		X											
16		X	X	X																							
17	X	X	X		X		X	X						X	X	X						X					
19	X		X																								
21	X	X	X																								
23	X	X	X	X	X	X	X				X		X			X		X		X							
24	X			X		X																					
26				X	X				X																		

Typhoid, Prophylaxis

	BAPT	TYPHOID	BRY	RHUS T	VER V
10	X				
11		X			
15	X		X	X	X
16	X	X			
21		X			

Typhoid, Relapsing

	ANT C	ARG N	ARS	BRY	CHINA	EUP PER	IPEC	NUX V
3	X						X	
6		X	X	X	X	X		X

Typhus Fever

	BRY	RHUS T	BAPT	HYOSC	ARS	MUR AC	PH AC	PHOS	BELL	CARB V	STRAM	GELS	OP	ACON	APIS	NIT AC	AGAR M	VER V	COCCUL	LACH	NUX V	CHIN S	MERC					
2		X	X		**X**	X	X	**X**		X					X		**X**					**X**	**X**					
8	X	X	X	X	X	X	X	X	X	X	X	X	X		X		X		X	X								
12	X	**X**	**X**	**X**	**X**	X	X	X	**X**	X	X	**X**	X	**X**		X		X										
13	X	**X**		**X**																	X							
15	**X**	**X**	**X**		X	X	X		X			X						**X**										
16	X	X	X	X	X	X	X	X	X	X	X	X		X														
17	X		X	X			X	X			X		X		X	X												
23	X					X																						
26	**X**	X	X	X	X	X	X	X	X	X	X		X	X		X			X	X	X							

Typhus Fever, Prophylaxis

	BAPT	HYOSC																										
12	X	X																										
16	X	X																										

Ulceration

	ARS	MERC	SIL	HEP	NIT AC	SULPH	LACH	CARB V	KALI BIC	CALEND	HYDRAST	GRAPH	MEZ	PAEONIA	BOR	CAUST	FL AC	LYC	PH AC	PHOS	PHYTO							
1			X	X		X		X			X			X		X	X			X								
2	**X**	**X**	**X**		**X**	**X**	**X**	**X**	**X**	**X**	**X**	X	**X**	**X**	X	X			X	**X**	X							
3		X	X			X					X		X															
5	X																											
6				X																								
7	**X**	**X**	**X**	X	**X**	X	**X**	**X**	**X**	X		X	X	X		X	X	X	X	X	**X**							
8	X	X	X	X	X	X	X	X	X	X		X	X		X	X	X	X	X	X	X							
9	X	X	X	X	X		X			X									X									
10	X	X		X													X											
12	X		X	X		X	X		X	E	X				E													
14	X	X		X	X				X	E				X	X													
15	X	X	X		X	**X**	X	X			X							X										
16		X							X																			
23					X						X	X		X	X		X											
24	X	X	X	X	X	X	X	X	X	X	X	X	X					X			X							
26	X	X	X	X	X	X	X	X				X				X		X	X									

E- External

Ulceration, Anus

	PAEONIA	AESC	CALC	CINA	HYDRAST	THUJA
1	X					
7	X		X		X	
8		X		X		
14						X

Ulceration, Arm

	ANANTH	RHUS T
7	X	
13		X

Ulceration, Bladder

	HYDRAST	RAN B
13		X
24	X	

Ulceration, Bone

	PHOS	ASAF	AUR	CALC FL	GETTY
1				X	
6	X				
8	X				X
17		X			
24			X		

Ulceration, Bowel

	BAPT	LACH	TEREB
1			X
14	X	X	

Ulceration, Breast

	PHYTO	AST R	HEP	PHOS	SIL	SULPH	CHIM	CON	LAC C	MERC I F	MERC
6	X										
7	X	X	X	X	X						
9	X							X	X	X	X
13			X	X	X	X					
14		X									
24	X					X	X				

Ulceration, Cervix

	HYDRAST	KREO	NIT AC	PHYTO	ALUMEN	ARG N	ARS	BUFO	CARB AC	CALEND	HELON	KALI BIC	SEP	SIL	THUJA
1		X			X	X	X		X						
8	X			**X**				X			X			X	
14		X											X		
15	X									X					
18	X		X									X			
26			X												X

Ulceration, Chronic

	LACH	CALC	CARB V	CAUST	GRAPH	SULPH
1				X		
3	X					
7		X		X	X	
8	**X**	X	X		X	**X**
9	X		X			

Ulceration, Conjunctiva

	ALUM	ARS	CHLOL	CROT T	HAM	HYDRAST	IPEC	MERC I F
6		X						
7	X		X	X		X	X	
8					X			
24								X

Ulceration, Cornea

	HEP	CALC	SIL	ARS	EUPHR	KALI BIC	GRAPH	AUR	LACH	MERC	SULPH	ARG N	CON	NIT AC	RHUS T	MERC I F	TUB	CROT T	MERC	MERC C	NAT CAR	NAT M	PSOR	PULS	ATROP
1	X		X				X												X					X	
2	X																X				X		X		
3												X	X				**X**	X							
4	**X**	**X**	X	X		X	**X**	X		X				X		**X**				X					
6	X	X	X	X	X	X	X	X			X	X	X	X	X	X		X	X			X			
7	X	X	X		X	X	X	X	X			X		X									X		**X**
8	X	X	X	X	X	X			X	X	X											X			
11					X	X		X							X					X					
13	X	X	X	X	X				X	X	X										X				
14	X	X	X																						
21	**X**									X			X		X									X	
24	X	X		X		X	X		X																
26	X	X		X	X						X														

Ulceration, Coccyx- See Ulceration, Os Coxae

Ulceration, Duodenum- See also Ulceration, Intestines

	KALI BIC	URAN N	ARG N	ARS	ANAC	NUX V	GRAPH	LYC	STRAM	ACET AC	ATROP	CARB V	CHAM	HAM	HYDRAST	MEDO	MORG P	ORNITHO	PHOS	SYMPH	TRILL P
1							X		X							X		X			
2	X	X																			
3	X	X	X	X	**X**		X	X						X	X				X		X
7	X	X	X																		
8	X	X		X																	
9	X	X	X	X	X	X					X										
11	X	X			X	X											X			X	
12		X	X	X																	
13										X											
14	X		X									X	X								
17		X																			
24	X								X												
27						X		X													

Ulceration, Duodenum, Perforated

	KALI BIC	LYC
3	X	
10		X

Ulceration, Ear

	CAMPH	BOV	KALI CAR	SIL	SULPH
6				X	X
13	**X**	X	X		

Ulceration, Eyelid

	MERC	ARS	SULPH	SPIG	STRAM	APIS	ARG N	EUPHR	GRAPH	HEP	KALI BIC	MERC C	NAT M
4								X					
7	X		X	X		X			X	X	X		
10	X	X											
13	X			**X**	**X**								X
14	X	X	X				X					X	
21			X										
27		X											

Ulceration, Face

	CON	PHYTO	PSOR	ANANTH	ARS	BROM	IOD	LACH
7	X	X	X	X				
8		X						
13	X		X		X		X	
24						X		X

Ulceration, Feet (Includes Ulceration, Soles)

	ARS	BAR C	GRAPH	HYDRAST	SEC	SULPH	AMBRA	ANANTH	BRY	CARB AC	CANTH	CAUST	IGN	IPEC	KREO	LACH	NAT C	NAT M	NAT SUL	PAEONIA	PHOS	PHYTO	PSOR	PULS	RUTA	SEP
1																				X						
4					X																					
7		X		X				X		X													X			
8			X																							
13	X	X	X		X	X	X		X		X	X	X	X	X	X	X	X	X		X			X	X	X
24	X			X		X																X				

Ulceration, Fingers (Includes Ulceration, Finger Joints)

	SEP	ANT T	BOR	SIL	PLAT	RAN B	ARS	BRY	CALC FL	CARB A	KALI CAR
3			X								
7	X	X						X	X		
8	X		X								
13	X			X	**X**	**X**				X	X
24		X		X			X				

Ulceration, Gastric- See Ulceration, Stomach

Ulceration, Genitalia, Female

	THUJA	NIT AC	AMM C	LAC C	LACH	MERC C	MUR AC	PHYTO	PSOR	SEP	SIL
7	X	X	X	X		X	X		X	X	
11		X									
14	X										
24	X				X			X			X

Ulceration, Genitalia, Male

	LACH	PHYTO	THUJA	ARS	HEP	NIT AC
7	X	X	X	X	X	
11						X
14			X			
24	X	X				

Ulceration, Glans Penis

	MERC	AUR M N	MERC C	NIT AC	SULPH
1	X	X			
7	X	X	X	X	X
8	X				

Ulceration, Gums

	MERC	NAT M	PHOS	CARB V	STAPHYS	HEP	NUX V	CALC	KREO	MERC C	BAPT	CAUST	LACH	LYC	SIL	BELL	KALI CAR	PSOR	SULPH	SULPH AC
1	X	X							X	X										
2	X		**X**																	
4											X									
6	X	X	X	X	X	X	X	X			X	X	X		X	X			X	
7	X	**X**	X	X	X	X	X	X	**X**	**X**			X	X	X			X		
8	**X**	X	X	X	X	X	X	**X**				X	X	X	X	X	X		X	X
10		X																		
11											X									
13	X	X	X	X	X		X		X	X				X			X	X		X
14	X																			
24						X														
26	X			X	X							X								

Ulceration, Hands

	ANANTH	ARS	HYDRAST	SEP	SIL
7	X		X		
13		X		X	X

Ulceration, Heel

	AMM M	ARS	CAUST	NAT CAR	SEP	ALL C	AMM C	GRAPH	KALI IOD	LAURO	NAT SUL
1				X							
3						X					
7			X								
8	X										
13	X	X	X	X	**X**		X	X	X	X	X
14		X									

Ulceration, Intestines See also Ulceration, Duodenum

	KALI BIC	ARG N	CALC	NIT AC	TEREB	CARB V	MERC C	ARS	COLOC	LYC	PYROG	SAL AC
1	X	X			X							
2	**X**						**X**				X	X
7	X	X	X		X	**X**		X	X	X		
8			X									
15				X								
26				X								

Ulceration, Larynx

	CALC	KALI BIC	KALI IOD	NIT AC	IOD	LYC	MERC C	ARG N	ARS	CARB V	CHLOR	CROT H	DROS	HEP	KREO	MANG	MERC	MERC I F	MERC I R	PHOS	SPONG	SULPH
1							X										X					
6		X	X	X	X	X												X				
7		X	X	X		X																
8	X	X	X	X	X		X	X	X	X	X		X	X	X	X			X	X	X	X
17	X											X										
24	X																					

Ulceration, Leg

	ARS	LYC	LACH	GRAPH	HYDRAST	RHUS T	ASAF	CARB V	MERC	PH AC	PHYTO	PSOR	SIL	SULPH	CALC
1		X													
4	X	X													
6	X	X	X	X	X	X			X					X	
7		X	X		X	X		X	X	X	X	X			
10	X														
12	X					B									
13	**X**	**X**	X	X			X	X		X		X	X	X	**X**
14			X												
24			X	X	X		X				X		X		

B- Both Internal and External

Ulceration, Lip

	SIL	NIT AC	ARS	MERC	BELL	CON	LYC	NAT M	SEP	SULPH	GRAPH	STAPHYS	CIC	HEP	KALI BIC	KALI CAR	PH AC	PSOR
3	X	X																
6							X										X	
7	X	X		X		X		X								X		X
8	X	X	X	X	X	X		X	X	X	X	X	X	X				
10	X		X	X			X		X									
13	**X**	**X**	X	**X**	X	X	X	X	X	X	**X**	**X**	X	X	X	X	X	X
24	X														X			
26	X		X		X					X								

Ulceration, Lungs

	KALI CAR	CALC	MERC	PHOS	SIL
1			X		
4	X				
17	X	X		X	X
24	X	X			

Ulceration, Mouth- See also Aphthae

	ARS	BOR	CON	KALI BIC	LACH
10			X		
11	X				
14		X			
24				X	X

Ulceration, Mouth, Outer

	HEP	NIT AC	RHUS T	AMM M	CALC	MERC	NAT M	PSOR	SIL
7	X	**X**	**X**	X		X	X	X	
24	X				X				X

Ulceration, Mucous Membranes

	NIT AC	CORNUS	HYDRAST	PHYTO	MERC	AMM M	ARS	BAPT	CARB V	CARB AC	LACH	MERC CY	NAT M	PAEONIA	SAL AC	THUJA
2		X														
6																X
7	X			X	**X**	X	X	X	X	X	X		X		X	
8		X	X											X		
12			B													
17												X				
18	X															
24				X												

B- Both Internal and External

Ulceration, Nails and Surrounds

	SIL	SULPH	SANG	HEP	ALUM	BAR C	CAUST	CON	IOD	MERC	NAT M	PHOS	PULS	SEP	TET
2			X									X			X
13	**X**	**X**	X	**X**	X	X	X	X	X	X	X		X	X	
24	X	X													

Ulceration, Nasal Cartilage/Septum

	KALI BIC	HIPPOZ	HYDRAST	AUR M	CAD S	CALC	FLAC	MERC I R	PENTHOR
1		X			X				
2		X							
3	X								
5	X		X						
8				X					
12								X	
14	X								
17		X	X				X		X
21			X						
24	X					X			

Ulceration, Nipples

	GRAPH	CALC	CAST EQ	RAT	SIL	HAM	MERC	PHYTO
1	X							
2			X					
3	E			X		E		
7		X	X		X		X	
8	X	X						
9				X				
14								X
21					X			

E- External

Ulceration, Nose/Nostrils- See also Ozaena

	CALC	AUR	KALI BIC	SULPH	ARS I	AUR M	CAUST	FL AC	GRAPH	KALI CAR	KALI IOD	PHOS	SEP	SIL
1			X					X					X	
6	X	X	X						X			X		
7			X	X				X			X		X	
8		X	X			X								
13			X	X						X				X
14	X	X			X									
17	X			X		X	X			X				X
19		X		X							X			
21	X				X									
24	X	X							X			X		
26	X						X							

Ulceration, Os Coxae

	ARG N	BAPT	CARB A	HYDRAST
1	X		X	
6		X		X

Ulceration, Palate

	KALI BIC	NIT AC	AUR	CINNAB	KALI CHL	LACH	MERC P	PH AC	PHYTO	SIL
7	X	X				X	X	X	X	
8			X							
11		X								
12					X					
14				X						
24	X									X

Ulceration, Penis- See also Chancre (Includes Ulceration, Prepuce)

	NIT AC	HEP	ARS	LACH	MERC	SEP	THUJA	ANANTH	AUR M N	CINNAB	COR R	KALI BIC	LAC C	PHYTO	SULPH
1	X			X				X							
6							X								
7	X	X	X	X	X	X	X		X	X		X	X	X	
11	X														
13	X		X		X	X					X				X
14	X	X													
24		X													

Ulceration, Peptic- See Ulceration, Stomach

Ulceration, Peptic, Perforated- See Ulceration, Stomach, Perforated

Ulceration, Perforated

	KALI BIC	LACH	LYC	SIL
4	X			
10			X	
14		X		
24				X

Ulceration, Pharynx

	KALI BIC	SULPH	CHLOR	KALI IOD	MERC I F	MERC P
1	X					
7	X	X				X
8		X				
17			X		X	
19				X		
24	X					

Ulceration, Pylorus

	URAN N	ORNITHO
1	X	X
8	X	

Ulceration, Rectum

	ALUMEN	HYDRAST	PHYTO	PHOS	ALUM	CALC	PAEONIA
6					X		
7	X	X	X			X	X
8	X			X			
24		X	X				

Ulceration, Sacrum- See Bedsores

Ulceration, Skin

	SULPH	HEP	STAPHYS	NIT AC	SIL	CALC	CARB V	LACH	ARS	CHAM	CIST	LYC	NUX M	PHOS	ASAF	MERC	PULS
1	X	X	X				X				X		X	X			
4				**X**													
7	X	X	X			X	X						X				
8	X	X	X	X	X	X		X		X		X					
10	X								X								
13	X	X	X	X	**X**	X	X	**X**	X	X	X	X		X	**X**	**X**	**X**
29*					X												

29* Fernandez I. M. Silica, a Drug of Great Utility in the Management of Chronic Skin Ulcers. Gaceta Homeopatica de Caracas, 2002, Jul- Dec, 20-23.

Ulceration, Soft Palate

	HEP	KALI BIC	PH AC
1	X		
6		X	X

Ulceration, Soles- See Ulceration, Feet

Ulceration, Stomach (Includes Ulceration, Gastric; Ulceration, Peptic)

	ARG N	ARS	KALI BIC	NUX V	PHOS	URAN N	LYC	ATROP	ANAC	GRAPH	HYDRAST	ORNITHO	MEZ	SEP	CARB V	SULPH	ACET AC	BAPT	CON	IRIS V	KREO	MERC C	SIL	SULPH AC	HAM	IPEC
1	X	X			X	X				X		X					X									
2	**X**	**X**	**X**			**X**		**X**				X													**X**	**X**
3	X	X	X			X					X	X	X				X	X				X		X		
4	X																									
5	X	X	X	X		X	X		X	X				X						X	X			X		X
6	X	X	X	X	X		X	X					X	X	X	X			X				X			
7	X		X	X	X						X		X								X					
8	X	**X**	X	**X**	**X**	X	X	X					X	X	X	X			X				X		X	
9	X	X	X	X		X		X	X																	
11	X	X	X	X	X	X		X		X	X	X										X				
12	X	X	X					X			X										X					
14	X	X	X		X										X		X	X		X						
15		X			X						X							X				X		X		
17						X																				
18	X	X	X	X	X		X		X	X										X						
19		X	X	X	X		X		X	X				X		X										
21	X	X	X		X		X		X	X																
23	X		X			X																				
24	X	X	X	X			X				X		X	X	X	X			X				X			
25	X	X		X	X	X	X		X			**X**														
27				X			X																			

Ulceration, Stomach, Perforated- See also Haematemesis; Ulceration, Stomach

	KALI BIC	PHOS	ACON	ARG N	ARS	ATROP	LYC	MERC	MERC C	NUX V
3	X									
6	X					X				
7		X		X						X
8	**X**							X	X	
10							X			
21			X							
24	X									
26		X			X					

Ulceration, Teeth, Roots Of

	MERC	FL AC	HEP	LACH	LYC	NAT M	NUX V	PHOS	STAPHYS	SULPH
4	X									
8	X	X	X	X	X	X	X	X	X	X

Ulceration, Throat

	MERC	LACH	NIT AC	MERC I F	IOD	ARS	HYDRAST	KALI BIC	KALI IOD	PHYTO	BAPT	BELL	CARB V	HEP	LYC	MERC C	THUJA	AILANTH	ALUM	ARG N	FL AC	IGN	MUR AC	SANG	KALI MUR
1		X							X					X							X				
4								X																	**X**
6	X	X	X	X	X		X	X	X		X			X	X		X		X					X	
7	X	**X**	X	X	X		X	X	X	X	X				X									X	
8	X	X	**X**	X								X					X		X			X			
12	X	X						X		X		X	X							X			X		
13	**X**			X	**X**							X		X	X	X						X			
14		X																							
15	X	X	X	X		X	X				X		X										X		
17					X	X				X							X	X		X	X				
18																X									
19						X			X							X									
21																		X							
24	X	X					X			X															
26	X		X			X							X												

Ulceration, Toes

	GRAPH	ARS	PLAT	SEP	SIL	SULPH	ANT T	BERB V	BRY	CARB V	CAUST	KALI IOD	PETR	THUJA
7	X	X							X					
13	**X**	X	**X**	**X**	**X**	**X**		X		X	X	X	X	X
24							X							

Ulceration, Toes, Webbing

	SANIC																											
1	X																											
3	X																											

Ulceration, Tongue (Includes Aphthae, Tongue)

	MERC	NIT AC	MUR AC	KALI BIC	LACH	NAT M	ARS	CIC	LYC	BAPT	BENZ AC	KALI IOD	PHYTO	SULPH AC	APIS	FL AC	AUR	BOV	BOR	CINNAB	DIG	GRAPH	KALI CHL	PSOR	ARG N			
1	X	X	X	X		X	X		X	X	X			X	X							X						
2		**X**								**X**					**X**	**X**		X							**X**			
3	X					X			X																			
6	X	X		X	X			X	X								X											
7	X	X	X	X	X			X				X									X			X				
8	X	X	**X**	X	X			X			X	X	X	X		X			X				X					
9			X																									
10		X	X			X				X			X				X											
11		X																										
12	X	X				X	X																X					
13	X		X	X	X	X		X	X		X	X	X					X		X	X	X						
14	X						X												X	X								
19																								X				
21	X																											
24				X	X		X							X														

Ulceration, Tonsils

	MERC	LYC	IGN	AUR	AILANTH	CALC	KALI BIC	LACH	NIT AC	AMM C	APIS	BELL	CAPS	CARB V	CINNAB	EUCAL	INDIUM	KALI MUR	MERC	MERC C	MERC I R	MERC P	MUR AC	PHYTO	SANIC			
1																			X									
4	X	X																										
5																							X					
6	X				X																							
7	X	X		X		X	X		X											X	X	X		X				
8	X	X		X		X				X					X		X											
9	X																											
10		X	X									X																
13		X	X	X				X																				
17																X									X			
18								X																				
19					X																							
22											X																	
24			X				X											X										
25	X																											
26	X		X						X				X	X														

Ulceration, Umbilicus

	NUX M	APIS	ARS
1	X		
3	X		
7		X	
24			X

Ulceration, Urethra

	NIT AC	ALUMEN	ARG N
1		X	
6	X		
7	**X**		X

Ulceration, Uterus

	HYDRAST	ALUMEN	ARG	ARG N	ARN	CALEND	HEP	HYDROC	SEP
1		X				X			
3									X
7		X	X	X	X			X	
8	**X**		X	X	X		X		
14								X	
15	X					B			X
24							X		

B- Both Internal and External

Ulceration, Uvula

	INDIUM	KALI BIC	IOD
2	X		
3			X
7		X	
8	X		
24		X	

Ulceration, Vagina

	HYDRAST	ALUMEN	ARG N	BAPT	NIT AC	SEP
1		X				
6	X			X		
7	X				X	X
8			X			

Ulceration, Varicose

	CARB V	HAM	LACH	PULS	SULPH	ARS	FL AC	CARD M	ARN	CALC	NIT AC	PYROG	SEC	SIL	AESC	CALC FL	CALEND	CAUST	CLEM	HYPER	KALI BIC	MERC	MEZ	PHOS	RHUS T	MERC C		
1					X		X					X																
2		X						X				X																
3		X					X					X																
5	X		X			X	X						X		X	X	E		E					X		**X**		
6								X											X									
7	X	**X**	X	**X**	**X**	X	X			X								X							X			
8	X	X	X	X	X	X		X		X							X	X							X			
9	X	X	X	X																E								
10							X																					
14	X			X	X		X						X															
15	X	X	X	X	X	X			X		X			X														
18	X		X			X			X		X		X		X	X					X	X	X					
19								X																				
21	X	**X**	X			X			X		X			X							X	X	X	X				
24	X				X																							
25	X	**X**	X	X																E								
26			X	X	X	X				X				X														

E- External

Ulceration, Varicose, Infected- See Infection, Skin

Ulceration, Vulva

	ANANTH	CAULO	KREO	SEC
1	X			
6				X
8		X		
9			X	

Ulcerative Colitis

	MERC C	ARG N	ARS	MERC	CROT H	NAT M	NIT AC	PH AC	PHOS	DYSENT C	PETR	SIULPH	AETHIOP	BAPT	BRY	CALC	COLOC	GAMBOG	GELS	GRAPH	HEP	IPEC	LACH	LYC	NUX V	ONENAN	SEP	SULPH
5	X	X	X			X	X																	X				
1'		**X**	X	**X**	X	X	X	X	X	**X**	**X**	**X**		X	X	X	X		X	X	X	X	X			X	X	
19	X			X														X										
2'	X		X						X																			
29*	X	X			X			X					X												X			X

29* Maas HPJA. Ulcerative Colitis treated with Homoeopathy. Brit Hom J, July 1993, 82, 179-185.

Undescended Testes- See Testes, Undescended

Uraemia

	CUPR AR	TEREB	ARS	OP	CARB AC	PHOS	AMM C	BELL	CANTH	HELL	HYDRAST	MORPH	PLUM	AUR	URT U	ASC S	CANN I	CUPR	DIG	GLON	LYC	NICOTIN	UREA	VER V				
1	X	X						X	X	X			X		X								X	X				
2	**X**	X		**X**	**X**		X								X	X	X						X					
3	**X**				X					X		X																
4	X		X										X					X										
6	**X**	**X**	**X**			**X**			X		X			**X**								X						
7		X	**X**			X		X								X												
8		X	X	X	X	X	X	X			X			X			X	X	X	X	X	X		X				
10			X			X																						
11	X	X		X	X		X	X	X	X		X								X								
12				X																								
14												X																
17	X	X		X	X		X			X	X	X	X						X									
23	X																											
27															**X**						X							

Urethra, Congestion (Includes Urethra, Catarrh)

	THUJA	CON	MERC	RHOD	BERB V	CARB V	HAM	HYDRAST	PARIERA	TEREB																		
5	X	X			X				X																			
7	X		X	X		X	X	X		X																		
13	X	X	X	X																								

Urethritis

	CANTH	CANN S	COP	APIS	ARG N	CUBEB	DORYPH	GELS	SULPH	TEREB	THUJA	ACON	ARS	CANN I	CLEM	HEP	MERC	MERC C	NIT AC	PETROS	NAT M							
1	X																X											
2			X	X			X																					
3		X									X																	
4	X											X			X													
5					X					X								X										
6													X															
7		X				X		X	X							X				X								
8						X		X																				
9	X			X						X																		
13	**X**	X	**X**		X			X	X							X												
14	**X**			X	X						X	X		X				X										
19	X	**X**					X				X		X	X	X				X	X								
20									X								X				**X**							
23		X	X			X	X			X									X									

Uricaemia- See also Gout

	BENZ AC	LYC	URT U	SEP	BERB V	LITH C	BRY	CUPR	FORMICA	NAT SUL	PULS	STAPHYS	ARG N	ARN
1	X					X			X	X				
3			X							X				
4			X											
5	X	X	X	X	X				X					
7	**X**			X				X			X	X		**X**
8	X	X		**X**	**X**	X	X	X			X	X	**X**	
10		X					X							
11	X													
16			X											
18		X			X									
25		X												

Urinary Tract Infection- See Nephritis

Urine, Alkaline

	BAPT	CANTH	KALI BIC	NAT M	ARS	BENZ AC	CAUST	FERR AC	FERR	FL AC	KALI AC	LACH	NUX V	PH AC
1	X	X		X										
2											X			
7	X	X	X	X		X			X	X				
8	**X**		X					X						
12		X					X						X	X
24					X							X		

Urine, Black- See also Haematuria

	LACH	COLCH	CARB AC	ARS	HELL	NAT M	PARIERA	TEREB	CHION	DIG	KALI CAR	KALI CHL	ARS H	BEN D	CANTH	ERIG	KALI ARS	PHOS
1	X	X	X					X										
2														X				
3		X																
6	X				X						X							
7	X	X	X	X	X	X	X	X	X	X	X		X		X			
8	X	X	X	X	X	X		X		X						X		
10	X											X					X	
12																		X
13	X	X				X												
14			X				X		X			X						
19				X														
24							X											

Urine, Milky

	PH AC	CINA	PHOS	APIS	LYC	AUR	COLOC	DULC	MUR AC	SULPH	ARN	AGAR M	AUR M	CARB V	HEP	IOD	LIL T	MERC	NIT AC	SPONG								
1	X		X	X		X	X					X				X	X			X								
2		X																										
3	X	X																										
5	X	X		X	X	X									X													
6	X				X					X																		
7	**X**	X	X	**X**	X		X	X	X	X	X	X	X		X	X	X		X	X								
8	X	X	X		X		X		X	X			X	X				X	X									
10	X					X																						
12		X																										
13		X		X				X			X							X										
14	X		X																									
15	X																											
16	X																											
24			X																									
26	X							X	X					X														

Urine, Mucoid

	CHIM	BERB V	PAREIRA	SARS	PULS	BENZ AC	CANTH	COLOC	DULC	EQUISET	KALI BIC	NAT M	ANT C	APOC	CANN I	MERC	MERC C	PH AC	SENEGA	UVA	SEP							
1	X		X			X											X											
2			X																									
4	X	X	X							X																		
5	X							X			X							X										
6	X		X		X		X	X	X		X				X				X	X	X							
7	X	X	X	**X**	**X**	X	X		X			**X**	X			X					**X**							
8	X	X		X	X		X	X	X	X		X	X			X		X	X									
10						X											X											
11	X	X		X										X	X													
13		**X**	X	X	X	X	X	X	X		X	**X**	X			X		X	X	X								
14	X	X	X								X			X	X													
16				X																								
17														X														
19			X		X					X							X											
20	X																											
21	X	X		X																X								
24			X	X																								
25		X								X																		

Urine, Offensive

	BENZ AC	NIT AC	CALC	SEP	BAPT	ARS	SULPH	BOR	MERC	VIOL T	PH AC	TEREB	DULC	CARB V	KREO	MOSCH	PULS	AUR
1	X	X		X	X			X				X				X		
2								X										
3	X	X		X														
4	**X**									X								
5	X	X	X	X							X							
6	X	X		X	X	X	X			X								
7	X	X	X	X	X	X	X	X	X	X	X	X	X	X		X	X	X
8	X	**X**		X		X	X		X	X	X		X	X		X	X	
10	X	X	X		X	X			X									
11	X	X	X		X							X						
13	**X**	**X**	**X**	X		X	X	**X**	**X**	**X**	X		**X**	X	X		X	**X**
14	X	X													X			
15		X			X													
17	X	X																
18	X			X														
19	X	X	X			X	X	X							X			
24		X	X		X		X		X			X						
27	X		X															

Urine, Offensive, Ammoniacal

	ASAF	MOSCH	NIT AC	IOD	AUR	FERR	PAREIRA	CARB V	CHIN S	DULC	LACH	PETR	STRONT	TUB
4							X							
5	X	X	X	X	X	X				X	X	X		X
7	X	X	X	X	X			X						
8	X	X	X											
13	**X**	X	X			X	X		X				X	
24				X										

Urine, Purulent

	ARS	CLEM	CANN S	CANTH	LYC	MERC	NIT AC	NUX V	PULS	SIL	SULPH	SABIN	BENZ AC	CALC	CHAM	CON	OCIM	SEP	UVA
6	X				X	X		X											
7	X	X	X	X			X	X											
8		X	X	X	X		X	X	X	X	X	X		X	X	X		X	
10	X									X			X				X		
11	X																		
13		**X**	X	X	X	X	X		X	X	X	**X**	X	X	X	X	X	X	**X**
24						X			X										
27											X								

Urine, Retention Of- See also Anuria; Urine, Scanty (Includes Ischuria; Urine, Suppression)

	OP	ACON	CAMPH	NUX V	APIS	BELL	ARS	CANTH	CAUST	ARN	STRAM	DIG	PULS	SULPH	HYOSC	PLUM	HELL	TEREB	CHIM	DULC	LYC	MERC C	CON	LAURO	RHUS T	AUR	EUP PUR	
1	X	X	X	X	X		X	X	X	X		X	X		X	X	X	X						X				
2	**X**	**X**	**X**												X			**X**									X	
3		X	X	X	X		X	X	X				X	X				X										
4		X	X	X				X				X					X					X						
5	X	X		X		X	X		X	X		X	X		X				X	X					X			
6	X	X	X	X	X	X	X	X			X			X	X	X							X			X		
7	**X**	**X**	X	X	**X**	X	X	**X**	X	X	X	X	X	X	X	X	X			X	X	X		X	X		X	
8	X	X	X	**X**	X	X	X	**X**	X	X	X	X	X	X	**X**	X	**X**			X	X		X	X	X	X	**X**	
9	X		X	X	X	X			X		X																	
10	X	X	X	X	X	X	X			X	X		X			X					X	X	X	X		**X**	X	
11	X				X	X											X		X		X	X						
12	X	X	X	X		X	X	X						X				X	X			X						
13	X	**X**	**X**	X		X	**X**	**X**	X	**X**	**X**	**X**	**X**	X	X	**X**				X	**X**	X	X	X	X			
14	X	X	X		X	X													X									
15				X							X			X														
16									X																			
17											X																	
19		X			X				**X**	X		X							X	X					X			
21	X							X		X								X										
22		X																										
23																			X									
24	X				X	X				X		X		X		X		X					X					
25	X		X	X	X	X			X		X																	
26	X	X	X	X			X						X				X			X								

Urine, Retention Of, Pregnancy, During- See Pregnancy, Urine, Retention

Urine, Scanty- See also Anuria; Urine Retention Of

	APIS	**ACON**	**TEREB**	**BRY**	**CANTH**	**ARS**	**BELL**	**LYC**	**HELL**	**COLCH**	**DIG**	**PHOS**	**EQUISET**	**MERC C**	**SARS**	**CHINA**	**LACH**	**CROT H**	**NIT AC**	**NUX V**	**OP**	**SULPH**						
1	X	X	X		X	X	X	X	X	X	X	X	X	X	X		X	X										
4	**X**	X	X		X			X			X	X	X	X		X						X						
5	X	X			X			X			X				X													
6	X	X	X	X	X	X		X	X	X		X				X	X		X		X							
7	**X**	X	X	X	**X**	X	X	X	**X**	X	X	X	**X**	**X**	**X**	X	X	**X**	**X**	**X**	**X**	**X**						
8	X	X	X	X	X	X	X		X	X	X	X				X	X		X	X	X	X						
9	X		X										X						X									
10	X		X	X		X			X			X			X	X	X	X										
11		X	X			X	X		X					X														
12		X																										
13	X		X	**X**	X		X			**X**	**X**										X	X						
14	X	X		X		X		X							X													
15	X			X		X	X																					
16							X	X																				
17	X																											
18					X									X														
19	**X**						X																					
21	X	X	X			X														X								
22	X	X		X																								
24	X	X	X	X	X		X	X	X	X								X										
25													X															
26				X				X												X								
27	X	X																										

Urination, Copious- See Polyuria

Urination, Disorders Of

	BENZ AC	**CAUST**	**CAPS**	**GRAPH**																								
2	**X**	**X**	**X**	**X**																								
8	X	X																										

Urination, Frequent- See also Polyuria

	APIS	**LYC**	**PH AC**	**CANTH**	**CAUST**	**KALI CAR**	**RHUS T**	**SULPH**	**BRY**	**NUX V**	**BAR C**	**CALC**	**MERC**	**PULS**
1	X													
2						**X**				**X**				
3			X		X					X				
4	X													
6												X		
7		**X**	X	X	**X**	X	X	X	X	**X**			X	**X**
8	X		X	X	X	X	X	X	X		X		X	X
9				X										
10								X						
11											X			
13	X	**X**	X	**X**	X	X	**X**	**X**	X		**X**	**X**	**X**	
14	X													
15									X					
18		X												
19							X							
21			X											
24		X										X		X

Urination, Profuse– See also Polyuria

	ACET AC	**ARG**	**PH AC**	**IGN**	**LAC AC**	**GELS**	**CANTH**	**VER A**	**MUR AC**	**PHOS**	**SARS**	**SULPH**	**VERBASC**	**CHEL**	**GLON**	**MOSCH**	**ARG N**	**NAT M**	**RHUS T**
1	X	X	X	X					X					X					
4		X		X	X	X							X			X			
5			X	X		X		X			X					X			
6		X		X			X		X										
7	**X**	**X**	X	X	**X**		X			**X**	X			X	X	X	X		
8	X		X	X	X		X	X	X				X				X	X	X
9	X														X				
10	X	X	X		X	X													
11	X	X	X		X	X													
13	X	X	**X**	X		X	X	X	**X**	X	**X**	**X**	X	X	X	X	**X**	**X**	**X**
14	X	X	X				X			X		X		X					
15				X				X		X									
17						X													
19					X						X								
24													X						
25															X				
26								X				X						X	X
27												X							

Urination, Urgent

	CANTH	NUX V	LYC	ACON	MERC	PULS	SEP	SULPH	THUJA	BELL	BERB V	DIG
1	X							X	X			
4	X											X
6		X	X	X	X		X	X		X		
7	X	X	X		X	X					X	
8	X						X					
9	X											
10	X			X								
11	X								X			
12	X											
14	X		X					X	X		X	X
18							X					
19		**X**		X			X			X		X
20	X				X							
21	X	X	X			X			X	X		
22	X	X										
24	X	X	X	X	X	X					X	
26		X				X		X				

Urticaria- See also Nettle Rash

	APIS	RHUS T	DULC	URT U	SULPH	ANT C	CALC	PULS	ARS	HEP	NAT M	ACON	BOV	SEP	CHLOR	BELL	BRY	COP	LYC	PSOR	ANAC	ASTAC F	CHLOL	IGN	NUX V	RUMEX	MEZ
1	**X**	X	X	X	X	X	X	X			X		X	X	X			X	X	X	X	X				X	
2		X		X	**X**		X			**X**			X		X			X								X	
3	X	X	X	X	X	X	X		X	X	X	X	X	X	X	X				X		X					
4	**X**	X	X		X	X	X	**X**	**X**		X	X	X	X													
5	X	X	X	X		X	X	X	X	X			X	X							X					X	
6	X	X	X	X	X	X	X	X	X	X	X			X		X	X	X	X	X	X			X			
7	**X**	**X**	X	**X**		X	X	X	**X**	X	**X**		X	**X**		X	X	X		X			**X**				X
8	**X**	**X**	X	X	X	X	**X**	X	**X**	X	X	X	X	X	**X**	X	X	X	X		X	X		X	X	X	**X**
9	X	X	X	X	X						X	X			X												
10	X	X	X				**X**	X	X	X		X				X	X		**X**						X		
12	**X**	X	X		X	X		X	**X**			**X**			**X**		X				X			X	X		
13	X	X	**X**	X	**X**	**X**	**X**	X	X	**X**	X	X		X		X	X	X	X					X	X		X
14	X	X	X		X	X		X		X		X	X														
15		**X**	X			X	X	X				**X**				X									X		
17			X																				X				
18	X			X	X						X								X	X							
19	**X**	**X**	X	**X**	X	X	X	X	X	X	**X**		X	X		X	X	X		X		X	**X**	X			X
20	**X**	X		X																							
21	X	X	X	X	X	X		X	X		X																
23	X			X		X							X									X	X			X	
25	X			**X**	X							X			X												
26	X	X	X	X			X	X	X	X							X										

Uterus, Anteversion- See also Uterus, Displacement Of

	HELON	LIL T	SEP	AUR	BELL	CALC	CALC PH	CAULO	CON	FERR	GRAPH	HAM	MERC	NUX M	NUX V	PLAT	STANN	TAR H
7	X	X	X						X			X						
8	X	X	X	X	X	X	X	X		X	X		X	X	X	X	X	X

Uterus, Congestion- See also Ailments from Labour (Includes Uterus, Catarrh)

	CALUO	SEP	APIS	BELL	NUX V	IGN	LACH	PULS	ALOE	ARAL	ARUNDO	CARB AC	CHAM	CHINA	GELS	FRAX	HEP	IOD	KALI MUR	SULPH	TEREB
6	X	X	X	X																X	
7	X	X	X	X	X		X	X			X			X	X		X				X
8	X	**X**	X			X	X		**X**	X		X						X	X		
10	X				X																
15				X	X	X		X					X								
18																X					

Uterus, Diseases Of

	CIMICI	SEP	PLAT	LIL T	MAG M	PULS	HYDRAST	BELL	CALC	HELON	CAULO	KREO	SABIN	SEC	APIS	AUR	CHAM	GELS	IOD	LYC	MUREX
1								X		X			X	X							
2	**X**		X	**X**	X	X	X	**X**	**X**	**X**		X		X		**X**	**X**	**X**	**X**		
4		X																			
6		X	X	X																	
7	**X**	**X**	X		**X**		X		X		X	X			**X**					**X**	**X**
8	X	X	X	X	X	X	X	X	X	X	X	X	X	X	X	X	X	X	X	X	X
9	X				X								X								
10		X																			
11	X																				
12			X			X	X														
14		X																			
15	X	X	X			X					X										
17			X	X																	
23	X			X	X	X															
25	X																				

Uterus, Displacement Of- See also Uterus, Anteversion

	SEP	AMM M	FERR IOD	LIL T	NUX M	BELL	CALC	LACH	NAT M
7	**X**	X	X	X	X	**X**	**X**	**X**	**X**
8		X			X				
15	X								
23			X	X					

Uterus, Enlargement

	CALC	CON	KALI IOD	SEP	USTIL	CAULO	FRAX	MITCH	POLYPOR
7	X	X	X	X	X				
8	X	X	X	X	X				
23							X	X	X
26						X			

Uterus, Hydatids- See Cysts, Hydatid, Uterus

Uterus, Prolapse- See Prolapse, Uterus

Uterus, Retroverted (Includes Uterus, Retroflexion)

	CAULO	SEP	FERR IOD	LIL T	CIMICI	HELON	AECS	AUR M	BELL	CALC	CALC PH	FERR	HEP	KALI CAR	LAC C	LACH	LYC	MUREX	NUX V	OVI G P	PLAT	SULPH	TAR H
1		X		X																			
2																				X			
4		X																					
6	X		X																				
7	X	X	X	X	X	X									X								
8	X	X	X	X	X	X	X	X	X	X	X	X	X	X		X	X	X	X		X	X	X
10	X																						

Uterus, Subinvolution

	CALC	CAULO	KALI BIC	LIL T	PULS	SEP	USTIL	BELL	BRY	CHINA	CIMICI	CYCL	HYDRAST	KALI BR	KALI CAR	KALI IOD	MILL	NAT HYPO	PLAT	POD	RUTA	SABIN	SEC	TANACET	TEREB
2																		X							
7	X	X	X	X	X	X	X	X					X			X									
8	X	X	X	X	X	X	X		X	X	X	X		X	X		X		X	X	X	X	X	X	X

Uvula, Diseases Of

	ALUMEN	ARG N	HYOSC	IGN	INDIUM	IOD	KALI BIC	LACH	NIT AC	NUX V	PHOS
2	X		X		X						
6		X		X		X	X	X	X	X	X
8	X	X	X	X	X	X	X	X	X	X	X

Uvula, Elongation Of

	HYOSC	ALUMEN	NAT M	IOD	APIS	KALI IOD	LACH	MANC	ALUM	BAPT	BAR M	BROM	CAPS	KALI CAR	MERC C	WYETHIA	CROT T	SULPH
1	X	X			**X**			X										
2	X														X			
3	X	X			**X**			X							X			
4			X						X							X		
6			X	X		X	X					X				X		
7	**X**	X	X	X		**X**	**X**			X			X	X			**X**	**X**
8	X	X	X	X				X					X					
9	X																	
10											X							
17	X	X	X	X		X	X			X	X	X		X				
24									X									
27		X																

Uvulitis- See also Uvula, Diseases Of

	CARB V	NUX V	BELL	CALC	MERC	COFF	PULS	SENEG	ACON	ALUMEN	APIS	ARG N	BAPT	CAPS	CAUST	COLCH	CROT H	GELS	IOD	KALI BIC	KALI NIT	LAC C	LYC	MERC C	NAT M	NAT SUL	NIT	SULPH
6												X																
7	X									X								X				X						
8	X	X	X	X	X	X	X								X				X				X		X			
10		X	X		X																							X
13	X	X		X	X	**X**	X	**X**								X				X						X	X	
15	X												X															
17	X	X	X	X					X		X			X			X				X			X				

Vaccinia

	BELL	VACCIN	ACON	APIS	PHOS	SULPH
2	**X**	**X**			X	
12	X		X	X		X

Vaccinosis- See Ailments from Vaccination

Vaccinosis, Prophylaxis

	THUJA	MALAND	NOSODE*
10	X	X	
16	X		
28			X

* A remedy made from the vaccine

Vagina, Congestion Of (Includes Vagina, Catarrh)

	ACON	BELL	PULS	THUJA
7	X	X	X	
8				X

Vagina, Dryness

	LYC	BELL	NAT M	SEP	ACON	GRAPH	FERR	CIMICI	ALUM	ARG N	ARS	BERB V	BRY	CALC	FERR PH	LYSS	SULPH
1	X		X	**X**													
4				X													
5	X	X	X	X	X	X	X				X	X					
6	X	X	X							X				X			X
7	X	X	X			X	X										
8	**X**	X	X		X	X		X									
9	X	X			X										X	X	
10	X																
13	**X**	X	X														
14	X																
17									X								
21	X	X	X										X				
27				X													

Vaginismus

	PLAT	CACT	BELL	IGN	LYC	PLUM	FERR PH	NAT M	BERB V	COFF	HAM	KREO	MAG PH	SEP	SIL	THUJA
2	X	X				X		X	X				X			X
6	X	X	X	X	X	X	X	X				X		X		
7	X	X	X	X	X	X	X				X		X		X	
8	X	X	X	X	X		X	X	X	X	X	X		X	X	X
9	X															
11	X															
14		X			X											
21		X	X	X		X				X						
23	X															

Vaginitis

	ACON	BELL	COCCUS	CURARE	KREO	NIT AC	HELON	ARS	AUR M	BOR	CALC	CAULO	CUBEB	FERR PH	GRAPH	HAM	HYDRAST	MAG PH	MERC	PULS	SEP	SULPH	TAR C	TAR H
2				X																				
4			X				**X**																	
5					X												X							
6								X																X
7	X	X	X	X												X			X					
8						X			X			X	X											
9	X	X												X				X				X		
10																							X	
20					X	X				X	X				X					X	X			

Varices

	CALC	NAT M	ZINC	ARN	CAUST	FERR	LYC	PULS	AMBRA	ARS	CARB V	GRAPH	KREO	LACH	MILL	SPIG	SULPH
2	X	X													X		
8	X	X	X	X	X	X	X	X	X	X	X	X	X	X	X	X	X
13	X	X	X	**X**	**X**	**X**	**X**	**X**	X	X	X	X	X	X		X	X
19			X														

Varicocele

	HAM	SULPH	PULS	ARN	BELL	COLLIN	LACH	LYC	NUX V	AMM M	AUR	CALC	CHINA	CLEM	FL AC	KALI CAR	PH AC	RUTA	SIL	STAPHYS	AESC	CANTH	CROT H	FERR PH	OSMIUM	PENTHOR	SEP	TAB
1	**X**	X	X	X	X		X			X			X	X		X				X								
2	X	X	X															X					X			X		X
6	X	X	X	X	X	X	X	X	X			X			X												X	
7	X	X	X	X		X	X	X	X		X	X					X		X									
8	X		X								X				X		X		X		X				X			
21	X		X																					X				
24		X		X	X					X			X	X								X						
27		X				X		X	X							X		X		X								

Varicose Ulcer- See Ulceration, Varicose

Varicose Veins (Includes Varicosis)

	PULS	HAM	FL AC	CARB V	LYC	SULPH	ARS	LACH	ARN	SEP	APIS	CALC FL	CARD M	NUX V	ZINC	CALC	SIL	AESC	VIP	BELL	GRAPH	ACON	AMBRA	FERR	MILL			
1	**X**	X	X			X	X	X						X					X	X					X			
2	**X**	**X**	X		X	X		**X**		X	X		X		X				X				X					
3		X	X															X	X	X			X					
5	X	X	X		X				X	X	X	X	X			X					X							
6	X				X					X																		
7	**X**	**X**	**X**		**X**	X	X			X	X			X		**X**				X				X				
8	X	X	X	X								X			X													
9	X	E	X	X													X	X				X						
10	**X**		X																									
11				X			X	X							X													
12	**X**	**B**	**X**			X	X				X			X			**X**			X		X						
13	**X**	B		X	X	X	X		X						X	X					X		X	X				
14	**X**		X	X		X	X	X				X													X			
15	X	X		X	X		X		X					X		X	X				X							
16	X	X																										
17			X																									
18	X	X	X	X	X	X		X	X	X	X	X	X	X	X			X	X		X							
19		X						X					X		X			X							X			
21	X	X		X																				X				
23	X	X	X									X							X									
25	X	E	X	X													X					X						
26	**X**	X		**X**	X	**X**			X																			
27		X	X	X					X	X			X															
28		X																										

B- Both Internal and External E- External

Varicose Veins, Genitals

	CARB V	ZINC	CALC	LYC	HAM	NUX V	PULS
7	X	X	X	X	X	X	
8		**X**	X				
10	X						
14	X			X			X

Varicose Veins, Nose

	CARB V
6	X
11	X
17	X

Varicose Veins, Pregnancy, From- See Pregnancy, Varicose Veins From

Varicose Veins, Prophylaxis

	PULS
14	X
16	X

Varicose Veins, Throat

	AESC	BAR M	CARB V	HAM	PULS
8			X	X	X
17	X	X			

Variola- See Smallpox

Varioloid- See Smallpox

Vegetations

	CALC	MANG	STAPHYS	MERC N
2				X
8	X	X	X	

Veins, Congestion Of (AKA Venous Congestion)

	CARB V	HAM	PULS	SEP	SULPH	PHOS	ACON	AESC	ANT T	CON	CONVAL	CYCL	GELS	GLON	GRAPH	HEP	LACH	LYC	MILL	OP	SANG	SEC	SIL	TUB	VER A	ZINC
4			X	X		X																				
5			X				X					X														
6	X			X	X				X	X					X		X	X					X		X	
8		X		X	X	X							X	X		X				X	X	X				X
10	X																									
11											X															
14																			X							
17								X																		
18	X		X																					X		
19					X																					
23		X																								
24		X																								

Veins, Diseases Of

	FL AC	HAM	ARN	BELLIS	CARB A	CARD M	CHIN S	OP	PULS	RUTA																		
2	**X**						X	X		X																		
4						X																						
5	X	X	X	X					X																			
15		X																										
17					X																							

Vertigo (Includes Dizziness, Giddiness)

	COCCUL	NUX V	GELS	CON	CHINA	PHOS	ACON	BRY	BELL	CALC	LACH	NAT M	PULS	SIL	SULPH	ARG N	THERID	ARN	GLON	CYCL	RHUS T	CAUST	LYC	PETR	BOR	OP		
1	**X**	X	X	X	X	X	X		X	X	X	X	X	X		X	X		X	X				X				
2	**X**	**X**	**X**	**X**	X		**X**	**X**	**X**	**X**	X	**X**		X	**X**		X			X					**X**			
3	X	X		X	X	X	X		X	X		X		X	X										X			
4	**X**	X	X	**X**	X	X	X	X		X	X		X			X	X				**X**	X		X		X		
5	X	X	X	X	X	X	X	X			X	X	X	X		X	X	X	X	X	X	X	X	X				
6	X	X	X	X	X	X	X	X	X	X	X	X	X	X	X	X	X	X	X	X	X	X	X		X	X		
7	X	X	X	X			**X**					**X**							X	X	X	X	**X**			X		
8	X	X	X	X	X	X	X	X	X	X	X	X	X	X	X	X	X	X	X	X	X	X	X	X	X	X		
9	X	X	X	X	X	X	X	X	X		X		X	X	X	X	X	X				X	X	X				
10		X	X	X	X	X	X	X	X	X	X		X	X	X			X	X			X	X			X		
11		X	X	X	X	X	X	X	X	X		X	X	X		X	X		X	X						X		
12	X	X	X		X	X		X	X										X									
13	**X**	**X**	X	**X**	X	**X**	**X**	X	**X**	**X**	X	**X**	**X**	X	**X**	X	X	**X**	X	X	**X**	X	X	**X**	X	X		
14	X	X	X	X	X	X	X	X		X	X	X	X	X				X	X						X			
15	X	X	X	X	X	X	X	X	X	X			X		X	X			X		X					X		
16					X																							
17	**X**	**X**	**X**	**X**	**X**	**X**	**X**	**X**	**X**	**X**	**X**	**X**	**X**	**X**	**X**	**X**	**X**	**X**	X	**X**	**X**		**X**	**X**	**X**	**X**		
18	X		X	X	X	X		X			X	X				X		X		X					X			
19	**X**	X	X	X	X	**X**	X	**X**	X	**X**	X	X	X	**X**	X	X	X	X	X	X	X	X		X	X			
20	X																							X				
21	X	X	X	X	X	X		X	X	X	X	X					X	X				X	X	X	X			
22		X																										
23	X		X	X			X		X																			
24	X	X	X			X	X	X	X	X					X					X	X							
25	X	X	X		X			X			X			X	X		X	X				X	X	X				
26	X	X		X		X	X		X	X	X		X	X	X						X	X	X			X		
27			X										X			X												

Vertigo, Auditory Nerve, From

	SAL AC	CAUST	CHENO	CHIN S	COLCH	GELS	NAT SIL	THER
1	X							
4		X		X		X	X	
8	X				X			X
24			X					

Vertigo, Senile

	ARN	RHUS T	AMBRA	CALC PH	CON	OP	PHOS	ALUM OX	FL AC	IOD	SULPH
1	X		X								
4		X	X		X					X	
5							X				
7		X		X							
8				X				X	X		
10	X				X	X					
14	X										
17		X				X					X
18							X				
24	X										

Vision, Diseases Of (Includes Blurred Vision; Colours, Spots, Mist or Veils before the Eyes; Dull Vision; Visual Flashes; Visual Floaters; Flickering or Indistinct Vision)

	GELS	PHOS	BELL	CHINA	CYCL	NAT M	NUX V	PULS	SIL	SULPH	HYOSC	IGN	KALI BIC	LACH	RUTA	ACON	AUR	CALC	CAUST	EUPHR								
1	X				X			X	X			X																
2																	X											
6	X	X	X	X	X	X	X	X	X		X	X	X		X	X	X	X	X	X								
7		X	X		X	X				X				X					X									
8	X	X	X	X		X	X	X	X	X	X	X		X	X		X	X	X	X								
9	X	X	X	X	X	X				X			X	X	X				X	X								
10			X			X	X									X												
11			X		X																							
12	X	X	X	X			X																					
13	X	X	X	X	X	X	X	X	X	X	X	X	X	X	X	X		X	X	X								
14	X	X		X	X					X			X	X			X	X										
15			X				X																					
17	X	X			X	X	X			X				X														
18	X			X	X								X															
19	X	X			X	X		X			**X**																	
20	X																											
21		X	X						X			X																
22				X									X															
24	X	X		X		X	X	X	X	X	X				X	X	X	X										
25	X	X		X											X					X								
26			X					X	X		X	X				X												
27		X																										

Vision, Left Side, Loss Of- See Hemianopia, Homonymous, Left Side
Vision, One Side Not Visible- See Hemianopia
Vision, Right Side, Loss Of- See Hemianopia, Homonymous, Right Side
Vision, Upper or Lower Half, Loss Of- See Hemianopia, Altitudinal

Vision, Weakness Of

	GELS	CAUST	BELL	AGAR M	LYC	PULS	CINA	CON	NAT M	RUTA	SULPH	AMM C	STRAM	BAR C	CALC	SEP	THUJA	ACON	CHINA	CROC	CYCL	OP	PHOS	SIL
1	X	X		X			X			X	X					X								
2										**X**														
5	X	X	X	X		X			X	X			X		X	X			X	X	X			X
6	X	X	X		X	X		X	X		X	X			X		X					X	X	
7	**X**	**X**	**X**	X	**X**	X	X	**X**	X			**X**	X						**X**		X	**X**		
8				X	X		X	X			X	X	X	X		X	X							
10	X	X	X			X					X							X						
13	**X**	X	X	**X**	**X**	**X**	X	**X**	X	**X**	X	X	**X**	X	X	X	X	**X**	X	**X**	**X**	X	**X**	**X**
15	X		X															X		X				
16														X										
17			X																					
20	X																							
24	X			X			X							X			X							
26		X			X				X						X	X							X	X

Vitamin A Deficiency Symptoms- See also Innutrition

	ARG N	AUR	EUPHR	KALI BIC	MERC C	BELL	CALC PH	NUX V	PH AC	PHOS	PHYSO
3							X		X	X	
11	X	X	X	X	X	X		X			X

Vitamin B3 Deficiency Symptoms- See also Innutrition; Pellagra

	BOV	HEP	ARS	GELS	PLUM IOD	SEC
11	**X**	**X**	X	X	X	X

Vitamin C Deficiency Symptoms- See also Innutrition

	AGAVE	KREO	MERC	TERM C	ARS	CARB V	CHINA	FERR PH	FIC REL	GRAPH	KALI PH	NIT AC	PHOS	SIL	STAPHYS
3						X				X	X			X	
11	**X**	**X**	**X**	**X**	X		X	X	X			X	X		X

Vitamin D Deficiency Symptoms- See also Innutrition; Osteoporosis; Rickets

	CALC PH	CALC	CALC HP	NAT M	NAT PH	PINUS S	SIL	ARS	ARS IOD	CALC FL	CALC SIL	FERR PH	FL AC	HECLA	IOD	KALI IOD	PH AC	PHOS	RHUS T	SANIC	SULPH	TUB	THUJA	THYROID
3	X									X									X					
11	**X**	**X**	**X**	**X**	**X**	**X**	**X**	X	X		X	X	X	X	X	X	X	X		X	X	X	X	X

Vitiligo- See also Discoloration of Skin

	ARS S FL	ARS	MERC	SEP	SIL	APIS	CALC	HYDROC	PHOS	SULPH	TUB	ALUMEN	ARS S R	BOR	CARB A	CARB V	KALI CAR	LED	MANG AC	NAT CAR	NAT M	NIT AC	PH AC	PSOR	SANIC	SEL	THUJA	
1	**X**	X				X		X			X			X			X							X				
6			X																									
7		**X**				**X**										X												
8		X	X	X	X		X		X	X		X			X							X	X					
9		X		X						X									X							X		
10	**X**																											
11	X	X			X								X					X										
14	**X**							X			X																	
19	X	X	X	X	X		X		X											X	X						X	
28																									X			

Vitreous Humor, Opacity

	PRUN S	AUR	CHOLEST	COCCUL	KALM
2	X		X		
6		X			X
8	X			X	

Vocal Cords, Weakness Of

	ARN	COCCUS	PHOS	STAPHYS
7		X		
8			X	X
18	X			

Voice, Diseases Of- See also Speech, Diseases Of; Voice, Hoarseness

	ARUM T	ARN	IOD	DROS	PHOS	SPONG	ANT C	OX AC	AUR M	BERB AQ	COCA	CROT H	HEP	LACH	MENTH P	NAT M	PRIM V	STAPHYS	STRAM
2	X	**X**	**X**				**X**	**X**	X	X	X				X		X	X	
6												X				X			
7	X	X	X	X	X	X													
9				X	X	X							X	X					X
24	X																		

Voice, Hoarseness (Note here that only the main remedies are used from 17)

	CAUST	PHOS	HEP	CARB V	ARUM T	DROS	ACON	BELL	SPONG	GELS	RHUS T	BRY	CALC	LACH	KALI BIC	CHAM	SENEG	SULPH	ARG N	ARN	ARS	BROM	EUP PER	GRAPH	STANN	MANG	NUX V	
1	X	X	X	X	X		X	X	X	X	X		X				X	X		X		X	X		X	X		
2			X		X									X									X					
3		X		X	X						X																	
4	X	**X**	X	**X**	**X**	X		X		X		X					X	X		X			X	X	X			
5	X	X	X	X	X	X	X		X						X						X	X						
6	X	X	X	X	X				X				X	X					X	X	X	X	X					
7	**X**	X	X	**X**	X	**X**	X	X	**X**	X	X	X	**X**	X	X	X	X	X	X		X	X	X		X	X	X	
8	X	X	X	X	X	X		X	X	X	X		X	X	X	X	X	X	X	X	X	X	X	X	X	X	X	
9	**X**	X	**X**	X		X	X	X				X			X				X	X		X						
10	X	X	X	X								X				X				X	X						X	
11	X		X				X	X				X	X		X		X		X				X					
12	X	X	X	X		X		X	X	X					X			X			X							
13	**X**	**X**	**X**	**X**		**X**	X	X	**X**	X	X	**X**	X	**X**	X	**X**	**X**	**X**		X	X	X		X	X	**X**	**X**	
14		X	X			X	X	X	X	X		X		X		X			X	X								
15	X	X	X	X		X	X	X	X	X		X	X	X		X		X									X	
16	X				X																							
17	X	X	X	X	X	X					X	X		X		X						X		X	X	X	X	
18	X	X			X		X				X								X					X				
19	X	X			X						X						X		X			X				X		
20		X									X																	
21	X			X	X		X			X																		
22			X							X					X													
24	X	X	X	X	X	X		X					X				X				X		X	X	X			
25	X	X	X	X			X		X						X													
26	X	X	X	X		X		X			X		X	X		X		X						X	X	X	X	
27	X						X																					

Voice, Hoarseness, From Singing (Includes Hoarseness, Public Speakers)

	ARG	ARUM T	FERR PH	HEP	ARG N	CAUST	SEL	GRAPH	RHUS T	ANT C	ARN	MANG AC	MANG	PHOS														
1	X	X			X								X															
4	X	X	**X**				X	X																				
6						X																						
7	**X**	X	X	X	X	X			**X**	X			X															
8		X	X		X	X	X	X		X																		
9				X																								
11	X				X	X						X																
12						X					X																	
17	X	X		X	X		X		X					X														
18	X											X																
23		X									X																	
24	X		**X**	**X**			X	X						X														
25				X																								

Vomiting (Includes Retching)

	IPEC	ARS	NUX V	BRY	VER A	PHOS	ANT C	IRIS V	PULS	ANT T	BELL	KREO	COCCUL	CUPR	AETHUSA	SANG	CALC	TAB	CHINA	SEP	CHAM	FERR	SULPH	PETR	CINA	LYC	EUP PER
1	**X**	X	X	X	X	X	X	X	X		X	X	X	X	X	X		X		X	X	X		X		X	X
2	**X**	**X**						X		**X**		X	**X**		**X**	X								**X**			
3	X	X	X	X	X	X	X	**X**	X		X	X			**X**		X	X	X	X	X		X	X	X	X	X
4	**X**	X	X	X		**X**	**X**	**X**			**X**	X			**X**		X		X				X				X
5	X	X	X	X	X	X	X	X	X	X		X		X		X	X	X	X	X	X	X			X	X	
6	X	X	X	X	X	X	X	X	X	X	X	X		X	X	X	X	X	X		X	X	X		X		X
7	**X**	**X**	**X**	**X**	**X**	**X**	**X**	X	**X**	**X**	**X**	X		**X**	X	X	X	X	X	X	**X**	**X**	**X**		X	X	**X**
8	X	X	X	X	X	X	X	X	**X**	X	X	X	X	X	X	X	X	X	X	X	X	**X**	**X**	X	X	X	X
9	X	X	X	X	X		X					X	X			X			X					X	X		
10	X	X	X	X	X	X	X		X		X	X			X	X	X		X	X	X		X				X
11	X	X	X	X	X	X		X	X		X						X		X	X		X					
12	X	X		X	X		X	X		X	X	X	X	X							X		X		X		
13	**X**	**X**	**X**	X	**X**	**X**	**X**	X	X	X	X	X	**X**	**X**		X	**X**	X	X	X	X	X	**X**	X	X	**X**	
14	**X**	X	X	X	X	X		X		X	X		X	X		X				X					X	X	
15	X	X	X	X	X		X	X	X	X	X		X	X							X		X				
16	X	X	X	X							X											X					
17									X	X					X	X		X						X			
18	X	X	X	X	X	X	X	X				X	X	X				X		X						X	
19	**X**	**X**	**X**	X	**X**	**X**	X	X	X	X		X	**X**	X	X	X		**X**	X	**X**	X	X		X		X	X
20		X		X	X	X		X	X		X		X					X									
21	X	X	X	X		X	X		X	X					X		X										
22	X	X	X	X	X	X	X	X								X											X
23	X	X			X							X	X	X				X									
24		X	X	X	X	X			X				X	X	X		X	X				X					
25	X	X	X		X	X	X			X		X					X		X					X	X		
26	**X**	X	**X**	X	X	X	X		X	X	X		X	X		X	X		X	**X**	X	X	**X**	X	X	X	
27	X																										

Vomiting, Bile

	ARS	IPEC	CHAM	IRIS V	BRY	EUP PER	PULS	NUX V	VER A	SEP	ANT C	BELL	COLCH	COLOC	LACH	LYC	PHOS	CUPR	SEC
6	X	X	X			X	X	X	X										
7	**X**	**X**	**X**	X	**X**	**X**	**X**	X	**X**	**X**	X	X	**X**	X	X	X	**X**	X	X
8	X	X	**X**	X		X	X	**X**	X	X	X	X		X	X	X	X	X	X
9		X		X															
10		X	X				X					X				X			
11	X			X	X	X													
12	X		X	X	X						X								
13	X	**X**	**X**	X	**X**	X	X	X	**X**	**X**	X	X	**X**	X	X	X	**X**	**X**	**X**
14	X	X		X															
15	X	X	X	X	X			X											
18													X						
19															X				
22	X				X	X													
24														X					
25		X		X						X									
26	X		X				X		X										

Vomiting, Faeces

	OP	PLUM	NUX V	BELL	CUPR	ACON	APOMOR	BRY	RAPH	SULPH	THUJA
1		X									
6	X				X						
7	**X**	X	X	X	X						
8	X	X	X	X		X	X	X	X	X	X
11	X										
13		X									
24	X	X	X								

Vomiting, Mucus

	IPEC	PULS	ARS	NUX V	ACON	ANT C	ANT T	BELL	CHAM	CON	DROS	SULPH	VER A	CINA	IGN	IRIS V	KALI BIC	SEC	SEP
7		X	X	X	X	X	X	X	X	X	X	X		X	X	X			
8		**X**	X	X	X	X		X	X	X	X	X	X	X	X	X		X	
10	X						X												X
11			X																
12	X					X							X					X	
13	X	X	X	X	X	X	X	X	X	X	X	X		X	X	X	X	X	
14	X																		
15	X	X		X					X				X						
17										X									
18																	X		
24																	X		X
25	X																		
26	X	X	X	X	X		X	X			X	X	X						X

Vomiting, Pregnancy Of- See Morning Sickness

Vulvitis

	COP	ITU	MERC	HELON	APIS	ARS	CANTH	CARB V	HYDRAST	KREO	PULS
2	X	X									
3	X	X									
4				**X**							
5			X						X	X	X
6			X			X					
8					X			X			
9							X				

Warts- See also Condylomata; Fig Warts

	THUJA	NIT AC	CAUST	DULC	ANT C	SEP	CALC	NAT CAR	STAPHYS	SULPH	NAT M	LYC	RHUS T	SABIN	SIL	NAT SUL	BAR C	CINNAB	FERR PIC	PH AC	KALI MUR	MEDO	ARS	LACH	RUTA	SARS	BELL	
1	X	X	X	X		X	X	X	X	X	X			X	X	X			X		X				X			
2	**X**	**X**	X	X	**X**	X	X	X	X	**X**	**X**	X	X				X	X	X	X	**X**	X		X	X	X		
3	X	X	**X**	X	X	X	X	X			X	X			X					X	X		X	X	X	X		
4	X	X							X																			
5	**E**	X	X	X	X	X	X	X	X					X	X	X		X				X						
6	X	X	X	X	X	X	X		X	X	X	X	X	X				X		X								
7	**X**	**X**	**X**	**X**												X	**X**				X		X	X			X	
8	X	X	X	X	X	X	X	X	X	X	X	X	X		X	X	X		X	X			X				X	
9	X	X	X		X				X					X														
10	X		X	X	X	X	X	X				X	X															
11	X	X	X	X	X		X	X							X				X									
12	B	X		X	X					X			B															
13	**X**	**X**	X	X		X	X	X	X	**X**	X	X	X		X		X			X			X	X	X	X	**X**	
14	X	X	X	X	X	X								X	X													
15	X		X							X																		
16																X												
17	X	X	X																									
18	X	X	X	X	X				X					X				X	X			X						
19	**X**	**X**	**X**	X		X	X	X	X		X	X		X		X	X	X				**X**				X		
20	X	X	X	X	X																							
21	X	X	X	X	X	X	X	X		X	X																	
22	X	X	X	X																								
24					X																							
26	**X**		**X**	**X**	**X**	**X**				X		X	X															
27	**X**	X																										
29*	X	X																										

B- Both Internal and External E- External

29* Manchanda RK, et al. Double Blind Placebo Controlled Clinical Trials of Homoeopathic Medicines in Warts and Molluscum contagiosum, CCRH Quarterly Bulletin, 1997, 19, 25-29.

Warts, Abdomen

	NAT SUL	SEP
5	X	
19		X

Warts, Anal

	THUJA	NIT AC	BENZ AC	CINNAB	EUPHR	LYC	NAT SUL	STAPHYS	AUR	COLOC	MERC C	MERC D	NAT PH	PETR	SABAD
1		X													
6				X	X						X				
7	**X**	X	X		X	X		X		X			X	X	
8	X		X				X								
9	X						X								
13	**X**	**X**						X							X
14												X			
19		**X**		X		X			X						
20	X														
24	X														

Warts, Arms

	CALC	SEP	CAUST	NAT CAR	SIL	NIT AC	SULPH	ARS	DULC	RHUS T	THUJA
7	X		X		X						X
8	X	X	X	X	X	X	X				
13	**X**	**X**	X	X	X	X	X	X	X	X	
19		X		X							

Warts, Cervix

	GRAPH	KREO	THUJA	NIT AC
7		X	X	X
8	X			
19			X	
26	X	X		

Warts, Chin

	LYC	THUJA
5	X	X
8	X	
19	X	
20		X

Warts, Ears

	BUFO	CALC	THUJA
19	X	X	
24			X

Warts, Eyelid

	CAUST	NIT AC	THUJA	ANT C	CINNAB
6	X		X		
7	X	X	X		X
8	X	X			
14	X				
19				X	
21	X				

Warts, Eyes, Around

	CAUST	CALC	SULPH	THUJA
1	X			
6	X			
8	X		X	
13	X			X
14	X			
19	X	X		

Warts, Face

	CAUST	CALC	DULC	NIT AC	THUJA	SEP	DULC	KALI CAR	MAG SUL
1	X								X
5	X	X		X	X			X	
7	X	X	X	X	X	X			
8	X	X	X	X	X	X			
10	X	X							
14	X								
19	X	X	X	**X**	**X**				
20	X		X						
21	X								
22			X						
26	X	X							
29*			X				X		

29* Manchanda RK, et al. Double Blind Placebo Controlled Clinical Trials of Homoeopathic Medicines in Warts and Molluscum contagiosum, CCRH Quarterly Bulletin, 1997, 19, 25-29.

Warts, Fingers

	CAUST	DULC	CALC	SEP	THUJA	RHUS T	NIT AC	ANT C	BAR C	BERB V	GRAPH	LACH	NAT CAR	NAT M	SULPH	ARG N	BUFO	CALC S	LAC C	LYC	NAT SUL	PETR	SIL
5	X	X		X	X			X			X		X								X		X
7	X	X	X	X	X		X		X					X									
8	X	X	X	X	X	X	X			X		X		X	X			X					
9	X																						
10	X	X	X	X	X	X							X										
13	X					X				X		X			X					X		X	
14	X																						
18											X												
19	X	X	X				X	X	X							X	X		X				
20	X	X																					
21	X																						
22	X																						
26		X	X	X	X	X																	
29*	X																						

29* Manchanda RK, et al. Double Blind Placebo Controlled Clinical Trials of Homoeopathic Medicines in Warts and Molluscum contagiosum, CCRH Quarterly Bulletin, 1997, 19, 25-29.

Warts, Genital

	THUJA	NIT AC	SABIN	MEDO	CINNAB	CALC	LYC	MERC D	STAPHYS	PH AC	CANN S	APIS	ARG N	CINNAB
1	X							X						
5	**X**	**X**	X	X	X	X								
6														X
7	X	**X**	X		**X**		X	X	X	X		X		
9	X			X										
12	X	X												
13	**X**	**X**	X				X		X	X	**X**			
14	X							X						
18			X											
19	**X**	**X**	X	X	X	X	X		X					
20	X	X												
29*	X			X		X							X	

29* Gimeno LQ. Homoeopathic Treatment of Human Papillomavirus infections previously treated by other methods. Brit Hom J, 1996, 85, 194-197.

Warts, Glans Penis (See also Warts, Genital)

	KALI MUR	LAC C	PH AC	STAPHYS	SULPH	THUJA	ANT T	AUR SUL	MEDO	NIT AC	SABIN	SEP
1	X		X		X	X		X				
7	X	X	X	X	X		X					X
13										X	X	
19		X		X		X			X			

Warts, Hands

	DULC	THUJA	CALC	NIT AC	NAT CAR	SEP	ANT C	CAUST	RHUS T	NAT M	BAR C	FERR PIC	LACH	SULPH	BERB V	BOR	BUFO	FERR	FERR M	FL AC	KALI MUR	LYC	MEDO	RUTA	SIL
1	X			X	X			X		X		X									X			X	
5	X	X	X	X	X	X	X	X			X							X		X					
7	**X**	**X**	X	X		X		X					X												
8	X	X	X	X	X	X			X	X				X											X
10	X	X	X		X	X			X			X													
12	X			X			X							X											
13	**X**	X	X	X	**X**	X			X	**X**			X		X	X			X			X			
14	X						X																		
19	X	X	X	X	X		X				X						X						X		
20	X																								
21	X	X																							
26	X	X	X			X			X																
29*								X																	

29* Manchanda RK, et al. Double Blind Placebo Controlled Clinical Trials of Homoeopathic Medicines in Warts and Molluscum contagiosum, CCRH Quarterly Bulletin, 1997, 19, 25-29.

Warts, Iris

	CINNAB	MERC	THUJA
6			X
19	X	X	

Warts, Lips

	CAUST	NIT AC	THUJA	CINNAB	MERC C
6				X	X
7	X	X			
19	X	X	**X**		

Warts, Mouth

	ANT C	ARG N	CAUST	CONDUR	NIT AC	PSOR
5	X		X		X	X
8				X		
19		X				

Warts, Mucous Membranes

	ARG N	MERC
19	**X**	X

Warts, Neck

	NIT AC	CALC	NAT CAR	SEP	SIL	THUJA
5	X		X		X	X
7				X		
8	X	X				

Warts, Nose

	CAUST	THUJA	NIT AC	NAT CAR
5	X	X	X	X
6	X			
7	X	X	X	
8	X	X		
9	X			
10	X	X		
13			X	
19	X	**X**	X	
22	X			

Warts, Palms

	NAT M	ANAC	RUTA	DULC	BERB V	CALC	NAT CAR	THUJA
1	X		X					
5	X	X	X	X	X	X	X	X
8	X	X						
14		X						
18	X							
19	X							
21	X							
22				X				

Warts, Penis- See also Warts, Genital

	CINNAB	THUJA	LYC	MEDO	SEP
1					X
19	X			X	
21	X	**X**	X		

Warts, Perineum

	MERC D	SABIN
7	X	
19		X

Warts, Plantar

	ANT C	THUJA	CALC	CAUST	MEDO	NIT AC	RUTA
18	X		X			X	
19	X	X			X		
20	X						
28	X	X		X			
29*							X

29* Manchanda RK, et al. Double Blind Placebo Controlled Clinical Trials of Homoeopathic Medicines in Warts and Molluscum contagiosum, CCRH Quarterly Bulletin, 1997, 19, 25-29.

Warts, Prepuce

	CINNAB	PH AC	SEP	CHIM	LYC	NIT AC	SABIN	THUJA
1		X	X					
5	X	X				X	X	
14			X	X				
19	X				X			X

Warts, Tongue

	AUR M	AUR	LYC
8	X		
17	X		
19	X	X	X
27	X		

Warts, Uterus

	CALC	KREO	MERC	NIT AC	THUJA	ANT T	GRAPH	LYC	STAPHYS
7	X	X	X	X					
8	X		X	X	X	X		X	X
10		X					X		
19	X				X				

Warts, Vagina

	STAPHYS	THUJA	ANT T	CALC	LYC	MEDO	MERC	NIT AC	PHOS
7									X
8	X	X	X	X	X		X	X	
19	X	X				X			

Waterbrash- See also Heartburn; Indigestion; Reflux

	NUX V	BRY	LYC	PULS	CALC	SIL	SULPH	SEP	CARB V	VER A	ARS	NAT M	PETR	PHOS	BAR C	DROS	LED	STAPHYS	CHINA	IPEC	MAG M	RHUS T	CARB A	SABAD				
1	X	X	X	X	X	X		X					X								X		X					
2	**X**	**X**	**X**							**X**											X							
3	X		X	X																								
4	X			X																								
7	**X**	**X**	**X**	X	X	**X**	**X**	X	**X**	X	X	X	X	X	**X**	X	X	**X**	X	X	X	X		**X**				
8	X	X	X		X	X	X	X	X	X	X	X	X	X	X	X	X	X		X		X		X				
10	X	X		X	X		X		X		X			X					X									
12			X																									
13	X	X	**X**	X	X	**X**	**X**	X	X	X	X	**X**	**X**	X	X	**X**	**X**	X	X	X		X	**X**					
15	X	X		X		X		X		X																		
19	X						X					X																
21		X																										
24	X				X																							
26	**X**	**X**	X	**X**	X	X	X	X	X		X																	

Weakness- See Fatigue for general weakness

Weakness, Abdomen

	PHOS	LACH	ALUM	ANAC	ANT C	ASAR	BAR C	CALC	CINNAB	CHINA	CLEM	CON	FERR ARS	MERC	NUX M	NUX V	OX AC	PETR	PH AC	POD	RHUS T	SULPH	THUJA	VER A				
5	X																											
7	X	X																X						X				
8							X							X														
10																				X								
13	X	X	X	X	X	X		X	X	X	X	X	X		X	X	X		X		X	X	X					

Weakness, Ankle

	NAT M	CALC PH	NAT CAR	CALC	CAUST	SIL	PINUS S	SULPH	CHAM	HAM	BRUC	CARB A	LAC D	MANCIN	MANG M	NAT	SEP	STRONT C	SULPH AC									
2		**X**	X	**X**		**X**	X			**X**				X	X													
3	X	**X**		X		X																						
4					X																							
7	X		X			**X**		X				X	X				X											
8	X	X	X	X	X		X	X			X					X			X									
9	X																											
10		X			X				X																			
11							X																					
13			X																									
14	X				X																							
17	X		X						X																			
19																		X										
21	X																											
25				X																								

Weakness, Arm, Left

	LACH	ALL C
10	X	
14		X
24	X	

Weakness, Arms (Includes Arms, Langour; Arms, Tired; Lameness, Arms)

	ACON	NAT M	NUX V	CARB V	AGAR M	ARS	CAUST	DIG	GELS	GLON	KALM	LACH	MAG PH	PETR	PH AC	PHOS	SEP	ANAC	ANGUST	NAT CAR
1	X	X							X											
5													X							
6	X																			
7	X	X		X		X		X	X	X	X	X		X	X	X	X			
9			X																	
11					X		X													
13	X	**X**	X	**X**	X	X	X			X	X	X		X	X	X	X	**X**	**X**	**X**
14		X											X							
17			X																	
19								X												

Weakness, Back- See also Weakness, Spine

	GRAPH	CALC	SIL	OX AC	CHINA	NAT M	KALI CAR	KALI PH	KALM	SULPH	CALC PH	IGN	SEP.
2			**X**		**X**						**X**	**X**	
4	X								X				
6	X			X									
7	X	**X**	X			**X**							**X**
8	X	X		X	X	X	X			X			
10									X				
11								X					
13			X	X									
18							X						
19		**X**								X			
20	X												
21								X					

Weakness, Back, Lower- See also Weakness, Spine, Lower

	HELON	KALI CAR	AESC	AGAR M	SEL	SEP	ZINC	AMM M	ARS	CALC	COCCUL	CON	CUPR AR	EUP PER	GRAPH	HYPER	KALI BIC	NUX M	PHOS	PULS	RUTA							
1			X																									
4	X																											
5		X		X	X	X		X												X								
6		X					X					X			X													
7	X	X	X	X	X		X		X	X			X	X		X	X	X			X							
8																			X									
14											X																	
19	X					X																						

Weakness, Bladder

	CAUST	HEP	MUR AC	ALUM	MAG M	ALL C	RHEUM	BELL	ALUM SIL	ARS	EQUISET	HYOSC	NUX V	PALLAD	PH AC	PHOS	RHUS T	SABAD										
1				X					X																			
2								**X**																				
3	X																											
4	X																											
7		**X**	**X**		X	X				X		X			X													
8			X	X	X		X				X																	
9	X												X															
10	X																X											
13			X	X	X	X	X							X														
14		X																										
19		X														X												
25	X																	X										

Weakness, Bones- See also Fractures; Osteomalacia, Osteoporosis, Rickets

	CALC PH	CALC	CALC IOD																									
1	X																											
11	X																											
24		X	X																									

Weakness, Brain

	BAR M	CAUST	FORMICA	GELS																								
1			X																									
8		X		X																								
10	X																											

Weakness, Chest

	STANN	PH AC	SULPH	HEP	KALI CAR	PHOS	SULPH AC	ALUMEN	ARG	ARS	CALC	CARB V	DIG	IOD	PLAT	RUTA
1	X			X												
4					X											
5									X							
6	X										X					
7	**X**		X	X		X	X			X						
8		X	X	X											X	
10	X	X	X			X		X								
11	X															
13	**X**	**X**	**X**	X	X	X	X					X	X	X	X	X
15		X									X					
17	X	X					X	X	X				X	X		X
19	X									X		X				
24					X											
26				X												

Weakness, Ciliary Muscles- See also Weakness, Eyes; Weakness, Vision

	ARG N	COCCUL	LACH	LIL T	PHYSO
1		X			
8	**X**				
9			X	X	X

Weakness, Digestion (Includes Digestion, Atony)

	HYDRAST	LYC	ANAC	CALC	CALC PH	CHINA	CYCL	MERC	NUX V	CARB V	KALI BIC	NAT CAR	NAT M	NUX M	SULPH	URAN N
1	X					X										X
6									X				X			
7	X	X	X			X	X	X	X							
8	X	X	X	X		X	X	X		X	X	X		X	X	
9				X									X			
10	X							X								X
11		X	X		X											
12		X														
13														X		
14					X					X						
15									X						X	
17												X				
21											X					
22					X											
25				X												
26							X									

Weakness, Digestion, Senile

	CARB V	NUX M
7		X
8	X	

Weakness, Extremities

	BUFO	CON	PLUM	ARG N	ARN	COCA	KALI PH	MAG PH	NUX V	PHOS	PIC AC	THUJA
1				X		X						
5								X				
6										X		
8	X		**X**									X
9					X				X			
11							X				X	
14	X	X										
17		X										

Weakness, Eyes- See also Weakness, Ciliary Muscles; Weakness, Vision

	NAT ARS	PHOS	RUTA	ZINC	ARS	LED	NAT M	PULS	THUJA
7	X	X			X				
8	X			X					
9			X			X	X		
10								X	
11		X							
24				X					X
25			X						

Weakness, Feet

	BELL	PULS	CHINA	OLEAND	OL AN	TAB
6	X					
7		X				
13	X	X	**X**	**X**	**X**	**X**

Weakness, Fingers (Includes Lameness, Fingers)

	CARB V	RHUS T	AMBRA	CARB A	HIPPOM	NAT M	NIT	PARIS	SEP	SIL	STRAM
1						X					X
7				X					X		
8	X										
13	X	X	X				X	X		X	
14		X									
17					X						

Weakness, Forearms

	RHUS T	CAUST	DIG	GELS	FL AC
1					X
5	X				
14	X	X		X	
19			X		

Weakness, Gall Bladder- See Liver, Torpidity

Weakness, Genital Organs- See also Impotence; Sterility

	DIG	SULPH	HELON	AGNUS	BAR C	BELLIS	BERB V	CALC PH	CARB A	DIOSC	GELS	HELL	HEP	MANG	MUR AC	NAT M	NUX M	PRUN P	SEP	STAPHYS
2																		X		
4			**X**			X														
7	X							X	X	X	X	X				X	X			X
8	X				X															
13		X		X			X						X	X	X				X	
27		X																		

Weakness, Hands

	BOV	ACON	ACT S	CAUST	KALI BIC	STANN	ZINC
1		X	X				
7					X	X	X
8			X				
13	X	X		X	X	X	X
14	X			X			
17	X						

Weakness, Heart (Includes Weakness, Pulse)

	DIG	STROPH	CRAT	ARN	CACT	CARB V	GELS	NAJA	ADONIS	AMM C	KALI CAR	LYCOP	ARS	CAFF	CAMPH	GRIND	HYDR AC	PHOS	RHUS T	CROT H	LACH
1		X			X		X			X			X			X					
4	X	X	X		X				X			X		X							
5	X	X	X	X		X	X	X	X	X	X					X					
6																	X				
7	X					X	X	**X**			X	X	X		X	X	X	X	X	**X**	**X**
8						X							X				X	X			
10		X	X	X		X		X		X								X			
11	X	X	X		X									X							
12	X						X												X		
14	X		X	X	X	X		X						X	X						
16																					X
17	X	X	X	X	X				X	X	X				X						
19		X					X		X		X	X							X		
24												X								X	
27	X			X																	

Weakness, Hip

	KALI CAR	CHINA	KREO	PIC AC	RUTA
6	X				
7	X			X	
10	X				
13		X	X		
17					X

Weakness, Intestines (Includes Atonic Constipation; Intestines, Torpidity)

	GRAPH	ALUMEN	CHAM	NAT M	NUX V	OP	RAPH
7	**X**	**X**	**X**	**X**	**X**	**X**	
18	X						
19							**X**

Weakness, Jaw

	ARS	LACH	LYC	OP	ARN	BAPT	CARB V	CAUST	HELL	KALI IOD	MUR AC	STRAM	VER V	ZINC
6	X	X	X	X		X		X			X		X	
7	X	X	X	X	X		X		X	X		X		X

Weakness, Joints

	RHUS T	BOV	CALC	CARB A	PULS	SEP	ALOE	ARN	BRY	NAT M	STAPHYS	ACON	KALI CAR	LYC	SULPH
3	X		X					X			X				
4					X										
7	**X**			X		X	X		X						
8	X	X		X	X					X					
13	**X**	**X**	X	X	X	**X**	X	X	X	X	X	**X**	**X**	**X**	**X**
14		X													
22			X												

Weakness, Kidneys- See also Urine, Scanty

	ADONIS	COLCH	CUPR AR	LYC	SER ANG	STRAM	TEREB	ZING
5				X				
7		X				X	X	X
14			X					
19	X				X			

Weakness, Knee

	NAT M	CALC	STAPHYS	CAUST	COCCUL	DIOSC	FERR	KALI CAR	MERC	NUX M	PHOS	CHINA	NIT AC	RUTA
1	X													
2					X									
3					X									
6		X												
7	**X**	X		X		X	X		X	X				
8			X			X								
13	X		**X**				X		X	X	X	**X**	**X**	**X**
14				X										
15		X												
17								X			X			
18								X						

Weakness, Larynx

	APIS	STANN	ARG	CANTH	CARB V	GELS	MANG AC	STANN IO
5			X			X	X	X
6	X							
7	X	X		X				
8		**X**						
10	X							
17					X			

Weakness, Legs

	ARG N	RHUS T	NUX V	PH AC	PULS	KALI CAR	PHOS	PLUM	ALUM	AGAR M	ALL C	ARG	BRY	COCCUL	FERR	KALM	KREO	NAT CAR	PIC AC	SULPH	TAR H	EUPHORB	MERC	NIT	OLEAND	STAPHYS		
1												X					X											
3																					X							
4	X						X									X												
6	X	X				X	X		X					X							X							
7	X	**X**	X	**X**		X	X	X		X			X	X	X			X		X								
8	X	X																										
9	X		X																									
10					X			X																				
13	X		X	X	**X**					X	X		X		X	X	X	X	X	X		**X**	**X**	**X**	**X**	**X**		
14		X									X	X							X									
15					X																							
18						X																						
19									**X**																			
24								X																				
25			X	X																								

Weakness, Ligaments (AKA Laxity, Ligaments)

	CALC FL	CALC PH
18	X	X
28	X	

Weakness, Limbs- See also Fatigue

	NUX V	GELS	CAUST	AMYL N	LED	ZINC	ARS	PHOS	SULPH	CALC	ANT C	BRY	CHAM	CHINA	CHIN S	CUPR	DULC	KALM	NAT M	PIC AC	PULS	STANN	VER A	MERC				
1			X	X		X										X												
4	X				X			X																				
5		X																										
6			X				X		X											X			X					
7	X		**X**	X		X	X	X		**X**	X	X	X	X	X	X	X	X	X		X	X	X	**X**				
8				X	X	**X**	X	X	X		X	X			X			X		X								
9	X	X																										
10	X	X							X					X														
14		X															X		X									
15	X									X											X							
17		X		X																		X						
21	X		X		X								X															
25					X																							

Weakness, Liver- See Liver, Torpidity

Weakness, Lungs

	ANT T	ARS	AMM C	CAMPH	CARB V	DROS	GRIND	MOSCH	SENEG	STANN IO	VER A
1	X						X				
5						X				X	
6								X			
7		X		X							X
14			X		X						
19	X	X							X		

Weakness, Mind

	CAUST	CON	ALET	AMM C	ANT T	BAPT	BAR C	CALC	CAULO	CHINA	IOD	LIL T	NAT M	NUX V	PH AC	PLUM
4												X				
6	X			X									X	X		
8	X		X		X	X		X	X						X	X
11											X					
14										X						
16		X														
17		X														
21							X									

Weakness, Mind, Senile

	AMBRA	ANAC	BUFO	LYC
8	X	X		
9				X
14			X	

Weakness, Muscles- See Amyotonia; Fatigue; Myasthenia; Weakness, Limbs

Weakness, Neck

	ABROT	VER A	COCCUL	GLON	PARIS	PLAT	ACON	ANT T	ARN	BRY	CALC PH	FL AC	KALI CAR	LYC	NAT M	PHOS	SIL	STANN	STAPHYS	SULPH
1	X											X								
3	X																			
5																X				
7		X	X	X	X															
8		X				X														
10											X									
11	X																			
13		X	X	X	X	X	X	X	X				X	X			X	X	X	X
14															X					
15										X										

Weakness, Pancreas

	IRIS V	NAT M
5	X	
6		X

Weakness, Pulse- See Weakness, Heart

Weakness, Rectum- See also Weakness, Intestines

	POD	GRAPH	IGN	SIL	ALUM	ANAC	ARN	BRY	CARB V	COCCUL	KALI CAR	NAT CAR	NUX V	OP	PULS	STAPHYS	SULPH	VER A	ZINC	ALUMEN
4	X																			
5						X														
7	X	X	X	**X**			X		X	X	X	X			X	X	X	X	X	**X**
8	X																			
10	X							X												
13			X		X	X	X		X	X	X		X	X	X	X	X	X	X	
14				X																
15			X																	
18		X			X			X						X						
24		X																		

Weakness, Sacrum

	SIL	ZINC	ARS	CALC PH	COLOC	MERC	NAT M	NUX M	PETR	SEP	SULPH
7	X	X		X							
13	X	X	X		X	X	X	X	X	X	X

Weakness, Senile

	AUR	AMBRA	ANAC	ANT T	BAR C	CHINA	CON	OP
6	X							
8	X	X	X	X	X	X	X	X

Weakness, Spine- See also Weakness, Back

	CALC PH	PHOS	AESC	AGAR M	CALC	CAST EQ	GELS	SEL	SIL	STRY PH	SULPH
1	X										
4	X	X									
5		X									
6							X				
7		X	X			X					
8	X	X			X				X		X
10	X										
14			X	X						X	
17								X			

Weakness, Spine, Lumbar- See also Weakness, Back, Lower

	CALC PH	KALI CAR
5		X
10	X	

Weakness, Stomach (Includes Atony, Stomach)

	DIG	SULPH	ARS	IGN	NUX V	SEP	VER A	ANT C
1		X				X		
5	X					X		
7	X			X			X	X
10		X						
13	X			X				
15			X		X			
17	X							
26	X	X	X		X		X	

Weakness, Tendon

	HYOSC	RUTA
4		X
9	X	
17	X	

Weakness, Thighs

	RUTA	ARS	CARB A	MUR AC	CHINA	MERC	PLAT	ACON	AGAR M	AMYL N	ANGUS	ARN	BRY	CALC	CON	CROC	GUAIAC	IRIS V	NUX V	OLEAND	PULS	RHEUM	SARS	STAPHYS				
1				X																								
7		X								X				X				X										
8	X		X																									
13	**X**	X	X	X	**X**	**X**	**X**	X	X		X	X	X			X	X		X	X	X	X	X	X				
17	X																											
19															X													

Weakness, Uterus- See also Labour

	CAUL	ALET	ARG	CARB V	SABIN	SEC	CALC PH	ERIG	FERR PH	FRAX	HELON	NAT M	NUX V	PALLAD	PITUIT	RHUS A	SULPH	THLASPI	USTIL									
1	X	X	X	X	X	X				X					X	X												
6	X											X																
7			X	X	X		X				X		X	X				X	X									
8						X											X											
9									X																			
14	X																											
16								X																				
19	X	X																										
27	X																											

Weakness, Vocal Cords- See also Weakness, Voice

	CAUST	PHOS	STANN	STAPHYS																								
1	X		X																									
8		X		X																								

Weakness, Voice- See also Weakness, Vocal Cords

	AMM C	BELL	CAUST	COCA	CROT H	HEP	SPONG	ANT C	ANT T	BROM	CAMPH	CANTH	CARB V	COCCUL	COCC C	ERIODYC	GELS	HELL	LYC	MANG AC	NAT M	PARIS	POP CAN	RHUS T	STANN	STAPHYS	STRAM	STRYCH
2				X																								
3																								X				
7		X	X	X	X	X	X	X	X		X	X	X	X				X	X			X			X	X	X	
8	X	X	X							X						X				X	X							
12						X	X																					
15																	X											
17	X				X										X								X					X

Weakness, Wrist

	PLUM	CAUST	CURARE
7		X	X
10	X		
14	X		

Wens- See Sebaceous Cyst, Scalp

Wheezing- See Dyspnoea

Whiplash

	BRY	CAUST	HYPER	RHUS T
19	X			
27	X	X	X	X

White Swelling- See Tuberculosis, Bone

Whitlow- See also Nails, Diseases Of; Panaritum (AKA Felon)

	HEP	SIL	LACH	LED	MERC	ARS	SULPH	MYRIST	AMM C	BELL	DIOSC	FL AC	CALC SUL	CALEND	PHOS	ACON	ALL C	BUFO	CALC	GRAPH	RHUS T
1	X	X		X				X			X						X				
2	X	**X**	**X**	X				X	X		X	X		**X**	**X**		X	X	X		
3	X	X					X		X			X	**X**								
5														E							
6				X	X																
8	X	X	X	X	X		X		X			X			X				X	X	X
9	X	X	X			X				X										X	
10	X	X	X		X	X	X														
12	X	X			X					X						X					
14	X	X		X				**X**													
15	X	X	X			X	X									X					X
16											X		X								
19																		X			
24				X																	
25	X	X	X		X	X				X											

E- External

Whooping Cough (AKA Pertussis)

	DROS	CUPR	BELL	IPEC	COCC C	COR R	ANT T	MEPH	ARN	CINA	ACON	HEP	KALI CAR	NAPHTH	BRY	PULS	CARB V	KALI BIC	NAT M	NUX V	VER A	ALL C	CASTAN V	MAG PH	SULPH	HYOSC	PERTUSS	SAMB
1	**X**	X	X	X	X	X		X					X	X				X	X			X					X	
2	**X**	X	**X**	**X**	**X**	**X**	**X**	X	**X**	X	**X**	**X**	**X**	X	X			X	X		X	X	X	X				X
3	X	X	X								X			**X**					X							X		
4	**X**	**X**	**X**	**X**	**X**	**X**	**X**	**X**		**X**				X				**X**					**X**	**X**			X	
5	**X**	X	X	X	X	X	X	X		X	X	X	X						X								X	X
6	X	X	X	X	X	X	X	X	X	X		X	X	X	X	X	X		X	X	X				X	X		
7	**X**	**X**	**X**	**X**	**X**	**X**	**X**	**X**	**X**	X		X	X		X	X	X	X	X	X	X	**X**	X	X	X	**X**		X
8	X	X	X	X	X	X	X	X	X	X	X	X	X	X	X	X	X	X	X	X	X	X	X		X	X		X
9	X	X	X	X	X	X		X			X			X									X				X	
10	X	X	X	X		X	X		X			X				X				X	X				X			
11	**X**	**X**	**X**	**X**	**X**	**X**	X	**X**	X	**X**		X		X										**X**		X	**X**	
12	**X**	**X**	**X**	X	X	X	**X**		X		**X**				X	X		X										
13	X	X		X	X	X	**X**	X	X	X		X			**X**	X	X		X	X	X				**X**	X		**X**
14	**X**	X	X	X	X						X											X						
15	X	X	X	X			X		X		X	X			X	X				X								
16	X	X			X	X		X					X				X						X				X	
17	X				X	X		X						X			X				X							X
18	X		X	X	X	X			X							X	X	X				X			X			
19	**X**	**X**	**X**	**X**	**X**	X	**X**	X	**X**	X			X		**X**	X	**X**					X						
21	X	X	X	X	X								X					X										
23	X	X	X	X	X	X		X		X				X									X	X				
24	X																											
26	X	X		X			X		X	X	X	X	X		X	X	X			X	X				X			
27	X																			X								

Whooping Cough, Prophylaxis

	PERTUSS	DROS	VACCIN
9	X		
10		X	X
11	X		
16	X	X	X
21	X		
29*	X		

29* English JM. Pertussin 30- Preventative for Whooping Cough? Homeopathy, 2007, 96, 125-127.

Worms- See also Oxyuriasis; Trichinosis; Worms, Hook; Worms, Pin; Worms, Round; Worms, Tape; Worms, Thread (Includes Helminthiasis)

	CINA	CALC	SPIG	SULPH	SIL	LYC	IGN	SANTIN	STANN	TEUCR	CIC	SABAD	NAT PH	ACON	DOLICH	CHINA	MERC	NUX V	TEREB	CALAD	HYOSC	NUX M	ARS
1		X	X					X	X				X							X			
2	X	**X**	**X**	**X**	X	**X**			X	**X**	X	X	X					X	X	X		X	**X**
3	X	X			X	X		X	X														
4	**X**	X	**X**				X		**X**			X								X			
5	X									X		X											
6	X	X		X	X	X	X				X			X	X		X		X				
7	**X**	**X**	**X**	**X**	X	X	X		X	X	X				X	**X**	**X**	**X**	**X**		X	X	
8						X									X				X	X			
9	X		X	X				X		X		X									X		
10	**X**				X	X	X				X			X		**X**		X			X		
11													**X**										
12		X		X	X		X	X						X			X	X					X
13															X							**X**	
14	X										X												X
15		X		X	X		X									X							
16	X	X		X		X								X									
17	X	X	X					X	X			X			X						X		
18	X	X																					
23	X		X					X				X											
24	X		X	X																			
25	X	X		X				X		X													
26	X	X	X		X	X	X				X			X			X						
27	**X**	X	X	X	X					X			X										

Worms, Hook (AKA Ancylostomiasis)

	THYMOL	CARB TET	CHENO	NAT PH	AESC	CINA	FERR M	NAPHTH	TEUCR	VIOL O
1	X	X	X							
11	X	**X**	X	**X**	X		X	X		X
12	X					X			X	

Worms, Pin (AKA Enterobiasis; Oxyuriasis)

	TEUCR	CINA	CUPR	NAT M	SULPH	CALC	EUPHORB	SABAD	SINAP	ACON	FERR	ABSINTH	ALL S	ARG N	CALC AC	CUPR OX	DOLICH	GRAPH	HEP	INDIG	PASS	PSOR	RAT	SANTON	SIL	SULPH IO	URT U	VIOL O
1	X								X																			
3	X																											
4	X								X																			
5	X	X	X	X		X		X				X				X		X		X	X	X			X	X		X
6							X																					
7		**X**	**X**	**X**	X	X		X		**X**	**X**		X	X			X		X				X					
8	X	X					X																					
9	X	X			X										X									X			X	
11	X																											
19		X																										

Worms, Round (AKA Ascarides; Ascaris)

	CINA	TUECR	CALC	ABROT	FERR	SIL	MERC	SPIG	SULPH	ACET AC	MAG C	SABAD	SEP	STANN	IGN	SULPH	TEREB	VALER										
1	X	X		**X**																								
2										X	X		X															
3		X																										
4		X																										
7	**X**	X	X		**X**	**X**	**X**		**X**	X	X	X	X				**X**											
9	X	X										X																
11	X			X				X																				
13	**X**	X	**X**		**X**	**X**		**X**						X	**X**	**X**		**X**										
14	X																											
15														X														
26	X		X				X		X																			

Worms, Tape (AKA Lumbricoides; Taenia)

	FILIX	SULPH	CALC	CINA	SABAD	KOUSSO	STANN	MERC	PLAT	PULS	CUCURB	GRANAT	SIL	CARB V	CUPR O N	GRAPH	CHINA	MAG CAR	MAG M	NUX V	PHOS	TEREB	VER A	CIC	SPIG
1	X	**X**		X		X					X				X		X			X		X	X		
2	X		X	X	X	X	X		X	X	X	X													
4															**X**										
6					X	X	X																		
7	**X**	**X**	**X**	X	X		X	**X**	X	X			**X**	**X**		**X**		X	X		X	X			
8	X	X	X		X		X		X	X			X	X		X	X	X	X	X	X		X		
10		X	X					X																	
11	X					X					X	X			X										
12	X			X																					
13	X	**X**	**X**	**X**	X		X	X	**X**	**X**			**X**	X		X	X	X	X	X	X	X	X	**X**	**X**
14	X																								
15	X					X		X																	
17												X													
23	X										X	X													
26	X		X	X		X																		X	X

Worms, Thread

	TEUCR	CINA	NAT PH	BAPT	SPIG	ARUM T	CHINA	INDIGO	SANTIN	SCHIRR	SINAP A	TELL	URT U
1		X	X									X	
2	**X**	X	**X**	**X**	**X**					X	X		
4								X					
6	**X**												
12	X						X						X
14		X											
15		X											
17	X					X							
21	X	X							X				

Wounds (Includes Wounds, Slow to Heal)

	CALEND	HYPER	ARN	LED	SIL	LACH	ACON	HEP	STAPHYS	BELL	PHOS	SULPH	CALC	CIC	MERC	MILL	RHUS T	APIS	ARS	BELLIS	CHINA	CON	NIT AC	RUTA	SULPH AC	SYMPH
1					X								X													
2	**X**	X	**X**	**X**		**X**				X	X							X	X							X
3	X	X																								
5	B																									
6						X																				
7				X		X					X					X										
8	X	X	X	X	X	X	X	X	X		X	X	X	X			X	X			X	X	X	X	X	
9		X			X	X	X	X	X	X					X				X							
10	B	B			X		X														X					
12	E		X		X		X	X		X																
13	X				X	X	X	X	X	X	X	X	X	X	X	X	X					X	X	X	X	
14	E																						X			
15	E	E	<u>**B**</u>	X	X		X			X		X		X			X			E	X					
16	X																									
18	B															X										
19	**X**	**X**	X	**X**	X	X	X	X	**X**		X	X		X	X	X		X	X	X						X
20	E	B																								
21	X	X	X	X					X																	
22	E	E	X	E				X																		
23	X	X		X																						
24	X	X	X	X	X	X	X	X	X						X		X			X		X		X	X	X
25		E		X																						
26	<u>**E**</u>		X		X			X				X	X													
29[1]					X																					
29[2]			X																							

B- Both Internal and External E- External

29[1] Oberbaum M, et al. Wound Healing by Homoeopathic Silica Dilutions in Mice. Journal of the Israeli Medical Association, 1992, Aug, 123, 3-4, 79-82.

29[2] Karow JH, Efficacy of Arnica montana D4 for healing of wounds after Hallux valgus surgery compared to diclofenac. J Altern Complement Med. 2008 Jan-Feb;14 (1):17-25.

Wounds, Bleeding

	PHOS	ARN	ARS	MILL
19	X			X
26	X	X	X	

Wounds, Dissecting

	ARS	LACH	APIS	CROT H	HAM	PYROG
7	**X**	**X**				
8			X	X	X	
19	X	X				X
26	X					

Wounds, Gun Shot

	ARN	HYPER	CALEND	EUPHR	NIT AC	PLUM	PULS	RUTA	SULPH	SULPH AC	SYMPH
2		X									X
4			X								
7	X	X			X						
8	X	X		X	X	X	X	X	X	X	
13	X			X		X	X	X	X	X	
24			X								

Wounds, Incisional (Includes Cuts)

	STAPHYS	CALEND	ARN	HYPER	SIL	HAM	HEP	SULPH	ACON	APIS	CALC S	CARB V	CIC	IOD	LACH	LED	NAT CAR	NIT AC	PLUM	SULPH AC
1	X																			
3	X																			
4	**X**																			
5	X			X																
7	**X**	X			X	X		X				X	X		X			X		
8	X	X				X								X						
9	X	B	X	E						X						X				
10	X	X																		
13	**X**		X		X			X									X		X	X
14	X										X									
16	X																			
18	X																			
19	X																			
22		X		E		X	X													
24	X																			
25		X	X		X	X	X		X											
28	X																			

B- Both Internal and External E- External

Wounds, Infected (Includes Wounds, Gangrenous; Wounds, Poisoned)

	ARS	LACH	SIL	ACON	BELL	HEP	HYPER	CALEND	AMM C	CARB V	CHINA	ECHIN	LED	PYROG	APIS	BROM	BUFO	EUPHORB	GALIUM	STAPHYS	SULPH	SULPH AC	VER V					
2												X																
3	X		X			X	X					E		X					X									
4		X													X													
8	X	X	X	X	X				X	X	X					X		X				X						
9			X	X	X	X	X																					
10	X																											
12	X																											
13	X	X	X	X	X				X	X	X																	
14																					X							
15																							X					
16								E																				
19	X							**X**					X	X			X											
21						X	X						X															
24		X																										
25			X	X	X	X	E													X								
26	X	X																										

E- External

Wounds, Inflamed

	SULPH AC	ACON	CALEND	CHAM	PULS	RHUS T	SULPH	ARN	ARS	BELL	BOR	GRAPH	HEP	HYPER	LACH	MERC	NIT AC	PLUM	SIL									
3	**X**													X														
4			B																									
8	X			X	X	X	X				X	X	X		X	X	X		X									
9		X								X																		
13	X	X	X	X	X	X	X		X									X										
26								X																				

B- Both Internal and External

Wounds, Lacerated

	CALEND	HYPER	ARN	HAM	STAPHYS	LACH	HEP	SIL	ACON	BELL	CHAM	LED	SULPH	SYMPH
1	X					X								
3		X												
4	**B**													
7	**X**	X		X								X		
8	X			X										
9	E	X	X				X	X	X	X				
14	X													
15	E						X	X			X		X	
16	E	X												
19			X		**X**									X
22	E	E												
24	B	X	**X**			X								
25	E		X	B										
26	X				X									

B- Both Internal and External E- External

Wounds, Puncture (Includes Splinters; Stab Wounds)

	LED	HYPER	APIS	ARN	SIL	HEP	ACON	CARB V	CIC	LACH	NIT AC	PHASEOL	ARAN D	ARS	BRY	CALEND	CON	GELS	PLUM	STAPHYS	SULPH	SYMPH
1	X																					
2	X		X									X	X									
3	X																					
4	**X**																					
6		X																				
7	**X**	**X**	**X**		X																	
8				X	X	X		X	X	X	X						X		X		X	
9	**X**		X																			
10	X																					
13				X	X	X	X	X	X	X	X											
14	X	X																				
15					X		X								X	X		X				
16	X											X										
17	X																					
19	**X**	X	**X**	X										X						X		X
20	**X**	B	X																			
21	X																					
22	E																					
24	X	X																				
25	**X**			E																		
26		X				X																

B- Both Internal and External E- External

Wounds, Suppurating

	SIL	HEP	BUFO	CALC	CALEND	CIC	GRAPH	HYPER	LED	MERC	PHOS	PYROG	STAPHYS	TAR C
1	X					X								
8			X	X							X			
9	X	X												
16								E						
19	**X**	X			X		X		X	X		X	X	X

E- External

Wrist, Diseases Of

	BOV	PRUN P
2		X
8	X	

Wrist Drop- See Weakness, Wrist

Wry Neck- See Torticollis

Xerostomia- See also Salivation, Deficient; Tongue, Dryness

	BELL	BRY	PULS	NUX M	ARS	ACON	NAT M	PHOS	CHAM	LACH	RHUS T	BOR	HYOSC	LYC	NUX V	SIL	SULPH	CHINA	KALI BIC	CAPS	CARB V	MUR AC	PLUM					
1		X	X	X	X			X		X		X	X		X					X	X							
4		X	X	**X**			X					X																
5	X	X	X	X	X	X				X	X	X		X														
6	X	X	X	X		X	X				X	X	X						X				X					
7		X	X	X	**X**	**X**	X	X	X					X		X		**X**		**X**	**X**	X	X					
8	X	X	X	X		X	X	X	X		X				X	X	X											
9			X	X			X			X									X									
10	X	X				X	X	X	X						X								X					
11	X	X			X																							
12	X				X		X						X															
13	**X**	**X**	X	X	X	**X**	X	X	**X**	**X**	**X**		**X**	**X**	**X**	**X**	**X**	**X**	X		X	**X**	**X**					
14	X	X	X		X	X																						
15		X							X										X			X						
17	X	X		X	X	X	X	X	X	X	X	X	X	X	X	X	X	X	X	X	X	X						
18	X			X																								
19	X		X								X						X											
20						X						X																
21	X	X		X	X	X	X													X								
22		X	X																									
24			X							X																		
26	X		X		X													X										
27	X																											
29*			X		X		X	X						X		X	X											

29* Haila S, et al. Effects of homeopathic treatment on salivary flow rate and subjective symptoms in patients with oral dryness: a randomized trial. Homeopathy. 2005 Jul, 94, 3, 175-81

Yellow Fever

	ARS	CROT H	ACON	CARB V	CAD S	BRY	BELL	LACH	IPEC	PHOS	ARG N	GELS	ALL C	ARS H	CAMPH	CUPR	RHUS T	VER A	CANTH	MERC	VER V	ANT T	NUX V	CIMICI				
1		X			X																							
2	**X**	**X**	**X**	X	X	**X**			X	X			X	X		X		X										
4	**X**	**X**	**X**	**X**			X	**X**	X	X	**X**	X			X													
6	**X**	X	**X**	**X**	X	**X**	**X**	**X**	X	X	X	**X**	X		X	X	X		X	X	**X**	X	X	**X**				
7	**X**	**X**	X	**X**	**X**	X	X	**X**		X	X	X	X	X	X	X	X	X	**X**	**X**	X	X	X					
8	**X**	**X**	X	X	X	X	X	**X**	X	X	X		X	X	X	X	X	X	X				X					
12	**X**	X	X		X	X	X		X			X								X		X		X				
14				X																								
15	X	X	X				X	X			X										X							
16	X				X				X																			
17				X																								
21	X		X			X																						
23		X			X									X														
26	X	X	X	X		X	X		X	X							X	X										

Yellow Fever, Prophylaxis

	ACON	ARS	BAPT	CIMICI																								
12	X		X	X																								
16		X																										

Zona- See Herpes

Zoster- See Herpes Zoster

Remedy Abbreviations

Abies c	Abies canadensis
Abies n	Abies nigra
Abrot	Artemisia abrotanum
Absinth	Artemisia absinthium
Acalyph	Acalypha indica
Acet ac	Acetic acid
Acetan	Acetanilidum
Acon	Aconitum napellus
Acon fe	Aconitum ferox
Acon l	Aconitum lycoctonum
Act r	See Cimici
Act sp	Actaea spicata
Adonis	Adonis vernalis
Adrenal	Adrenalin
Aethusa	Aethusa cynapium
Aesc	Aesculus hippocastanum
Aethiop	Aethiops antimonialis
Agar m	Agaricus muscarius
Agaricin	Agaricinum
Agave a	Agave americana
Agnus	Agnus castus
Agraph	Agraphis nutans
Ailanth	Ailanthus grandulosa
AKA	Also Known As
Alcohol	Alcohol (Ethanol)
Alet	Aletris farinosa
Alfalfa	Alfalfa
All c	Allium cepa
All s	Allium sativum
Alnus	Alnus rubra
Aloe	Aloe socotrina
Alston	Alstonia constricta
Alum	Alumina
Alumen	Alumen
Alum o	Aluminium oxydatum
Alum sil	Alumina silicata
Ambra	Ambra
Ambros	Ambrosia
Am benz	Ammonium benzoicum
Amm c	Ammonium carbonicum
Amm cau	Ammonium causticum
Amm m	Ammonium muriaticum
Amm pic	Ammonium picricum
Amphis	Amphisbaena vermicularis
Amyg p	Amygdalus persica
Amyl n	Amyl nitrite
Anac	Anacardium orientalis
Anag	Anagallis arvensis
Ananth	Anantherum muricatum
Angust	Angustura vera
Anhal	Anhalonium lewinii
Anil	Anilinum
Anise	Anise stellatum
Anthrac	Anthracinum
Anthrok	Anthrakokali
Ant c	Antimonium crudum
Ant iod	Antimonium iodatum
Ant m	Antimonium muriaticum
Ant s a	Antimonium sulph auratum
Ant t	Antimonium tartaricum
Antipyr	Antipyrinum
Apis	Apis mellifica
Apoc	Apocynum cannabinum
Apomor	Apomorphinum
Aq mar	Aqua marina
Aquileg	Aquilegia vulgaris
Aralia	Aralia racemosa
Aran d	Aranea diadema
Arg	Argentum metallicum
Arg n	Argentum nitricum
Arist cl	Aristolochia clematitis
Arist m	Aristolochia milhomens
Arn	Arnica montana
Ars	Arsenicum album
Ars br	Arsenicum bromatum
Ars h	Arsenicum hydrogenisatum
Ars iod	Arsenicum iodatum
Ars s fl	Arsenicum sulfuratum flavum
Ars s r	Arsenicum sulfuratum rubrum
Art v	Artemisia vulgaris
Arum dr	Arum dracontium
Arum t	Arum triphyllum
Arundo	Arundo mauritanica
Asaf	Asafoetida
Asar e	Asarum europaeum
Asc s	Asclepius syriaca/cornuti
Asc t	Asclepius tuberosa
Aspara	Asparagus officionalis
Aspido	Aspidosperma quebracho
Astac f	Astacus fluviatilis
Ast r	Asterias rubens
Atrop	Atropine
Atrop s	Atropinum sulphuricum
Aur	Aurum metallicum
Aur fl	Aurum fluoratum
Aur m	Aurum muriaticum
Aur m n	Aurum mur natronatum
Aur s	Aurum sulphuratum

Avena	Avena sativa
Bacilin	Bacillinum
Bac test	Bacillinum testinum
Bad	Badiaga
Bals	Balsamum peruvianum
Bapt	Baptisia tinctoria
Bar c	Baryta carbonica
Bar iod	Baryta iodata
Bar m	Baryta muriatica
Bell	Belladonna
Bellis	Bellis perenis
Benzin	Benzinum
Ben d	Benzinum dinitricum
Ben n	Benzinum nitricum
Benz ac	Benzoic acid
Berb aq	Berberis aquifolium
Berb v	Berberis vulgaris
Beryl	Beryllium metallicum
Bism	Bismuth subnitricum
Blatta	Blatta orientalis
Bolet	Boletus laricis
Bor	Borax
Bothr	Bothrops lanceolatus
Bov	Bovista lycoperdon
Brach	Brachyglottis repens
Brass	Brassica napus
Brom	Bromium
Bruc	Brucea antidysenterica
Bry	Bryonia alba
Bufo	Bufo rana
Bunga	Bungarus fasciatus
Cact	Cactus grandiflorus
Cad	Cadmium metallicum
Cad s	Cadmium sulphuratum
Caff	Caffeine
Cajuput	Cajuputum
Calabar	See Physo
Calc ars	Calcarea arsenicosa
Calc	Calcarea carbonica
Calc ca	Calcarea caustica
Calc chl	Calcarea chlorinate
Calc fl	Calcarea fluorica
Calc hp	Calcarea hypophosphorosa
Calc iod	Calcarea iodata
Calc m	Calcarea muriatica
Calc o t	Calcarea ovi testae
Calc ph	Calcarea phosphorica
Calc ren	Calcarea renalis
Calc sil	Calcarea silicata
Calc sul	Calcarea sulphurica
Calend	Calendula officionalis
Calo	Calotropis gigantea
Caltha	Caltha palustris
Camph	Camphora
Cand a	Candida albicans
Cann i	Cannabis indica
Cann s	Cannabis sativa
Canth	Cantharis vesicatora
Caps	Capsicum annum
Carb a	Carbo animalis
Carb ac	Carbolic acid
Carb s	Carboneum sulphuratum
Carb tet	Carbon tetrachloride
Carb v	Carbo vegetalis
Carc	Carcinosum Foubister
Card m	Cardus marianus
Casc	Cascarilla
Cassia s	Cassia sophora
Cast eq	Castor equi
Castan v	Castanea vesca
Caul	Caulophyllum thalictroides
Caust	Causticum
Ceanoth	Ceanothus americanus
Cedron	Cedron
Cenchr	Cenchris contortrix
Cer ox	Cerium oxydatum
Cerato	Cerato
Cetrar	Cetraria islandica
Cham	Chamomilla matricaria
Cheir	Cheiranthis cheiri
Chel	Chelidonium majus
Chen oil	Chenopodium oil
Cheno	Chenopodium anthelminticum
Cheno v	Chenopodium vulvaria
Chim	Chimaphilla umbellata
China	China officionalis
Chin ars	China arsenicosum
Chin m	Chininum muriaticum
Chin s	Chininum sulphuricum
Chio	Chionanthus virginica
Chiro	Chironex fleckeri
Chlf	Chloroform
Chlol	Chloral hydrate
Chlor	Chlorum aqua
Cholest	Cholesterinum
Chr ac	Chromic acid
Chr ox	Chromium oxydatum
Chrys a	Chrysophanic acid
Cic	Cicuta virosa
Cimex	Cimex lectularius

Cimic	Cimicifuga racemosa
Cina	Cina artemisia
Cinerar	Cineraria maritima
Cinnab	Cinnabaris
Cinnam	Cinnamomum zeylanicum
Cist	Cistus canadensis
Citrus l	Citrus limon
Clem	Clematis erecta
Cobalt	Cobaltum metallicum
Coca	Coca erythroxylon
Coccin	Coccinella
Coccul	Cocculus indicus
Coccus	Coccus cacti
Cochl	Cochlaeria armoracia
Codein	Codeine
Coff	Coffea cruda
Coff t	Coffea tosta
Colch	Colchicum autumnale
Coli	Escherichia coli
Colibac	Colibaccilinum
Collin	Collinsonia
Coloc	Colocynthis
Colocin	Colocynthinum
Com	Comocladia dentata
Condur	Condurango
Con	Conium maculatum
Conval	Convallaria majalis
Cop	Copaiva
Cor r	Corallium rubrum
Cornus	Cornus circinata
Corn f	Cornus florida
Coto	Coto bark
Cotyl	Cotyledon umbilicus
Crat	Crataegus oxycantha
Cresol	Cresol
Croc	Crocus sativa
Crot c	Crotalus cascavella
Crot h	Crotalus horridus
Crot t	Croton tiglium
Cubeb	Cubeba officionalis
Cucurb	Cucurbita pepo
Culex	Culex musca
Cund	See Condur
Cupr	Cuprum metallicum
Cupr ar	Cuprum arsenicosum
Cupr o n	Cuprum oxydatum nigrum
Cupr sul	Cuprum sulphuricum
Cupre l	Cupressus lawsoniana
Curar	Curare
Cycl	Cyclamen
Cyprip	Cypripedium
Damian	Damiana aphrodisiaca
Daphne	Daphne indica
Diadem	See Aran d
Dig	Digitalis purpurea
Diosc	Dioscorea villosa
Diphther	Diphtherinum
Dolich	Dolichos pruriens
Doryph	Doryphora decemlineata
Dros	Drosera rotundifolia
Dub	Duboisinum
Dubo m	Duboisia myoporoides
Dulc	Dulcamara
Dysent c	Dysentaria bacillus
Echin	Echinacea angustifolia
Elae	Elaeis guineensis
Elaps	Elaps corollinus
Elat	Elaterium officinarium
Electr	Electricitas
Emetine	Emetine
Epigea	Epigea repens
Epilob	Epilobium palustre
Epipheg	Epiphegus virginiana
Equiset	Equisetum hyemale
Ergotin	Ergotinum
Erig	Erigeron Canadensis
Eriodyc	Eriodyctyon californicum
Erod	Erodium cicutarium
Eryng a	Eryngium aquaticum
Erythrin	Erythrinus
Eserin	Eserine physostigminum
Ether	Ether
Eucal	Eucalyptus globulus
Eugen	Eugenia jambos
Euon	Euonymus atropurpura
Eup per	Eupatorium perfoliatum
Eup pur	Eupatorium purpureum
Euph c	Euphorbia corollata
Euph pil	Euphorbia pilulifera
Euph po	Euphorbia polycarpa
Eupg pr	Euphorbia prostata
Euphorb	Euphorbium officinarum
Euphr	Euphrasia officionalis
Eupion	Eupionum
Fel	Fel tauri
Ferr	Ferrum metallicum
Ferr ars	Ferrum arsenicosum
Ferr iod	Ferrum iodatum
Ferr m	Ferrum muriaticum
Ferr ma	Ferrum magneticum

Ferr per	Ferrum pernitricum
Ferr ph	Ferrum phosphoricum
Ferr pic	Ferrum picricum
Ferr py	Ferrum pyrophosphoricum
Ferr sul	Ferrum sulphuricum
Fic rel	Ficus religiosa
Filix	Filix mas
Fl ac	Fluoric acid
Folic	Folliculinum
Formica	Formica rufa
Frag	Fragaria vesca
Frax	Fraxinus americana
Fucus	Fucus vesiculosus
Fum	Fumaria officionalis
Gadus	Gadus morrhua
Gall ac	Gallic acid
Galph	Galphimia glauca
Gambog	Gambogia
Gastein	Gastein aqua
Gels	Gelsemium sempervirens
Gent	Gentiana lutea
Ger mac	Geranium maculatum
Getty	Gettysburg aqua
Geum	Geum rivale
Giardia	Giardia lamblia nosode
Ginseng	Ginseng
Glan fe	Glandular fever nosode
Glon	Glonoine
Glycerin	Glycerine
Gnaph	Gnaphalium
Gossip	Gossypium
Granat	Granatum
Graph	Graphites naturalis
Grat	Gratiola officionalis
Grind	Grindelia robusta
Grind sq	Grindelia squarrosa
Guaco	Guaco
Guaiac	Guaiacum officionale
Guaran	Guarana
Guarea	Guarea trichloides
Gummi	See Gambog
Gunpow	Gunpowder
Gymnem	Gymnema sylvestre
Ham	Hamamelis virginiana
Hecla	Hecla lava
Hedeom	Hedeoma pulegipoides
Hedera	Hedera helix
Helianth	Helianthus anuus
Hell	Helleborus niger
Helod	Heloderma suspectum
Helon	Helonias dioica
Hep	Hepar sulphuris
Hippom	Hippomanes
Hippoz	Hippozaeninum
Hirudo	Hirudo medicinalis
Hist	Histamine hydrochloricum
Hoang	Hoang nan
Homar	Homarus
Hura	Hura brasiliensis
Hydrang	Hydrangea arborescens
Hydrast	Hydrastis canadensis
Hydroc	Hydrocotyle asiatica
Hydr ac	Hydrocyanic acid
Hyos	Hyoscyamus niger
Hyosc h	Hyoscine hydrochloride
Hyosin	Hyosciamine
Hyper	Hypericum
Hypoth	Hypothalamus
Iber	Iberus amara
Icthyol	Icthyolum
Ign	Ignatia amara
Ilex a	Ilex aquafolium
Ilex p	Ilex paraguayensis
Illicium	Illicium anisatum
Indig	Indigo tinctoria
Indium	Indium metallicum
Influenz	Influenzinum nosode
Inula	Inula helenium
Insulin	Insulin
Iod	Iodum purum
Iodofor	Iodoformum
Ipec	Ipecacuanha
Ipomoea	Ipomoeia purpura
Irid	Iridium metallicum
Iris f	Iris foetidissima
Iris t	Iris tenax
Iris v	Iris versicolor
Itu	Itu
Jab	Jaborandi
Jac car	Jacaranda caroba
Jac g	Jacaranda gualandai
Jatr	Jatropha curas
Jatr u	Jatropha urens
Jug c	Juglans cinerea
Jug r	Juglans regia
Juni c	Juniperus communis
Juni v	Juniperus virginianus
Kali ars	Kali arsenicosum
Kali bic	Kali bichromicum
Kali br	Kali bromatum

Kali car	Kali carbonicum
Kali chl	Kali chloricum
Kali cy	Kali cyanatum
Kali hp	Kali hypophosphoricum
Kali iod	Kali iodatum
Kali man	Kali permanganicum
Kali mur	Kali muriaticum
Kali nit	Kali nitricum
Kali ph	Kali phosphoricum
Kali sul	Kali sulphuricum
Kalm	Kalmia latifiolia
Kaolin	Kaolin
Kissing	Kissingen aqua
Kousso	Kousso
Kreo	Kreosotum
Lac ac	Lactic acid
Lac c	Lac caninum
Lac d	Lac defloratum
Lac fel	Lac felinum
Lac v d	Lac vaccinum defloratum
Lach	Lachesis muta
Lachn	Lachnanthes tinctoria
Lact v	Lactuca virosa
Lapis	Lapis albus
Lappa	Lappa arctium
Lath	Lathyrus sativus
Latro h	Latrodectus hasselti
Latro k	Latrodectus katipo
Latro m	Latrodectus mactans
Lauro	Laurocerasus
Lecithin	Lecithin
Led	Ledum
Lem min	Lemna minor
Lepid	Lepidium bonariense
Lept	Leptandra virginica
Lesp c	Lespedeza capitata
Lil t	Lilium tigrinum
Limul	Limulus cyclops
Linum u	Linum usitatissimum
Lith c	Lithium carbonicum
Lith m	Lithium muriaticum
Lob dor	Lobelia dortmanna
Lob i	Lobelia inflata
Lob pur	Lobelia purpurascens
Lob syph	Lobelia syphilitica
Lol t	Lolium temulentum
Lonicer	Lonicerum xylosteum
Luffa	Luffa operculata
Lupul	Lupulus humulus
Lyc	Lycopodium clavatum
Lycop	Lycopus virginicus
Lysid	Lysidium
Lyss	Lyssinum
Macrot	Macrotinum
Mag	Magnesium metallicum
Mag car	Magnesia carbonica
Mag m	Magnesia muriatica
Mag p ar	Magnetis polus arcticus
Mag p au	Magnetis polus australis
Mag ph	Magnesia phosphorica
Mag sul	Magnesia sulphurica
Magn gr	Magnolia grandiflora
Maland	Malandrinum
Malaria	Malaria officionalis
Manc	Mancinella
Mandra	Mandragora officinarium
Mang	Manganum metallicum
Mang ac	Manganum aceticum
Mang m	Manganum muriaticum
Mang ox	Manganum oxydatum
Medo	Medorrhinum
Mela	Melastoma ackermanni
Melilot	Melilotus officionalis
Menisp	Menispermum canadense
Menth p	Mentha piperita
Meny	Menyanthes trifoliata
Meph	Mephitis putorius
Merc	Mercurius vivus/solubilis
Merc ac	Mercurius aceticus
Merc au	Mercurius auratus
Merc c	Mercurius corrosivus
Merc cy	Mercurius cyanatus
Merc d	Mercurius dulcis
Merc I f	Mercurius iodatus flavus
Mec I r	Mercurius iodatus rubus
Merc n	Mercurius nitrosus
Merc p	Mercurialis perennis
Merc ph	Mercurius phosphoricus
Merc p r	Mercurius precip. ruber
Merc su	Mercurius sulphuricus
Meth bl	Methylene blue
Mez	Mezereum
Mill	Millefolium achillea
Mitch	Mitchella repens
Morbil	Morbillinum
Morg g	Morgan-Gaertner bacillus
Morg p	Morgan pure bacillus
Morgan	Morgan bacillus
Morph	Morphine
Morph s	Morphinum sulphuricum

Mosch	Moschus moschiferus
Mur ac	Muriatic acid
Murex	Murex purpureus
Mygal	Mygale lasiodora
Myrica	Myrica cerifera
Myrist	Myristica sebifera
Myrtus	Myrtus communis
Naja	Naja tripudians
Naphtha	Naphthalene
Nat	Natrum metallicum
Nat acet	Natrum aceticum
Nat ars	Natrum arsenicosum
Nat car	Natrum carbonicum
Nat hypo	Natrum hypochlorosum
Nat m	Natrum muriaticum
Nat nit	Natrum nitricum
Nat ph	Natrum phosphoricum
Nat sal	Natrum salicylicum
Nat sel	Natrum selenicum
Nat sul	Natrum sulphuricum
Nepenth	Nepenthe
Nicc sul	Niccolum sulphuricum
Niccol	Niccolum metallicum
Nicotin	Nicotine
Nit	Nitrogen
Nit ac	Nitric acid
Nit s d	Nitri spiritus dulcis
Nm x	Nitro-muriatic acid
Nuph	Nuphar
Nux m	Nux moschata
Nux v	Nux vomica
Ocim	Ocimum canum
Oenanth	Oenanthe
Oleand	Oleander
Ol an	Oleum animale
Ole jec a	Oleum jecoris aselli
Ol san	Oleum Santali
Onos	Onosmodium virginianum
Oophor	Oophorinum
Op	Opium
Opercul	Operculina turpenthum
Origan	Origanum majorana
Ornitho	Ornithogalum umbellatum
Oscillo	Oscillococcinum
Osmium	Osmium metallicum
Ovi g p	Ovi gallinae pellicula
Ox ac	Oxalic acid
Oxytrop	Oxytropis lamberti
Paeonia	Paeonia officionalis
Pallad	Palladium metallicum

Pancr	Pancreatinum
Paraf	Paraffinum
Parathy	Parathyroidinum
Pareira	Pareira brava
Paris	Paris quadrifolia
Parotid	Parotidinum
Parthen	Parthenium hysterophorus
Pass	Passiflora incarnata
Paull	See Guaran
Penthor	Penthorum sedoides
Pepsin	Pepsin
Pertuss	Pertussinum nosode
Petiver	Petiveria tetranda
Petr	Petroleum
Petros	Petroselinum sativum
Phaseol	Phaseolus nanus
Phell	Phellandrinum aquaticum
Ph ac	Phosphoric acid
Phos	Phosphorus
Phos hy	Phosphorus hydrogenatus
Physal	Physalia
Physo	Physostigma venenosum
Phyto	Phytolacca decandra
Pic ac	Picric acid
Pilo	Pilocarpine
Pilo m	Pilocarpinum muriaticum
Pinus s	Pinus sylvestris
Piper m	Piper methysticum
Piper n	Piper nigrum
Piscid	Piscidia
Pituit	Pituitary gland
Pix	Pix liquida
Plantag	Plantago major
Platan	Platanus occidentalis
Plat	Platina metallicum
Plat m	Platinum muriaticum
Plect	Plectranthus fruiticosus
Plum	Plumbum metallicum
Plum iod	Plumbum iodatum
Pneumoc	Pneumococcinum
Pod	Podophyllum peltatum
Polyg	Polygonum aviculare
Polypor	Polyporus pinicola
Pop can	Populus candicans
Pop t	Populus tremuloides
Pothos	Ictodes foetidus
Prednis	Prednisone
Prim o	Primula obconica
Prim v	Primula veris
Prop	Propylaminum

Proteus	Proteus bacillus
Prun p	Prunus padus
Prun s	Prunus spinosa
Psor	Psorinum
Ptel	Ptelea trifoliata
Pulmo v	Pulmo vulpis
Puls	Pulsatilla
Puls n	Pulsatilla nuttaliana
Pyrog	Pyrogenium
Pyrus	Pyrus americanus
Quebr	Quebracho aspidosperma
Quer g s	Quercus glandium spiritus
Quin	Quinidine
Rad br	Radium bromatum
Ran b	Ranunculus bulbosus
Ran s	Ranunculus scleratus
Raph	Raphanus sativus
Rat	Ratanhia peruviana
Rauwolf	Rauwolfia serpentina
Rhamn c	Rhamnus californica
Rhamn f	Rhamnus frangula
Rheum	Rheum palmatum
Rhod	Rhododendron chrysanthum
Rhus ar	Rhus aromatica
Rhus g	Rhus glabra
Rhus t	Rhus toxicodendron
Rhus v	Rhus venata
Ricin	Ricinus communis
Robin	Robinia pseudacacia
Rosa c	Rosa canina
Rumex	Rumex crispus
Ruta	Ruta graveolens
Sabad	Sabadilla officionalis
Sabal	Sabal serrulata
Sabin	Sabina
Sac lac	Saccharum lactis
Sacch	Saccharum officionale
Sal ac	Salicylic acid
Salix n	Salix nigra
Samb	Sambuccus nigra
Samb c	Sambuccus canadensis
Sang	Sanguinaria canadensis
Sang n	Sanguinarium nitricum
Sanic	Sanicula aqua
Santin	Santonin
Sapo	Saponaria officionalis
Sarc ac	Sarcolactic acid
Saro	Sarothamnus
Sarr	Sarracenia purpurea
Sars	Sarsaparilla offiicionalis
Sassaf	Sassafras officionalis
Scarlet	Scarlet fever nosode
Schin	Schinus molle
Scill	See Squilla
Scirr	Scirrhinum
Scroph	Scrophularia nodosa
Scut	Scutellaria laterifolia
Sec	Secale cornutum
Secretin	Secretin
Sel	Selenium
Sela	Selaginella apus
Semp	Sempervivum tectorum
Senec	Senecio aureus
Seneg	Polygala senega
Sepia	Sepia succus
Ser ang	Serum anguillae
Sil	Silica terra
Sil mar	Silica marina
Sinap a	Sinapis alba
Sinap	Sinapis nigra
Skook	Skookum chuck
Slag	Slag
Sol	Sol
Sol c	Solanum carolinense
Sol n	Solanum nigrum
Sol o	Solanum oleraceum
Sol t a	Solanum tub aegrotans
Solan	Solaninum
Solid	Solidago virgaurea
Sphing	Sphingurus martini
Spig	Spigelia anthelmintica
Spig m	Spigelia marylandica
Spira	Spiranthes autumnalis
Spirae	Spiraea ulmaria
Spong	Spongia tosta
Squilla	Squilla maritima
Stann	Stannum metallicum
Stann io	Stannum iodatum
Staphyl	Staphylococcinum
Staphys	Staphysagria
Stell aq	Stellaria aquatica
Stell m	Stellaria media
Stercul	Sterculia acuminata
Sticta	Sticta pulmonaria
Stig	Stigmata maydis
Stilling	Stillingia silvatica
Stram	Stramonium
Stront	Strontium metallicum
Stront b	Strontium bromatum
Stront c	Strontium carbonate

Stront i	Strontium iodatum	Triost	Triosteum perfoliatum
Stroph	Strophanthus hispidus	Trit r	Triticum repens
Strych	Strychnine	Tromb	Trombidium muscae
Stry ars	Strychninum arsenicosum	Tub	Tuberculinum
Stry ph	Strychninum phosphorica	Tub av	Tuberculinum aviaire
Stry val	Strychninum valerianicum	Tussil	Tussilago petasites
Succin	Succinum	Upas	Upas tieute
Sulfon	Sulfonal	Uran n	Uranium nitricum
Sulo ac	Sulphurosum acidum	Urea	Urea pura
Sulph	Sulphur	Uric ac	Uric acid
Sulph ac	Sulphuric acid	Urin	Urinum humanum
Sulph io	Sulphur iodatum	Urotrop	Urotropinum
Sumbul	Sumbulus moschatus	Urt u	Urtica urens
Symph	Symphytum officionale	Ustil	Ustilago maydis
Symphor	Symphoricarpus racemosus	Uva	Uva ursi
Syph	Syphilinum	Vaccin	Vaccininum
Syzigium	Syzigium jambolanum	Valer	Valeriana officionalis
Tab	Tabacum	Vanad	Vanadium metallicum
Tamus	Tamus communis	Variol	Variolinum
Tanacet	Tanacetum vulgare	Ver a	Veratrum album
Tannin	Tannic acid	Ver v	Veratrum viride
Tar c	Tarentula cubensis	Verbasc	Verbascum thapsus
Tar h	Tarentula hispanica	Verbena	Verbena hastata
Tarax	Taraxacum officionale	Verin	Veratrinum
Tart ac	Tartaric acid	Vermic	Vermiculite
Taxus	Taxus baccata	Vesicar	Vesicaria communis
Tell	Tellurium metallicum	Vespa	Vespa crabro
Tereb	Terebinthina	Vib op	Viburnum opulus
Term c	Terminalia chebula	Vib p	Viburnum prunifolium
Tet	Tetradymite	Vinca	Vinca minor
Teucr	Teucrium marum	Viol o	Viola odorata
Teucr s	Teucrium scorodonia	Viol t	Viola tricolor
Thallium	Thallium metallicum	Vip	Vipera berus
Thea	Thea chinensis	Vip red	Vipera aspis
Ther	Theridion curassavicum	Vip t	Vipera torva
Thev	Thevitia nerifolia	Visc a	Viscum album
Thio	Thiosinaminum	Weis	Weisbaden aqua
Thlaspi	Thlaspi bursa pastoris	Wildbad	Wildbad aqua
Thuja	Thuja occidentalis	Wyethia	Wyethia helenoides
Thymol	Thymol	X-ray	X-ray
Thyroid	Thyroidinum	Xanth	Xanthoxylum fraxineum
Tilea	Tilea europea	Xero	Xerophyllum
Titanium	Titanium metallicum	Yersin	Yersinia pestis nosode
Tongo	Tongo	Yohimb	Yohimbinum
Toxicop	Toxicophis pugnax	Zinc	Zincum metallicum
Trac d	Trachinus draco	Zinc m	Zincum muriaticum
Trifol p	Trifolium pratanse	Zinc ph	Zincum phosphoricum
Trifol r	Trifolium repens	Zinc sul	Zincum sulphuricum
Trill p	Trillium pendulum	Zing	Zingiber officionale
		Ziz	Zizia aurea

Rubric Index

www.ingramcontent.com/pod-product-compliance
Ingram Content Group UK Ltd.
Pitfield, Milton Keynes, MK11 3LW, UK
UKHW051029041026
15470UKWH00015B/1792

9 780958 079822